Hughes Syndrome

Springer
London
Berlin
Heidelberg
New York
Barcelona
Hong Kong
Milan
Paris
Singapore
Tokyo

M. A. Khamashta (Ed.)

Hughes Syndrome
Antiphospholipid Syndrome

With a Foreword by Eng M. Tan

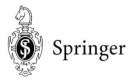 Springer

M. A. Khamashta, MD, MRCP, PhD
Deputy Head, Lupus Research Unit, St Thomas' Hospital,
Lambeth Palace Road, London, SE1 7EH

ISBN 1-85233-232-8 Springer-Verlag London Berlin Heidelberg

British Library Cataloguing in Publication Data
Hughes syndrome : antiphospholipid syndrome
  1. Antiphospholipid syndrome
  I. Khamashta, Munther A.
  616'.0798
  ISBN 1852332328

Library of Congress Cataloging-in-Publication Data
Khamashta, Munther A.
  Hughes syndrome : antiphospholipid syndrome / M.A. Khamashta.
    p. cm.
  Includes bibliographical references and index.
  ISBN 1-85233-232-8 (alk. paper)
  1. Antiphospholipid syndrome. I. Title.
  RC600.K48 2000
  616.97'8–dc21   99-087170

Typeset by EXPO Holdings, Malaysia
Printed and bound at: Kyodo Printing Co (S'Pore) Pte Ltd, Singapore
28/3830-543210 Printed on acid-free paper SPIN 10747442

To my daughter Leila

Foreword

I am very happy to be asked by Dr. Munther Khamashta to write a Foreword to this first comprehensive description of the many facets of the antiphospholipid syndrome (APS). Although I have been an interested and long-time participant in studies to elucidate the nature of some human diseases associated with immunological abnormalities, I have not had a personal involvement with work on the APS. I have however watched with great fascination the evolution of this field from initial observations of clinical symptoms to studies defining the pathophysiological abnormalities.

The APS began with reports in 1983, 1984 and 1985 (see Khamashta: Hughes Syndrome, A History) on a number of clinical symptoms which appeared to have an underlying common pathogenic mechanism – vascular thrombotic episodes. These included peripheral vascular thromboses, cerebral vascular infarctions, livedo reticularis, spontaneous abortions and portal and pulmonary hypertension. A striking feature of this unfolding story was that already in 1983, suspicion was cast on the likely association of anti-cardiolipin/phospholipid antibodies with the clinical syndromes. Continuing studies on the pathophysiology have helped to fine-tune the immunological abnormalities. Most investigators believe that proteins complexed to phospholipids such as β-2–glycoprotein-1 are the primary targets of the autoantibodies but there appears to be continuing evidence that phospholipids themselves are also target antigens. The argument here may hinge on the fact that the immunogen itself might be a complex of phospholipid and protein and the humoral immune response is directed at different component parts of this complex, depending on the "immunogenicity" of different components to a genetically susceptible host. In fact, many autoantigens in lupus and other autoimmune diseases are complexes of nucleic acids and proteins, a classical example being the Sm antigens comprising complexes of small nuclear RNAs and small nuclear ribonucleoproteins.

In autoimmune diseases like lupus, we have advanced the notion that the humoral antibody responses are antigen-driven and that the antigens are self proteins rendered immunogenic due to a variety of reasons, including overexpression, ectopic localization and structural alterations of various kinds such as mutagenesis or complexing with foreign materials. An interesting aspect of the APS story is the diverse nature of clinical symptoms which involve totally different organ systems but rarely involve more than one organ system at a time. This is in contrast to lupus which is also a multi-system disease, but the individual patient often has multiple organ system involvement. It is possible that the APS might fall into the following mechanistic scenario:

Different inciting agents → → → Thrombosis in different organ systems → → → antigenic modification of procoagulant phospholipid-protein → → → humoral antibody responses → → → in-situ antigen-antibody complex formation → → → inflammation, further thrombosis, recruitment of cellular immune infiltrates → → → perpetuation of repeated cycles of thrombosis, inflammation and immune responses.

The diversity of the APS could be explained on the uniqueness of the initial inciting event leading to pro-coagulation occurring in specific organ systems and thus would not have to invoke aberrant immune responses manifesting the great variety of clinical syndromes. One of the challenges in the future would be to explain or identify the different inciting agents for the different syndromes encountered.

One of the issues which has been raised is that the anti-phospholipid syndrome is a misnomer since the major target antigen appears to be the protein or the lipoprotein complex. Many investigators are inclined towards keeping the original moniker of the APS because of both historical and common usage reasons. The history of clinical medicine and biomedical research is replete with examples where original designations have been retained in spite of subsequent studies showing that the designation was not totally correct. The important thing is that the essence of the original observations in the APS was correct.

It is rare that an investigator and his colleagues have the opportunity to open up a new field in clinical medicine and biomedical research. This has happened with the anti-phospholipid syndrome. Graham Hughes and his colleagues deserve enormous kudos for recognizing that a number of clinical syndromes shared a common feature of vascular thrombosis and for carrying this into consolidation of the clinical observations with laboratory analysis. Much clinical and basic research by many investigators worldwide have resulted from these beginnings. This volume stands as a tribute to Hughes and his colleagues.

Eng M. Tan, M.D.
The Scripps Research Institute
La Jolla, California 92037
U.S.A.

Prologue

Memory loss, migraine, strokes, accelerated atheroma, recurrent miscarriages – some of the features which make the antiphospholipid syndrome (APS) so important to patients and clinicians worldwide.

The finding that simple and reproducible assays can identify patients at risk both for venous *and* arterial thrombosis has opened up new avenues for treatment across may specialities.

From the early days in the late 1970's and early 1980's, I had felt strongly that the syndrome would one day outstrip lupus in frequency. Indeed my colleagues and I were often impatient at the seemingly slow acceptance of the syndrome by the medical (and obstetric) community in the early years. All that has changed. The number of papers and meetings relating to the syndrome has become a flood, and there is widespread realisation that this may, in fact be one of *the* most common and important auto-immune diseaes.

My grateful thanks to my colleagues, mentors and friends, especially Dr Tan and Charles Christian, whose guidance I have always valued, and to Nigel Harris and Aziz Gharavi, who not only worked with me in the early days of the syndrome, but have become world leaders in APS research.

Most of all, my grateful thanks to Munther Khamashta, my colleague and friend for a decade.

His reputation in this field is truly international. It is a testimony to his personal qualities that he has been able to persuade the world leaders in APS to contribute to this volume.

Graham Hughes

Contents

Contributors

Olga Amengual
Lupus Research Unit
The Rayne Institute
St. Thomas' Hospital
London SE1 7EH, UK

Paul Ames
Department of Haematology
St Thomas' Hospital
London SE1 7EH, UK

Mary-Carmen Amigo
Department of Rheumatology
Instituto Nacional de Cardiologia
I. Chávez
Universidad Nacional Autónoma de
México
Juan Bdiano 1
Tlalpan
Mexico City 14080
Mexico

Eduardo Anglés-Cano
Director of Research, INSERM U. 143,
Hémostase-Biol. Vasculaire
84,rue du Général Leclerc
Bicêtre, 94276-Cedex, France

Jef Arnout
Center for Molecular and Vascular
Biology
University of Leuven
Herestraat 49
B-3000 Leuven, Belgium

Tatsuya Atsumi
Department of Medicine II
Hokkaido University School of Medicine
Kita 5, Nishi 7, Kita-ku
Sapporo 060-8635, Japan

Tiziano Barbui
Divisione di Ematologia
Ospedali Riuniti di Bergamo
Largo Barozi 1
24128 Bergamo, Italy

Carlos Battagliotti
Department of Internal Medicine and
Therapeutics
National University of Rosario
Boulevard Oroño 568
Rosario, Santa Fe 2000, Argentina

H. Michael Belmont
Lupus Clinic, Hospital for Joint
Diseases
301 East 17th Street
New York, NY 10021, USA

Jackob Ben-David
Department of Otolaryngology
The Bnai-Zion Medical Centre
47 Golomb Avenue, PO box 4940
Haifa, 31048, Israel

Maria Laura Bertolaccini
Lupus Research Unit,
The Rayne Institute,
St. Thomas' Hospital
London, SE1 7EH, UK

Susan Bewley
Consultant Obstetrician
Department of Obstetrics and
Gynaecology
St. Thomas' Hospital
London SE1 7EH, UK

Miri Blank
Research Unit of Autoimmune
Diseases, Department of Medicine "B"
Sheba Medical Center, Tel-Hashomer
52621 Sackler Faculty of Medicine
Tel Aviv University
Tel Aviv, Israel

D. Ware Branch
Professor of Obstetrics and Gynaecology
University of Utah Health Sciences
Center
Room 2B200
50 N Medical Drive
Salt Lake City, UT 84132, USA

Robin L. Brey
Department of Medicine (Neurology),
The University of Texas Health Science
Center at San Antonio
7703 Floyd Curl Drive
San Antonio, TX 78229-3900, USA

Roberto Caporali
Servizio di Reumatologia
Policlinico S. Matteo
Piazzale Golgi 2
I-27100, Pavia, Italy

Luis Carreras
Favaloro University
Division of Haematology
Solis 453
Buenos Aires, Argentina

Cristina Castañon
Chief of Department of Opthalmology,
Instituto Nacional de Cardiologica
Ignacio Chavez
Juan Badiano 1, Tlalpan
Section XVI Mexico DF 14080, Mexico

Ricard Cervera
Systemic Autoimmune Diseases Unit,
Hospital Clinic
Villarroel 170
08036 Barcelona, Spain

María-José Cuadrado
Lupus Research Unit
The Rayne Institute
St. Thomas' Hospital
London SE1 7EH, UK

David D'Cruz
Bone and Joint Research Unit
Arthritis and Rheumatism Council
Building
Royal London Hospital
25–29 Ashfield Street
London E1 2AD, UK

Nicoletta Del Papa
Pad. Granelli, IRCCS Policlinico
Via Francesco Sforza, 35
20122 Milan, Italy

Ronald H. W. M. Derksen
Department of Rheumatology and
Clinical Immunology
University Hospital Utrecht
PO Box 85500
3508 GA Utrecht, The Netherlands

Pablo M. Dobado-Berrios
Unidad de Investigación
Hospital Universitario Reina Sofía
Córdoba, Spain

Siobhán Donohoe
Haemostasis Research Unit
Haematology Department
University College London
98 Chenies Mews
London WC1E 6HX

Keith B. Elkon
Department of Medicine
The Hospital for Special Surgery
Cornell University Medical College
535 East 70th Street
New York, NY 10021, USA

Josep Font
Systemic Autoimmune Diseases Unit,
Hospital Clinic
Villarroel 170
08036 Barcelona, Spain

Ricardo R. Forastiero
Favaloro University
Division of Haematology
Solis 453
Buenos Aires, Argentina

Monica Galli
Divisione di Ematologia
Ospedali Riuniti di Bergamo
Largo Barozi 1
24128 Bergamo, Italy

Romeo Garcia-Torres
Department of Pathology
Instituto Nacional de Cardiologia
I. Chávez
Juan Badiano 1, Tlalpan
Mexico City 14080, Mexico

Azzudin E. Gharavi
Department of Medicine,
Morehouse School of Medicine
720 Westview Dr SW
Atlanta, GA 30310-1495, USA

Tim Godfrey
Lupus Research Unit
St Thomas' Hospital
London SE1 7EH, UK

Theo-Dou Golan
Division of Clinical Immunology
The Bnai-Zion Medical Centre
47 Golomb Avenue, PO Box 4940
Haifa 31048, Israel

Philip G. de Groot
Department of Haematology
University Hospital Utrecht
PO Box 85500
3508 GA Utrecht, The Netherlands

E. Nigel Harris
Dean and Senior VP Academic Affairs,
Morehouse School of Medicine
720 Westview Dr SW
Atlanta, GA 303310-1495, USA

Graham R. V. Hughes
Head, Lupus Research Unit
The Rayne Institute
St Thomas' Hospital
London SE1 7EH, UK

Beverley J. Hunt
Departments of Haematology and
Rheumatology
Guy's and St Thomas' Hospital Trust
London SE1 7EH, UK

David Isenberg
Bloomsbury Rheumatology Unit/Centre
for Rheumatology
Arthur Stanley House
Middlesex Hospital
50 Tottenham Street
London W1P 9PG, UK

Aharon Kessel
Division of Clinical Immunology,
The Bnai-Zion Medical Centre
47 Golomb Avenue, PO Box 4940
Haifa. 31048, Israel

Munther Khamashta
Deputy Head, Lupus Research Unit
The Rayne Institute
St Thomas' Hospital
London SE1 7EH, UK

Takao Koike
Department of Medicine II
Hokkaido University School of
Medicine
Kita 15, Nishi 7, Kita-ku
Sapporo 060-8635, Japan

Ilan Krause
Research Unit of Autoimmune Diseases
Department of Medicine "B"
Sheba Medical Center
Tel-Hashomer 52621
Sackler Faculty of Medicine
Tel Aviv University, Tel Aviv, Israel

Robert G. Lahita
Chief of Rheumatology
Saint Vincent's Medical Center
153 West 11th Street, NR1 202
New York, NY 10011, USA

Lorin Lakasing
Foetal Health Research Group
Department of Obstetrics and
Gynaecology
St Thomas' Hospital
London SE1 7EH, UK

Richard M. Leach
Department of Intensive Care,
St Thomas' Hospital
London SE1 7EH, UK

Steven R. Levine
Department of Neurology
Wayne State University
4201 St. Antoine
Detroit, MI 48201, USA

Michael D. Lockshin
Barbara Volcker Center for Women &
Rheumatic Disease
Hospital for Special Surgery
Cornell Medical Center, 535E 70th Street
New York, NY 10021, USA

Chari López-Pedrera
Unidad de Investigación
Hospital Universitario Reina Sofía
Córdoba, Spain

Samuel J. Machin
Department of Haematology,
University College Hospital
Gower Street
London WC1E 6AU, UK

Ian Mackie
Haemostasis Research Unit,
Department of Haematology,
University College London
98 Chenies Mews
London WC1E 6HX

Charles G. Mackworth-Young
Kennedy Institute of Rheumatology
1 Aspenlea Road
London W6 8LH, UK

Gale A. McCarty
Associate Professor of Medicine,
Indiana University Medical Center
Rheumatology Division
541 Clinical Drive, Room 492
Indianapolis, IN 46202-5103, USA

Marta E. Martinuzzo
Favaloro University
Division of Haematology
Solis 453, Buenos Aires, Argentina

Pier Luigi Meroni
Pad. Granelli, IRCCS Policlinico
Via Francesco Sforza, 35
20122, Milan, Italy

Carlomaurizio Montecucco
Servizio di Reumatologia
Policlinico S. Matteo
Piazzale Golgi 2
1-27100, Pavia, Italy

M. Gina Navarrete
Department of Medicine (Neurology),
The University of Texas Health Science
Center at San Antonio
7703 Floyd Curl Drive
San Antonio, TX 78229-3900, USA

Catherine Nelson-Piercy
Consultant in Obstetric Medicine
Department of Obstetrics
Guy's and St Thomas' Hospital Trust
London SE1 7EH, UK

Ann L. Parke
Department of Rheumatology
University CT Health Ctr
Farmington CT 06030-1310, USA

Michelle Petri
Division of Rheumatology
Johns Hopkins University School of
Medicine
1830E. Monument Street, Suite 7500
Baltimore, MD 21205, USA

Silvia S. Pierangeli
Department of Medicine
Morehouse School of Medicine
720 Westview Dr SW
Atlanta, GA 30310-1495, USA

Jean-Charles Piette
Service de Médecine Interne
Groupe Hospitalier Pitié-Salpetrière
83 Boulevard de l'Hôpital
75651 Paris, Cedex 13, France

T. Flint Porter
Assistant Professor of Obstetrics and
Gynecology
LDS Hospital Perinatal Center
8th Avenue and C Street
Salt Lake City, UT 84143, USA

Anisur Rahman
Specialist Registrar in Rheumatology
Bloomsbury Rheumatology Unit
Arthur Stanley House
40–50 Tottenham Street
London W1P 9PG, UK

Elena Raschi
Pad. Granelli, IRCCS Policlinico
Via Francesco Sforza 35
20122 Milan, Italy

Joan Carles Reverter
Haemotherapy and Haemostasis Service
Hospital Clinic Barcelona
Villarroel 170, 08036 Barcelona, Spain

Pedro A. Reyes
Instituto Nacional de Cardiologia
Ignacio Chavez
Juan Badiano 1, Tlalpan
Section XVI Mexico DF 14080, Mexico

Robert Roubey
Division of Rheumatology and
Immunology, CB 7280
Room 3330 Thurston Building
University of North Carolina
Chapel Hill, NC 27599, USA

Lisa R. Sammaritano
Associate Professor of Medicine
Cornell University
Hospital for Special Surgery
535 East 70th Street
New York, NY 10021, USA

Matthias K. Schneider
Department of Rheumatology
Heinrich-Heine University/MNR-Clinic
Moorenstr 5
Duesseldorf D-40225, Germany

Yehuda Shoenfeld
Research Unit of Autoimmune Diseases
Department of Medicine "B"
Sheba Medical Center, Tel-Hashomer
52621, Sackler Faculty of Medicine
Tel Aviv University, Tel Aviv, Israel

Mario Siebler
Department of Neurology
Heinrich-Heine University/MNR-Clinic
Moorenstr 5
Duesseldorf D-40225, Germany

Robert M. Silver
Associate Professor of Obstetrics and
Gynecology
University of Utah Health Services Center
Room 2B200, 50 N Medical Drive
Salt Lake City, UT 84132, USA

Christof Specker
Department of Rheumatology
Heinrich-Heine University/MNR-CliniC
Moorenstr 5
Duesseldorf D-40225, Germany

Dolors Tàssies
Haemotherapy and Haemostasis Service
Hospital Clinic Barcelona
Villarroel 170
08036 Barcelona, Spain

Angela Tincani
Servizio di Immunologia Clinica,
Ospedali Civile di Brescia
Brescia, Italy

Elias Toubi
Director, Division of Clinical
Immunology
The Bnai-Zion Medical Centre
47 Golomb Avenue, PO Box 4940
Haifa, 31048, Israel

Akito Tsutsumi
Department of Medicine II
Hokkaido University School of Medicine
Kita 15, Nishi 7, Kita-ku
Sapporo 060-8635, Japan

Lori B. Tucker
Division of Pediatric Rheumatology
Room 1A-21
British Colombia's Children's Hospital
4480 Oak Street
Vancouver, BC V6H 3V4, Canada

Outi Vaarala
Department of Biochemistry
National Public Health Institute
Mannerheimintie 166
00300 Helsinki, Finland

Francisco Velasco
Servicio de Hematologia y Hemoterapia
Hospital Universitario Reina Sofía
Córdoba, Spain

Jos Vermylen
Center for Molecular and Vascular
Biology
University of Leuven
Herestraat 49
B-3000 Leuven, Belgium

Tonia Vincent
Kennedy Institute of Rheumatology
1 Aspenlea Road
London W6 8LH, UK

Frances M. K. Williams
ARC Clinical Research Fellow
Lupus Research Unit
The Rayne Institute
St. Thomas' Hospital
London SE1 7EH, UK

Wendell A. Wilson
Professor of Medicine, Department of
Medicine
LSU Medical Center
1542 Tulane Avenue
New Orleans, LA 70112, USA

Section 1
Clinical Aspects

1 Hughes Syndrome: History

M. A. Khamashta

In the 17 years since Graham Hughes's detailed description of the antiphospholipid syndrome (APS), the condition has come to be regarded as one of the most common autoimmune diseases. The impact of the description has been enormous – for example, the recognition that some individuals with connective tissue diseases require anticoagulation rather than steroids or anti-inflammatory treatment has brought about a fundamental change in medical practice. In obstetrics, APS is now regarded as the most important prothrombotic cause of recurrent pregnancy loss – with pregnancy success improving from below 20% to a current live birth rate of over 70% [1].

In neurology, Hughes syndrome may be associated with up to 20% of strokes in the under 40-year-olds – a striking figure not least in terms of medical economics, let alone in potentially preventable suffering.

In vascular disease, Hughes syndrome may well provide insights into immunological factors in the pathogenesis of atheroma [2].

In short, the syndrome links immunology with thrombosis and vascular disease. The mechanisms are complex and our current knowledge will be detailed in this volume. Suffice to say that the antibodies probably bind not simply to phospholipid – nor simply to phospholipid cofactor. In view of this increasing complexity, colleagues at the Sixth APS meeting in Louvain put forward the eponym *Hughes syndrome* in honour of the physician who fully described the condition – an eponym with which most colleagues working in the field – and those contributing to this volume, are content.

Graham Hughes's description of the condition was not, as is sometimes the case, based on a single case report, or a small series. It was a truly comprehensive and lifetime work – starting in the world of lupus. The 1983 description of the syndrome was the culmination of a decade of work in which careful clinical observations were combined not only with scientific studies, but also with a sharing of information. His ward rounds were and are famous for the cross-fertilization of ideas.

In 1983–86, Dr Hughes and his team described the association of antiphospholipid antibodies (aPL) with *arterial* as well as venous thrombosis, with neurological disease, especially stroke, with pulmonary hypertension, with livedo, with occasional thrombocytopenia, and with recurrent miscarriages. More significantly, he recognized that this syndrome, which he initially named the anticardiolipin syndrome and later the primary antiphospholipid syndrome, was separable from lupus. My colleague, Aziz Gharavi, remembers at the 1985 American College of Rheumatology meeting in New Orleans, hearing Graham forecast that the "primary" APS would one day outstrip lupus in prevalence, and that in the world of obstetrics, anticoagulation would replace steroids in the management of recurrent fetal loss in this disease. Both forecasts are proving correct. In the early 1980s Graham Hughes's team, led initially by Drs Nigel Harris and Aziz Gharavi, and later by myself, instituted collaborative workshops and, in 1984, the first international APS meeting – a meeting which has become a regular fixture, and which culminated in the most recent 8th International Symposium on Antiphospholipid Antibodies in Sapporo, Japan, organized by Takao Koike, in which preliminary consensus classification criteria for Hughes Syndrome were established [3, 4].

The following extract is, with permission, taken from Dr Hughes's own account of the description of the APS [5]:

> The description of the syndrome in 1983 came after a number of years of study of lupus, of myelopathy (especially so-called Jamaican neuropathy) and of atypical forms of connective tissue disease. We had become interested in the association of a false-positive VDRL with transverse myelopathy, and hypothesized, probably wrongly, that anticardiolipin antibodies might cross-react with neuronal phospholipids including cephalin and sphingomyelin [6].

> With our large clinic population, it is relatively easy to spot subsets of disease and it soon became apparent that the presence of anticardiolipin antibodies (also the lupus anticoagulant) – hence antiphospholipid antibodies, were strongly associated with thrombosis and miscarriage. From a clinical point of view, the association with thrombosis related not merely to venous thrombosis, but – differentiating it from almost all other prothrombotic conditions – *arterial* thrombosis, especially strokes.

> In 1983, I was invited to present my findings to a British dermatology society meeting – the "Prosser White oration" [7]. The following extract, taken from that paper, highlights, I believe both the clinical features of the syndrome, and the recognition of a "Primary" antiphospholipid syndrome:

> Although many of these patients fall under the general heading of lupus, or lupus-like disease, I believe that the group is sufficiently homogeneous, and in some ways (such as the frequently negative ANA serology) sufficiently different from typical systemic lupus erythematosus (SLE) to warrant separate consideration. The manifestations of this syndrome are thrombosis (often multiple) and, frequently, spontaneous abortions (often multiple), neurological disease, thrombocytopenia and livedo reticularis. The livedo reticularis is often most florid on the knees. This may or may not be associated with mild to moderate Raynaud's phenomenon.

> These patients' blood pressure often fluctuates, apparently correlating with the severity of the livedo, suggesting a possible renovascular aetiology. However, this group of patients rarely has primary renal disease.

> The cerebral features are prominent and of three varieties: headaches – often migrainous and intractable; epilepsy (or abnormal EEGs) – often going back to early teenage. Fortunately, severe or difficult-to-control epilepsy is infrequent. Some patients have chorea. Cerebro-vascular accidents – sometimes transient and seemingly attributable to migraine, are frequently progressive.... The patients may develop transient cerebral ischaemic attacks or visual field defects, or, more significantly, progressive cerebral ischaemia.

> Two other features of the syndrome are a tendency to multiple spontaneous abortions and peripheral thrombosis, often with multiple leg and arm vein thrombosis. We have also seen Budd–Chiari syndrome and renal vein thrombosis in some of these patients.

> We have, of course, tended to group these patients under the diagnostic umbrella of systemic lupus, though an alternative label of "primary" Sjögren's syndrome covers other patients, and characteristic dry Schirmer's tests and lymphocytic infiltration of the minor salivary glands have been found in a number (though not all) of this group of patients. To

my mind, however, the most striking, and often the most serious feature of the disease is the tendency to thrombosis, particularly cerebral thrombosis. So prominent has this feature been that we have some patients in their 40s and 50s who had been diagnosed as primary cerebrovascular disease or – when the labile hypertension has been observed – as hypertensive cerebrovascular disease. The finding that many of these patients may have high titres of circulating anti-cardiolipin antibodies leads us to believe that a new line of investigation may be possible in such patients.

In the early 1980s my team then at Hammersmith, collected large numbers of patients who had the syndrome, yet did not meet the classification criteria for lupus – we called these patients "anticardiolipin syndrome" – and changed the name to the antiphospholipid syndrome when it was clear that these patients' sera were also cross-reactive with other phospholipids such as phosphatidylserine [8–10].

So, in the few years between 1983 and 1987, our description of the syndrome included recurrent fetal loss [11], livedo [7], renal thrombosis [12], strokes [13], liver thrombosis including Budd–Chiari syndrome [14], myelopathy [15], chorea [16], bowel infarction [17], thrombocytopenia [18], pulmonary hypertension [19] and dementia [20].

The clinical collaborators included Margaret Byron, Bernie Colaco, Genevieve Derue, Mee-Ling Boey, later joined by Charles Mackworth-Young, Sozos Loizou, Bupendra Patel, John Chan, Keith Elkon, Mark Walport and Ron Asherson. In the laboratory, two research fellows, Aziz Gharavi, and later Nigel Harris, spearheaded the development of immunoassays culminating in the first (*Lancet*) paper on the assay for anticardiolipin antibodies [21] which paved the way for the development of the enzyme-linked immunosorbent assay (ELISA) [22] and the widespread testing and recognition of the syndrome.

In his 1983 Prosser-White lecture, Graham Hughes emphasized his view that many of the patients did not have classic lupus, and deserved separate consideration as a syndrome [7]. His group, in the early 1980s, published a number of reports which associated aPL with the syndrome *outside* of systemic lupus. He reported aPL in Behçet's disease, idiopathic transverse myelopathy and Guillain–Barré syndrome [23], idiopathic thrombocytopenia [18], migraine, epilepsy [24], heart valve disease [25] and Addison's disease [26].

Graham Hughes's view was that this was most certainly a "distinct" syndrome which occurs in ANA-negative lupus erythematosus (LE) patients, atypical lupus patients and, as expected, individuals with no lupus at all [7]. In 1987 his group was the first to introduce the term "antiphospholipid syndrome" and "primary antiphospholipid syndrome" [10] and 2 years later, in 1989, two large series of patients were published, one by his group [27] and another by the group in Mexico [28], which confirmed and detailed the earlier clinical descriptions.

1990 heralded the next major advance, when three groups [29–31] reported that aPL required a plasma protein "cofactor" to bind cardiolipin on ELISA plates. β_2-glycoprotein I was identified as this cofactor. Since then, a number of "cofactors", including prothrombin, have been described [32]. The binding of antibodies to the antigen site is clearly complex and dependent on molecule configuration. Studies using monoclonal antibodies have, for example, suggested binding to a trimolecular site including phospholipid, protein C and cofactor [33]. It is now felt that the cumbersome term "phospholipid-cofactor syndrome" is probably wrong.

From Osler on, many observers of lupus have recognized thrombosis as a feature in some patients. Similarly, many other features, including thrombocytopenia and recurrent miscarriage, are well recognized as features of the disease. Historically, the "oldest" immunological finding in SLE is the Wasserman reaction. In 1952, Moore and Mohr recognized that their false positive (BFP-STS) syphilis tests could occur in lupus [34]. In 1957, Laurell and Nilsson [35] found that the "lupus inhibitor" was frequently associated with BFP-STS.

Bowie et al [36] in clinical studies of lupus, reported thrombotic lesions in patients with a circulating anticoagulant. Beaumont et al in 1954 [37] were the first to report a patient with lupus anticoagulant and recurrent abortions. This was followed by similar observations by Nilsson et al [38], 20 years later and by Soulier and Boffa [39] 5 years later.

This volume acknowledges the many who have worked so hard to bring recognition to the syndrome. To Nigel Harris and Aziz Gharavi – involved from the early days – to the dozens of research fellows who have trained in our laboratory, and whose names are associated with so much of the APS literature; to Donato Alarcon-Segovia, for his enthusiasm in endorsing the syndrome with his surveys of his own lupus patients; to Takao Koike, for providing so much to the studies of β_2-glycoprotein I; to Marie Claire Boffa, for her collaboration and organizing ability in setting up collabortive workshops, and to Yehuda Shoenfeld for contributing so much momentum, especially through his animal model studies, to our knowledge of the syndrome.

This syndrome is common. Many physicians ask "where were all these patients before?". They were always there – in lupus clinics, in migraine clinics, in anticoagulant clinics with strokes, with multiple sclerosis, and with a gamut of vascular problems. It is also probable that many, many patients – notably those with memory loss or subtle neurological deficit, remain undiagnosed.

The description of the APS by Graham Hughes has had an impact on patients in all corners of medical practice.

References

1. Khamashta MA, Mackworth Young C. Antiphospholipid (Hughes) syndrome – a treatable cause of recurrent pregnancy loss. Br Med J 1997;314:244.
2. Harats D, George J, Levy Y, Khamashta MA, Hughes GRV, Shoenfeld Y. Atheroma: links with antiphospholipid antibodies, Hughes syndrome and lupus. Quart J Med 1999;92:57–59.
3. 8th International Symposium on Antiphospholipid Antibodies, Sapporo, Japan (1998). Lupus 7 (Suppl 2): 1–234.
4. Wilson WA, Gharavi AE, Koike T et al. International consensus statement on preliminary classification criteria for definite antiphospholipid syndrome. Report of an international workshop. Arthritis Rheum 1999;42:1309–1311.
5. Hughes GRV. Hughes syndrome – the syndrome behind the name (otherwise known as antiphospholipid syndrome). Isr Med Ass J 1999;1:100–103.
6. Wilson WA, Hughes GRV. Aetiology of Jamaican neuropathy. Lancet 1975;i:240.
7. Hughes GRV. Connective tissue disease and the skin. The 1983 Prosser-White oration. Clin Exp Dermatol 1984;9:535–544.
8. Hughes GRV. The anticardiolipin syndrome. Clin Exp Rheumatol 1985;3:285.
9. Harris EN, Baguley E, Asherson RA, Hughes GRV. Clinical and serological features of the antiphospholipid syndrome. Br J Rheumatol 1987;26:19 (abstract).
10. Mackworth-Young CG, David J, Loizou S, Walport MJ. Primary antiphospholipid syndrome: features in patients with raised anticardiolipin antibodies and no other disorders. Br J Rheumatol 1987;26:94 (abstract).
11. Derue GJ, Englert HJ, Harris EN et al. Fetal loss in systemic lupus: association with anticardiolipin antibodies. J Obstet Gynaecol 1985;2:207–209.
12. Hughes GRV, Asherson RA. Formes atypiques du lupus erythemateux dissemine. In: Crosnier J, Funck-Brentano JL, Brack JF, Grungeld JP, editors. Actualites nephrologiques. Flammarion Medicine: Paris, 1984.

13. Harris EN, Gharavi AE, Asherson RA, Boey ML, Hughes GRV. Cerebral infarction in systemic lupus. Association with anticardiolipin antibodies. Clin Exp Rheumatol 1984;2:47–51.
14. Mackworth-Young CG, Gharavi AE, Boey ML, Hughes GRV. Portal and pulmonary hypertension in a case of systemic lupus erythematosus: possible relationships with clotting abnormality. Eur J Rheumatol Inflamm 1984;7:72–74.
15. Harris EN, Gharavi AE, Mackworth-Young CG, Patel BM, Derue G, Hughes GR. Lupoid sclerosis: a possible pathogenetic role for antiphospholipid antibodies. Ann Rheum Dis 1985;44:281–282.
16. Asherson RA, Hughes GRV. Antiphospholipid antibodies and chorea. J Rheumatol 1988;15:377–379.
17. Asherson RA, Morgan SH, Harris EN, Gharavi AE, Kraus T, Hughes GRV. Arterial occlusion causing large bowel infarction in SLE. Reflection of clotting diathesis. Clin Rheumatol 1986;5:102–106.
18. Harris EN, Gharavi AE, Hegde U et al. Anticardiolipin antibodies in autoimmune thrombocytopenic purpura. Br J Haematol 1985;59:231–234.
19. Asherson RA, Mackworth-Young CG, Boey ML et al. Pulmonary hypertension in systemic lupus erythematosus. Br Med J 1983;287:1024–1025.
20. Asherson RA, Mercy D, Philips G et al. Recurrent stroke and multi-infarct dementia in systemic lupus erythematosus associated with antiphospholipid antibodies. Ann Rheum Dis 1987;46:605–611.
21. Harris EN, Gharavi AE, Bowie ML et al. Anticardiolipin antibodies: detection by radioimmunoassay and association with thrombosis in SLE. Lancet 1983;ii:1211–1214.
22. Harris EN, Gharavi AE, Patel SP et al. Evaluation of the anticardiolipin antibody test: report of a standardisation workshop held on April 4th, 1986. Clin Exp Immunol 1987;58:215–222.
23. Harris EN, Englert H, Derue G et al. Antiphospholipid antibodies in acute Guillain–Barré syndrome. Lancet 1983;ii:1361–1362.
24. Herranz MT, Rivier G, Khamashta MA, Blaser KU, Hughes GRV. Association between antiphospholipid antibodies and epilepsy in patients with systemic lupus erythematosus. Arthritis Rheum 1994;37:568–571.
25. Khamashta MA, Cervera R, Asherson RA et al. Association of antibodies against phospholipids with heart valve disease in systemic lupus erythematosus. Lancet 1990;335:1541–1544.
26. Asherson RA, Hughes GRV. Addison's disease and primary antiphospholipid syndrome. Lancet 1989;ii:874.
27. Asherson RA, Khamashta MA, Ordi-Ros J et al. The "primary" antiphospholipid syndrome: major clinical and serological features. Medicine (Baltimore) 1989;68:366–374.
28. Alarcon-Segovia D, Sanchez-Guerrero J. Primary antiphospholipid syndrome. J Rheumatol 1989;16:482–488.
29. Matsuura E, Igarashi Y, Fujimoto M, Ichikawa K, Koike T. Anticardiolipin co-factor(s) and differential diagnosis of autoimmune disease. Lancet 1990;336:177–178.
30. Galli M, Comfurius P, Maassen C et al. Anticardiolipin antibodies (ACA) are directed not to cardiolipin but to a plasma protein co-factor. Lancet 1990;335:1544–1547.
31. McNeil HP, Simpson RJ, Chesterman CN, Krilis SA. Antiphospholipid antibodies are directed against a complex antigen that includes a lipid-binding inhibitor of coagulation: $_2$-glycoprotein I (apolipoprotein H). Proc Natl Acad Sci USA 1990;87:4120–4124.
32. Roubey RAS. Auto-antibodies to phospholipid binding proteins: a new view of lupus anticoagulants and other "antiphospholipid" antibodies. Blood 1994;84:2854–2867.
33. Atsumi T, Khamashta, MA, Amengual O et al. Binding of anticardiolipin antibodies to Protein C via β_2-glycoprotein I (β_2-GPI): a possible mechanism in the inhibitory effect of antiphospholipid antibodies on the Protein C system. Clin Exp Immunol 1998;112:325–333.
34. Moore JE, Mohr CF. Biologically false positive serological test for syphilis. Type, incidence and cause. J Am Med Ass 1952;150:467–473.
35. Laurell AB, Nilsson IM. Hypergammaglobulinaemia, circulating anticoagulant and biological false positive Wasserman reaction: a study of 2 cases. J Lab Clin Med 1957;49:694–707.
36. Bowie EJW, Thompson Jr JH, Pascuzzi CV, Owen CA. Thrombosis in systemic lupus erythematosus despite circulating anticoagulant. J Lab Clin Med 1983;62:416–430.
37. Beaumont JL. Syndrome hemorrhagique acquis du a un anticoagulant circulant. Sang 1954;25:1–15.
38. Nilsson IM, Astedt B, Hedner U et al. Intrauterine death and circulating anticoagulant ("antithromboplastin"). Acta Med Scand 1975;197:153–159.
39. Soulier JP, Boffa MC. Avortements a repetition thromboses et anticoagulant circulant anti-thromboplastine. Nouv Press Med 1980;9:859–864.

2 Antiphospholipid Syndrome: General Features

T. Godfrey and D. D'Cruz

Introduction

The first papers on the antiphospholipid syndrome (APS) described recurrent arterial and venous thromboses and fetal losses. These remain the characteristic clinical features of this syndrome although the spectrum of associated symptoms and signs has broadened considerably over the last 15 years. The aim of this chapter is to give a clinical overview and preliminary classification criteria for the APS by way of introduction to the more detailed chapters that follow.

Demographics

APS has been recognized largely as a disease of young women due to the association with systemic lupus erythematosus (SLE), and pregnancy loss. In our experience approximately 50% of patients with APS do not have an underlying systemic disease and are labeled primary APS (PAPS). The age of first thrombosis in PAPS has been shown to range between 32 and 45 years [1]. There are problems with reporting bias, with young patients with thrombosis, and pregnancy loss more likely to be investigated, hence skewing the results. However, antiphospholipid antibodies (aPL) are being increasingly recognized in a diverse number of conditions and in older subjects.

The prevalence of APS in SLE increases with duration of follow up and on the number of samples tested for aPL. In a cohort of 667 patients with SLE (15% definite APS and 21% probable APS), with a mean follow up of 3.1 years, the prevalence of definite APS increased from 5 to 15% as the number of samples tested increased from 1–3 to 7–10 [2].

Racial differences have been noted with immunoglobulin A (IgA) anticardiolipin antibodies (aCL) more common in Afro-Caribbeans [3]. Histocompatibility genes associated with APS also show genetic differences. HLA-DR4 seems more important in Anglo-Saxons, whereas DR7 emerges in populations of Latin origin [4].

Definition and Classification of APS

An international consensus statement on classification criteria for definite antiphospholipid syndrome was published after a workshop in 1998 (Table 2.1) [5].

Table 2.1. Preliminary criteria for the classification of the antiphospholipid syndrome.

Clinical criteria

1. Vascular thrombosis:
   One or more clinical episodes of arterial, venous, or small vessel thrombosis, in any tissue or organ. Thrombosis must be confirmed by imaging or Doppler studies or histopathology, with the exception of superficial venous thrombosis. For histopathologic confirmation, thrombosis should be present without significant evidence of inflammation in the vessel wall.

2. Pregnancy morbidity
   a) One or more unexplained deaths of a morphologically normal fetus at or beyond the 10th weeks of gestation, with normal fetal morphology documented by ultrasound or by direct examination of the fetus, or
   b) One or more premature births of a morphologically normal neonate at or before the 34th week of gestation because of severe pre-eclampsia or eclampsia, or severe placental insufficiency or
   c) Three more unexplained consecutive spontaneous abortions before the 10th week of gestation, with maternal anatomic, or hormonal abnormalities and paternal and maternal chromosomal causes excluded.

Laboratory criteria

1. Anticardiolipin antibody of IgG and/ or IgM isotype in blood, present in medium or high titre, on two or more occasions, at least 6 weeks apart, measured by a standard enzyme linked immunosorbent assay for β_2-glycoprotein 1-dependent anticardiolipin antibodies.
2. Lupus anticoagulant present in plasma on two or more occasions at least 6 weeks apart, detected according to the guidelines of the International Society on Thrombosis and Hemostasis.

Definite APS is considered to be present if at least one of the clinical and one of the laboratory criteria are met.

The purpose of the classification criteria was to facilitate studies of treatment and causation, and focused on defining a category of "definite" APS. Probable or possible categories were excluded due to lack of supportive prospective studies or experimental evidence. The workshop acknowledged that thrombosis may be multifactorial and other contributing factors and comorbidities should be identified.

Other features of APS such as thrombocytopenia, hemolytic anemia, transient cerebral ischaemia, transverse myelopathy or myelitis, livedo reticularis, cardiac valve disease, multiple sclerosis-like syndrome, chorea, and migraine were felt by the workshop to not have as strong an association and were excluded as classification criteria. This should not deter the practicing clinician from making the diagnosis or administering therapy if other causes of such features have been excluded.

Piette has urged clinicians to be aware of suspicious symptoms. Fever and weight loss are unusual in APS and suggest infection or malignancy. Splenomegaly is not a feature of PAPS unless complicated [6]. Human immunodeficiency virus (HIV) infection is the syphilis of the late 20th century and can be a great mimicker, including the production of aPL, although thrombosis associated with aPL in these patients is rare.

When Should aPL Be Measured?

In the past 15 years it has become increasingly recognized that hereditary or acquired defects in anticoagulant mechanisms may predispose to thrombosis. The requirement for thrombophilia screening in patients who develop a thrombotic event must be assessed on an individual patient basis. Indications for screening are

Table 2.2. Indications for the measurement of aPL.

- Connective tissue disease especially SLE
- Venous/arterial thrombosis before the age of 45 years
- Thrombosis after trivial provocation
- Association of arterial and venous thrombosis
- Association of thrombosis and fetal loss
- Recurrent events
- Family history
- Thrombosis in an unusual site: retinal vein, portal, cerebral venous, renal vein
- Recurrent superficial thromophlebitis
- Recurrent miscarriage
- Coumarin-induced skin necrosis

listed in Table 2.2. The prevalence of aPL in SLE ranges between 30 and 50%; therefore a search for these antibodies is mandatory [7, 8]. aPL have also been found in a variety of other systemic autoimmune disorders including Sjögren's syndrome, myositis, vasculitis and rheumatoid arthritis [9].

The timing of measurement may be important. It has been suggested that aPL may be consumed during a thrombotic episode, or alternatively due to endothelial activation and exposure of cryptic antigens they may become positive after thrombosis: "epiphenomenon" [10]. For these reasons aPL should be measured between 6 weeks and 3 months post-thrombosis to confirm results. Steroid therapy and the development of the nephrotic syndrome may also be associated with a falsely negative result [11–13].

What Should Be Measured?

It is generally agreed that both IgG and IgM aCL isotypes should be tested in addition to lupus anticoagulant (LA). The significance of IgA aCL antibodies is however debated. Several studies have found an increased prevalence in Afro-Caribbean or Afro-American patients with SLE [14]. However the thrombotic risk is unclear. In contrast, in Spanish patients a very low prevalence was found, 2% in SLE patients and no cases of PAPS were positive [15]. A London-based study found a low frequency in a SLE population (13%) and in only 3/18 of these was IgA the only aCL isotype [16]. Molina et al found a correlation with hemolytic anemia, but not with thrombosis, in Hispanics [3]. Lopez, however, found a significant association of IgA aCL with thrombosis and thrombocytopenia in SLE patients that was more significant than IgM or IgG [17]. McCarty found IgA aCL to be the only isotype in 28 patients with APS [18].

IgA aCL has been associated with infection including human T-cell lymphotrophic virus (HTLV-1). An elevated total IgA level in sera of patients with HTLV-1 suggests that the IgA aCL in this population may represent polyclonal B-cell activation [19]. Tsutsumi measured IgA anti-β_2-glycoprotein I (anti-β_2GPI) in 124 SLE patients, and found 25% were positive and a significant relationship to thrombosis was observed [20].

Anti-β_2-glycoprotein I assays have shown a higher specificity for APS than aCL in 120 patients with PAPS, SLE with APS and SLE without APS. Anti-β_2GPI were detected in 53.5% of APS patients but only 4.1% of SLE patients [21].

Prevalence of aPL

General Population

What is the prevalence of aPL in the general population? Nencini et al in 1993 studied 55 healthy volunteers with a mean age of 40 years; only one patient had a positive aCL or LA [22]. In 543 blood donors under 65 years Fields et al found a prevalence of 2% for aCL [23]. The Antiphospholipid Antibodies in Stroke Study (APASS) Group also found a prevalence of aCL in 4.3% of 257 hospitalized patients (non stroke) with mean age 66, which was similar to the prevalence in 1014 in-patients studied by Schved et al with a mean age of 66.7 years with the most frequent association carcinoma or alcohol abuse [24, 25]. Ginsberg in a population of 179 patients, mean age 55 years in whom DVT had been excluded found a prevalence of aCL in 18% and LA in 2% [26].

Venous Thromboembolism

In patients with venous thromboembolism(VTE): the prevalence of aCL varies from 3% to 17% and LA 3–14%. The lowest rates were found by Kearon et al in a study of "idiopathic" VTE. The highest figures were found by Schulman et al who examined 897 patients with VTE, with a follow up of 4 years, in whom aCL were tested 6 months post-deep vein thromboembolism (DVT). Interestingly, of 20 recurrent episodes aCL was negative in 14 at the time of the recurrent episode [26–29].

Systemic Lupus Erythematosus

The highest prevalence of aPL occurs in patients with SLE, with estimates varying between 30 and 63%. Ghirardello et al found 51.4% of SLE patients were positive for aCL and 8.6% for LA, whilst in Horbach's retrospective study IgG aCL were found in 64% of patients with a history of thrombosis and 41% in those without thrombosis; LA were found in 25.1% [30, 31].

Arterial Thrombosis

In the situation of stroke Nencini et al found 18% of young patients, mean age 38 years, were positive for aPL (LA and aCL) whereas APASS found 9.7% of first stroke patients had a positive aCL. In myocardial infarction the prevalence of aCL is between 5 and 15% [22, 24, 32].

Elderly

Many autoantibodies become more prevalent with increasing age and aPL is no exception. Fields found that 12% of 300 healthy elderly, those older than 65, had IgG or IgM aCL antibodies and that there was an association with positive antinuclear antibodies (ANA) but not rheumatoid factor [23]. Schved found a prevalence of 7% [25]. However, it is unclear whether this is a result of the increasing prevalence of associated conditions in the elderly such as malignancy, and drug treatment. The significance of such antibodies in the elderly remains unclear although they have been found to be a risk factor for ischemic stroke in both the young and elderly.

Risk of Positive aPL Tests

What is the risk of having these antibodies in the above groups of patients? In VTE Bongard compared 107 patients with DVT to 186 without DVT and found no association with aCL [33]. Ginsberg, in 1995, studied patients with a first episode of venous thromboembolism. A strong association with LA was found with an odds ratio of 9.4 but no significant association was found with aCL, even when only those patients with high levels (greater than 50 G phospholipid (GPL) units) were studied [26]. Simioni also found a significant association with the LA with an odds ratio of 10.7 [29]. Schulman in 1998 examined the incidence of recurrent DVT in patients who were aCL positive. The risk ratio for further venous thrombosis was 2.1 [28]. A similar risk was found by Kearon in 1999 who looked at recurrence rates in 162 patients with "idiopathic" DVT where the risk was 2.3 for aCL and 6.8 for LA [27]. In a meta-analysis Wahl in 1998 examined the risk of venous thromboembolism in aPL positive patients without autoimmune disease or previous thrombosis. The odds ratio was 11.1 for LA and 1.6 for aCL. However, that risk rose to 3.21 if higher titers of aCL were examined [34]. There were 90 DVTs in the American Physicians Health Study and aCL levels greater than the 95th percentile (greater than 33 GPL units) had a relative risk of venous thromboembolism of 5.3 [35].

In terms of arterial disease the American Physicians Study did not find a significant association of aCL with CVA. A study of community-dwelling elderly by Schmidt, found no association between MRI findings and aCL status but there was an association with neuropsychological performance [36]. Nencini and coworkers in 1993 found 18% of young strokes were positive for aPL tested at 99 days post-CVA compared to 2% of controls. They also found that the recurrence rate for stroke was higher in the aPL group compared to a group of stroke patients that were negative [22]. The APASS group compared first stroke to a control population of non-stroke hospitalized patients. ACL were studied and were positive in 24 of 248 of the stroke patients compared to 11 of 257 control patients. The odds ratio for stroke in patients who were aCL positive was calculated at 2.33. There was no correlation between time of blood drawn after first stroke and aCL status. In addition they found that the prevalence of aCL was only slightly higher in patients with prior stroke compared with those with first stroke. They concluded that it was unlikely that stroke causes a positive aCL status i.e. is an epiphenomenon [24]. This was supported in a study by Chakravarty et al who found that none of initial antibody-negative stroke patients became positive when sera were retested after 6 months [37]. The APASS group concluded that aCL were a risk factor for first ischemic stroke and the extent of association was comparable to that between stroke and hypertension. Kittner, who reviewed several epidemiological studies concluded that the strength of association between aCL and stroke, in patients over 50 years, was comparable to hypertension with an odds ratio of 2.2. In a young population < 50 years the odds ratio may rise to 8.3 [38].

Further information on arterial disease is obtained from the Helsinki heart study. In this study healthy men with a low-density lipoprotein (LDL) cholesterol greater than 5.2 mmol/l, with a mean age of 49 years, were studied for cardiac end points. In the highest quartile of aCL patients, the odds ratio for myocardial infarct was significant at 2.0. In multivariate analysis the risk was independent of other risk factors and interestingly aCL levels were higher in smokers [32].

In SLE, Ghirardello et al found that thrombosis was associated with LA and to a lesser extent with IgG aCL [30]. Horbach et al found that LA was a significant risk factor for both VTE and arterial events (odds ratio 6.55 and 9.77, respectively) but only IgM aCL greater than 20 M phospholipid (MPL) units were associated with venous events (odds ratio 3.90). There was no association of aCL with arterial disease [31]. Abu Shakra et al studied 390 lupus patients and found no association of aCL with thrombosis, but there was an association with Coombs positive status and thrombocytopenia. LA was associated with thrombosis with odds ratio of 7.9 [39]. Wahl performed a meta-analysis of the risk of venous thromboembolism and examined 26 studies comprising 2249 patients. The odds ratio for LA and venous events was 6.32 and 2.17 for aCL. When recurrent venous events were examined these ratios increased to 11.6 and 3.91, respectively [40].

A significant impact on survival has also been noted by several authors. In a retrospective study of 52 patients with aCL followed over 10 years, 29% of APS patients (31 patients) had recurrent events and in the asymptomatic group (21 patients) half developed APS. Mortality was 10% [41]. The negative impact on survival of aCL has been reported by several authors. Jouhikainen et al compared 37 SLE patients, LA positive, with 37 age and sex matched SLE patients without LA. During a median follow up of 22 years, 30% in the LA group died in contrast to 14% in the control group [42]. Among patients with VTE (major associated disease excluded) the mortality in Swedish patients was 15% at 4 years in those with aCL and 6% in those without antibodies ($P = 0.01$) [28].

In summary, the following observations can be made. aPL are present in approximately 2–4% of the normal population and the prevalence increases with age. A high prevalence amongst SLE patients is seen. There is an association with both venous and arterial thrombosis but the strength of association varies amongst studies. This probably reflects on different population groups, study designs i.e. retrospective versus prospective, different assays used and definitions of thrombosis. In several studies the risk of thrombosis appears to be higher with LA and the data suggests a true association rather than epiphenomenon. In a given patient, both aCL and LA should be measured. A significant impact on long-term survival has been noted. The positive predictive value of individual tests will need to be evaluated in future studies.

Risk Factors for Thrombosis in APS

In a cohort of 360 patients in the Italian aPL Registry (patients identified by either previous thrombosis, abnormal coagulation study suggestive of LA, or suffering with a disease known to be associated with aPL) followed prospectively for a median of 3.9 years, with either a positive LA or aCL, 34 patients developed a thrombotic event (26 spontaneously). This was a total incidence of 2.5%/patient-year, with a rate of 5.4%/patient-year in those with a previous thrombosis and 0.95%/patient-year in asymptomatic subjects [43]. Clearly the mere presence of aPL is not sufficient for an event. Patients with aCL > 40 units and previous thrombosis were important risk factors for future events. The importance of previous thrombosis as a risk factor was highlighted by the recurrence rate in our patients at St. Thomas' Hospital, where those with APS and previous thrombosis, had a recurrence rate of 20%/patient-year of follow-up [44]. In pregnancy, patients with a prior history of miscarriages or vascular occlusions have a significantly higher rate of adverse pregnancy outcome [43].

Emlen was also concerned about the low positive predictive value of current aPL assays and reminded us of the many risk factors for thrombosis in lupus patients [45]. Most centers dealing with large numbers of SLE patients are now focussing on the increased prevalence of arterial disease and aiming to correct risk factors in individual patients including hypertension, lipids and homocysteinemia in the hope of preventing late morbidity, which is often vascular in origin.

Several studies have shown that risk factors can be additive. In venous thrombosis in the young, Rosendaal found that the risk of thrombosis rose sharply with the number of risk factors and that fewer factors were required for thrombosis in older subjects (greater than 55 years) [46]. The coincidental presence of other coagulation abnormalities such as factor V Leiden in patients with APS has been reported by several groups. Factor V Leiden and aCL can both cause the activated protein C resistance phenotype and not surprisingly the combination has been associated with severe thrombosis [47–50]. Methylenetetrahydrofolate reductase $C^{677} \rightarrow T$ substitution (increased homocystinuria) may also have an effect on age at first occlusive event [49]. Furthermore, Peddi reported the development of catastrophic APS in a patient with SLE, aCL and antithrombin III deficiency [51].

Conditions Associated with Secondary APS

It has been estimated that up to one half of patients with APS do not have an associated systemic disease [52]. A large number of conditions have however been reported in association with aPL. These are listed in Table 2.3. In most of these conditions apart from SLE, thrombosis i.e. APS is unusual. In a prospective study Merkel found 16% of rheumatoid arthritis and SLE patients had either IgG or IgM aCL compared with 4.0% of blood donors. Patients with scleroderma, myositis, undifferentiated connective tissue disease and systemic vasculitis did not differ in prevalence from the control blood donors [9].

Table 2.3. aPL in other conditions.

• Connective tissue disorders	• Drugs
• Systemic vasculitis	Chlorpromazine
• Malignancy	Quinine/quinidine
• Crohn's disease	Hydralazine
• Infection	Procainamide
Syphilis/Lyme	Phenytoin
Human immunodeficiency virus	Interferon-α
Hepatitis C	
Cytomegalovirus	
Mycoplasma	

The manifestations of APS are not usually seen in infection- or drug-associated aCL although occasional reports of the development of thrombosis in infections such as acquired immune deficiency syndrome (AIDS) and cytomegalovirus (CMV) has prompted people to recommend searching for infections in patients developing manifestations of APS [53, 54]. Procainamide has been shown to produce β_2-glycoprotein 1-dependent antibodies that are potentially pathogenic [55].

Differences Between Primary and Secondary APS

Vianna et al found that PAPS and APS secondary to SLE had similar clinical features, but heart valve disease, autoimmune hemolytic anemia, lymphopenia, neutropenia, and low C4 levels were more common in patients with SLE [56]. Anti-dsDNA or antibodies to extractable nuclear antigens were not found in PAPS and their presence should suggest a secondary cause. The distinction between PAPS and APS due to SLE can sometimes be difficult. Features such as thrombocytopenia, anemia, renal, and central nervous system (CNS) disease may be seen in both conditions. Piette has been a strong advocate of exclusion criteria for PAPS and these are listed in Table 2.4 [57].

There do not appear to be any differences in rates of arterial or venous thrombosis, or fetal loss [43, 56, 58]. Shah et al found IgM aCL more commonly in SLE than PAPS (22/42 versus 1/10) but no difference in thrombotic rates [41].

Descriptions of families with multiple family members affected have suggested a familial association. Not all studies in SLE have found an association with HLA class 2 alleles though several studies have shown an association with HLA DR4, HLA-DR7 and HLA-DRw53. There appear to be ethnic differences with HLA-DR4 more important in Anglo-Saxons and HLA DR7 in populations of Latin extraction. At this stage no clear pattern of differences between PAPS and secondary APS has emerged [4, 50, 59].

The number of cases reported in the literature of patients with PAPS evolving into SLE is small. Silver et al and Mujic et al have reported the evolution in small numbers (7/71 and 3/80, respectively) but Asherson et al and Vianna et al did not find any [52, 56, 60, 61]. The short period of follow-up may have been responsible for the latter result (5 and 2 years, respectively) as several patients have developed the syndrome after 10 years. The presence of high titer of ANA (> 1:320) and lymphopenia may be predictive [62].

Table 2.4. Exclusion criteria to distinguish SLE associated APS from PAPS.

- Malar or discoid rash
- Oral, pharyngeal, or nasal ulceration
- Frank arthritis
- Pleurisy/pericarditis
- Persistent proteinuria > 0.5 g/day, due to biopsy proven immune complex related glomerulonephritis
- Lymphopenia < 1000 cells/μl
- Antibodies to dsDNA (crithidia or radioimmunoassay), or ENA
- ANA > 1:320
- Treatment with drugs known to produce aPL
- Follow up < 5 years from the initial clinical manifestation.

Clinical Features

Clinical features will be covered extensively in following chapters. The definite associations are with arterial and venous thrombosis, recurrent miscarriage and thrombocytopenia. The latter is generally mild and occurs in 20–40% of patients with APS. Severe thrombocytopenia is unusual [63]. Cardiac valve abnormality is also seen in up to 35% of patients, usually regurgitation and the mitral valve is affected more often than the aortic. Valve thrombi, subendothelial deposits of immunoglobulins, including aCL have been noted in deformed valves [64]. Diastolic dysfunction and cardiomyopathy perhaps related to subclinical myocardial damage has also been reported [65]. Avascular necrosis is of interest to rheumatologists and most cases

Table 2.5. Clinical associations.

CNS	Bone
Chorea	Avascular necrosis
Migraine	Bone marrow necrosis
Psychosis	
Epilepsy	**Obstetric**
CVA/TIA	Recurrent miscarriage
Hypoperfusion on SPECT scanning	Pre-eclampsia
Sensorineural hearing loss	Growth retardation
Transverse myelopathy	HELLP syndrome
Cognitive impairment	
Pseudotumor cerebri	**Renal**
Cerebral vein/artery thrombosis	Glomerular thrombosis
Retinal venous thrombosis	Renal artery stenosis
Multiple sclerosis like syndrome	Renal insufficiency
	Renal artery thrombosis
	Renal vein thrombosis
Gastrointestinal	
Hepatic necrosis	**Pulmonary**
Acalculous cholecystitis	Pulmonary embolism
Budd–Chiari	Pulmonary hypertension
Intestinal ischemia	ARDS
Vascular disease	**Endocrine**
Atherosclerosis	Adrenal failure
Cardiac valvular disease	Hypopituitarism
Acute myocardial infarction	
Failed angioplasty	**Hematological**
Diastolic dysfunction	Thrombocytopenia
Intracardiac thrombosis	Autoimmune hemolytic anemia
Cardiomyopathy	
Buerger's disease	
Skin	
Livedo reticularis	
Cutaneous ulcers	
Dego's Disease	
Splinter hemorrhages	
Superficial thrombophlebitis	
Distal cutaneous ischemia	

CVA, cerebrovascular accident; TIA, transient ischemic attack; SPECT, single position emission computerized tomography; HELLP, hemolytic anaemia, elevated liver function tests and low platelets; ARDS, adult respiratory distress syndrome.

are seen in patients taking steroids. However, although avascular necrosis has been reported in small number of patients with PAPS, studies in patients with SLE have not shown a definite association with aPL. Numerous other associations have been reported and these manifestations are listed in Table 2.5. Whether these will all stand the test of time remains to be determined.

Conclusion

The APS has been clearly defined with distinct clinical and serological features. Early recognition of this syndrome by clinicians in a variety of specialties is crucial in improving the risk of morbidity and mortality in these patient populations.

References

1. Piette JC, Cacoub P. Antiphospholipid syndrome in the elderly: caution. Circulation 1998;97:2195–2196.
2. Perez-Vazquez ME, Villa A, Drenkard C, Cabiedes J, Alarcon-Segovia D: Influence of disease duration, continued follow up and further antiphopholipid testing on the frequency and classification category of antiphospholipid syndrome in a cohort of patients with SLE. J Rheumatol 1993;20:437–42.
3. Molina JF, Gutierrez-Urena S, Molina J et al. Variability of anticardiolipin antibody isotype distribution in 3 geographic populations of patients with systemic lupus erythematosus. J Rheumatol 1997; 1997;24:291–296.
4. Sebastiani GD, Galeazzi M, Morozzi G, Marcolongo R: The immunogenetics of the antiphospholipid syndrome, anticardiolipin antibodies,and lupus anticoagulant. Semin Arthritis Rheum 1996;25:414–420.
5. Wilson WA, Gharavi AE, Koike T et al. International consensus statement on preliminary classification criteria for definite antiphospholipid syndrome. Report of an International Workshop. Arthritis Rheum 1999;42:1309–1311.
6. Piette JC: Criteria for the antiphospholpid syndrome. Lupus 1998;7(Suppl 2):S149–S157.
7. Cervera R, Font J, Lopez-Soto A et al. Isotype distribution of anticardiolipin antibodies in SLE, prospective analysis of 100 patients. Ann Rheum Dis 1990;49:109–113.
8. Alarcon-Segovia D, Deleze M, Oria CV et al. Antiphospholipid antibodies and the antiphospholipid syndrome in SLE. A prospective analysis of 500 consecutive patients. Medicine 1989;68:353–365.
9. Merkel P, Chang Y, Pierangeli S, Convery K, Harris N, Polisson R. The prevalence and clinical associations of anticardiolipin antibodies in a large inception cohort of patients with connective tissue diseases. Am J Med; 1996; 101: 576–583.
10. Petri M. Update on antiphospholipid antibodies. Curr Opin Rheumatol 1998;10:426–430.
11. Perez-Vazquez ME, Cabiedes J, Cabral AR, Alarcon-Segovia D. Decrease in serum antiphospholipid antibodies upon development of the nephrotic syndrome in patients with SLE: relationship to urinary losses of IgG and other factors. Am J Med 1992;92:357–363.
12. Silveira LH, Jara LJ, Espinoza LR. Transient disappearance of serum antiphospholipid antibodies can also be due to prednisolone therapy. Clin Exp Rheumatol 1996; 14: 217–226.
13. Drenkard C, Sanchez-Guerrero J, Alarcon-Segovia D. Fall in antiphospholipid antibody at time of thrombooclusive episodes in SLE. J Rheumatol 1989;16:614–617.
14. Faghiri Z, Taheri F, Wilson WA et al. IgA is the most prevalent isotype of anticardiolipin and anti-β_2 glycoprotein-1 antibodies in Jamaican and African–American SLE patients. Lupus 1998; 7(Suppl 2):S185.
15. Selva-O'Callaghan A, Ordi-Ros J, Monegal-Ferran F, Martinez N, Cortes-Hernandez F, Vilardell-Tarres M. IgA anticardiolipin antibodies – relation with other antiphospholipid antibodies and clinical significance. Thromb Haemost 1998;79:282–285.
16. Bertolaccini ML, Atsumi T, Amengual O, Katsumata K, Khamashta MA, Hughes GRV. IgA anticardiolipin antibody testing does not contribute to the diagnosis of antiphospholipid syndrome in patients with SLE. Lupus 1998;7(Suppl 2): S184.
17. Lopez LR, Santos ME, Espinoza LR, La Rosa FG. Clinical significance of IgA versus IgG and M anticardiolipin antibodies in patients with SLE. Am J Clin Pathol 1992;98:449–454.

18. McCarty GA, Freeland E,Wagenknecht DR, McIntyre JA. Antiphospholipid antibody syndrome in 28 patients with IgA as the sole antibody isotype. Lupus 1998;7(Suppl 2):S186.
19. Wilson WA, Morgan OC, Barton EN et al. IgA antiphospholipid antibodies in HTLV1 associated tropical spastic paraparesis. Lupus 1995;4:138-141.
20. Tsutsumi A, Matsuura E, Ichikawa K et al. Ig A class anti β_2 glycoprotein 1 in patients with SLE. J Rheumatol 1998;25:74-78.
21. Amengual O, Atsumi T, Khamashta MA, Koike T, Hughes GR. Specificity of ELISA for antibody to beta 2 glycoprotein 1 in patients with antiphospholpid syndrome. Br J Rheumatol 1996;35:1239-1243.
22. Nencini P, Baruffi M, Abbate R, Massai G, Amaducci L, Inzitari D. Lupus anticoagulant and anticardiolipin antibodies in young adults with cerebral ischaemia. Stroke 1992;23:189-193.
23. Fields R, Toubbeh H, Searles R, Bankhurst A. The prevalence of anticardiolipin antibodies in a healthy elderly population and its association with antinuclear antibodies. J Rheumatol 1989;16:623-625.
24. Antiphospholipid Antibodies in Stroke Study Group. Clinical, radiological, and pathological aspects of cerebrovascular disease associated with antiphospholipid antibodies. Stroke 1993;24(Suppl 1):S1-123.
25. Schved JF, Dupuy-Fons C, Biron C, Quere I, Janbon C. A prospective epidemiological study on the occurrence of antiphospholipid antibody: the Montpellier Antiphospholipid (MAP) Study. Haemostasis 1994;24:175-182.
26. Ginsberg J, Wells P, Brill-Edwards P et al. Antiphospholipid antibodies and venous thromboembolism. Blood 1995;86:3685-3691.
27. Kearon C, Gent M, Hirsh J, Weitz J et al. A comparison of three months of anticoagulation with extended anticoagulation for a first episode of idiopathic venous thromboembolism. N Engl J Med 1999;340:901-907.
28. Schulman S, Svenungsson E, Granqvist S and the Duration of Anticoagulation Study Group. Anticardiolipin antibodies predict early recurrence of thromboembolism and death among patients with venous thromboembolism following anticoagulant therapy. Am J Med 1998;104:332-338.
29. Simioni P, Prandoni P, Zanon E et al. Deep venous thrombosis and lupus anticoagulant. A case–control study. Thromb Haemost 1996;76:187-189.
30. Ghirardello A, Doria A, Ruffatti A et al. Antiphospholipid antibodies (aPL) in systemic lupus erythematosus. Are they specific tools for the diagnosis of aPL syndrome. Ann Rheum Dis 1994;53:140-142.
31. Horbach DA, van Oort E, Donders RC et al. Lupus anticoagulant is the strongest risk factor for both venous and arterial thrombosis in patients with systemic lupus erythematosus – comparison between different assays for the detection of antiphospholpid antibodies, Thromb Haemost 1996;76:916-924.
32. Vaarala O, Puurunen M, Manttari M et al. Anticardiolipin antibodies and risk of myocardial infarction in a prospective cohort of middle-aged men. Circulation 1995;91:23-27.
33. Bongard O, Reber G, Bounameaux H, deMoerloose P. Anticardiolipin in acute venous thromboembolism. Thromb Haemost 1992;67:724.
34. Wahl DG, Guillemin F, de Maistre E, Perret-Guillaume C, Lecompte T, Thibaut G. Meta-analysis of the risk of venous thrombosis in individuals with antiphospholipid antibodies without underlying autoimmune disease or previous thrombosis. Lupus 1998;7:15-22.
35. Ginsburg K, Liang M, Newcomer L et al. Anticardiolipin antibodies and the risk for ischemic stroke and venous thrombosis. Ann Intern Med 1992;117:997-1002.
36. Schmidt R, Auer-Grumbach P, Fazekas F, Offenbacher H, Kapeller P. Anticardiolipin antibodies in normal subjects. Neuropsychological correlates and MRI findings. Stroke 1995;26:749-754.
37. Chakravaty KK, Byron MA, Webley M et al. Antibodies to cardiolipin in stroke: Association with mortality and functional recovery in patients without systemic lupus erythematosus. Q J Med 1991;79:397-405.
38. Kittner S, Gorelick P. Antiphospholipid antibodies and stroke: an epidemiological perspective. Stoke 1992;23(Suppl 1):1-19, 1-22.
39. Abu-Shakra M, Gladman DD, Urowitz MB, Farewell V. Anticardiolipin antibodies in systemic lupus erythematosus: clinical and laboratory correlations. Am J Med 1995;99:624-628.
40. Wahl DG, Guillemin F, de Maistre E, Perret C, Lecompte T, Thibaut G. Risk for venous thrombosis related to antiphospholipid antibodies in systemic lupus erythematosus. A meta-analysis. Lupus 1997;6:467-473.
41. Shah NM, Khamashta MA, Atsumi T, Hughes GRV. Outcome of patients with anticardiolipin antibodies: a 10 year follow up of 52 patients. Lupus 1998;7:3-6.
42. Jouhikainen T, Stephansson E, Leirisalo-Repo M. Lupus anticoagulant as a prognostic marker in systemic lupus erythematosus. Br J Rheumatol 1993;32:568-573.

43. Finazzi G, Brancaccio V, Moia M et al. Natural history and risk factors for thrombosis in 360 patients with antiphospholipid antibodies. A four year prospective study from the Italian Registry. Am J Med. 1996;100:530–536.
44. Khamashta M, Cuadrado M, Mujic F, Taub N, Hunt B, Hughes GRV. The management of thrombosis in the antiphospholipid–antibody syndrome. N Engl J Med 1995;332:993–997.
45. Emlen W. Antiphospholipid antibodies: new complexities and new assays. Arthritis Rheum 1996;39:1441–1443.
46. Rosendaal F. Thrombosis in the young: epidemiology and risk factors. A focus on venous thrombosis. Thromb Haemost 1997;78:1–6.
47. Brenner B, Vulfsons SL, Lanir N, Nahir M. Coexistence of familial antiphospholipid syndrome and factor V Leiden: impact on thrombotic diathesis. Br J Haematol 1996;94:166–167.
48. Alarcon-Segovia D, Ruiz-Arguelles GJ, Garces-Eisele J, Ruiz-Arguelles. Inherited activated protein C resistance in a patient with familial primary antiphospholipid syndrome. J Rheumatol 1996;23:2162–2165.
49. Ames P, Tommasino C, D'Andrea G, Iannaccone L, Brancaccio V, Margaglione M. Thrombophilic genotypes in subjects with idiopathic antiphospholpid antibodies – prevalence and significance. Thromb Haemost 1998;79:46–49.
50. Schutt M, Kluter H, Hagedorn-Greiwe M, Fehm HL, Wiedemann GJ. Familial coexistence of primary antiphospholipid syndrome and factor V Leiden. Lupus 1998;7:176–82.
51. Peddi VR, Kant KS. Catastrophic secondary antiphospholipid syndrome with concomitant antithrombin III deficiency. J Am Soc Nephrol 1995;5:1882–1887.
52. Asherson RA, Khamashta MA, Ordi-Ros J et al. The primary antiphospholipid syndrome: major clinical and serological features. Medicine 1989;68:366–374.
53. Soweid AM, Hajjar RR, Hewan-Lowe KO, Gonzalez EB. Skin necrosis indicating antiphospholipid syndrome in patient with AIDS. S Med J 1995;88:786–778.
54. Labarca J, Rabaggliati R, Radrigan F et al Antiphospholipid syndrome associated with cytomegalovirus infection: case report and review. Clin Infect Dis 1997;24:197–200.
55. Merrill JT, Shen C, Gugnani M, Lahita RG, Mongey AB. High prevalence of antiphospholipid antibodies in patients taking procainamide. J Rheumatol 1997;24:1083–1088.
56. Vianna JL, Khamashta MA, Ordi-Ros J et al. Comparison of the primary and secondary antiphospholipid syndrome: a European multicenter study of 114 patients. Am J Med 1994;96:3–9.
57. Piette JC, Weschler B, Frances C, Papo T, Godeau P. Exclusion criteria for primary antiphospholipid syndrome. J Rheumatol 1993;20:1802–1804.
58. Krnic-Barrie S, O'Connor CR, Looney S, Pierangeli S, Harris N, Phil M. A retrospective review of 61 patients with antiphospholipid syndrome. Analysis of factors influencing recurrent thrombosis. Arch Intern Med 1997;157:2101–2108.
59. Granados J, Vargas-Alarcon G, Drenkard C et al. Relationship of anticardiolipin antibodies and antiphopholipid syndrome to HLA-DR7 in Mexican patients with SLE. Lupus 1997;6:57–62.
60. Silver RM, Draper MJ, Scott JR, Lyon JL, Reading J, Branch DW. Clinical consequences of antiphospholipid antibodies. An historic cohort study. Obstet Gynecol 1994;83:372–377.
61. Mujic F, Cuadrado MJ, Lloyd M et al. Primary antiphospholipid syndrome evolving into SLE. J Rheumatol 1995;22:1589–1592.
62. Seisdedos L, Munoz-Rodriguez F J, Cervera R, Font J, Ingelmo M. Primary antiphospholipid syndrome evolving into SLE. Lupus 1997;6:285–286.
63. Galli M, Finazzi G, Barbui T. Thrombocytopenia in the antiphospholipid syndrome: pathophysiology, clinical relevance and treatment. Ann Med Interne 1996;147(Suppl 1):24–27.
64. Hojnik M ,George J, Ziporen L, Schonfeld Y. Heart valve involvement in the antiphopsholipid sydrome. Circulation 1996;93:1579–1587.
65. Coudray N, de Zuttere D, Bletry O et al. M mode and Doppler echocardiographic assessment of left ventricular diastolic function in primary antiphospholipid syndrome. Br Heart J 1995;74:531–535.

3 Hemocytopenias in Antiphospholipid Syndrome

C. Montecucco and R. Caporali

Thrombocytopenia is included among the features of the human antiphospholipid syndrome (APS) [1] and is present in some animal models [2]. Hemolytic anemia can also be found in APS although less frequently than thrombocytopenia [1].

These hemocytopenias are mainly due to autoimmune mechanisms as supported by the presence of bone marrow megakaryocytes and platelet-associated immunoglobulins (Igs) for thrombocytopenia and by increased reticulocytes and positive direct Coombs' test for hemolytic anemia. However antiphospholipid antibodies (aPL) were also reported in association with thrombotic thrombocytopenia and microangiopathic hemolytic anemia.

The present chapter deals with the clinical feutures of aPL-associated cytopenia either autoimmune or thrombotic/microangopathic. The last part includes other aPL-associated hemocytopenias which are either less frequent or less well documented.

Autoimmune Thrombocytopenia

Prevalence in Primary and Secondary APS

A correlation between thrombocytopenia and aPL is well documented in spite of differences related to the criteria of patient selection and the methods employed to detect aPL. Thrombocytopenia was found in 26% of cases in a series of 319 patients with positive test for either lupus anticoagulant (LA) or anticardiolipin antibodies (aCL) collected from the Italian Registry of aPL [3]. This series included 112 patients with SLE and 207 with primary APS or without any clinical syndrome. In 70 patients with established primary APS, thrombocytopenia was reported in about 30% of cases [4]. A multicenter study by Vianna et al [5] showed thrombocytopenia in 40% of patients with either primary APS or APS secondary to SLE.

In SLE, thrombocytopenia was found in about 40% of LA-positive patients compared with 15% of LA-negative patients [6]. In 37 SLE patients with positive LA followed up for a median of 22 years, thrombocytopenia was more common and appeared earlier than in a comparable series of SLE without LA [7]. By pooling the results of different studies performed by measuring aCL, thrombocytopenia was reported in 32% of aCL-positive SLE and 11% of aCL-negative SLE [6]. In a more recent study carried out on 390 SLE patients from a single center, thrombocytopenia was found much less frequently even though it remained highly associated with aCL [8]. The patients with both LA and high aCL show the highest frequency of thrombocytopenia [9].

Several cases of pediatric APS were reportedly associated with thrombocytopenia [10, 11]; however a trend toward a positive correlation between aCL and thrombocytopenia in pediatric SLE was either confirmed [12] or denied [13]. The relatively small number of patients studied probably accounts for these discrepancies [14].

A close correlation with thrombocytopenia was reported for other markers of APS such as antimitochondrial antibodies type-M5 [15, 16] and antibodies reacting to thromboplastin in a solid phase assay [17]. On the contrary the antibodies to oxidated low-density lipoproteins do not correlate with thrombocytopenia [18]. A strong relationship between APS features, including thrombocytopenia, and antibodies to β_2-glycoprotein I (β_2-GPI) has been reported by different groups [19, 20]. Anti-β_2-GPI seems to show higher specificity but lower sensitivity for thrombocytopenia with respect to aCL or LA [21–23].

Many papers have addressed the relationship between aCL specific idiotypes and thrombocytopenia. Most of these studies showed a stronger correlation with IgG [24–27], a few others with IgA [28, 29].

Higher than normal levels of aPL also have been reported in many autoimmune diseases other than SLE and primary APS; however the features of APS are rarely found in these patients [30–33] and it is difficult to establish any clinical association [6].

Clinical Features

APL-related thrombocytopenia is a chronic, usually mild form and is seldom associated with hemorrhagic complications. Values lower than 50×10^9 platelets/L are uncommon, although platelet counts can fluctuate with time. Among the patients enrolled in the Italian Registry of aPL [3], 32 (11%) had severe thrombocytopenia and only two experienced bleeding. It should be kept in mind that bleeding may be related to several causes other than thrombocytopenia: including high-intensity oral anticoagulation for thromboembolic disease, hypoprothrombinemia, which has been reported in patients with LA and hemorrhagic complications [34] and acquired defects of platelet function which are frequently associated with aPL [35]. Severe thrombocytopenia is likely to act as an additional risk factor for bleeding complications in these patients and it might explain a higher than expected incidence of life-threatening bleeding events in APS patients on high-intensity warfarin therapy [36].

Arterial and/or deep venous thrombosis in APS may occur despite very low platelet counts; however two retrospective studies showed that the frequency of aPL-associated thrombotic events is significantly lower when the platelet count is less than 50×10^9/l [3, 37].

aPL and Anti-platelet Antibodies

The pathogenic role for aPL in thrombocytopenia was first suggested by Harris et al [38] and is still controversial. aPL may occasionally bind to unactivated platelets [39, 40]. However, since anionic phospholipids are concentrated in the inner leaflet of the cell membrane and exposed only after platelet activation [41], aPL binding is more likely to occur following platelet activation induced by other mechanisms. Accordingly, several groups have found that aPL can bind to pre-activated platelets in a β_2-GPI dependent way, inducing further platelet activation [42–44]. Therefore, aPL may have a role in thrombocytopenia but they are not the only actor on the scene [36]. Indeed, many studies failed to detect any antiphospholipid activity in eluates from platelets of patients with aPL-related thrombocytopenia [45–47].

Galli et al [45] found antibodies to the specific platelet membrane glycoproteins (GP) IIb/IIIa and Ib/IX in 40% of aPL-positive patients as well as a significant correlation between these antibodies and thrombocytopenia. Antiplatelet GP antibodies are pathogenetically linked to idiopathic thrombocytopenic purpura (ITP) and the frequency found in aPL-associated thrombocytopenia (59%) was similar to that in ITP [45]. In recent years several other studies reported increased levels of specific antibodies directed to internal platelet antigens [48] or to specific membrane GP [47, 49] in aPL-related thrombocytopenia. In a recent study, Godeau et al [46] showed antibodies to a large panel of platelet GP in the sera from 11 of 15 thrombocytopenic patients with APS.

The role of antibodies to platelet membrane GP is supported by the following data: (a) anti-GP are rarely found in SLE and APS with normal platelet counts [49]; (b) anti-GP, but not aCL or LA, can usually be eluted from platelets of patients with aPL-associated thrombocytopenia [45, 46]; (c) anti-GP in thrombocytopenic patients do not cross-react with phospholipids or β_2-GPI [45, 50, 51]; (d) treatment with glucocorticoids increases platelet number and reduces anti-GP titer but not aPL titer [50]. It remains to be elucidated why aPL are associated so frequently with anti-platelet GP antibodies.

aPL in ITP and Other Autoimmune Thrombocytopenias

ITP is usually associated with antiplatelet antibodies reacting to specific membrane GP. Nevertheless, higher than normal titers of aCL have been detected in 25% to 30% of ITP patients by different groups [25, 38]. Combining aCL assay and LA testing by kaolin clotting time and dilute Russell's viper venom time, Stasi and colleagues [52] were able to find either LA or aCL in 46% of ITP, and both LA and aCL in 16%.

Two questions are raised by these data: are aPL pathogenic in ITP and can aPL identify a subset of ITP with peculiar clinical features and a tendency to develop APS? Although aPL binding to platelet membrane cannot be excluded, the same anti-platelet GP antibody profile was seen in aPL-positive thrombocytopenia and classic ITP [45, 50]. Furthermore, aPL levels are neither influenced by therapy nor related to the disease activity [50]. In 149 patients with ITP [52], aPL were not associated with age, sex, platelet count, platelet-associated Igs or severity of hemorrhages. Also, no significant difference between patients with normal and elevated aPL was found as for clinical course and response to therapy. These data do not support the view that aPL be pathogenic in ITP or may select a category with different outcome. However since SLE and APS may occasionally develop in patients presenting as ITP [38, 53, 54], we believe that a careful search for other signs of APS, including direct Coombs' test (see below), should be performed in patients with high-titer aCL and LA.

Heparin-induced thrombocytopenia and thrombosis (HIT) are related to specific antibodies directed to the complex of platelet factor 4 (PF4) and heparin. Although pathophysiological and clinical homologies between HIT and APS have been suggested [55], the occurrence of HIT together with aPL was reported only occasionally [56]. Recently Lasne et al [57] showed low-titer anti-PF4/heparin antibodies and/or heparin dependent anti-platelet activity in sera from two of 20 patients with primary APS, and borderline values in four more patients. The clinical relevance of this association should be further investigated.

Pseudothrombocytopenia is the phenomenon of spuriously low platelet counts due to in vitro platelet clumping in the presence of platelet antibodies and ethylene diamine tetra-acetic acid (EDTA)or other anticoagulants. EDTA-dependent anti-platelet antibodies are directed against membrane GP and seem to recognize cryptic antigens on the GP IIb [58]. A positive test for aCL was reported in 56 of 88 cases of pseudothrombocytopenia [59] but the frequency of EDTA-dependent pseudo-thrombocytopenia in APS has not been assessed.

Autoimmune Hemolytic Anemia (AIHA)

Many different studies have noted the frequent occurrence of positive direct Coombs'test in SLE patients with LA, aCL, and anti-M5 [16, 17, 60–64]; aPL were also associated with a positive Coombs' test occasionally found in healthy blood donors [65]. In primary APS a positive Coombs' test was reported in ten of 70 patients (14%) and AIHA in three (4%) [4].

Higher frequency was observed in APS secondary to SLE [5]. In two different series, direct Coombs' test was positive in 31% and 49.5% of aCL-positive SLE as compared with 2 and 13% of aCL-negative SLE [8, 60]. The association with AHIA is less evident probably due to its relative rareness and the mutifactorial origin of anemia in SLE. Nevertheless, a significant correlation between aPL and hemolytic anemia was reported by different groups in large series of patients with SLE and related disorders [66–68]. As for the specific isotypes, IgM were mainly correlated with AIHA in some studies [17, 27, 67–69], even though other studies found a correlation with immunoglubin G (IgG) [4, 5]. Genetic and racial factors may partially account for these discrepancies [70].

A number of investigators found aCL in eluates from erythrocytes of patients with aCL-associated AIHA [25, 60, 71–74]. A direct binding of aPL to red blood cell membrane in these patients is supported by the following data: (a) aCL were not found in eluates obtained from red blood cells in aCL-negative AIHA or aCL-positive SLE without AIHA [60, 73]; (b) a correlation between serum aCL titers and hemolytic activity has been found in one case [73]; (c) anti-red blood cell binding activity present in eluates can be inhibited by absorption on phospholipid micelles [72, 74]; (d) anti-cardiolipin binding activity present in eluates can be inhibited by absorption on fixed red blood cell membranes [60].

The antigen recognized on the erythrocyte surface by aPL remains undefined. Cardiolipin is not present on red blood cell membrane and other negatively charged phospholipids are present only in the inner leaflet. In some patients with AIHA, IgM aCL displayed extensive cross-reactivities with different negative and neutral phospholipids including phosphatidylcholine that is exposed on bromelain-treated red blood cell surface [71]. Red blood cell membrane phosphatidylcholine might be a candidate target for aPL as it has been found in mice [75]. To date, however, the mechanisms underlying aPL-associated AIHA are not fully understood and we cannot exclude that other factors, such as immune complexes fixed on red blood cells, may have a role [76]. ACL were found to be enriched in circulating immune complexes from patients with APS [77]. Also the presence of other anti-erythrocyte antibodies cannot be ruled out [78]. In a patient with splenic lymphoma and mono-clonal IgM aCL, direct Coombs' test was positive for IgG1 and IgG2 antibodies [79]. This is not surprising as AIHA associated with B-cell malignancies is not due to monoclonal antibodies, but is mostly related to T-cell impairment.

aPL in Idiopathic AIHA and Evans' Syndrome

IgM aCL reacting with a broad spectrum of negative and neutral phospholipids were found in four of 14 patients with idiopathic AIHA by Guzman et al [80]. Six of these patients also had IgG aCL, while only one of the 14 control patients with non-autoimmune hemolytic anemia had IgG aCL, and none IgM aCL. A recent study by Lang et al [81] confirmed the presence of aPL in idiopathic AIHA as well as in AIHA associated with SLE. These authors also demonstrated that both IgG and IgM aCL titers were increased in warm-type AIHA and in cold-agglutinin disease as well. This finding is in keeping with a previous report of IgG aCL showing cold-agglutinin activity [74] and it may have clinical relevance when cardiopulmonary surgery requiring hypothermia is needed (Barzaghi N. et al, manuscript in preparation).

The eponymic Evans' syndrome is used to define the clinical association of autoimmune thrombocytopenic purpura with AIHA. Many of these patients have SLE or will develop SLE or SLE-like disease [53, 69]. Evans' syndrome was found in 5% of patients with SLE, mainly in association with high aCL levels [26], and in 10% of patients with primary APS [4]. Ten of 12 patients with SLE and Evans' syndrome studied by Delezé and colleagues [53] had positive tests for aPL. The two patients who did not have evidence of aPL were studied at the onset of SLE with active hemolysis and the authors raised the possibility of a transient seronegativity due to absorption of aPL on cell membranes [53]. In a previously published paper, we had found a positive aCL assay in six of seven patients suffering from Evans' syndrome without overt SLE [25]; the only aCL-negative patient had a positive immuno-fluorescent assay for anti-M5 antibodies, i.e. a marker of APS that do not cross-react with phospholipids and cofactors [15]. It could be of interest for readers to know that four of these patients developed overt APS, including one case of chorea and one transverse myelitis, in the following 10 years.

Thrombotic and Microangiopathic Hemocytopenia

Thrombotic thrombocytopenic purpura (TTP) is a rare hematologic syndrome due to an occlusive microangiopathy. It is characterized by the presence of microangio-pathic schistocytic hemolytic anemia, consumption thrombocytopenia with often severe hemorragic complications, fluctuating central nervous system symptoms, fever, and, less frequently, renal impairment. Similar features can be found in other thrombotic microangiopathies such as hemolytic uremic syndrome (HUS) which is usually found in children following intestinal infections and is characterized by

Table 3.1. Comparison of the main clinical and laboratory features associated with thrombocytopenia and hemolytic anemia in antiphospholipid syndrome and thrombotic microangiopathy.

	APS	CAPS	TTP	DIC
Renal involvement	+ −	+ +	+ −	+ −
CNS involvement	+ −	+ +	+ +	+ −
Multiorgan failure	+ −	+ +	+ +	+ −
Hemorrhages	− −	± −	+ −	+ +
Anti-platelet antibodies	+ −	+ −	− −	− −
Direct Coombs' test	+ −	+ −	− −	− −
Schistocytes	− −	± −	+ +	+ −
Low plasma fibrinogen	− −	± −	− −	+ +
Prolonged partial prothrombin time	+ − *	+ − *	− −	+ + †
Fibrin degradation products	− −	+ −	− −	+ +
Low serum complement	+ −	+ −	− − ‡	− − §
Antinuclear antibodies	+ −	+ −	− − ‡	− − §
Anticardiolipin antibodies	+ +	+ +	− − ‡	− − §

APS = antiphospholipid syndrome; CAPS = catastrophic APS; TTP = thrombotic thrombocytopenic purpura; DIC = disseminated intravascular coagulation.
* Negative mixing test (lupus anticoagulant);
† Positive mixing test;
‡ TTP may be associated with SLE;
§ DIC may be associated with CAPS.

prominent renal involvement, and the HELLP syndrome (hemolysis, elevated liver enzymes and low platelet count) occurring in pregnancy. Thrombocytopenia and microangiopathic hemolytic anemia are also present in disseminated intravascular coagulation (DIC).

The differential diagnosis between thrombotic microangiopathy and APS is often a clinical challenge (Table 3.1). The following points should be taken into account: (a) a minor degree of thrombocytopenia in APS could be related to increased platelet activation and consumption [82]; (b) many clinical and laboratory features may be shared by SLE and TTP [83]; (c) TTP may develop in patients with SLE and vice versa [84]; (d) aPL may be present in some cases of TTP, HUS and HELLP syndrome [84–87]; (e) DIC can occur in the catastrophic APS [88].

aPL in TTP and Related Disorders

aPL have not been commonly detected in primary TTP [89]; however, some definite cases of TTP were reported in patients with primary APS [85]. TTP may occur in SLE; traditional estimates range from 1 to 4% [83], though postmortem studies may suggest higher percentages [90]. On the other hand, four cases of SLE were found among 175 TTP patients gathered by the Italian Cooperative Group for TTP [83, 91].

In their excellent review, Musio and colleagues [84] reported on 41 cases of TTP in association with SLE. In 30 cases TTP followed SLE, in six TTP preceded SLE and in five TTP and SLE occurred simultaneously. A positive test for aCL was found in eight of 17 patients tested and LA in two of 14. Several more cases, reported in papers published in 1998, were not associated with aCL and/or LA [92, 93]. Therefore, a positive aCL assay was found in about 40% of SLE with TTP, and LA in about 15%, i.e, a figure similar to that expected for unselected SLE patients [63].

Nevertheless, one can not exclude that aPL, as well as other autoantibodies, may concur to cause endothelial injury resulting in TTP [83, 84]. TTP associated with aCL was recently reported in a 38-year-old man with a 12-year history of non-insulin dependent diabetes (Type II diabetes) and rapidly progressive diabetic vasculopathy [94]. APL have not been commonly found in long-lasting diabetes [95], but it seems likely that aPL may have acted as "second hit" on vascular endothelium to induce TTP in this case. Finally, two recently reported cases of chronic recurrent TTP were proven to be negative for aCL and positive for anti-phosphatidylinositol or phosphatidylserine antibodies [96]. Whether other aPL may be relevant in aCL-negative TTP remains to be ascertained.

A positive assay for IgG aCL was found in eight of 17 children with classic HUS [97]. Because this condition is triggered by intestinal infections, only further studies addressed to β_2-GPI binding will clarify the nature of these antibodies.

HELLP syndrome does usually complicate severe pre-eclampsia, i.e., a disorder characterized by endothelial damage different from that induced by aPL [98]. It seems likely that a further endothelial damage induced by aPL may switch on thrombotic microangiopathy. In recent years, several cases of postpartum HUS and HELLP syndrome associated with aPL have been reported [86, 87]. A case of catastrophic APS occurring in a patient who had had HELLP syndrome 31 years before was also reported [99]. Most cases of HELLP syndrome are however aPL-negative.

aPL in DIC

Though DIC has been rarely found in both primary and secondary APS, a full-blown picture of DIC was observed in 14 of the 50 reviewed cases of catastrophic APS [88], as well as in one case of catastrophic APS in childhood [100]. Schistocytes were reported in 8% of cases with catastrophic APS [88]. We have described a patient with aPL and quiescent SLE who developed DIC with thrombocytopenia, severe anemia with rare schistocytes and a clinical picture of purpura fulminans characterized by widespread cutaneous thromboses [101]. The relative sparing of internal organ vessels did not allow the diagnosis of catastrophic APS in this case.

Other Hemocytopenias

Monoclonal antibodies to β_2-GP1 may bind neutrophils [102] and a few studies have reported a clinical association between neutropenia and aCL in patients with SLE [67]. Lymphopenia does not correlate with aPL.

aPL have been reported in a number of patients suffering from hematologic malignancies [63], and hemocytopenias related to the development of non-Hodgkin lymphomas may be observed in APS [3].

Bone marrow necrosis is a rare syndrome leading to severe pancytopenia associated with poor outcome. It has been reported in patients with malignancies, severe infections, sickle cell anemia and, more recently, APS [103–105].

Sickle cell anemia is associated with changes in membrane lipid phase which may contribute to the generation of aPL [106]. aPL were found in a significant though variable percentage of patients with homozygous disease [107, 108]. APL did not correlate with the hematological and clinical features, even though APS has been reported in one case [109].

Patients with human immunodeficiency virus [HIV] infection may develop thrombocytopenia and show increased level of aCL. However, the presence of aCL does not correlate with thrombocytopenia in these patients [25, 110–112].

In 1988 we studied a series of patients with non-A–non-B chronic hepatitis who had aCL-associated thrombocytopenia [25]. Some of these patients had true autoimmune hepatitis while others were subsequently proven to have hepatitis C virus [HCV] infection. More recently, aCL with the characteristics of infection-related aPL were found in about 20% of patients with HCV [113]. A trend of higher incidence of thrombocytopenia among aCL-positive patients with HCV infection was reported in some studies [114, 115].

References

1. Hughes GRV. The antiphospholipid syndrome. Ten years on. Lancet 1993;324:341–344.
2. Aron AL, Cuellar RL, Brey RL, Maceown S, Espinoza LR, Shoenfeld Y. Early onset of autoimmunity in MRL/++ mice following immunization with beta 2 glycoprotein I. Clin Exp Immunol 1995;101:78–81.
3. Finazzi G. The Italian Registry of antiphospholipid antibodies. Haematologica 1997;82:101–5.
4. Asherson RA, Khamashta MA, Ordi-Ros J, Derksen RH, Machin SJ, Barquinero J et al. The "primary" antiphospholipid syndrome: major clinical and serological features. Medicine (Baltimore) 1989;68:366–74.
5. Vianna JL, Khamashta MA, Ordi-Ros J, Font J, Cervera R, Lopez-Soto A et al. Comparison of the primary and secondary antiphospholipid syndrome: a european multicenter study of 114 patients. Am J Med 1994;96:3–9.
6. Love PE, Santoro SA. Antiphospholipid antibodies: anticardiolipin and the lupus anticoagulant in systemic lupus erythematosus (SLE) and in non-SLE disorders. Prevalence and clinical significance. Ann Intern Med 1990;112:682–698.
7. Jouhikainen T, Stephansson E, Leirisalo-Repo M Lupus anticoagulant as a prognostic marker in systemic lupus erythematosus. Br J Rheumatol 1993;32:568–573.
8. Abu-Shakra M, Gladman DD, Urowitz MB, Farewell V. Anticardiolipin antibodies in systemic lupus erythematosus: clinical and laboratory correlations. Am J Med 1995;99:624–628.
9. Nojima J, Suehisa E, Kuratsune H, Machii T, Toku M, Tada H. High prevalence of thrombocyto-penia in SLE patients with a high level of anticardiolipin antibodies combined with lupus anti-coagulant. Am J Hematol 1998;58:55–60.
10. Ravelli A, Caporali R, Bianchi E, Viola S, Solmi M, Montecucco C, Martini A. Anticardiolipin syn-drome in childhood: a report of two cases. Clin Exp Rheumatol 1990;8:95–98.
11. Falcini F, Taccetti G, Tragani S, Tafi L, Petralli S, Matucci-Cerinic M. Primary antiphospholipid syndrome: a report of two pediatric cases. J Rheumatol 1991;18:1085–1087.
12. Ravelli A, Caporali R, Di Fuccia G, Zonta L, Montecucco C, Martini A. Anticardiolipin antibodies in pediatric systemic lupus erythematosus. Arch Pediatr Adolesc Med 1994;148:398–402.
13. Seaman DE, Londino AV Jr, Kwoh CK, Medsger TA Jr, Manzi S. Antiphospholipid antibodies in pediatric systemic lupus Erythematosus. Pediatrics 1995;96:1040–1045.
14. Ravelli A, Caporali R, Montecucco C, Martini A. The antiphospholipid syndrome in childhood. J Rheumatol 1996;23:1121–1122.
15. La Rosa L, Covini G, Galperin C, Catelli L, Del Papa N, Reina GL et al. Anti-mitochondrial M5 type antibody represents one of the serological markers for anti-phospholipid syndrome distinct from anti-cardiolipin and anti-beta2-glycoprotein I antibodies. Clin Exp Immunol 1998;112:144–151.
16. Laperche S, Abuaf N, Meyer O, Carsique R, Deschamps A, Rajoely B et al. Association of antimito-chondrial antibodies type 5 and anti-beta 2 glycoprotein I antibodies in the antiphospholipid syn-drome. J Rheumatol 1994;21:1678–1683.
17. Font J, Lopez-Soto A, Cervera R, Casals FJ, Reverter JC, Munoz FJ et al. Antibodies to thromboplas-tin in systemic lupus erythematosus: isotype distribution and clinical significance in a series of 92 patients. Thromb Res 1997;86:37–48.
18. Cuadrado MJ, Tinahones F, Camps MT, de Ramon E, Gomez-Zumaquero JM, Mujic F et al. Antiphospholipid, anti-beta 2-glycoprotein I and anti-oxidized-low-density-lipoprotein antibodies in antiphospholipid syndrome. Quart J Med 1998;91:619–626.

19. Cabiedes J, Cabral AR, Alarcon-Segovia D. Clinical manifestations of the antiphospholipid syndrome in patients with systemic lupus erythematosus associate more strongly with anti-beta 2-glyco-protein-I than with antiphospholipid antibodies. J Rheumatol 1995;22:1899–1906.
20. Amengual O, Atsumi T, Khamashta MA, Koike T, Hughes GR. Specificity of ELISA for antibody to beta 2-glycoprotein I in patients with antiphospholipid syndrome. Br J Rheumatol 1996;35:1239–1243.
21. Day HM, Thiagarajan P, Ahn C, Reveille JD, Tinker KF, Arnett FC. Autoantibodies to beta2-glyco-protein I in systemic lupus erythematosus and primary antiphospholipid antibody syndrome: clinical correlations in comparison with other antiphospholipid antibody tests. J Rheumatol 1998;25:667–674.
22. Sanfilippo SS, Khamashta MA, Atsumi T, Amengual O, Bertolaccini ML, D'Cruz Det al. Antibodies to beta2-glycoprotein I: a potential marker for clinical features of antiphospholipid antibody syn-drome in patients with systemic lupus erythematosus. J Rheumatol 1998;25:2131–2134.
23. Ravelli A, Caporali R, Ballardini G, Scatola C, Montecucco C, Martini A. Relationship between anti-cardiolipin and anti-beta 2 glycoprotein I antibodies in pediatric systemic lupus erythematosus. Arthritis Rheum 1996;39:S 190.
24. Harris EN, Gharavi AE, Boey ML, Patel BM, Mackworth-Young CC, Loizou S et al. Thrombocytopenia in SLE and related autoimmune disorders: association with anticardiolipin antibody. Br J Haematol 1985;59:227–230.
25. Caporali R, Longhi M, De Gennaro F, Di Lauro M, Carnevale R, Montecucco C. Antiphospholipid antibody-associated thrombocytopenia in autoimmune dieases. Med Sci Res 1988;16:537–539.
26. Alarcon-Segovia D, Delezé M, Oria CV, Sanchez-Guerrero J, Gomez-Pacheco L, Cabiedes J. Antiphospholipid antibodies and the antiphospholipid syndrome in systemic lupus erythemato-sus. A prospective analysis of 500 consecutive patients. Medicine 1989;68:353–365.
27. Sachse C, Luthke K, Hartung K, Liedvogel B, Kalden JR, Peter HH et al. Significance of antibodies to cardiolipin in unselected patients with systemic lupus erythematosus: clinical and laboratory asso-ciations. The SLE Study Group. Rheumatol Int 1995;15:23–29.
28. Lopez LR, Santos ME, Espinoza LR, La Rosa FG. Clinical significance of immunoglobulin A versus immunoglobulins G and M anti-cardiolipin antibodies in patients with systemic lupus erythemato-sus. Correlation with thrombosis, thrombocytopenia and recurrent abortion. Am J Clin Pathol 1992;98:449–454.
29. Tajima C, Suzuki Y, Mizushima Y, Ichikawa Y (1998) Clinical significance of immunoglobulin A antiphospholipid antibodies: possible association with skin manifestations and small vessel vas-culitis. J Rheumatol 1998;25:1730–176.
30. Caporali R, Ravelli A, De Gennaro F, Neirotti G, Montecucco C, Martini A. Prevalence of anti-cardiolipin antibodies in juvenile chronic arthritis. Ann Rheum Dis 1991;50:599–601.
31. Cervera R, Garcia-Carrasco M, Font J, Ramos M, Reverter JC, Munoz FJ et al. Antiphospholipid antibodies in primary Sjogren's syndrome: prevalence and clinical significance in a series of 80 patients. Clin Exp Rheumatol 1997;15:361–365.
32. D'Annunzio G, Caporali R, Montecucco C, Vitali L, Alibrandi A, Stroppa P et al. Anticardiolipin antibodies in first-degree relatives of type 1, insulin dependent diabetic patients. J Pediatr Endocrinol Metab 1998;11:21–25.
33. Caporali R, Ravelli A, Romenghi B, Montecucco C, Martini A. Antiphospholipid antibody-associated thrombosis in juvenile chronic arthritis. Arch Dis Child 1992;67:1384–1386.
34. Peacock NW, Levine SP. Case report: The lupus anticoagulant-hypoprothrombinemia syndrome. Am J Med Sci 1994;307:346–349.
35. Orlando E, Cortellazzo S, Marchetti M, Sanfratello R, Barbui T. Prolonged bleeding time in patients with lupus anticoagulant. Thromb Haemost 1992;68:495–499.
36. Galli M, Finazzi G, Barbui T. Thrombocytopenia in the antiphospholipid syndrome. Br J Haematol 1996;93:1–5.
37. Lechner K, Pabinger-Fasching I. Lupus anticoagulants and thrombosis. A study of 25 cases and review of the literature. Haemostasis 1985;15:254–262.
38. Harris EN, Gharavi AE, Hedge V, Derue G, Morgan SH, Englere H et al. Anticardiolipin antibodies in autoimmune thrombocytopenic purpura. Br J Haematol 1985;59:231–234.
39. Hasselaar P, Derksen RHWM, Blokzijl L, de Groot P. Crossreactivity of antibodies directed against cardiolipin, DNA, endothelial cells and blood platelets. Thromb Haemost 1990;63:169–173
40. Out HJ, de Groot PG, van Vliet M, de Gast GC, Nieuwenhuis HK, Derksen RH. Antibodies to platelets in patients with anti-phospholipid antibodies. Blood 1991;77:2655–2659.
41. Bevers EM, Smeets EF, Confurius P, Zwaal RFA. Physiology of membrane lipid asymmetry. Lupus 1994;3:235–240.
42. Robbins DL, Leung S, Miller-Blair DJ, Ziboh V. Effect of anticardiolipin/beta2-glycoprotein I com-plexes on production of thromboxane A2 by platelets from patients with antiphospholipid syn-drome. J Rheumatol 1998;25:51–56.

43. Arvieux J, Roussel B, Pouzol P, Colomb MG. Platelet activating properties of murine monoclonal antibodies to beta 2 glycoprotein I? Thromb Haemost 1993;70:336–341.
44. Vazquez-Mellado J, Llorente L, Richaud-Patin Y, Alarcon-Segovia D. Exposure of anionic phospholipids upon platelet activation permits binding of beta 2 glycoprotein I and through it that of IgG antiphospholipid antibodies.Studies in platelets from patients with antiphospholipid syndrome and normal subjects. J Autoimmun 1994;7:335–348.
45. Galli M, Daldossi M, Barbui T. Anti-glycoprotein Ib/IX and IIb/IIIa antibodies in patients with antiphospholipid antibodies. Thromb Haemost 1994;71:571–75.
46. Godeau B, Piette JC, Fromont P, Intrator L, Schaeffer A, Bierling P. Specific antiplatelet glycoprotein autoantibodies are associated with the thrombocytopenia of primary antiphospholipid syndrome. Br J Haematol 1997;98:873–879.
47. Panzer S, Gschwandtner ME, Hutter D, Spitzauer S, Pabinger I. Specificities of platelet autoantibodies in patients with lupus anticoagulants in primary antiphospholipid syndrome. Ann Hematol 1997;74:239–242.
48. Fabris F, Steffan A, Cordiano I, Borzini P, Luzzatto G, Randi ML et al. Specific antiplatelet autoantibodies in patients with antiphospholipid antibodies and thrombocytopenia. Eur J Haematol 1994;53:232–236.
49. Macchi L, Rispal P, Clofent-Sanchez G, Pellegrin JL, Nurden P, Leng B et al. Anti-platelet antibodies in patients with systemic lupus erythematosus and the primary antiphospholipid antibody syndrome: their relationship with the observed thrombocytopenia. Br J Haematol 1997;98:336–341.
50. Lipp E, von Felten A, Sax H, Muller D, Berchtold P. Antibodies against platelet glycoproteins and antiphospholipid antibodies in autoimmune thrombocytopenia. Eur J Haematol 1998;60:283–288.
51. Shi W, Chong BH, Chesterman CN. Beta 2 glycoprotein I is a requirement for anticardiolipin binding to activated platelets: differences with lupus anticoagulants. Blood 1993;81:1255–1262.
52. Stasi S, Stipa E, Masi M, Oliva F, Sciarra A, Perotti A et al. Prevalence and clinical significance of elevated antiphospholipid antibodies in patients with idiopathic thrombocytopenic purpura. Blood 1994;84:4203–4208.
53. Deleze M, Oria CV, Alarcon-Segovia D. Occurrence of both hemolytic anemia and thrombocytopenic purpura (Evans' syndrome) in systemic lupus erythematosus. Relationship to antiphospholipid antibodies. J Rheumatol 1988;15:611–615.
54. Stasi R, Stipa E, Masi M, Cecconi M, Scimò MT, Oliva F et al. Long term observation of 208 adults with chronic idiopathic thrombocytopenic purpura. Am J Med 1995;98:437–442.
55. Arnout J. The pathogenesis of the antiphospholipid syndrome: a hypothesis based on parallelisms with heparin-induced thrombocytopenia. Thromb Haemost 1996;75:536–541.
56. Jackson J, McDonald M, Casey E, Kelleher S, Murray A, Temperley I et al. Mixed connective tissue disease with arterial thrombosis, antiphospholipid antibodies and heparin induced thrombocytopenia. J Rheumatol 1990;17:1523–1524.
57. Lasne D, Saffroy R, Bachelot C, Vincenot A, Rendu F, Papo T. Test for heparin-induced thrombocytopenia in primary antiphospholipid syndrome. Br J Rheumatol 1997;97:939.
58. Fiorin F, Steffan A, Pradella P, Bizzaro N, Potenza R, De Angelis V. IgG platelet antibodies in EDTA-dependent pseudothrombocytopenia bind to platelet membrane glycoprotein Iib. Am J Clin Pathol 1998;110:178–183.
59. Bizzaro N, Brandalise M. EDTA-dependent pseudothrombocytopenia. Association with antiplatelet and antiphospholipid antibodies. Am J Clin Pathol 1995;103:103–107.
60. Hazeltine M, Rauch J, Danoff D, Esdaile JM, Tannenbaum H. Antiphospholipid antibodies in systemic lupus erythematosus: evidence of an association with positive Coombs' and hypocomplementemia. J Rheumatol 1988;15:80–86.
61. Tincani A, Meroni PL, Brucato A, Zanussi C, Allegri F, Mantelli P et al. Anti-phospholipid and anti-mitochondrial type M5 antibodies in systemic lupus erythematosus. Clin Exp Rheumatol 1985;3:321–326.
62. Gharavi AE, Harris EN, Asherson RA, Hughes GRV. Anticardiolipin antibodes: isotype, distribution and phospholipid specificity. Ann Rheum Dis 1987;46:1–6.
63. Montecucco C, Longhi M, Caporali R, De Gennaro F . Hematological abnormalities associated with anticardiolipin antibodies. Haematologica 1989;74:195–204.
64. Mueh JR, Herbst KD, Rappaport SI (1980) Thrombosis in patients with lupus anticoagulant. Ann Int Med 1980;92:156–159.
65. Win N, Islam SI, Peterkin MA, Walker ID. Positive direct antiglobulin test due to antiphospholipid antibodies in normal healthy blood donors. Vox Sang 1997;72:182–184.
66. Merkel PA, Chang Y, Pierangeli SS, Convery K, Harris EN, Polisson RP. The prevalence and clinical associations of anticardiolipin antibodies in a large inception cohort of patients with connective tissue diseases. Am J Med 1996;101:576–583.

67. Cervera R, Font J, Lopez-Soto A, Casals F, Pallares L, Bove A et al. Isotype distribution of anti-cardiolipin antibodies in systemic lupus eErythematosus: prospective analysis of a series of 100 patients. Ann Rheum Dis1990;49:109–113.
68. Deleze M, Alarcon-Segovia D, Oria CV, Sanchez-Guerrero J, Fernandez-Dominguez L, Gomez-Pacheco L et al. Hemocytopenia in systemic lupus erythematosus. Relationship to antiphospholipid antibodies. J Rheumatol 1989;16:926–930.
69. Fong KY, Loizou S, Boey ML, Walport MJ. Anticardiolipin antibodies, haemolytic anaemia and thrombocytopenia in systemic lupus erythematosus. Br J Rheumatol 1992;31:453–455
70. Molina JF, Gutierrez-Urena S, Molina J, Uribe O, Richards S, De Ceulaer C et al. Variability of anti-cardiolipin antibody isotype distribution in 3 geographic populations of patients with systemic lupus erythematosus. J Rheumatol 1997;24:291–96.
71. Cabral AR, Cabiedes J, Alarcon-Segovia D. Hemolytic anemia related to an IgM autoantibody to phosphatidylcholine that bind in vitro to stored and to bromelain-treated human erythrocytes. J Autoimmun 1990;3:773–787.
72. Arvieux J, Scweizer B, Roussel B, Colomb MG. Autoimmune hemolytic anemia due to anti-phospholipid antibodies. Vox Sang 1991;61:190–195.
73. Sthoeger Z, Sthoeger D, Green L, Geltner. D. The role of anticardiolipin autoantibodies in the pathogenesis of autoimmune hemolytic anemia in systemic lupus erythematosus. J Rheumatol 1993;20:2058–2061.
74. Del Papa N, Meroni PL, Barcellini W, Borghi MO, Fain C, Khamashta M et al. Antiphospholipid antibodies cross-reacting with erythrocyte membranes. A case report. Clin Exp Rheumatol 1992;10:395–399.
75. Arnold LW, Haughton G. Autoantibodies to phosphatidylcholine. The murine antibromelain RBC response. Ann N Y Acad Sci 1992;651:354–359.
76. Hammond A, Rudge AC, Loizou S, Bowcock SJ, Walport MJ. Reduced numbers of complement receptor type 1 on erythrocytes are associated with increased levels of anticardiolipin antibodies. Arthritis Rheum 1989;32:259–264.
77. Arfors L, Lefvert AK. Enrichment of antibodies against phospholipids in circulating immune complexes (CIC) in the anti-phospholipid syndrome (APLS) Clin Exp Immunol 1997;108:47–51.
78. Alarcon-Segovia D, Mestanza M, Cabiedes J, Cabral AR. The antophospholipid/cofactor syndromes. II. A variant in patients with systemic lupus erythematosus with antibodies to beta2-glycoprotein I but no antibodies detectable in standard antiphospholipid assays. J Rheumatol 1997;24:1545–1551.
79. Sawamura M, Yamaguchi S, Murakami H, Amagai H, Matsushima T, Tamura J. Multiple autoanti-body production in a patient with splenic lymphoma. Ann Hematol 1994;68:251–54.
80. Guzman J, Cabral AR, Cabiedes J, Pita-Ramirez L, Alarcon-Segovia D. Antiphospholipid antibodies in patients with idiopathic autoimmune haemolytic anemia. Autoimmunity 1994;18:51–56.
81. Lang B, Straub RH, Weber S, Rother E, Fleck M, Peter HH. Elevated anticardiolipin antibodies in autoimmune haemolytic anaemia irrespective of underlying systemic lupus erythematosus. Lupus 1997;6:652–655.
82. Machin SJ. Platelet and antiphospholipid antibodies. Lupus 1996;5:386–387.
83. Porta C, Bobbio-Pallavicini E, Centurioni R, Caporali R, Montecucco C. Thrombotic thrombocy-topenic purpura in systemic lupus erythematosus. J Rheumatol 1999;20:1625–1626.
84. Musio F, Bohen EM, Yuan CM, Welch PG. Review of thrombotic thrombocytopenic purpura in the setting of systemic lupus erythematosus. Semin Arthritis Rheum 1998;28:1–19.
85. Durand JM, Lefevre P, Kaplanski G, Soubeyrand J. Thrombotic microangiopathy and the antiphos-pholipid antibody syndrome. J Rheumatol 1991;18:1916–1918.
86. Huang JJ, Chen MW, Sung JM, Lan RR, Wang MC, Chen FF. Postpartum hemolytic uremic syn-drome associated with antiphospholipid antibody. Nephrol Dial Transplant 1998;13:182–186.
87. McMahon LP, Smith J. The HELLP syndrome at 16 weeks gestation: possible association with antiphospholipid syndrome. Aust N Z J Obstet Gynaecol 1997;37:313–314.
88. Asherson RA, Cervera R, Piette JC, Font J, Lie JT, Burcoglu A et al. Catastrophic antiphospholipid syndrome. Clinical and laboratory features of 50 patients. Medicine 1998;77:195–207.
89. Montecucco C, Di Lauro M, Bobbio-Pallavicini E, Longhi M, Caporali R, DeGennaro F et al. Anti-phospholipid antibodies and thrombotic thrombocytopenic purpura. Clin Exp Rheumatol 1987;5:355–358.
90. Devinsky O, Petito CK, Alonso DR. Clinical and neuropathological findings in systemic lupus ery-thematosus: the role of vasculitis, heart emboli, and thrombotic thrombocytopenic purpura. Ann Neurol 1988;23:380–384.
91. Porta C, Caporali R, Montecucco C Thrombotic thrombocytopenic purpura and autoimmunity: a tale of shadow and suspects. Haematologica 1999;84:260–269.

92. Jorfen M, Callejas JL, Formiga F, Cervera R, Font J, Ingelmo M. Fulminant thrombotic thrombo-cytopenic purpura in systemic lupus erythematosus. Scand J Rheumatol 1998;27:76–77.
93. Caramaschi P, Riccetti MM, Pasini AF, Savarin T, Biasi D, Todeschini G. Systemic lupus erythe-matosus and thrombotic thrombocytopenic purpura. Report of three cases and review of the liter-ature. Lupus 1988;7:37–41.
94. Morita H, Suwa T, Daidoh H, Takeda N, Ishizuka T, Yasuda K. Case report: diabetic microangio-pathic hemolytic anemia and thrombocytopenia with antiphospholipid syndrome. Am J Med Sci 1996;311:148–151.
95. Lorini R, d'Annunzio G, Montecucco C, Caporali R, Vitali L, Pessino P et al. Anticardiolipin anti-bodies in children and adolescents with insulin-dependent diabetes mellitus. Eur J Pediatr 1995;154:105–108.
96. Trent K, Neustater BR, Lottenberg R. Chronic thrombotic thrombocytopenic purpura and antiphospholipid antibodies: a report of two cases. Am J Haematol 1997;54:155–159.
97. Ardiles LG, Olavarria F, Elgueta M, Moya P, Mezzano S. Anticardiolipin antibodies in classic pedi-atric hemolytic–uremic syndrome: a possible pathogenic role. Nephron 1998;78:278–283.
98. Porta C, Buggia I, Bonomi I, Caporali R, Scatola C, Montecucco C. Nitrite and nitrate plasma levels, as markers of nitric oxide synthesis, in antiphospholipid antibodies-related conditions and in thrombotic thrombocytopenic purpura. Thromb Haemost1997;78:965–967.
99. Neuwelt CM, Daikh DI, Linfoot JA, Pfister DA, Young RG, Webb RL et al. Catastrophic antiphos-pholipid syndrome: response to repeated plasmapheresis over three years. Arthritis Rheum 1997;40:1534–1539.
100. Falcini F, Taccetti G, Ermini M, Trapani S, Matucci-Cerinic M. Catstrophic antiphospholipid anti-body syndrome in pediatric systemic lupus erythematosus. J Rheumatol 1997;24:389–392.
101. Gamba G, Montani N, Montecucco C, Caporali R, Ascari E. Purpura fulminans as clinical mani-festation of atypical SLE with antiphospholipid antibodies: a case report. Haematologica 1991;76:426–428.
102. Arvieux J, Jacob MC, Roussel B, Bensa JC, Colomb MG. Neutrophil activation by anti-beta 2 glyco-protein I monoclonal antibodies via Fc gamma receptor II. J Leukocyte Biol 1995;57:387–394.
103. Paydas S, Kocak R, Zorludemir S, Baslamisli F. Bone marrow necrosis in antiphospholipid syn-drome. J Clin Pathol 1997;50:261–262.
104. Moore J, Ma DD, Concannon A. Non-malignant bone marrow necrosis: a report of two cases. Pathology 1998;30:318–320.
105. Bulvik S, Aronson I, Ress S, Jacobs P. Extensive bone marrow necrosis associated with antiphos-pholipid antibodies. Am J Med 1995;98:572–574.
106. Westerman MP, Unger L, Kucuk O, Quinn P, Lis LJ. Phase changes in membrane lipids in sickle red cell shed-vesicles and sickle red cells. Am J Hematol 1998;58:177–182.
107. De Ceulaer K, Khamashta MA, Harris EN, Serjeant GR, Hughes GR. Antiphospholipid antibodies in homozygous sickle cell disease. Ann Rheum Dis 1992;51:671–672.
108. Kucuk O, Gilman-Sachs A, Beaman K, Lis LJ, Westerman MP. Antiphospholipid antibodies in sickle cell disease. Am J Haematol 1993;42:380–383.
109. Yeghen T, Benjamin S, Boyd O, Pumphrey C, Bevan DH. Sickle cell anemia, right atrial thrombosis, and the antiphospholipid antibody. Am J Hematol 1995;50:46–48.
110. Montecucco C, Caporali R, De Gennaro F, Sacchi P, Gamba G, Minoli L. Autoanticorpi circolanti nell'infezione da virus dell'immunodeficienza umana (HIV). Reumatismo 1989;41:177–185.
111. Intrator L, Oksenhendler E, Desforges L, Bierling P. Anticardiolipin antibodies in HIV infected patients with or without thrombocytopenic purpura. Br J Haematol 1988;68:269.
112. MacLean C, Flegg PJ, Kilpatrick DC. Anti-cardiolipin antibodies and HIV infection. Clin Exp Immunol 1990;81:263–266.
113. Cacoub P, Musset L, Amoura Z, Guilani P, Chabre H, Lunel F et al. Anticardiolipin, anti-beta2-glycoprotein I, and antinucleosome antibodies in hepatitis C virus infection and mixed cryoglobu-linemia. Multivirc group. J Rheumatol 1997;24:2139–2144.
114. Prieto J, Yuste JR, Beloqui O, Civeira MP, Riezu JI, Aguirre B et al. Anticardiolipin antibodies in chronic hepatitis C: implication of hepatitis C virus as the cause of the antiphospholipid syndrome. Hepatology 1996;23:199–204.
115. Leroy V, Arvieux J, Jacob MC, Maynard-Muet M, Baud M, Zarski JP. Prevalence and significance of anticardiolipin, anti-beta2 glycoprotein I and anti-prothrombin antibodies in chronic hepatitis C. Br J Haematol 1998;101:468–474.

4 Cardiac Manifestations in the Antiphospholipid Syndrome

J. Font and R. Cervera

Introduction

A variety of cardiac manifestations have been found in association with antiphospholipid antibodies (aPL), both in patients with systemic lupus erythematosus (SLE) and with the "primary" antiphospholipid syndrome (APS). They mainly include valvular and coronary artery diseases as well as intracardiac thrombus and cardiomyopathy.

Valvular Disease

Heart valve lesions are the most common cardiac manifestations described in patients with aPL. The introduction of two-dimensional and Doppler echocardiography has revealed a high prevalence of valvular abnormalities, such as thickening, stenosis, regurgitation, and vegetations, in patients with SLE. Additionally, it appears that, since the introduction of corticosteroid therapy, valvular involvement has become more prevalent among patients with SLE due to their increased longevity [1]. In several studies, these valvular lesions have been associated with the presence of aPL [2–6]. More recently, valvular lesions have also been described in patients with the "primary" APS [7–9]. Although most cases are symptomless, an increasing number of papers report cases with severe valvular dysfunction resulting in cardiac failure, sometimes requiring valve replacement [2–9].

Echocardiographic Findings

Valve Dysfunction and Thickening

Nesher et al [10] have recently performed a meta-analysis of 13 studies on valvular involvement in SLE, as documented by Doppler echocardiography, and they have found valvulopathy in 35% of SLE patients. The mitral valve was involved most commonly, and lesions included leaflet thickening, vegetations, regurgitation, and stenosis. Most of these studies also looked at the possible relationship of valvulopathy to the presence of aPL. Although several studies documented a statistically significant association between aPL and valvulopathy [2–6], others found no significant difference in aPL-positive and aPL-negative patients [11, 12]. The meta-analysis of these studies showed that 48% of aPL-positive SLE patients had valvulopathy, compared with only 21% of aPL-negative SLE patients. Additionally, Nesher et al [10], in an analysis of studies involving patients with "primary" APS, found that 36% had valvulopathy.

Thickening of the valve leaflets is the most common lesion detected by echocardiography in both SLE and "primary" APS patients. Valve thickness increases by two- to threefold or more, compared with normal valves [7–9]. The mitral valve is involved most commonly, followed by the aortic valve. Most thickened valves develop hemodynamic abnormalities, so that thickening as the sole abnormality is uncommon. Analysis of data from multiple studies [10] show that mitral regurgitation is the most common hemodynamic dysfunction, occurring in 22 and 26% of all patients with "primary" APS and SLE, respectively. Aortic regurgitation is less common, occurring in 6 and 10%, respectively. Mitral and aortic stenosis are uncommon, and usually accompany valvular regurgitation. Involvement of right-sided valves is also uncommon, and probably reflects pulmonary hypertension secondary to mitral or aortic regurgitation. In many cases, two or more valves are involved.

The valvular abnormalities associated with aPL may resemble those seen in cases of rheumatic fever. However, several echocardiographic differences have been observed. In APS-related cases, valve thickening is generally diffuse, and when localized thickening is noted, it involves the leaflets' mid-portion or base. Chordal thickening, fusion, and calcification is rarely seen and, when present, is not prominent. In contrast, valve thickening is typically confined to the leaflets' tips in rheumatic fever, and chordal thickening, fusion, and leaflet calcification is prominent in these cases [10] (Table 4.1).

Vegetations

Early reports of the link between aPL and SLE vegetations -the so-called "Libman–Sacks endocarditis" – date back to the mid 1980s when isolated reports of the association started appearing in the literature [2, 3]. Several recent echocardiographic

Table 4.1. Differential diagnosis between APS-related valve lesions, rheumatic fever and infective endocarditis.

Features	APS-related	Rheumatic fever	Infective endocarditis
Fever	+/–	+/–	+
Leucocytosis	–	–	+
C-reactive protein	–	–	+
Blood cultures/Serologies	–	–	+
aPL	+	–	–
Echocardiography	Diffuse valve thickening (if localized, it involves the leaflets' midportion or base) Chordal thickening, fusion and leaflet calcification are rare and minimal	Localized valve thickening involving the leaflets' tips. Chordal thickening, fusion and leaflet calcification are common and prominent	Mobile mass localized on the auricular surface of the auriculoventricular ventricular valves or aortic surface of aortic valve. Valve abscess and rupture are common.

+ present; – absent.

studies with larger numbers of patients have confirmed that SLE patients possessing aPL have a significantly higher prevalence of vegetations, particularly on the mitral valve, than those without [4–6, 13]. Information on the histological appearance of these lesions in patients with aPL derives from anecdotal reports of individual cases and systematic studies are clearly lacking.

Pathogenesis

The pathogenesis of valvular abnormalities in APS is not entirely clear. It has been postulated that in APS the aPL directly cause valvular or endothelial injury unrelated to clinical severity of the disease. Ziporen et al [1] have shown positive staining for human immunoglobulins and for complement compounds in the subendothelial ribbon-like layer along the surface of the leaflets and cups. Recently, Amital et al [14] reported similar findings with the deposition of anticardiolipin antibodies (aCL) in the subendothelial layer of the valve. These findings clearly indicate that the deposition of aPL on the valves resembles the deposition of immune complexes in the dermo-epidermal junction or in the kidney basement membrane in patients with SLE.

García-Torres et al [15] hypothesized that interaction of circulating aPL with local factors in the valves may lead to endocardial damage, resulting in superficial thrombosis and subendocardial mononuclear-cell infiltration, causing fibrosis and calcification. Alternatively, the initial event could be intravalvular capillary endothelial damage caused by aPL interacting with local antigens. This can lead to intracapillary thrombosis, focal inflammation, and the development of fibrosis and scarring. Both pathways may result in valvular deformities which can be hemodynamically significant. Thus, the initial event could be binding of aPL to valvular endothelial cells, leading to local inflammatory reaction, resulting in valve deformities. This proposed mechanism may be supported by the hemodynamic and echocardiographic improvement observed in several patients following treatment with prednisone, which probably diminishes the valvular inflammatory reaction [10].

As postulated by Hojnik et al [16], the above data suggest that aPL play a pathogenetic role in the development of valvular lesions rather then being elicited by the antigens expressed in the damaged valve tissue or merely being an epiphenomenon. Thrombotic tendency may not be the only mechanism whereby aPL may mediate valve damage. At present, there is no explanation for an apparently selective vulnerability of the endocardium to the action of aPL.

Clinical Manifestations

Most cases are clinically silent and detected by either chest auscultation, echocardiography, or at autopsy. Nevertheless, 4 to 6% of all SLE and "primary" APS patients develop severe mitral or aortic regurgitation, and valve replacement surgery has been performed in half of these patients [10] (Fig. 4.1).

Patients with severe valvular regurgitation present with symptoms of congestive heart failure such as fatigue, shortness of breath, and orthopnea. A murmur is present in most cases. It is sometimes difficult to differentiate this from valvulitis associated with rheumatic fever. However, antistreptococcal antibodies are not present, and the echocardiographic presentation is different, as previously described.

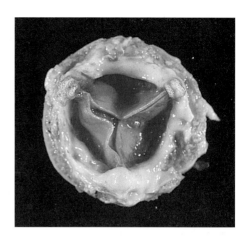

Figure 4.1. Valvular thickening and thrombosis in a prosthetic mitral valve of a patient with primary APS.

Hemodynamic abnormalities and symptoms may progress over a period of several weeks or months, remain stable, or improve.

Although infective endocarditis has been described in several patients with SLE, it is a very uncommon complication of this disease. However, several SLE patients have been reported presenting with the following combination of signs and serology: (i) fever; (ii) cardiac murmurs with echocardiographic demonstration of valve vegetations; (iii) splinter hemorrhages (Fig. 4.2); (iv) serological evidence of SLE activity (e.g., high titers of antibodies to dsDNA and low serum complement levels); (v) moderate to high elevations of aPL; and (vi) repeatedly culture-negative blood samples [17]. All these manifestations are explicable on the basis of SLE activity and complications associated with the APS. Interestingly, similar features were reported by our group [18] in a patient with "primary" APS. Three simple laboratory tests

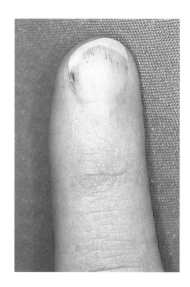

Figure 4.2. Splinter hemorrhages in a patient with valve vegetations and aPL.

may also assist in making a differential diagnosis between true infective endocarditis and SLE activity with "pseudoinfective endocarditis" in a patient with the above combination of signs: (a) the white cell count: if low, would point to SLE activity alone, if high, to an infective etiology; (b) the C-reactive protein: SLE patients are usually unable to mount a response of this protein to disease activity alone and elevation would imply infection; and (c) the aCL level: if it is negative or low positive only, this would be in keeping with infective endocarditis, rather than clot deposition on valve alone without infection. It has recently been shown that patients with simple infective endocarditis, e.g. on rheumatic valves, or valves congenitally abnormal, may in fact demonstrate aCL, but the levels are never high positive [19]. A moderate or high positive level would also usually point towards SLE activity rather than infection (Table 4.1).

A further problem in patients with aPL and valve lesions is the development of embolic cerebrovascular complications such as transient ischemic attacks, strokes, or multi-infarct dementia. Early reports [20–22] suggested a relationship between the presence of aPL, valve disease and ischemic cerebral events, indicating an embolic source for these episodes. Although clinical studies of embolic stroke are limited by the inability to diagnose cardiogenic stroke with certainty, the Antiphospholipid Antibodies in Stroke Study (APASS) found that one-third of stroke patients who had elevated aCL levels had abnormal echocardiograms [23].

Coronary Artery Disease

Unstable Angina

Isolated unstable angina has been reported occasionally in patients with the APS [24, 25]. Additionally, some patients with myocardial infarction and aPL presented with angina before or after the acute infarction. Díaz and Becker [26] found aCL in 8 out of 22 (36.4%) patients with unstable angina and, as Hamsted et al [27] that found a high incidence of aCL in young patients with myocardial infarction, they were unable to identify an association between aCL positivity and either the severity of angiographic coronary disease or an adverse clinical outcome. Thus, aCL does not appear to act independently of the usual coronary risk factors or alter the morphological features of atherosclerotic coronary narrowing as determined angiographically.

Myocardial Infarction

Myocardial Infarction in Individuals with aPL

In a prospective cohort of 4081 healthy middle-aged men, Vaarala et al [28] found that the presence of a high aCL level was an independent risk factor for myocardial infarction or cardiac death. The risk was estimated with logistic regression analysis using a nested case–control design with 133 patients (individuals from the cohort who developed myocardial infarction or cardiac death during the study) and 133 control subjects. Subjects with the aCL level in the highest quartile of distribution had a relative risk for myocardial infarction of 2.0 compared with the remainder of the population. This risk was independent of confounding factors, such as age, smoking, systolic blood pressure, low-density lipoprotein (LDL), and high-density lipoprotein. There was a correlation between the levels of aCL and antibodies to oxidized LDL, and their joint effect was additive for the risk. Antibodies to oxidized LDL have been associated with the progression of carotid atherosclerosis. It is possible that part of the effect of aPL could be mediated via a cross-reacting property directed against oxidized LDL [28]. As suggested by Matsuura et al [29], this interaction may lead to an enhanced uptake of oxidized LDL by macrophages.

Myocardial Infarction in Patients with the APS

Several cases of myocardial infarction have been documented both in patients with APS associated with SLE and in the "primary" APS [30–46]. Asherson et al [47] reported a series of 13 patients with this complication. Six suffered from classic SLE, three from "lupus-like" disease ("probable" SLE) and four from a "primary" APS. Five had suffered from myocardial infarction under the age of 30 years and four were in their early 20s. Nine of the 13 had suffered from previous thrombo-embolism. Warfarin discontinuation or unsatisfactory coagulation control was a precipitating factor in several patients. The left anterior descending coronary artery is most frequently involved and there is usually no evidence of atherosclerosis in vessels affected.

The real prevalence of myocardial infarction in patients suffering from APS is, however, relatively low. In the "primary" APS, prevalence ranges between 0 and 7% in the largest series [24, 25, 48–51]. Asherson et al [24]found a history of myocardial infarction in five of 70 (7%) patients in their multicenter study while our group [50] reported one out of 23 (4%) patients with this complication. Although other authors [25, 48, 51] however have not documented any patients with myocardial infarction in larger series, isolated cases have been published. In the APS associated with SLE, the prevalence of myocardial infarction is similarly low [52, 53].

aPL in Patients with Myocardial Infarction

Although patients without any evidence of an autoimmune disease suffering from myocardial infarctions do not usually demonstrate elevations of aPL when tested within 24 hours of the acute episode [54], it has been reported that a percentage of these patients, when followed for several months, might develop aPL elevations. However, prevalence of aPL varies between 3 and 80% in different series of patients with myocardial infarctions [27, 55–64]. This wide range of variation may be because of differences in the sensitivity of laboratory assays, or may reflect the effects of patient selection. Sletnes et al [57], in the largest study of aPL in patients surviving an acute infarct, found that 13.2% of 597 patients were positive for aPL compared with 4.4% of a reference population. However, in a multivariate analysis, adjusted for major cardiovascular risk factors, aPL were not found to be an independent risk factor for mortality, reinfarction, or non-hemorrhagic stroke. These aPL might arise because of vascular injury and exposure of neoantigens and might in fact be different idiotypes from those pathogenic idiotypes demonstrable in patients with SLE or "primary" APS.

Interestingly, Hamsten et al [27], in a series of 62 young survivors of myocardial infarction (under the age of 45 years), found an increase in recurrent thrombotic events in those with aPL. Specifically, in eight out of 13 patients with elevated aPL levels, recurrent cardiovascular thombotic events occurred. Thromboses included cerebral infarction, arterial occlusion of the lower limbs, new myocardial infarction, pulmonary embolus and deep vein thrombosis. However, these results have not been verified by other authors [56, 57, 60].

It seems that several subspecificities of aPL may occur in patients with myocardial infarctions and some evidences suggest that these antibodies may contribute to the development of myocardial infarction. As Vaarala [65] suggests, it is possible that aPL are initiated as a consequence of the underlying systemic arterial inflammatory disease and reflect the spreading of the autoimmune response against several antigens modified in the atherosclerotic vessel wall. Furthermore, a recent study from George et al [66] provides the first direct evidence for the proatherogenic effect of β_2-glycoprotein I immunization and establishes a new model for immune-mediated atherosclerosis.

Thus, aPL are associated with myocardial infarction but in non-SLE populations cannot be used for screening of individuals with increased risk for myocardial infarction. However, selective aPL estimations should be undertaken in: (i) younger patients (under 45 years of age); (ii) those with a previous history of venous or arterial thrombosis or recurrent fetal losses; and (iii) those with a family history of an autoimmune disease, especially if lupus related. The presence of other risk factors such as atherosclerotic disease, hypertension, excessive smoking, etc., should not prevent one from ordering this test, as multiple risk factors may be present [67, 68].

Coronary Bypass Graft and Angioplasty Occlusions

There is a substantial failure rate following aortocoronary venous bypass grafting. Early graft occlusions (10–20%) seems to be due to technical and hemodynamic factors, including the caliber of the graft and anastomosis and unsatisfactory distal run-off. Subsequently, other grafts become occluded as they become arterialized, smooth muscle proliferates, and coronary arteriosclerosis continues. Interestingly, Morton et al [69], in a series of 83 patients who underwent coronary bypass graft surgery, found that aCL levels were elevated in those patients with late bypass graft occlusions. The same group [70] have also reported a very powerful association of aCL with coronary artery bypass graft occlusion in a placebo group not treated with aspirin. The rise in aCL observed following bypass surgery has been greater among individuals with a history of previous myocardial infarction. These findings raise the possibility that aCL represent an immune response to myocardial injury.

Additionally, Eber et al [71], in a series of 65 men with coronary artery disease treated with percutaneous transluminal coronary angioplasty, have reported increased IgM aCL levels in patients with restenosis.

Intracardiac Thrombus

The endocardial surface may also be an important site for thrombus formation in patients with aPL. Primary intracardiac mural thrombi have been reported in these patients [72, 73]. It is important to stress that their presence may lead to diagnostic confusion; on occasion there may be difficulty in differentiation from a cardiac tumor, e.g., atrial myxoma, using non-invasive imaging techniques.

Cardiomyopathy

Acute Cardiomyopathy

Brown et al [74] described a 22-year-old female with SLE who succumbed within 24 hours of admission with profound hypotension and peripheral circulatory collapse and who at necropsy demonstrated the presence of microthrombi in multiple organs, including the heart (cardiac "microvasculopathy"). An essentially similar patient, a male with a "primary" APS, who had previously suffered a myocardial infarction, transient ischemic attacks, stroke, aortic regurgitation, and who had extensive livedo reticularis, was described by Murphy and Leach [75]. He died suddenly and multiple platelet thrombi within the intramyocardial arteries were found at autopsy. Kattwinkel et al [76] also reported a patient with a "primary" APS, myocardial infarction being caused by cardiac microvasculopathy. Angiography in these patients may reveal normal coronary arteries as the disease involves the microcirculation.

Chronic Cardiomyopathy

Patients with aPL and chronic myocardial dysfunction, unexplained in the context of valve abnormalities or other obvious causes, have been documented. Leung et al [13] in a study of 75 consecutive SLE patients found that aPL were significantly associated with left ventricular (global/isolated) dysfunction. Four of five patients with isolated left ventricular dysfunction had positive aPL.

Conclusions

It can be seen from the previous described studies that: (a) aPL-associated cardiac manifestations could be found in up to 40% of patients with APS, although significant morbidity, however, appears in only 4 to 6% of these patients; (b) most of these manifestations are explicable on the basis of thrombotic lesions, either on valves or in the myocardial circulation; and (c) they may mimic other similar conditions, such as rheumatic fever, infectious endocarditis, etc. For this reason, the estimation of aPL in cardiological practice assumes considerable importance.

References

1. Ziporen L, Goldberg I, Arad M, et al. Libman–Sacks endocarditis in the antiphospholipid syndrome: immunopathogenic findings in deformed heart valves. Lupus 1996;5:196–205.
2. Ford PM, Ford SE, Lillicrap DP. Association of lupus anticoagulant with severe valvular heart disease in systemic lupus erythematosus. J Rheumatol 1988;15:597–600.
3. Anderson D, Bell D, Lodge R, Grant E. Recurrent cerebral ischemia and mitral valve vegetation in a patient with lupus anticoagulant. J Rheumatol 1987;14:839–841.
4. Nihoyannopoulos P, Gomez PM, Joshi J, Loizou S, Walport MJ, Oakley CM. Cardiac abnormalities in systemic lupus erythematosus. Association with raised anticardiolipin antibodies. Circulation 1990;82:369–375.
5. Khamashta MA, Cervera R, Asherson RA, Font J, Gil A, Coltart D. et al. Association of antibodies against phospholipids with heart valve disease in systemic lupus erythematosus. Lancet 1990;335:1541–1544.

6. Cervera R, Font J, Paré C, Azqueta M, Pérez-Villa F, López-Soto A et al. Cardiac disease in systemic lupus erythematosus: prospective study of 70 patients. Ann Rheum Dis 1992;51:156–159.
7. Cervera R, Khamashta MA, Font J, Reyes PA, Vianna JL, López-Soto A et al. High prevalence of significant heart valve lesions in patients with the "primary" antiphospholipid syndrome. Lupus 1991;1:43–47.
8. Brenner B, Blumenfeld Z, Markiewicz W, Reisner SA. Cardiac involvement in patients with primary antiphospholipid syndrome. J Am Coll Cardiol 1991;18:931–936.
9. Galve E, Ordi J, Barquinero J, Evangelista A, Vilardell M, Soler-Soler J. Valvular heart disease in the primary antiphospholipid syndrome. Ann Intern Med 1992;116:293–298.
10. Nesher G, Ilani J, Rosenmann D, Abraham AS. Valvular dysfunction in antiphospholipid syndrome: Prevalence, clinical features, and treatment. Semin Arthritis Rheum 1997;27:27–35.
11. Metz D, Jolly D, Graciet-Richard J, Nazeyrollas P, Chabert JP, Maillier B et al. Prevalence of valvular involvement in systemic lupus erythematosus and association with antiphospholipid syndrome: a matched echocardiographic study. Cardiology 1994;85:129–136.
12. Roldan CA, Shively BK, Lau CC, Gurule FT, Smith EA, Crawford MH. Systemic lupus erythematosus valve disease by transesophageal echocardiography and the role of antiphospholipid antibodies. J Am Coll Cardiol 1992;20:1127–1134.
13. Leung W-H, Wong K-L, Lau C-P, Wong C-K, Cheng C-H. Association between antiphospholipid antibodies and cardiac abnormalities in patients with systemic lupus erythematosus. Am J Med 1990;89:411–419.
14. Amital H, Langevitz P, Levy Y, Afek A, Goldberg I, Pras M et al. Valvular deposition of antiphospholipid antibodies in the antiphospholipid syndrome: a clue to the origin of the disease. Clin Exp Rheumatol 1999;17:99–102.
15. García-Torres R, Amigo MC, de la Rossa A, Moron A, Reyes PA. Valvular heart disease in primary antiphospholipid syndrome: clinical and morphological findings. Lupus 1996;5:56–61.
16. Hojnik M, George J, Ziporen L, Shoenfeld Y. Heart valve involvement (Libman–Sacks endocarditis) in the antiphospholipid syndrome. Circulation 1996;93:1579–1587.
17. Asherson RA, Gibson DG, Evans DW, Baguley E, Hughes GRV. Diagnostic and therapeutic problems in two patients with antiphospholipid antibodies, heart valve lesions and transient ischaemic attacks. Ann Rheum Dis 1988;47:947–953.
18. Font J, Cervera R, Paré C, López-Soto A, Pallarés L, Azqueta M et al. Haemodynamically significant non-infective verrucous endocarditis in a patient with "primary" antiphospholipid syndrome. Br J Rheumatol 1991;30:305–307.
19. Asherson RA, Tikly M, Staub H, Wilmshurst A, Coltart DJ, Khamashta MA et al. Infective endocarditis, rheumatoid factor, and anticardiolipin antibodies. Ann Rheum Dis 1990;49:107–108.
20. Young SM, Fisher M, Sigsbee A, Errichetti A. Cardiogenic brain embolism and lupus anticoagulant. Ann Neurol 1989;26:390–392.
21. D'Alton JG, Preston DN, Bormanis J et al. Multiple transient ischemic attacks, lupus anticoagulant and verrucous endocarditis. Stroke 1985;16:512–514.
22. Levine SR, Kim S, Deegan MJ, Welch KMA. Ischemic stroke associated with anticardiolipin antibodies. Stroke 1987;18:1101–1106.
23. The Antiphospholipid Antibodies in Stroke Study Group. Clinical and laboratory findings in patients with antiphospholipid antibodies and cerebral ischaemia. Stroke 1990;21:1268–1273.
24. Asherson RA, Khamashta MA, Ordi-Ros J, Derksen RHWM, Machin SJ, Barquinero J et al. The "primary" antiphospholipid syndrome: major clinical and serological features. Medicine (Baltimore) 1989;68:366–374.
25 Camps MT, Guil M, Grana MI, de Ramón E. Manifestaciones clínicas y analíticas del síndrome antifosfolípido primario. Med Clin (Barc) 1995;104:37–38.
26. Díaz MN, Becker RC. Anticardiolipin antibodies in patients with ustable angina. Cardiology 1994;84:380–384.
27. Hamsten A, Norberg R, Bjorkholm M, DeFirre U, Holm G. Antibodies to cardiolipin in young survivors of myocardial infarction: an association with recurrent cardiovascular events. Lancet 1986;1:113–116.
28. Vaarala O, Mänttäri M, Manninen V, Tenkanen L, Puurunen M, Aho K et al. Anti-cardiolipin antibodies and risk of myocardial infarction in a prospective cohort of middle-aged men. Circulation 1995;91:23–27.
29. Matsuura E, Kobayashi K, Yasuda T, Koike T. Antiphospholipid antibdodies and atherosclerosis. Lupus 1998;7 (Suppl 2):S135–S139.
30. Asherson RA, Mackay KR, Harris EN. Myocardial infarction in a young male with systemic lupus erythematosus, deep vein thrombosis and antibodies to phospholipid. Br Heart J 1986;56:190–193.

31. Staub HL, Harris EN, Khamashta MA et al. Antibody to phosphatidylethanolamine in a patient with lupus anticoagulant and thrombosis. Ann Rheum Dis 1989;48:166–169.
32. Asherson RA, Harris EN, Gharavi AE, Hughes GRV. Myocardial infarction in SLE and "lupus-like" disease. Arthritis Rheum 1985;29:1292–1293.
33. Bingley PJ, Hoffbrand BI. Antiphospholipid antibody syndrome: a review. J R Soc Med 1987;80:445–448.
34. Hodges JR. Chorea and the lupus anticoagulant. J Neurol Neurosurg Psychiatr 1987;50:368–369.
35. Vermylen J, Blockmans D, Spitz B, Deckmyn H. Thrombosis and immune disorder. Clin Haematol 1986;15:393–412.
36. Waddell CC, Brown JA. The lupus anticoagulant in 14 male patients. JAMA 1982;248:2493–2495.
37. Jungers P, Lioté F, Dautzenberg MD et al. Lupus anticoagulant and thrombosis in systemic lupus erythematosus. Lancet 1984;1:574–575.
38. Harpaz D, Glikson M, Sidi Y, Hod H. Successful thrombolytic therapy for acute myocardial infarction in a patient with the antiphospholipid antibody syndrome. Am Heart J 1991;122:1492–1495.
39. Mills TJ, Safford RE, Kazmier FJ. Myocardial infarction, persistent coronary artery thrombosis and lupus anticoagulant. Int J Cardiol 1988;21:190–194.
40. Ghirardello A, Doria A, Ruffatti A, Rigoli AM, Vesco P, Calligaro A et al. Antiphospholipid antibodies (aPL) in systemic lupus erythematosus. Are they specific tools for the diagnosis of aPL syndrome? Ann Rheum Dis 1994;54:140–142.
41. Shaley Y, Green L, Pollak A, Bentwich Z. Myocardial infarction with central retinal artery occlusion in a patient with antinuclear antibody-negative systemic lupus erythematosus. Arthritis Rheum 1985;85:1185–1187.
42. Bick RL, Baker WF. Anticardiolipin antibodies and thrombosis. Hematol Oncol Clin North Am 1992;6:1287–1299.
43. Asherson RA, Chan JKH, Harris EN, Gharavi AE, Hughes GRV. Anticardiolipin antibody, recurrent thrombosis, and warfarin withdrawal. Ann Rheum Dis 1985;44:823–825.
44. Exner T, Koutts J. Autoimmune cardiolipin-binding antibodies in oral anticoagulant patients. Aust N Z J Med 1988;18:669–673.
45. Shortell CK, Ouriel K, Green RM, Condemi JA, DeWeese JA. Vascular disease in the antiphospholipid syndrome: A comparison with the patient population with atherosclerosis. J Vasc Surg 1992;15:158–166.
46. Rosove MH, Brewer PMC. Antiphospholipid thrombosis: clinical course after the first thrombotic event in 70 patients. Ann Intern Med 1992;117:303–308.
47. Asherson RA, Khamashta MA, Baguley E, Oakley CM, Rowell NR, Hughes GRV. Myocardial infarction and antiphospholipid antibodies in SLE and related disorders. Quart J Med 1989;73:1103–1115.
48. Alarcón-Segovia D, Sánchez-Guerrero J. Primary antiphospholipid syndrome. J Rheumatol 1989;16:482–488.
49. Mackworth-Young CG, Loizou S, Walport MJ. Primary antiphospholipid syndrome: features of patients with raised anticardiolipin antibodies and no other disorder. Ann Rheum Dis 1989;48:362–367.
50. Font J, López-Soto A, Cervera R et al. The "primary" antiphospholipid syndrome: antiphospholipid antibody pattern and clinical features of a series of 23 patients. Autoimmunity 1991;9:69–75.
51. Martínez-Vázquez C, Albo C, Ribera A, Bordón J, Rodríguez A, Sopeña B et al. Síndrome antifosfolípido primario. Aspectos clínico-evolutivos de 24 casos. Rev Clin Esp 1994;194:164–169.
52. Cervera R, Font J, López-Soto A et al. Isotype distribution of anticardiolipin antibodies in systemic lupus erythematosus. Prospective analysis of a series of 100 patients. Ann Rheum Dis 1990;49:109–113.
53. Alarcón-Segovia D, Delezé M, Oria CV, Sánchez-Guerrero J, Gómez-Pacheco L, Cabiedes J et al. Antiphospholipid antibodies and the antiphospholipid syndrome in systemic lupus erythematosus: a prospective analysis of 500 consecutive patients. Medicine (Baltimore) 1989;68:353–374.
54. Sletnes KE, Larsen EW, Stokland O, Wisloff F. Antiphospholipid antibodies detected as anticephalin and anticardiolipin antibodies in patients with acute myocardial infarction: immunological response to myocardial necrosis? Thromb Res 1990;59:675–680.
55. Klemp P, Cooper R, Jordan E, Przybojewski N. Anti-cardiolipin antibodies in ischaemic heart disease. Clin Exp Immunol 1988;74:254–257.
56. De Caterina R, D'Ascanio A, Mazzone A, Gazzaetti P, Bernini W, Neri R et al. Prevalence of anti-cardiolipin antibodies in coronary artery disease. Am J Cardiol 1989;65:922–923.
57. Sletnes KE, Smith P, Abdelnoor M, Arnesen H, Wisloff F. Antiphospholipid antibodies after myocardial infarction and their relation to mortality, reinfarction, and non-haemorrhagic stroke. Lancet 1992;339:451–453.
58. Cortellaro M, Cofrancesco E, Boschetti C. Cardiolipin antibodies in survivors of myocardial infarction. Lancet 1993;342:192.

59. Edwards T, Thomas RD, McHugh NJ. Anticardiolipin antibodies in ischaemic heart disease. Lancet 1993;342:989.
60. Phadke KV, Phillips RA, Clarke DT, Jones M, Naish P, Carson P. Anticardiolipin antibodies in ischaemic heart disease: marker or myth? Br Heart J 1993;69:391–394.
61. Yilmaz E, Adalet K, Yilmaz G, Badur S, Erzengin F, Koylan N et al. Importance of serum anticardiolipin antibody levels in coronary heart disease. Clin Cardiol 1994;17:117–121.
62. Raghavan C, Ditchfield J, Taylor RJ, Haeney MR, Barnes PC. Influence of anticardiolipin antibodies on immediate patient outcome after myocadial infarction. J Clin Pathol 1993;46:1113–1115.
63. Gavaghan TP, Krilis SA, Daggard GE, Baron DE, Hickie JB, Chesterman CN. Anticardiolipin antibodies and occlusion of coronary artery bypass grafts. Lancet 1987;2:977–978.
64. Bick RL. The antiphospholipid-thrombosis syndromes. Fact, fiction, confusion, and controversy. Am J Clin Pathol 1993;100:477–480.
65. Vaarala O. Antiphospholipid antibodies and myocardial infarction. Lupus 1998;7 (Suppl 2):S132–S134.
66. George J, Afek A, Gilburg B, Blank M, Levy Y, Aron-Maor A et al. Induction of early atherosclerosis in LDL-receptor-deficient mice immunized with β-2-glycoprotein I. Circulation 1998;98:1108–1115.
67. Asherson RA, Cervera R. Antiphospholipid antibodies and the heart. Lessons and pitfalls for the cardiologist. Circulation 1991;84:920–923.
68. Asherson RA, Cervera R. Antiphospholipid and the heart: reply. Circulation 1992;85:2332.
69. Morton KE, Gavaghan TP, Krilis SA, Daggard GE, Baron DW, Hickie JB et al. Coronary artery bypass graft failure: an autoimmune phenomenon? Lancet 1986;2:1353–1356.
70. Gavaghan TP, Krilis SA, Daggard GE, Baron DE, Hickie JB, Chesterman CN. Anticardiolipin antibodies and occlusion of coronary bypass grafts. Lancet 1987;2:977–978.
71. Eber B, Schumacher M, Auer-Grumbach P, Toplak H, Klein W. Increased IgM anticardiolipin antibodies in patients with restenosis after percutaneous transluminal coronary angioplasty. Am J Cardiol 1992;69:1255–1258.
72. Lubbe WF, Asherson RA. Intracardiac thrombus in systemic lupus erythematosus associated with lupus anticoagulant. Arthritis Rheum 1988;31:1453–1454.
73. Leventhal LJ, Borofsky MA, Bergey PD, Schumacher HR Jr. Antiphospholipid antibody syndrome with right atrial thrombosis mimicking an atrial myxoma. Am J Med 1989;87:111–113.
74. Brown JH, Doherty CC, Allan DC, Morton P. Fatal cardiac failure due to myocardial microthrombi in systemic lupus erythematosus. Br Med J 1989;298:525.
75. Murphy JJ, Leach IA. Findings at necropsy in the heart of a patient with anticardiolipin syndrome. Br Heart J 1989;62:61–64.
76. Kattwinkel N, Villanueva AG, Labib SB, Aretz T, Walek JW, Burns DL et al. Myocardial infarction caused by cardiac microvasculopathy in a patient with the primary antiphospholipid syndrome. Ann Intern Med 1992;116:974–976.

5 Cerebral Disease in the Antiphospholipid Syndrome

M. G. Navarrete, R. L. Brey and S. R. Levine

Introduction

Antiphospholipid antibody syndrome (APS) has been associated with central nervous system (CNS) involvement in a large number of patients. However, not all studies have found a significant correlation between antiocardiolipin (aCL) levels and neurological/neuropsychiatric manifestations of APS [1]. Clinical manifestations of APS associated with the CNS include arterial thrombotic events, psychiatric manifestations and a variety of other non-thrombotic neurological syndromes [2] (see Table 5.1). In fact, some of the most debilitating clinical aspects of APS are the neurological and neuropsychiatric manifestations. Nevertheless, the specific role of antiphospholipid antibodies (aPL) in the CNS remains one of the least understood aspects of this syndrome, which is partly due to the heterogeneity of its symptomatology. Patients may present with diffuse or global dysfunction, including coma, grand mal seizures, and cognitive dysfunction, psychosis, affective disorders, as well as focal symptoms attributable to lesions to a specific area of the brain. A majority of cognitive disorders associated with aPL area are probably the result of thrombotic events; however, there may be other aPL-mediated mechanisms, as well [3].

Table 5.1. Neurologic syndromes associated with antiphospholipid antibodies.

Cerebrovascular ischemia	Chorea
Stroke	Transverse myelopathy
Transient ischemic attack	Guillain–Barré syndrome
Cerebral venous sinus thrombosis	
Ocular ischemia	Diabetic peripheral neuropathy
Dementia	Sensorineural hearing loss
Acute ischemic encephalopathy	Sudden onset
With Sneddon's syndrome	Progressive
Without Sneddon's syndrome	Transient global amnesia
Atypical migrainous-like events	Psychiatric disorders
Seizures	Orthostatic hypotension

Cerebral Ischemia

Cerebral ischemia associated with aPL is the most common arterial thrombotic manifestation [4, 5]; however, the importance of aPL as a cardiovascular risk factor is controversial. Many studies have found that aPL are associated with an increased risk for incident [6–10] and recurrent [11] episodes of cerebral ischemia, but some have not [12–14].

The average age of onset of aPL-associated cerebral ischemia is several decades younger than the typical cerebral ischemia population [11]. Regardless of age, patients with cerebral ischemia often have other risk factors for cerebrovascular disease [6, 8, 9, 11]. A higher than expected frequency of coronary artery [10, 15] and peripheral arterial [16] graft occlusion has also been noted in patients with aPL. These clinical observations coupled with recent findings of endothelial cell activation by aPL [17, 18] support the hypothesis that aPL may act in concert with other vascular risk factors that damage endothelial cells.

Cerebral ischemic events can occur in any vascular territory (see Fig. 5.1) [19]. Angiography typically demonstrates intracranial branch or trunk occlusion or is normal in about one third of patients so studied [20]. A variety of cardiac valvular lesions have been associated with aPL. Cardiac emboli are therefore another possible cause of cerebrovascular disease symptoms in some patients. Echocardiography (primarily two-dimensional, transthoracic) is abnormal in one-third of patients, typically demonstrating non-specific left-sided valvular (predominantly mitral) lesions, characterized by valve thickening [21, 22]. These may represent a potential cardiac source of stroke [21–24]. In a large consecutive autopsy series, a higher inci-

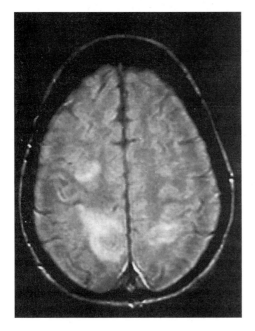

Figure 5.1. Brain magnetic resonance imaging study (MRI) showing multiple strokes in a young woman with antiphospholipid antibodies, strokes and seizures.

dence of cardiac valvular abnormalities and "bland" (non-vasculitic) thromboembolic lesions were found in patients with aPL (see Fig. 5.2) [25]. Microthrombotic
occlusive disease of multiple small vessels ("thrombotic microangiopathy") has
been reported in a large number of patients with catastrophic APS [26]. Clinical
events consistent with multiple small vessel occlusion occurred in these patients
within a short time period of days to weeks.

Recurrent stroke and thromboembolic events in patients with aPL have been
reported to occur both early (within the first week to year of an index episode
of cerebral ischemic) [11, 27] and late (5–10 years) [4, 5]. The initial type of the

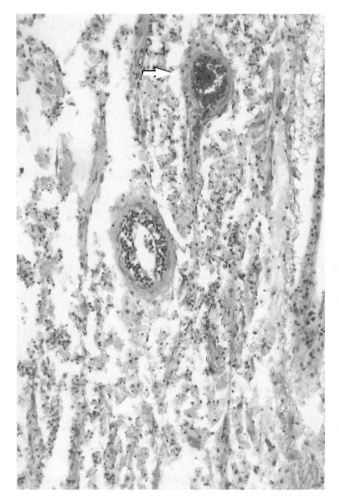

Figure 5.2. Hematoxylin and eosine stained section of post-mortem brain tissue from a patient with antiphospholipid antibodies and the catastrophic antiphospholipid antibody syndrome. Arrow indicates a small cerebral blood vessel with thrombus, but no inflamation.

thromboembolic event (i.e., arterial, venous, miscarriage) appears to be the most likely type of event to recur in a given patient in some [28] but not all studies [5, 29]. Shah and colleagues studied patients with both primary and secondary APS over a 10-year period and found recurrent thromboembolic events to be common in both groups [4]. In their series of 52 patients with aPL, 9/31 (29%) patients with APS developed recurrent thrombotic episodes and 11/21 (52%) patients with aPL but without clinical manifestations developed them over the follow-up period. Of the 12 patients who initially presented with cerebral ischemia, four had new events over the follow-up period. Seven additional episodes of cerebral ischemia occurred in patients with aPL but without initial clinical manifestations. Krnic-Barrie and colleagues [5] retrospectively evaluated 61 patients with primary and secondary APS for an average of 6.4 years to identify risk factors for the development of recurrent thrombosis. Of the patients with initial arterial thrombotic events, 26 out of 44 (59%) resulted in cerebral ischemia. There was no difference between patients with primary and secondary APS regarding recurrent arterial or venous events (arterial: 55 versus 38% and venous: 47 versus 50%). In patients with primary and secondary APS recurrent arterial events were associated with Caucasian race and venous events with the puerperium or oral contraceptive use. High titers of aCL have been associated with recurrent events in patients with primary [11, 27, 30] and secondary APS [31, 32]. In a case study of 141 patients with secondary APS, the presence of both aCL and lupus anticoagulants (LA) were associated with thrombotic events [33]. In this study 84% of patients with an abnormal aCL IgG level and LA had a thrombotic event as compared to 16% with an abnormal aCL IgG only, 9.1% with LA only, and 3.8% with neither. All patients with high levels of aCL and LA and none of the patients without LA had an arterial thrombosis. The correlation between a high level of aCL and LA has been previously reported, however, Verro and colleagues did not find a similar relationship between very high titer and risk for recurrent thrombotic events [34]. A greater risk for thrombosis has been associated with aPL having the following features: cardiolipin or β_2-glycoprotein 1 immunoreactivity of the IgG-2 isotype [35–37] and phosphatidylserine immunoreactivity [35]. In addition, Specker and colleagues have shown that cerebral microemboli detected by transcranial Doppler are found in patients with APS and that they correlate with a history of cerebral ischemia [38, 39].

There are no data to suggest that the severity of the thromboembolic event, including stroke, influences aCL titer. aCL do not appear to be a result of the thrombotic event in the brain [8, 11] or elsewhere [31]. In a case–control study of patients with giant cell arteritis the prevalence of abnormal aCL levels was higher in patients with temporal arteritis than in controls (20.7 versus 2.9%). The prevalence was even higher in patients who also had positive temporal artery biopsies than in patients with normal biopsies (31.2 versus 16.7%) [40]. Both aCL and a positive biopsy were associated with thrombosis in univariate analyses; however, only a positive biopsy remained predictive of thrombosis in multivariate analyses. Further, nearly half of biopsy positive patients with high aCL levels at the time of diagnosis had normal levels when retested after 10 days of corticosteroid treatment. The authors speculate that in giant cell arteritis, the aCL produced may be a consequence of severe endothelial damage and have no relationship to thrombosis. No further analysis of aCL subtype or other phospholipid specificities were performed, thus it is possible that nonpathogenic antibodies are formed in this situation, similar to those found in response to drugs or infections [41].

Venous Sinus Thrombosis

A recent review suggests that aPL may be an important factor contributing to cerebral venous sinus (CVT) thrombosis even in the presence of other potential risk factors for thrombosis [42] including the syndrome of activated protein C resistance due to factor V Leiden mutation [43]. The onset of CVT in patients with aPL occurs at a younger age and has more extensive superficial and deep cerebral venous system involvement than CVT without aPL. In addition, a higher rate of post-CVT migraine and more infarctions on brain imaging studies may possibly be seen in patients with aPL than in those without them [42].

Dementia and Other Cognitive Dysfunction

Cognitive deficits associated with primary or secondary APS can vary from mild neurocognitive disorders to more severe vascular dementia [44]. Despite the increased interest within the last few years, research in this area is limited and few formal neuropsychological studies have been conducted thus far to assess the prevalence and nature of cognitive deficits in APS. Although many studies evaluating neurocognitive deficits in patients with aPL have been anecdotal [45, 46], several cross-sectional and prospective studies have been recently published [47–50]. There is no specific pattern of cognitive dysfunction that has been consistently identified; however, there are many similarities in the deficits found in aPL positive patients across different studies (refer to Table 5.2).

When cognitive dysfunction is milder, patient complaints include forgetfulness, attention deficits, difficulty concentrating on tasks, and other deficits that mildly interfere with everyday function. These mild changes in the cognitive status may be the only clinical manifestation of APS [51]. Formal neuropsychological testing may be the most sensitive tool to measure small cognitive changes that might not be obvious on brief bedside examinations such as the Mini Mental Status Examination [52]. In addition, cognitive functioning assessed by these tests may provide an accurate index of the patient's general CNS status [52, 53].

Table 5.2. Neurocognitive dysfunction associated with antiphospholipid antibodies.

Authors	Number of subjects	Indexes measured (only indexes correlated with deficits)	Neurocognitive deficits found
Hanly et al, 1999 [48]	51	Persistent aCL IgG elevations Persistent aCL IgA elevations	Psychomotor speed Conceptual reasoning and executive functioning
Menon et al, 1999 [50]	45	Persistent aCL IgG elevations	Psychomotor speed, attention, and concentration
Denburg et al, 1997 [47]	61	LA-positivity	Verbal memory, verbal fluency, cognitive flexibility, and psychomotor speed
Schmidt et al, 1995 [54]	53	aCL IgG elevations	Mnemonic skills, visuopractical abilities, attention and concentration

There are many documented cases of neurocognitive deficits secondary to APS that are not related to cerebrovascular disease [45, 46, 54]. For example, Mikdashi and Kay [45] reported four patients who exhibited psychomotor retardation and had the same deficit pattern, including decreased visual attention, word retrieval problems, executive function difficulties, and impairment of both verbal and non-verbal memory skills. None of these patients had a history of stroke.

Sneddon's Syndrome and Other aPL-associated Dementia

Recurrent stroke in patients with livedo reticularis (Sneddon's syndrome) has been associated with aPL [55]. The frequency of aPL in patients with Sneddon's syndrome has ranged from 0 to 85% [55–57]. This syndrome is also frequently accompanied by dementia, most likely on the basis of multiple infarctions. Sneddon's original patients all had focal neurological deficits, which he considered to be "limited and benign," leaving little residual disability [58]. Subsequent descriptions of the syndrome have revealed a spectrum of clinical neurological manifestations. Zelzer and colleagues described three stages of neurological involvement: (1) "prodromal" symptoms such as dizziness or headaches preceding focal neurological deficits by years; (2) recurrent focal neurological deficits due to recurrent cerebral ischemia, also lasting years; and (3) progressive cognitive impairment leading to severe dementia [56]. Tourbah and colleagues correlated the magnetic resonance imaging (MRI) abnormalities found in 26 patients with Sneddon's syndrome with disability, presence of cardiovascular risk factors, cardiac valvular abnormalities on echocardiogram and titer of aPL [57]. Disability (defined by memory disturbance or ability to perform activities of daily living) was found in 50% of the patients. Severe disability, which was consistent with dementia, was present in over half of the patients with disability. Systemic hypertension was present in 65%, cardiac valvular abnormalities in 61% and aPL in 42% of patients with no correlation found between any of these and MRI abnormalities. The presence of disability was correlated with increasing severity of MRI lesions.

An aPL-associated dementia without the other features of Sneddon's syndrome has also been described. In many patients this appears to be due to multiple cerebral infarctions [59]. In addition, the catastrophic APS can present with an acute organic brain syndrome characterized by fulminant encephalopathy [60]. Asherson reported that in a group sample of 50 patients with catastrophic APS over 50% had CNS involvement [26].

aPL-Associated Cognitive Dysfunction: Secondary APS

aPL positivity has been associated with several different patterns of cognitive dysfunction in patients with secondary APS, depending on the study. Verbal memory deficits, decreased psychomotor speed, and decreased overall productivity have been significantly correlated to elevated aPL levels [47, 48, 50]. Denburg and colleagues [47] found LA-positive patients to score significantly lower than LA-negative patients on measures of verbal memory, cognitive flexibility and psychomotor speed. In addition, the cognitive deficits were noted even in patients who had no past or present clinical neuropsychiatric event, suggesting a specific association between the antibodies and cognitive functioning. Several recent studies have also reported cognitive dysfunction with increased IgG aCL titers [48, 50]. Menon and colleagues [50] reported that systemic lupus erythematosus (SLE) patients with consistently elevated IgG aCL levels over a period of 2–3 years performed significantly worse than SLE patients with occasionally elevated or never elevated titers on a variety of neuropsychological tests. These results were not observed with anti-DNA antibody titers or C3 levels. Attention and concentration, as well as psychomotor speed, were the domains most affected. Hanly and colleagues [48] followed 51 female SLE patients over a 5-year period and found that persistent aCL IgG elevations were associated with decreased psychomotor speed, while persistent aCL IgA elevations were correlated with problems with executive functioning and reasoning abilities. They also found no association between cognitive deficits and anti-DNA antibodies.

apL-Associated Cognitive Dysfunction: Primary APS

An association between high aCL titers and cognitive dysfunction has also been found in patients without SLE. For example, Schmidt and colleagues found subtle neuropsychological dysfunction in otherwise normal elderly people with increased levels of aCL IgG [54]. This correlation with aCL IgG titers was significant despite the lack of evidence of any anatomic abnormalities on MRI or correlation of aCL positivity with MRI. De Moerloose and colleagues evaluated the prevalence of aCL in 192 elderly patients [61]. The overall prevalence of aCL was 10.9% and decreased by decade in patients 70–99 years of age from 18 to 10 to 7%, whereas the prevalence of antinuclear antibody (ANA) positivity increased by decade from 22 to 32 to 42%. There was no association between the presence of aCL and decreased survival. In contrast, and in keeping with previous findings, Cesbron found a trend towards an increased prevalence of aCL by decade in 1042 elderly subjects between the ages of 60 and 99 years [62]. In addition, high aCL levels were associated with increased physical disability in this population independent of age, gender, visual or hearing abnormalities, Mini Mental Status Examination scores, or history of cerebrovascular or cardiovascular disease.

Medication-induced Cognitive Dysfunction

Another issue in defining the cognitive manifestations of APS is the possible effect that medications used for its treatment may have on cognitive functioning. Although some studies have found no adverse effect on cognitive functioning from medications such as corticosteroids [63, 51], many studies have reported an adverse effect [64–66]. Carbotte and colleagues found no association between the use of steroids and significant cognitive impairment in a group of 74 patients with either SLE or RA, as compared to 35 normal controls [63]. However, only significant cognitive impairment was assessed and all patients were on very low doses of steroids. Several researchers, however, have reported that most cognitive difficulties are seen with high-dose treatment or chronic use by making the hippocampal neurons more vulnerable to metabolic insults [64–66]. Some of the more common possible manifestations of this treatment are diminished attention and concentration, as well as explicit memory problems. Although these cognitive problems were initially thought to be transient and dose dependent, long-term effects have been reported [65, 66]. Thus, cognitive difficulties are a potential problem with secondary antiphospholipid antibody syndrome as patients with illnesses such as systemic lupus erythematosus are often treated with corticosteroids. A particular dilemma is the differentiation of cognitive deficits due to the illness itself versus medication side-effects, since the former requires the increase of medication and the later may warrant taking the patient off the medication.

Psychosis and Major Affective Disorders

Psychiatric problems such as mood alteration and psychosis are perhaps the most misunderstood manifestations of antiphospholipid antibody syndrome. This is due to the lack of research in this area, as well as the complexity of the subject. The wide diversity of potential etiologies combined with numerous clinical manifestations makes any psychiatric diagnosis secondary to APS very difficult. For example, behavioral complications such as psychosis and mood disorders may manifest independently of cognitive loss, although in many cases the two occur concurrently. It is also extremely difficult to determine whether or not the psychiatric symptoms are mostly due to a psychological reaction of suffering from a major chronic illness. In addition, medications such as corticosteroids, which are often prescribed for the management of some of the symptoms of primary and secondary APS, may induce psychiatric symptoms themselves [65, 67]. Steroid-induced psychiatric symptoms may include depression, hypomania, irritability, restlessness and anxiety, and to a lesser extent psychosis [65].

Although depression and psychosis have been associated with aPL, it remains unclear to what extent this finding is simply related to the development of medication-induced aPL [68]. Schwartz and colleagues demonstrated an association between aCL, LA and psychosis in 34 unmedicated patients without known autoimmune disorder admitted to the hospital with a first acute episode of psychosis [68]. Thirty-four percent of patients had aCL IgG and nine percent had LA, neither of which was present in 20 normal control subjects. Patients were treated with a variety of neuroleptics and reassessed for the presence of these antibodies 3–9 months later. Although one patient developed aCL IgM and four developed aCL IgG after treatment, three patients who were aCL IgG positive prior to treatment were negative for these antibodies post-treatment. There was no relationship between the presence of aCL or LA and thrombotic manifestations, response to antipsychotic therapy or type of neuroleptic used. The authors speculated that aPL might be causally related to the development of psychosis in some patients on an autoimmune basis and concluded that their presence cannot be assumed to simply be the result of antipsychotic treatment.

West and colleagues reported that systemic lupus erythematosus patients with diffuse neuropsychiatric manifestations such as depression and psychosis did not have significantly higher levels of aPL when compared to other SLE patients [69]. However, aPL antibodies and lupus anticoagulant were detected at a greater frequency in patients who had focal or complex neuropsychiatric manifestations of SLE.

Migraine

The prevalence of aPL in patients with migraine does not appear to be increased, even in an SLE population in whom the prevalence of both migraine and aPL are increased over the general population [70]. Tietjen and colleagues studied 68 young people with transient focal neurologic events (with and without migraine) and found aPL immunoreactivity to be present in 29 of them [71]. Distinguishing features of the group with aPL were a lower frequency of a family headache history and a higher frequency of retinal and hemisensory deficits.

The largest case control study to date has failed to demonstrate an association of aCL immunoreactivity in patients under 60 years of age with either migraine with aura, migraine without aura, or transient focal neurologic events compared to controls [70]. However, in patients with transient focal neurological events, aCL were associated with diabetes mellitus, a negative family history of stroke and briefer spells. Neuroimaging studies in patients with aCL suggest that permanent focal damage may be more common in this group despite the transient nature of their symptoms. Interestingly, the short-term risk of stroke or other thromboembolic events in association with aCL was not similarly increased. As discussed previously, however, this lack of association could be due to a follow-up period that was too brief.

Although migrainous stroke is rare, Silvestrini and colleagues found aPL immunoreactivity in 6/16 patients with migranous cerebral infarction [72]. None of these patients had SLE, but all had other risk factors for stroke. These data highlight the importance of considering the presence of aPL in migrainous stroke.

Seizures

Antiphospholipid antibodies have been reported with increased frequency in SLE patients with epilepsy by some [73, 74] but not all [75] investigators. The etiology of seizures in SLE patients may be aPL-associated cerebral infarction [73, 74]. Brey and colleagues did not find either aCL immunoreactivity or LA in a small group of young epileptic patients without SLE who served as controls in a study of aPL and cerebral ischemia [8]. Verrot and colleagues conducted a study with the general epilepsy population to find a relationship between aPL and epilepsy [76]. Similar to studies with SLE patients, the authors found a high correlation between aCL antibodies and epilepsy. There are some animal data that support the possibility of a primary immunologic basis for seizures associated with aPL [3, 77]. aPL have been demonstrated to bind directly to cat brain [3], and aPL have been shown to reduce a γ-aminobutyric acid (GABA) receptor-mediated chloride current in snail neurons [77]. This inhibitory effect suggests a direct and reversible mechanism through which antiphospholipid antibodies might lower seizure threshold.

Chorea

Cervera and colleagues reviewed chorea in adults and children with APS [78]. Chorea can occur in both primary and secondary APS [79, 80] and is often the presenting clinical feature. Of the 50 patients described and reviewed by Cervera, six developed chorea with estrogen-containing oral contraceptive use, and four in association with pregnancy or the post-partum period [78], highlighting the potential role of estrogen in this disorder. The chorea was bilateral in 55% of patients and, fortunately, reversible in most patients with treatment with haloperidol, cortico-steroids or the discontinuation of oral contraceptives. In patients with persistent chorea, aPL-associated striatal ischemia has been postulated. However, in patients with reversible chorea, dysfunction related to striatal binding of aPL is quite plaus-ible. This hypothesis, first suggested by Asherson et al [79], is supported by several recent case reports describing patients with aPL-associated chorea studied serially using positron emission tomography (PET). Transient hypermetabolism in the con-tralateral basal ganglia was seen in all patients [81, 82], suggesting an underlying excitatory rather than ischemic pathophysiologic mechanism.

Transverse Myelopathy

Harris and colleagues [83] were the first to describe a patient with transverse myelitis, aPL immunoreactivity and a "lupus-like" disease. Lavalle and colleagues [84] described 12 SLE patients with transverse myelitis and found all of them to have aPL immunoreactivity. Six also had other APS clinical manifestations (thrombocytopenia, thrombosis, livedo reticularis and leg ulcers). Transverse myelitis only occurs in 1% of patients with SLE [84], therefore, the number of patients described in this report is remarkable. Ruiz-Arguelles and colleagues recently described a patient with re-fractory hiccup as the heralding symptom of transverse myelitis in association with aCL [85]. This patient was successfully treated with corticosteroids. Cross-linked fibrin derivatives (an indicator of ongoing thrombosis) were negative during the time of maximal neurologic deficit. The pathophysiology of spinal cord damage in aPL-associated myelopathy is uncertain; however, both ischemia and an antibody-mediated interaction have been suggested. In the case presented by Ruiz-Arguelles, the response to corticosteroids and the lack of evidence acutely for ongoing thrombo-sis suggest that either inflammation or an antibody-mediated interaction with spinal cord phospholipids may be more likely.

Other Neurologic Syndromes

Guillain–Barré Syndrome

Several studies suggest an association between aPL and Guillain–Barré Syndrome [86, 87]. One suggests that a failure of plasma exchange to normalize the aPL levels may be predictive of eventual relapse [86]. Shigeta and colleagues studied the asso-ciation of antibodies against sulfatide and phospholipid in 68 non-insulin depend-ent diabetes mellitus (Type II diabetes) patients with diabetic neuropathy [88]. Both antibodies were more common in patients with moderate to severe neuropathic symptoms and anti-sulfatide antibodies were more commonly associated with slower sural nerve conduction velocity suggesting that autoimmune nerve dysfunc-tion may be involved in diabetic neuropathy.

Sensorineural Hearing Loss

Toubi and colleagues studied the association between aCL and sudden or progres-sive sensorineural hearing loss in 30 patients and matched normal controls. None of the control group had aCL, whereas 27% of the patient group had aCL in low-moderate titers [89]. Of the patients with aCL, five of eight had sudden deafness. In addition, two of five patients with sudden deafness patients and aCL relapsed as compared with none of six patients without them. Naarendorp and Spiera reported six patients with SLE or a lupus-like syndrome with sudden sensorineural hearing loss, all of which had aCL or LA [90]. The authors suggest that sudden sensorineural hearing loss may be a previously unrecognized manifestation of APS, that the mechanism is likely to be vascular and speculate that the appropriate treatment for these patients may be anticoagulant therapy.

Transient Global Amnesia

Transient global amnesia (TGA), a syndrome of sudden, unexplained memory loss has been associated with aPL immunoreactivity [91]. The etiology of TGA in patients without aPL is controversial and thought to be related to ischemia or epileptiform activity in bilateral hippocampal areas. As both cerebral ischemia and epilepsy have been associated with aPL, either could play a role in aPL-associated TGA.

Ocular Syndromes

Many reports of stroke and TIA associated with aPL include some patients with ocular ischemia as well [92, 93]. The ophthalmologic ischemic manifestations commonly associated with aPL include anterior ischemic optic neuropathy, branch and central retinal artery occlusions, cilioretinal artery occlusions, combined artery and vein occlusions and amaurosis fugax [93]. These manifestations are found in patients with both primary and secondary APS.

Neuroimaging Studies

Brain magnetic resonance imaging (MRI) studies in patients with APS (primary or secondary) have revealed small foci of high signal in subcortical white matter scattered throughout the brain [94–96]. This type of pattern is seen in many other disease processes and is, as such, non-specific. The correlation between MRI lesions in patients with aPL and clinical nervous system symptoms is reported to be high by some investigators [70, 94–96] and not by others [54, 97].

Toubi and colleagues [96] found aPL immunoreactivity in 53/96 (55%) SLE patients with CNS manifestations as compared to 20/100 (20%) of SLE patients without them. In this study, 53 patients with CNS manifestations underwent MRI imaging and 33 showed high-intensity lesions that were interpreted as "suggestive of vasculopathy". MRI abnormalities were seen more frequently in patients with as compared to those without aPL immunoreactivity. Some of these patients with MRI abnormalities had seizures or psychiatric disturbances and not stroke. This suggests that in some cases, aPL-associated neurologic manifestations may be due to an aPL–brain phospholipid interaction whereas in other the underlying pathogenic feature may be thrombotic. Although useful in demonstrating structural lesions such as infarcts and hemorrhages in the brains of patients with focal lesions, imaging techniques are poorly correlated with diffuse or global dysfunction. For example, the status of aCL titers in a group of 233 normal elderly participants was found to have no influence in the MRI results [54]. Using brain MRI and PET imaging, neuropsychological testing, a neurological examination and serum testing for aPL antibodies and antineuronal antibodies, Sailer and colleagues [97] studied 35 SLE patients, whose disease was inactive. Twenty patients had neurological deficits, three had psychiatric symptoms and ten had cognitive impairment. No differences in global glucose utilization by PET imaging were seen between SLE patients with, as compared to those without, neurological or cognitive abnormalities. On MRI imaging, the number and size of the white matter lesions correlated with the presence of neurological deficit, but were unrelated to the severity of cognitive impairment. Large lesions (8 mm or greater) were associated with high aCL IgG levels. Tietjen also found an association between MRI lesions and aCL levels in young patients with migraine associated transient focal neurologic events [70]. In a study evaluating the association between neuropsychologic abnormalities and aPL in an elderly population no association between aCL and MRI lesions was found, supporting Sailer's findings in the group with cognitive impairment only [54].

Hachulla and colleagues performed brain MRI in patients with primary and secondary APS [98]. Both cerebral atrophy and white matter lesions were more common in both groups in comparison with control subjects. The number and volume of white matter lesions were increased in patients with primary and secondary APS who also had neurologic symptoms. Only a weak correlation was found between the presence of LA and cerebral atrophy.

Treatment

Treatment of the APS can be directed towards preventing thromboembolic events by using antithrombotic medications or towards modulating the immune response with immunotherapy (see Table 5.3). In the case of thrombotic manifestations, both approaches have been used [37, 99, 100]. Treatment of non-thrombotic neurologic manifestations such as seizures, chorea, dementia unassociated with multiple cerebral infarctions or transverse myelitis has usually been limited to immunotherapy in combination with other symptomatic treatment.

Unfortunately, the mechanism by which aPL lead to thrombosis is unclear, and is probably heterogeneous. A variety of prothrombotic effects on platelets, coagulation proteins, prostaglandins, and endothelial cells have been associated with aPL [6, 7]. It is likely that the most appropriate therapeutic choice for a given patient may depend on which of these effects caused the patient's thromboembolic

Table 5.3. Treatment for thrombosis associated with antiphospholipid antibodies.

Anti-thrombotic therapy	Immune system modulation
Aspirin	Intravenous immunoglobulin therapy
Dipyridamole	Plasmaphoresis
Warfarin	Corticosteroids
Low-molecular-weight heparin	Cyclophosphamide
	Azathiaprine

episode. For platelet or prostaglandin abnormalities aspirin or other antiplatelet therapy might be expected to be beneficial whereas for thrombomodulin, protein C, protein S or cardiac valvular abnormalities anticoagulation might be needed. This may provide a partial explanation for the discrepant findings in the aPL treatment literature on thromboembolic manifestations.

Therapies aimed at modulating the immune response in preventing both thrombotic and non-thrombotic neurologic manifestations of APS also have variable success [37, 99, 100]. In patients with primary (and probably secondary) APS, corticosteroid therapy has not been beneficial in preventing recurrent thromboembolic events [100]. As with aPL-associated thrombosis, a more precise definition of the nature of the aPL-target tissue interaction would help guide more rational therapeutic decision making.

References

1. Emmi L, Bergamini C, Spinelli A, Liotta F, Marchione T, Caldini A et al. Ann New York Acad Sci 1997;823:188–200.
2. McNeil HP, Chesterman CN, Krilis SA. Immunology and clinical importance of antiphospholipid antibodies. Adv Immunol 1991;49:193–280.
3. Kent M, Vogt E, Rote NS. Monoclonal antiphosatidylserine antibodies react directly with feline and murine central nervous system. J Rheumatol 199724:1725–1733.
4. Shah NM, Khamashta MA, Atsumi T, Hughes GRV. Outcome of patients with anticardiolipin antibodies: a 10 year follow-up of 52 patients. Lupus 1998;7:3–6.
5. Krnic-Barrie S, Reister O'Connor C, Looney SW, Pierangeli SS, Harris EN (1997). A retrospective review of 61 patients with antiphospholipid syndrome. Arch Intern Med 157:2101–2108.
6. Antiphospholipid Antibodies in Stroke Study (APASS) Group. Anticardiolipin antibodies are an independent risk factor for first ischemic stroke. Neurology 1993;43:2069–2073.
7. Camerlingo M, Casto L, Censori B, Drago G, Frigeni A, Ferraro B. Anticardiolipin antibodies in acute non-hemorrhagic stroke seen within six hours after onset. Acta Neurol Scand 1995;92:60–71.
8. Brey RL, Hart RG, Sherman DG, Tegeler CT. Antiphospholipid antibodies and cerebral ischemia in young people. Neurology 1990;40:1190–1196.
9. Levine SR, Deegan MJ, Futrell N, Welch KMA. Cerebrovascular and neurologic disease associated with antiphospholipid antibodies: 48 cases. Neurology 1990;40: 1190–1196.
10. Brey, RL, Abbott RD, Sharp DS et al. Beta-2-glycoprotein 1-dependent anticardiolipin antibodies are an independent risk factor for ischemic stroke in the Honolulu heart cohort. Stroke 1999;30:250.
11. Levine SR, Brey RL, Sawaya KL, Salowich-Palm L, Kokkinos J, Kostrzema B et al. Recurrent stroke and thrombo-occlusive events in the antiphospholipid syndrome. Ann Neurol 1995;38:119–124.
12. Montalban J, Khamashta M, Davalos A, Codina M, Swana GT, Calcagnotto ME et al. Value of immunologic testing in stroke patients: a prospective multicenter study. Stroke 1994;25:2412–2415.
13. Ginsburg KS, Liang MH, Newcomer L, Goldhaber SZ, Schur PH, Hennekens CH et al. Anticardiolipin antibodies and the risk for ischemic stroke and venous thrombosis. Ann Intern Med 1992;117:997–1002.
14. Antiphospholipid Antibody in Stroke Study Group (APASS).Anticardiolipin antibodies and the risk of recurrent thrombo-occlusive events and death. Neurology 1997;48:91–94.
15. Klemp P, Cooper RC, Strauss FJ et al. Anticardiolipin antibodies in ischemic heart disease. Clin Exp Immunol 1988;89:411–419.
16. Ciocca RG, Choi J, Graham AM. Antiphospholipid antibodies lead to increased risk in cardiovascular surgery. Am J Surg 1995;170:198–200.
17. Del Papa N, Raschi ER, Catelli L, Khmashta MA, Ichikawa K, Tincani A. Endothelial cells as a target for antiphospholipid antibodies: role of anti-beta-2-glycoprotein 1 antibodies. AJRI 1997;38:212–217.
18. Del Papa N, Guidali L, Sala A, Buccellati C, Khamashta MA, Ichikawa K. Endothelial cells as target for antiphospholipid antibodies. Arthritis Rheumatol 1997;40:551–561.
19. Coull BM, Levine SR, Brey RL. The role of antiphospholipid antibodies and stroke. Neurol Clin 1992;10:125–143.

20. Antiphospholipid Antibodies in Stroke Study (APASS) Group. Clinical and laboratory findings in patients with antiphospholipid antibodies and cerebral ischemia. Stroke 1990;21:1268–1273.

21. Ford SE, Lillicrap DM, Brunet D, Ford PM. Thrombotic endocarditis and lupus anticoagulant, a pathogenetic possibility for idiopathic rheumatic type valvular heart disease. Arch Pathol Lab Med 1989;113:350–353.

22. Khamashta MA, Cervera R, Asherson RA et al. Association of antibodies against phospholipids with valvular heart disease in patients with systemic lupus erythematosus. Lancet 1990;335:1541–1544.

23. Badui E, Solorio S, Martinez E, Bravo G, Enciso R, Barile L et al. The heart in the primary antiphospholipid syndrome. Arch Med Res 1995;26:115–120.

24. Nesher G, Ilany J, Rosenmann D, Abraham AS. Valvular dysfunction in antiphospholipid syndrome: prevalence, clinical features and treatment. Semin Arthritis Rheum 1997;27:27–35.

25. Ford SE, Kennedy LA, Ford PM. Clinico-pathological correlations of antiphospholipid antibodies. Arch Path Lab Med 1994;118:491–495.

26. Asherson RA. The catastrophic antiphospholipid syndrome, 1998. A review of the clinical features, possible pathogenesis and treatment. Lupus 1998;7 (Suppl 2):55–62.

27. Levine SR, Salowich-Palm L, Sawaya KL, Perry M, Spencer HJ, Winkler HJ et al. IgG anticardiolipin antibody titer >40 GPL and the risk of subsequent thrombo-occlusive events and death. Stroke 1997;28:1660–1665.

28. Rosove MH, Brewer PMC. Antiphospholipid thrombosis:clinical course after the first thrombotic event in 70 patients. Ann Intern Med 1992;117:303–308.

29. Triplett DA, Brandt JT, Musgrave KA, Orr CA. The relationship between lupus anticoagulants and antibodies to phospholipids. JAMA 1988;259:550–554.

30. Levine SR, Brey RL, Salowich-Palm L, Sawaya KL, Havstad S. Antiphospholipid antibody associated stroke: prospective assessment of recurrent event risk. Stroke 1993;24:188–204.

31. Alarcon-Segovia D, Deleze M, Oria CV et al. Antiphospholipid antibodies and the antiphospholipid syndrome in systemic lupus erythematosus: a prospective analysis of 500 consecutive patients. Medicine 1989;68:353–365.

32. Escalante A, Brey RL, Mitchell BD, Dreiner U. Accuracy of anticardiolipin antibodies in identifying a history of thrombosis among patients with systemic lupus erythematosus. A, J Med 1995;98:559–567.

33. Nojima J, Suehisa E, Akita N, Toku M, Fushimi R, Tada H et al. Risk of arterial thrombosis in patients with anticardiolipin antibodies and lupus anticoagulant. Br J Haematol 1997;96:447–450.

34. Verro P, Levine SR, Tietjen GE. Cerebrovascular ischemic events with high positive anticardiolipin antibodies. Stroke 1995;26:160.

35. Inanc M, Radway-Bright EL, Isenberg DA. Beta-2-glycoprotein 1 and anti-beta-2-glycoprotein I antibodies: where are we now? Br J Rheumatol 1997;36:1247–1257.

36. Sammaritano LR, Ng S, Sobel R, Kong Lo S, Simantov R, Furie R et al. Anticardilipin subclass: association of IgG2 with arterial and/or venous thrombosis. Arthritis Rheumatol 1998;1998–2006.

37. Vasquez-Mellado J, Llorente L, Richaud-Patin Y, Alarcon-Segovia D. Exposure of anionic phospholipids upon platelet activation permits binding of beta-2-glycoprotein 1 and through it that of IgG antiphospholipid antibodies. J Autoimmunity 1994;7:335–348.

38. Specker Ch, Rademacher J, Sohngen D, Sitzer M, Janda I, Siebler M et al. Cerebral microemboli in patients with antiphospholipid syndrome. Lupus 1997;6:638–644.

39. Specker C, Perniok A, Brauchmann W, Siebler M, Schneider M. Detection of cerebral microemboli in APS-Introducing a novel investigation method and implications of analogies with carotid artery disease. Lupus 1998;7 (Suppl 2): 75–80.

40. Duhaut P, Berruyer M, Pinede L, Demolombe-Rague S, Loire R, Seydoux D et al. Anticardiolipin antibodies and giant cell arteritis: a prospective, multicenter case–control study. Arthritis Rheumatol 1998;41:701–709.

41. Drouvalakis KA, Buchanan TTC. Phospholipid specificity of autoimmune and drug induced lupus anticoagulants; association of phosphatidylethanolamine reactivity with thrombosis in autoimmune disease. J Rheumatol 1998;25:290–295.

42. Carhuapoma JR, Mitsias P, Levine SR. Cerebral venous thrombosis and anticardiolipin antibodies. Neurology 1997;28:2363–2369.

43. Descheins M-A, Conard J, Horellou MH, Ameri A, Preter M, Chendru F et al. Coagulations studies, factor V Leiden, and anticardiolipin antibodies in 40 cases of cerebral venous sinus thrombosis. Stroke 1996;27:1724–1730.

44. Coull BM, Goodnight, SH. Antiphospholipid antibodies, prethrombotic states, and stroke. Stroke 1990;21:1370–1374.

45. Mikdashi JA, Kay GG. Neurocognitive deficits in antiphospholipid syndrome. Neurology 1996;46:A359 (June).

46. Van Horn G, Arnett FC, Dimachkie MM. Reversible dementia and chorea in a young woman with the lupus anticoagulant. Neurology 1996;46:1566–1603.
47. Denburg SD, Carbotte, RM, Ginsberg, JS, Denburg, JA. The relationship of antiphospholipid antibodies to cognitive function in patients with systemic lupus erythematosus. J Int Neuropsychol Soc 1997;3:377–386.
48. Hanly JG, Hong C, Smith S, Fisk JD. A prospective analysis of cognitive function and anticardiolipin antibodies in systemic lupus erythematosus. Arthritis Rheum 1999;42:728–734.
49. Long AA, Denburg SD, Carbotte RM, Singal DP, Denburg JA. Serum lymphocytotoxic antibodies and neurocognitive function in systemic lupus erythematosus. Ann Rheum Dis 1990;49: 249–253.
50. Menon S, Jameson-Shortall E, Newman SP, Hall-Craggs MR, Chinn R, Isenberg DA. A longitudinal study of anticardiolipin antibody levels and cognitive functioning in systemic lupus erythematosus. Arthritis Rheum 1999;42:735–741.
51. Denburg SD, Carbotte, RM, Denburg, JA. Cognition and mood in systemic lupus erythematosus. Ann N Y Acad Sci 1997;823:45–59.
52. Lezak MD. Neuropsychological assessment, 3rd edn. Oxford: Oxford University Press, 1998;18.
53. Spreen O, Strauss E. A compendium of neuropsychological tests: administration, norms, and commentary (Chapter 8). New York: Oxford University Press, 1991.
54. Schmidt R, Auer-Grumbach P, Fazekas F, Offenbacher H, Kapeller P. Anticardiolipin antibodies in normal subjects. Neuropsychological correlates and MRI findings. Stroke 1995;26:749–754.
55. Kalashnikova LA, Nasonov EL, Kushekbaeva AE, Gracheva LA. Anticardiolipin antibodies in Sneddon's syndrome. Neurology 1990;40:464–467.
56. Zelzer B, Sepp N, Stockhammer G, Dosch E, Hilty E, Offner D et al. Sneddon;s syndrome; A long term follow-up of 21 patients. Arch Dermatol 1993;129:437–444.
57. Tourbah A, Peitte JC, Iba-Zizen MT, Lyon-Caen O, Godeau P, Frances C. The natural course of cerebral lesions in sneddon syndrome. Arch Neurol 1997;54:53–60.
58. Sneddon IB. Cerebral vascular lesions in livedo reticularis. Br J Dermatol 1965;77:180–185.
59. Coull BM, Bourdette DN, Goodnight SH, Briley DP, Hart R. Multiple cerebral infarctions and dementia associated with anticardiolipin antibodies. Stroke 1987;18:1107–1112.
60. Chinnery PF, Shaw PI, Ince PG, Jackson GH, Bishop RI. Fulminant encephalopathy due to the catastrophic primary antiphospholipid syndrome. J Neurol 1997;Neurosurg Psych 62:300–301.
61. de Moerloose P, Boehlen F, Reber G. Prevalence of anticardiolipin and antinuclear antibodies in an elderly hospitalized population and mortality after a 6-year follow-up. Age Ageing 1997;319–321.
62. Cesbron J-Y, Amouyel Ph, Masy E. Anticardiolipin antibodies and physical disability in the elderly. Ann Intern Med 1997;126:1003.
63. Carbotte RM, Denburg, SD, Denburg, JA. Prevalence of cognitive impairment in systemic lupus erythematosus. J Nerv Mental Dis 1986;174:357–364.
64. Wolkowitz OM, Reus VI, Weingartner, H, Thompson K, Breier A, Doran A, et al. Cognitive effects of corticosteroids. Am J Psychiatry.1990;147:1297–1303.
65. Wolkowitz OM, Reus VI, Canick J, Levin B, Lupien S. Glucocorticoid medication, memory and steroid psychosis in medical illness. Ann N Y Acad Sci 1997;823:81–96.
66. Keenan PA, Jacobson MW, Soleymani RM, Mayes MD, Stress ME, Yaldoo DT. The effect on memory of chronic Prednisone treatment in patients with systemic disease. Neurology 1996;47:1396–1402.
67. Ling MHM, Perry PH, Tsuang MT. Psychiatric side effects of corticosteroid therapy. Arch Gen Psychiatry 1981;38:471–477.
68. Schwartz M, Rochas M, Weller B, Sheinkman A, Tal I, Golan D et al. High association of anticardiolipin antibodies with psychosis. J Clin Psychiatry 1998;59:20–23.
69. West SG, Emlen W, Wener MH, Kotzin BL. Neuropsychiatric lupus erythematosus: a 10-year experience on the value of diagnostic tests. Am J Med 1995;99:153–163.
70. Tietjen GE, Day M, Norris L, Aurora S, Halvorsen A, Schultz L et al. Role of anticardiolipin antibodies in young persons with migraine and transient focal neurologic events. Neurology 1998;50:1433–1440.
71. Tietjen GE, Levine SR, Brown E et al. Factors which predict antiphospholipid immuno-reactivity in young people with focal neurologic deficits. Arch Neurol 1993;50:833–836.
72. Silvestrini M, Matteis M, Troisi E, Cupini LM, Zaccari G, Bernardi G. Migrainous stroke and the antiphospholipid antibodies. Eur Neurol 1994;34:316–319.
73. Herranz MT, Rivier G, Khamashta MA, Blaser KU, Hughes GRV. Association between antiphospholipid antibodies and epilepsy in patients with systemic lupus erythematosus. Arthritis Rheum 1994;37:586–571.
74. Inzelberg R, Korczyn AD. Lupus anticoagulant and late onset seizures. Acta Neurol Scand 1989;79:114–118.
75. Formiga F, Mitjavila F, Pac M, Moga I. Epilepsy and antiphospholipid antibodies in systemic lupus erythematosus patients. Lupus 1997;6:486.

76. Verrot D, San-Marco M, Dravet C et al. Prevalence and significance of antinuclear and anticardi-
    olipin antibodies in patients with epilepsy. Am J Med 1997;103:33–37.
77. Liou HH, Wang CR, Chou HC et al. Anticardiolipin antisera from lupus patients with seizures
    reduce a GABA receptor-mediated chloride current in snail neurons. Life Sci 1994;54:1119–1125.
78. Cervera R, Asherson RA, Font J, Tikly M, Pallares L, Chamorro A et al. Chorea in the antiphospho-
    lipid syndrome: clinical, radiologic, and immunologic characteristics of 50 patients from our clinics
    and recent literature. Medicine 1997;76:203–212.
79. Asherson RA, Hughes GRV. Antiphospholipid antibodies and chorea. J Rheumatol 1988;15:377–379.
80. Hatron PY, Bouchez B, Wattel A et al. Chorea, systemic lupus erythematosus, circulating lupus
    anticoagulants. J Rheumatol 1987;14:991–993.
81. Furie R, Ishikawa T, Dhawan V, Eidelberg D. Alternating hemichorea in primary antiphospholipid
    syndrome: evidence for contralateral striatal metabolism. Neurology 1994;44:2197–2199.
82. Sunden-Cullberg J, Tedroff J, Aquilonius S-M. Reversible chorea in primary antiphospholipid syn-
    drome. Movement Dis 1998;13:147–149.
83. Harris EN, Gharavi AE, Mackworth CG et al. Lupoid sclerosis: a possible pathogenic role for
    antiphospholipid antibodies. Ann Rheum Dis 1985;44:281–283.
84. Lavalle C, Pizarro S, Drenkard C et al. Transverse myelitis: a manifestation of systemic lupus ery-
    thematosus associated with antiphospholipid antibodies. J Rheumatol 1990;17:34–37.
85. Ruiz-Arguelles GJ, Guzman-Ramos J, Flores-Flores J, Garay-Martinez J. Refractory hiccough
    heralding transverse myelitis in the primary antiphospholipid syndrome. Lupus 1998;7:49–50.
86. Jackson C, Brey RL, Barohn R et al. Anticardiolipin antibodies in Guillain–Barré Syndrome. Clin
    Exp Rheumatol 1992;10:657.
87. Harris EN, Englert H Derue G et al. Antiphospholipid antibodies in acute guillain-barre syndrome.
    Lancet 1983;2:1361–1362.
88. Shigeta H, Yamaguchi M, Nakano K, Obayashi H, Takemura R, Fukui M et al. Serum autoanti-
    bodies against sulfatide and phospholipid in NIDDM patients with diabetic neuropathy. Diabetes
    Care 1997;20:1896–1899.
89. Toubi E, Ben-David J, Kessel A, Podoshin L, Golan TD. Autoimmune aberration in sudden sen-
    sorineural hearing loss: association with anticardiolipin antibodies. Lupus 1997;6:540–542.
90. Naarendorp M, Spiera H. Sudden sensorineural hearing loss in patients with systemic lupus erythe-
    matosus or lupus-like syndromes and antiphospholipid antibodies. J Rheumatol 1998;25:589–592.
91. Montalban J, Arboix A, Staub H, Barquinero J, Marti-Vilalta J, Codina A et al. Transient global
    amnesia and antiphospholipid antibodies. Clin Exp Rheumatol 1989;7:85–87.
92. Rafuse PE, Canny CLB. Initial identification of antinuclear antibody-negative systemic lupus ery-
    thematosus on ophthalmic examination: a case report with discussion of the ocular significance of
    anticardiolipin (antiphospholipid) antibodies. Can J Ophthalmol 1992;27:189–193.
93. Labutta RJ. Ophthalmic manifestations in the antiphospholipid syndrome. In: Asherson RA,
    Cervera R, Piette JC, Shoenfeld Y, editors. The antiphospholipid syndrome. Boca Raton, FL: CRC
    Press, 1996; 213–218.
94. Molad Y, Sidi Y, Gornish M et al. Lupus anticoagulant: correlation with magnetic resonance
    imaging of brain lesions. J Rheumatol 1992;19:556–561.
95. Provenzale JM, Heinz ER, Ortel TL, Macik BG, Charles LA, Alberts MJ. Antiphospholipid antibodies in
    patients without systemic lupus erythematosus: neuroradiologic findings. Radiology 1994;192:531–537.
96. Toubi E, Khamashta MA, Panarra A, Hughes GRV. Association of antiphospholipid antibodies with
    central nervous system disease in systemic lupus erythematosus. Am J Med 1995;99:397–401.
97. Sailer M, Burchert W, Ehrenheim C, Smid HGOM, Haas J, Wildhagen K et al. Positron emission
    tomography and magnetic resonance imaging for cerebral involvement in patients with systemic
    lupus erythematosus, J Neurol 1997;244:186–193.
98. Hachulla E, Michon-Pasturel U, Leys D, Pruvo J-P, Queyrel V, Masy E et al. Cerebral magnetic
    imaging in patients with or without antiphospholipid antibodies. Lupus 1998;7:124–131.
99. Deschiens MA, Conrad J, Horellou MH, Ameri A, Preter M, Chendru F et al. Coagulations studies,
    factor V Leiden, and anticardiolipin antibodies in 40 cases of cerebral venous sinus thrombosis.
    Stroke 1996;27: 1724–1730.
100. Brey RL, Levine SR. Treatment of neurologic complications of the antiphospholipid syndrome.
    Lupus 1996;5:473–476.

6 Skin Manifestations of the Antiphospholipid Antibody Syndrome

C. A. Battagliotti

Several skin manifestations have been described in patients with antiphospholipid antibody syndrome (APS) (Table 6.1) [1–3]. The most frequent skin lesions are livedo reticularis and skin ulcers.

Vascular occlusion is generally the first and most frequent manifestation observed in patients with antiphospholipid antibodies (aPL) accounting for 41% of the cases. Forty percent of these patients present with other multisystem thrombotic phenomena during the course of the disease, underscoring the significance of skin lesions as a diagnostic marker and predictor of systemic involvement.

In spite of the association of skin lesions with different isotypes of immunoglobulins, the presence of IgA anticardiolipin antibodies has been reported as an independent predictive factor of skin lesions (skin ulcers, chilblains lupus and vasculitis) [4].

Livedo Reticularis

Livedo reticularis is the commonest skin manifestation in patients with APS, characterized by a dark purple reticular pattern usually involving the upper and lower limbs [3, 6].

The skin normally receives its blood supply through a vascular system arranged in the form of cones with their base towards the skin surface. Each cone is supplied by an arteriole. The pattern of livedo reticularis corresponds to areas of anastomosis

Table 6.1. The skin and the antiphospholipid syndrome .

- Livedo reticularis
- Sneddon's syndrome
- Skin ulcers
- Necrotizing vasculitis
- Livedoid vasculitis
- Cutaneous gangrene
- Superficial thrombophlebitis
- Pseudovasculitic lesions. Nodules, papules, pustules, palmar–plantar erythema
- Subungual bleeding

Table 6.2. Livedo reticularis and associated diseases.

- Antiphospholipid syndrome
- Systemic lupus erythematosus (with or without aPL)
- Systemic vasculitis (polyarteritis nodosa, cryoglobulinemia)
- Pseudovasculitic syndromes (cholesterol embolization)
- Overlapping syndromes
- Scleroderma
- Infectious diseases (syphilis, tuberculosis)

between two cones where diminished blood flow is associated with the dilatation of venules and capillaries. Therefore, the alteration in arterial blood flow caused by the livedo may result from:

- Blood inflow obstruction
- Blood hyperviscosity
- Blood outflow obstruction.

Livedo may be observed in normal subjects, specially women, after exposure to cold, displaying a symmetrical and regular mottled pattern. However, the relationship with a large number of pathological conditions (Table 6.2) is very important. A detailed examination of the features of the reticular pattern, including location, extension, symmetry and regularity and the presence of associated skin lesions will contribute to the differential diagnosis [3, 5, 7, 8].

The pattern of involvement associated with APS is generally disseminated, with incomplete circular segments, non-infiltrated, persistent or irregular with wide ramifications (livedo racemosa). Some patients present a fine, regular and complete network. (Fig. 6.1).

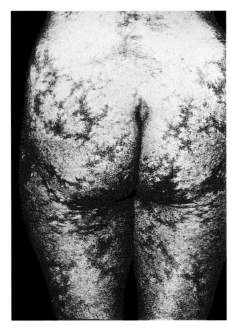

Figure 6.1. Livedo reticularis of the gluteal region and both thighs of a patient with SLE and APS.

Sneddon's Syndrome

In 1965, Sneddon described the association between livedo reticularis and stroke [9]. Later on, the presence of aPL in some of the patients that carry the syndrome suggests that a subset of patients might have the APS [10–12].

Although there are differences in the terminology used for the Sneddon syndrome livedo, its features are very clear. The skin lesions are extensive, patchy, persistent and do not disappear with skin heating. Usually, this is the pattern observed in patients with a prior condition that accounts for the vascular lesion (secondary Sneddon's syndrome), such as autoimmune or thrombophilic diseases.

Beyond the initial description, there are numerous reports of cardiac and renal involvement, development of hypertension as well as gynecological and obstetrical complications [13, 14]. There are no laboratory tests that contribute to a definite diagnosis; however, 35% of patients with Sneddon's syndrome have anti-endothelial cell antibodies as opposed to patients with stroke and no livedo reticularis [15]. Prognosis is variable, mainly depending on the extension and progression of brain lesions that might lead to a severe and definite mental deterioration.

The pathological study of livedo reticularis shows endothelitis and obliterating endarteritis without necrotizing vasculitis [12]. In some cases the characteristics of the APS overlap so that in all patients affected with livedo reticularis with non-inflammatory small vessel thrombosis in their biopsy, the measurement of aPL is mandatory.

Skin Ulcers

Lower limb ulcers are one of the most frequent skin manifestations in patients with APS. They have been observed in 20–30% of patients. The prevalence of skin ulcers is very high when associated with aCL in systemic lupus erythematosus (SLE) [3, 6].

Although characteristics are variable, ulcers are painful, small (0.5–3.0 cm in diameter), with stellate, oval or irregular borders surrounded by a purple-brownish and recurrent purple halo. They are generally located in the ankles, legs and feet. Healing is difficult; when accomplished it results in a white scar with a pigmented halo [16, 17] (Fig. 6.2).

Giant ulcers and cases resembling gangrenous pyoderma have been reported, although in the latter case, the characteristic undercut borders of pyoderma are absent. Post-phlebitic ulcers are seldom seen though an increased prevalence of aPL has been described in elderly patients with venous ulcers (Figs 6.2 and 6.3).

Necrotizing Vasculitis and Livedoid Vasculitis

Generally, no inflammatory changes are observed in the biopsies taken from skin lesions of patients suffering from the APS. The association with vasculitis might reflect the coexistence of two diseases, most commonly SLE.

In 1967, Bard and Winkelmann described a group of patients with chronic and recurrent livedoid-like lesions circumscribed to the lower limbs and with histological images of hyalinizing segmentary vasculitis of the dermis vessels related to

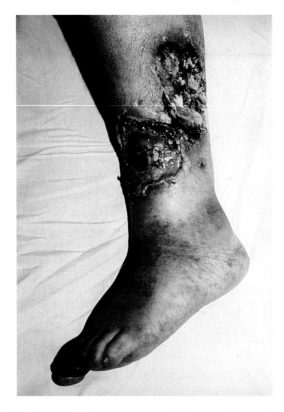

Figure 6.2. Patient with primary APS that presents necrotic ulcers on the leg and necrosis of the toes.

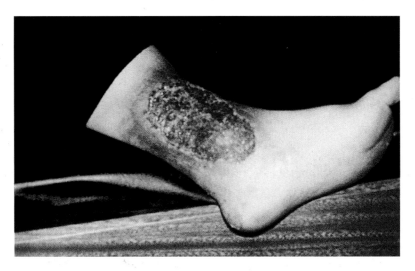

Figure 6.3. Primary APS with skin giant ulcer on the left leg refractory to anticoagulant and fibrinolytic treatment.

thrombotic occlusion and lymphocytic infiltration. This disorder was termed livedoid vasculitis or segmentary hyalinizing vasculitis. These cases presented with livedo lesions, purpura with a trend towards ulceration that became covered with dark crusts and inflammatory borders. After months or weeks they healed forming porcelain-white star-like scars, atrophic with telangiectasis and hyperpigmented borders. These latter lesions have been termed white atrophy and some authors consider it as a disorder per se. The term was coined by Milian in 1929 who attributed its formation to a previous ulceration with a probable syphilitic or tuberculous etiology. There is consensus in that there are different stages in the evolution of the same process that leads to livedoid vasculitis. Other authors believe that "white atrophy" is the end stage of different disorders that result in a stellate porcelain-like scar [18–20].

Livedoid vasculitis predominates in young women with characteristic lesions on the lower limbs; it recurs with seasonal exacerbations. Its presentation might be primary or idiopathic. However, it is sometimes related to SLE, Sjögren's syndrome, APS, polyarteritis nodosa, rheumatoid arthritis, scleroderma, Raynaud's phenomenon, cryoglobulinemia, macroglobulinemia, venous vascular pathology and diabetes [19, 21].

Controversy exists as to the pathogenesis but possible suggested mechanisms include imbalance of the coagulation and fibrinolysis system and alteration of platelet function.

Skin lesions typically found are: erythematosus plaques, petechial purpura, livedo, painful ulcers of different sizes, white atrophy, telangiectases and hyperpigmentation. In some patients, direct immunofluorescence of skin vessels reveals IgG, IgM, IgA, fibrin and to a lesser degree, deposits of complement [22].

Histological characteristics of livedoid vasculitis overlap with the vascular changes seen in the APS. Segmental hyalinization and non-inflammatory occlusion of the dermal arterioles leading to skin ulceration is observed.

Cutaneous Gangrene and Necrosis

Digital gangrene is a well-recognized manifestation in patients with APS [2, 3]. The process starts with erythematous macules, cyanosis or pseudocellulitis ending in necrosis. In patients with SLE or other autoimmune diseases, aPL quite often coexists with other pathogenic factors such as cryoglobulins, antiendothelial cell antibodies or hepatitis viruses. Patients who are smokers, hypertensive or are on oral contraceptives have an increased risk of necrosis. (Figs 6.4, 6.5 and 6.6) Angiographic images show occlusion or severe stenosis of middle and large sized vessels.

Some patients develop extensive superficial skin necrosis (3%) generally involving the limbs, head and buttocks. The onset is sudden, with an extensive and painful purpuric lesion followed by a necrotic plaque with purpuric and active edges and bullous lesions. The thrombosing microangiitis seen in examined tissues is characteristic [2, 23].

Superficial Thrombophlebitis

Thrombotic episodes in the deep veins of the lower limbs are common. Similar mechanisms might lead to the involvement of the superficial venous territory [3].

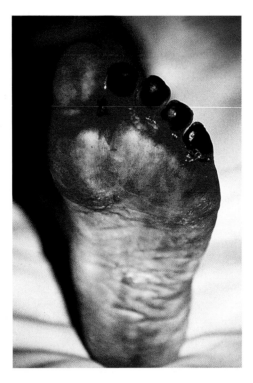

Figure 6.4. Evolution to gangrene with distal necrosis of the left foot toes in the patient carrier of primary APS shown in Fig. 6.3.

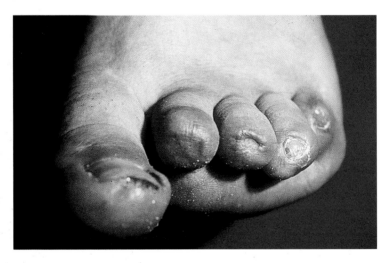

Figure 6.5. Cure by spontaneous amputation of the left foot toes affected with gangrene in a patient with a primary APS.

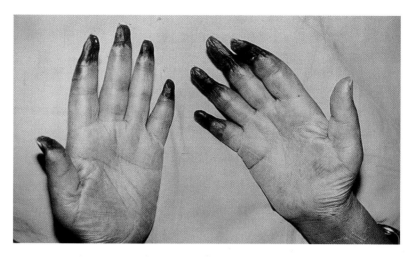

Figure 6.6. Digital necrosis with gangrene of the fingers of a patient with SLE and APS.

Pseudo-vasculitic Lesions: Nodules, Papules, Pustules, Palmar–Plantar Erythema

A wide variety of skin lesions might be included under the term pseudo-vasculitic, erythematous macules, painful nodules and purpura, among others. The APS accounts for the microthrombosis observed in skin vessels [3, 24] (Figs 6.7 and 6.8).

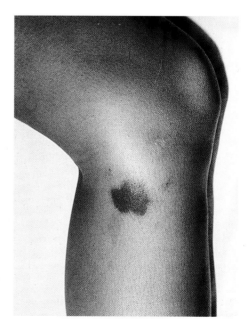

Figure 6.7. SLE along with APS presenting with papuloerythematosus skin lesion (irregular borders) on the lower limb.

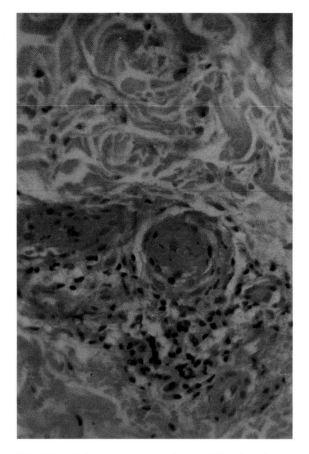

Figure 6.8. Biopsy of skin with non-inflammatory vascular thrombosis (venular) of a patient with SLE and APS.

Subungual Hemorrhages

Chip-like subungual hemorrhages are longitudinally distributed, small reddish to black linear lesions which persist after ungual compression. They are not exclusively associated with the APS because ungual trauma can be seen in healthy subjects as well as patients with infectious endocarditis. They are caused by thrombotic or embolic phenomena. *It is worth pointing out that the presence of these lesions in several fingers is related to an underlying pathological process* [3, 6].

What Do Skin Lesion Biopsies of Patients with APS Show? [3, 25]

The main histopathological picture is: non-inflammatory thrombosis in small arteries and/or veins of the dermis and hypodermis. A pattern that might be associated or be the only one observed is that of obliterating endarterial occlusion, character-ized by narrowing of the vessel lumen with endothelial cell proliferation and fibro-hyalinization of the vessel wall. The absence of vasculitis is characteristic. Lymphocytic or lymphoplasmocytic infiltrating isolates might be observed. Based on skin involvement, the following histologic pattern is observed [25].

- Gangrenous lesion
    Vascular thrombosis
    Dermal hemorrhage
    Obliterating endarteritis
    Epidermal necrosis
- Ulcerous lesion
    Vascular thrombosis
    Capillary proliferation
    Obliterating endarteritis
    Dermal hemorrhage
    Deposit of hemosiderin
- Livedo reticularis
    Center of the reticular pattern (apparently normal skin)
        Normal biopsy
        Obliterating endarteritis in deep arterioles of the dermis or hypodermis
    Tissue of the reticulate (involved segment of the skin):
        Hyperplasia of dermal vessels.

Wherever the site of biopsy in livedo reticularis, thrombosis is rare except in the case of catastrophic APS or in the presence of ulcers or necrosis.

Association of Skin Lesions with Different Organ Involvement

It should be remembered that 41% of patients with APS begin their disease with skin manifestations and that 40% of patients will develop multisystem thrombotic phe-nomena during the course of the disease. The association of livedo reticularis with cerebrovascular involvement has already been pointed out (Sneddon's syndrome). The presence of multiple subungual hemorrhages might coincide with thrombotic events of other organs such as the brain, skin, adrenal glands, kidney, etc.

Entities Associated with APS

Different pathologic entities have been described to occur in association with APS. It should be underscored that patients affected with inflammatory bowel disease (ulcer-ative colitis, Crohn's disease) are susceptible to thrombosis during the active stage of the disease in relation to aPL. Up to 10% of patients will develop ischemic lesions of the central nervous system and embolic events, including peripheral necrosis [26, 27]. Skin lesions observed in this life-threatening syndrome are livedo reticularis, acro-cyanosis, extensive skin necrosis, palmar erythema and gangrene [28].

Treatment

It is hard to predict if the patient who only has a skin lesion will later develop an extra cutaneous thrombotic event. However, it is worth remembering that 40% of patients that begin with skin lesions will eventually undergo systemic involvement. Hence, it is important to consider extensive skin necrosis and digital ischemia as major thrombotic events; in these cases, patients should received long term anticoagulant treatment [29, 30, 31]. The approach to minor skin manifestations is less clear. It is yet to be defined whether platelet antiaggregation is enough or whether it will be necessary to attempt the use of more aggressive treatments.

Alternative treatments should be developed for patients resistant to standard approaches [32]. Thrombolytic agents in low dose have been proposed in patients with skin lesions where the thrombotic events account for the clinical picture (i.e., livedoid vasculitis). Thrombolitic agents not only accomplish the patency of involved arteries but also play a significant role by increasing microcirculation [33].

Some patients have been treated with streptokinase or urokinase with or without heparin with varying responses. The intravenous infusion of rTPA (recombinant tissue plasminogen activator) at a dose of 20 mg/day diluted in saline solution during 8 hours for 10 days resulted in the healing of ulcer lesions. Unwanted effects such as bleeding that might threaten the patient's life should be considered. This therapeutic modality should be selected when all the other alternatives have failed. It is critical to test coagulation status prior to and during infusion; treatment should be withdrawn as soon as minimum bleeding is noticed [33, 34].

Conclusion

Antiphospholipid antibodies are strongly related to thrombotic events. It is the most common acquired coagulation defect among the ones accountable for procoagulant states.

Skin involvement might be the first manifestation of the APS (41%) and over a third of these patients will develop multisystem thrombotic events during the course of the disease.

References

1. Battagliotti CA. Síndrome de anticuerpos antifosfolipídicos. In: Battagliotti C, Greca A et al, editors. Temas seleccionados de terapéutica clínica. UNR Editora. 1996;328–334.
2. Alegre VA, Gastineau DA, Winkelmann RK. Skin lesions associated with circulating lupus anticoagulant. Br J Dermatol 1989;120:419–429.
3. Gibson GE, Daniel Su WP, Pittelkow MR. Antiphospholipid syndrome and the skin. J. Am Acad Dermatol 1997;36:970–982.
4. Tajima C, Suzuki Y, Mizushima Y, Ichikawa Y. Clinical significance of immunoglobulin A apl. Possible association with skin manifestations and small vessel vasculitis. J Rheumatol 1998;25:1730–1736.
5. Naldi L, Locati F, Marchesi L et al. Cutaneous manifestations associated with antiphospholipid antibodies in patients with suspected primary APS: a case control study. Ann Rheum Dis 1993;52:219–222.
6. Eng AM. Cutaneous expressions of antiphospholipid syndromes. Semin Thromb Hemost 1994;20:71–78.
7. Asherson RA, Mayou SC, Merry P et al. The spectrum of livedo reticularis and anticardiolipin antibodies. Br J Dermatol 1989;120:215–221.

8. Weinstein C, Miller MH, Axtens R et al. Livedo reticularis associated with increased titers of anti-cardiolipin antibodies in systemic lupus erythematosus. Arch Dermatol 1987;123:596–600.
9. Sneddon JB. Cerebrovascular lesions and livedo reticularis. Br J Dermatol 1965;77:180–185.
10. Martínez Hernandez PL, López Guzmán A, Espinosa Arranz E, Monereo Alonso A, Arnalich Fernández F. Síndrome de Sneddon: valor diagnóstico de los anticuerpos antifosfolipídicos. Rev Clin Esp 1991;189:272–274.
11. Tourbach A, Piette JC, Iba-Zizen MT, Lyon-Caen O, Godeau P, Francés C. The natural course of cerebral lesion in Sneddon syndrome. Arch Neurol 1997; 54: 53–60.
12. Stephens CJM. Sneddon's syndrome. Clin Exp Rheumatol. 1992;10:489–492.
13. Macario F, Macario MC, Ferro A, Goncalves F, Campos M, Marques A. Sneddon's syndrome: a vascular systemic disease with kidney involvement? Nephron 1997;75:94–97.
14. Ohtani H, Imai H, Yasuda T et al. A combination of livedo racemosa, occlusion of cerebral blood vessels and nephropathy: kidney involvement in Sneddon's syndrome. Am J Kidney Dis 1995;26:511–515.
15. Frances C, le Tonqueze M, Slohzin KV et al. Prevalence of anti-endothelial cell antibodies in patients with Sneddon's syndrome. J Am Acad Dermatol 1995;33:64–68.
16. Rattan CE, Burton JL. Antiphospholipid syndrome and cutaneous vasoocclusive disorders. Semin Dermatol 1991;10:152–159.
17. Reyes E, Alarcón-Segovia D. Leg ulcers in the primary antiphospholipid syndrome. Report of a case with a peculiar proliferative small vessel vasculopathy. Clin Exp Rheumatol 1991;9:63–66.
18. Leroux B, Barón E, Garrido G, Alonso A, Bergero A, Fernandez Bussy R. Vasculitis livedoide: nuestra experiencia. Dermatol Argent 1998;2:121–126.
19. Winkelman R, Schroeter A, Kierland R, Ryan T. Clinical studies of livedoid vasculitis. Mayo Clin Proc 1994;49:746–750.
20. Kern A. Atrophie blanche. J Am Acad Dermatol 1982;6:1048–1053.
21. Stephansson EA, Niemp KM, Jouikainen T, Vaarala O, Polosue T. Lupus anticoagulant and skin. Acta Dermato Venereol 1991;71:416–422.
22. Hassan ML, Di Fabio NA, Martinez Aquino E, Schroh R, Kien C, Magnin PH. Vasculitis livedoide. Estudio clínico, histopatológico y laboratorial de 10 casos. Rev Arg Derm 1987;68:311–319.
23. Dodd HJ, Sarkany I, O'Shayghnessy D. Widespread cutaneous necrosis associated with lupus anticoagulant. Clin Exp Dermatol 1985;10:581–586.
24. Asherson RA, Jacobelli S, Rosemberg H, McKee P, Hughes GRV. Skin nodules and macules resembling vasculitis in the antiphospholipid syndrome – a report of two cases. Clin Exp Dermatol 1992;17:266–269.
25. Alegre VA, Winkelmann RK. Histopathologic and immunofluorescence study of skin lesions associated with circulating lupus anticoagulant. J Am Acad Dermatol 1988;19;117–124.
26. Martinovic Z, Perisic K, Pejnovic N, Lukacevic S, Rabrenovic L, Petrovic M. Antiphospholipid antibodies in inflammatory bowel diseases. Vojnosanit Pregl 1998;55:47–49.
27. Mevorach D, Goldberg Y, Gomori JM, Rachmilewitz D. Antiphospholipid syndrome manifested by stroke in a patient with Crohn's disease. J Clin Gastroenterol 1996;22:141–143.
28. Asherson RA, Cervera R, Piette JC, Font J, Lie JT, Burcoglu A et al. Catastrophic antiphospholipid syndrome. Clinical and laboratory features of 50 patients. Medicine 1998;77:195–207.
29. Lockshin MD. Which patients with antiphospholipid antibody should be treated and how? Rheum Dis Clin NA 1993;19:235–251.
30. Derksen RH, De Groot PH, Kater L et al. Patients with antiphospholipid antibodies and venous thrombosis should receive lifelong anticoagulant treatment. Clin Exp Rheumatol 1992;10:662–668.
31. Khamashta MA, Cuadrado MJ, Mujic F, Taub NA, Hunt BJ, Hughes GRV. The management of thrombosis in the antiphospholipid antibody syndrome. N Engl J Med 1995;332:993–997.
32. Curwin J, Kyung Jang I, Fuster V. Expanded use of thrombolytic therapy. Mayo Clin Proc 1992;332:993–997.
33. Klein KL, Pittelkow MR. Tissue plasminogen activator for treatment of livedoid vasculitis. Mayo Clin Proc 1992;67:923–933.
34. Gertner E, Lie JT. Systemic therapy with fibrinolytic agents and heparin for recalcitrant nonhealing cutaneous ulcer in the antiphospholipid syndrome. J Rheumatol 1994;21:2159–2161.

7 Kidney Disease in Antiphospholipid Syndrome

M. C. Amigo and R. García-Torres

Even though the kidney is a major target organ in the antiphospholipid syndrome (APS), until recently the renal manifestations associated with antiphospholipid antibodies (aPL) have received scarce attention. This can be explained because APS was first described in patients with systemic lupus erythematosus (SLE) and such research studies were focussed on the immune-complex-mediated glomerulonephritis rather than renal vascular lesions that could be secondary.

In addition, because of the frequent occurrence of thrombocytopenia and systemic hypertension, renal biopsy in APS patients would often be considered a high-risk procedure to be discouraged if not formally contraindicated [1].

Nevertheless, knowledge about renal vascular involvement in APS has slowly acquired a critical mass and it is now clear that large vessels, both arterial and venous, as well as the intraparenchymatous arteries and microvasculature may all be affected with the clinical consequences shown in Table 7.1.

Renal Artery Lesions

Large- and medium-size vessel occlusion has been associated with APS in the context of SLE as well as in its primary form [2, 3]. Renal artery occlusion/stenosis has been reported in patients with positive assays for aPL. Some of these patients

Table 7.1. Renal vascular involvement in APS.

Vascular lesion	Clinical consequences
Renal artery lesions: (trunk or main branches) Thrombosis/occlusion/stenosis?	Renovascular hypertension (severe) Renal infarcts (silent, painful, hematuria)
Glomerular capillary thrombosis leading to glomerular sclerosis (studied mainly in SLE)	Increased likelihood of renal insufficiency
Renal thrombotic microangiopathy (glomerular capillaries, afferent arterioles and interlobular arteries) with/without focal or diffuse necrosis (cortical necrosis)	Systemic hypertension (usually severe) Renal failure (mild to end-stage), Proteinuria (mild to nephrotic range) Cortical atrophy
Renal vein thrombosis (unilateral or bilateral)	Renal failure (if bilaterally compromised)

had autoimmune rheumatic conditions, mainly SLE, while others had the primary antiphospholipid syndrome (PAPS).

An early observation by Ostuni et al [4] described a 13-year-old girl with SLE and severe systemic hypertension. Bilateral renal artery stenosis/thrombosis resulted in a poorly perfused kidney and cortical irregularities were present in the contralateral kidney. Hernández et al [5] reported on a young woman with sudden, severe hypertension and a renal infarction who, 14 years later, developed SLE. Asherson et al [6] described a young man with PAPS, arterial hypertension, and a right renal artery stenosis with renal infarction which was thought to be caused by thrombotic occlusion. Ames et al [7] reported an instance of bilateral renal artery occlusion in a patient with PAPS and an unclear systemic disease. Rossi et al [8] reported two cases of renovascular hypertension with renal artery stenosis and suggesting a pathogenetic link between renal artery stenosis, thrombosis, fibromuscular dysplasia, and aPL. Similar considerations were independently made by Mandreoli and coworkers [9, 10]. Particularly interesting is a report by Poux et al [11] on an athletic 35-year-old man with PAPS who suddenly developed arterial hypertension and a left renal infarction. Angiographic studies revealed complete thrombosis of the aorta below the renal arteries plus an extensive colateral circulation arising from the superior mesenteric artery.

In the presence of aPL, renal infarctions result from partial or total, transient or permanent occlusion of renal arteries [4, 5, 8, 9, 12, 13]. Such occlusion may be caused by diverse mechanisms such as in situ thrombosis/stenosis of a renal artery or an embolic event originating on a verrucous cardiac valve. In other cases the cause of a renal infarction was not found [14].

Clinically, severe systemic hypertension, pain in the renal area, hematuria, and renal failure are common forms of presentation of major vessel involvement in PAPS. As commented by Hughes et al [15], arterial hypertension may be labile in early disease. Occasionally, a silent infarct is fortuitously discovered on computed tomography. It cannot be overemphasized that in cases of renal artery stenosis of unknown origin, APS must be excluded. Renal scintigraphy and selective renal angiography are useful procedures to confirm diagnosis and determine the extent of damage.

Succesful treatment with antihypertensive drugs [8, 12], aspirin [13], anticoagulant therapy [4, 7, 9, 12] as well as transluminal angioplasty [6] has been reported. However, adverse outcomes may occur [5]. The sooner an arterial lesion causing arterial hypertension is relieved, the likelier is a successful outcome.

Glomerular Capillary Thrombosis

Hyaline thrombi have been described in patients with active, usually proliferative lupus nephritis. The prevalence and significance of this finding have been carefully studied by Kant et al [16] and Glueck et al [17]. They found an overall rate of capillary thrombosis of near 50% in cases of proliferative glomerulonephritis including 78% in patients with detectable lupus anticoagulant (LA) and only 38% in those without. The presence of glomerular thrombi in the initial biopsy was a strong predictor of glomerular sclerosis. Other studies, however, have not shown an association between aPL and prognosis in lupus nephritis [18–20].

Intrarenal Vascular Lesions

Thrombotic Microangiopathy

The association of the distinctive lesion known as thrombotic microangiopathy (TMA) with aPL was initially described in patients with SLE [21–23]. In another clinical setting, Kincaid-Smith and coworkers [24] showed acute or healed TMA in 22 biopsies obtained in 12 patients with LA and pregnancy-related renal failure. Subsequently, isolated cases of TMA in patients with PAPS were reported [25, 26]. In 1992, at a time in which some still doubted the very existence of Hughes' syndrome, we had the opportunity of studying five patients who had renal disease and arterial hypertension among 20 consecutive patients with PAPS [27]. Mild renal failure was present in three patients while two had end-stage renal failure requiring hemodialysis. Proteinuria from mild to nephrotic range was also present. Biopsy findings in all five patients were consistent with TMA. Some biopsies showed diffuse damage while others had only focal parenchymatous lesions. Microangiopathy involved both the vascular tree and the glomerular tufts (Fig. 7.1).

Recent and recanalized thrombi were observed (Figs 7.2 and 7.3), as if acute lesions were superimposed on the chronic, healed damage (Table 7.2). Ultrastructural studies showed electron-lucent subendothelial deposits and ischemic obsolescence of glomeruli in the absence of histologic and immunohistochemical findings suggestive of SLE. We concluded that in PAPS, depending on the degree and extension of damage, patients could have isolated hypertension, severe proteinuria, and renal

Table 7.2. PAPS-associated nephropathy/main histologic features.

Acute lesions	Chronic lesions
Glomerular	
Mesangial expansion	Basement membrane thickening
Mesangiolysis	Cellular vanishing
Glomerular capillary collapse	Glomerular tuft retraction
Basement membrane wrinkling	Bowman's space widening
"Double contours" with mesangial interposition	Ischemic obsolescence
Translucent subendothelial deposits	Segmental or global glomerular sclerosis
Intracapillary thrombi	
Hemorrhagic infarction	
Necrosis	
Arterioles	
Recent occlusive thrombi	Mural organized thrombi
Laminar thrombi	Recanalizing occlusive thrombi
Endothelial edema/degeneration	Microaneurysms
Subendothelial mucoid edema	Plexiform lesions
Necrosis	Subendothelial fibrosis
	Concentric and muscular hyperplasia
	Myofibroblastic proliferation
	Diffuse fibrosis
Leads to	
TMA with/without focal necrosis	Ischaemic atrophy

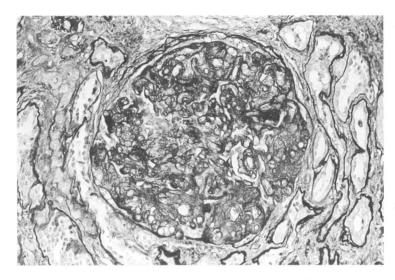

Figure 7.1. Severe and advanced glomerular thrombotic microangiopathy. Capillary lumina are occluded by severe mesangiolysis and deposition of heterogeneous subendothelial material, leading to a segmental "double contour" aspect (PAS).

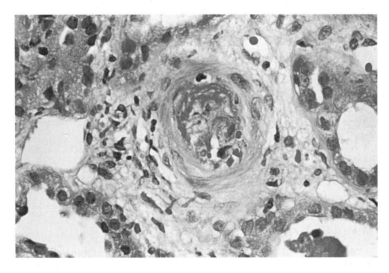

Figure 7.2. A small arteriole with a recent, almost occlusive, partially laminated thrombus. Some complete and fragmented white and red cells are seen (hematoxylin/eosin).

failure including cortical necrosis. In chronic cases, fibrosis and focal atrophy could be found as well as arterial and arteriolar fibromuscular hyperplasia (Figs 7.4 and 7.5).

Subsequent isolated cases or small series have confirmed our findings [28–30]. TMA is the characteristic histologic lesion of the microvasculature in the PAPS-related

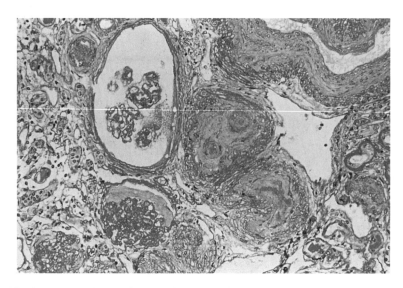

Figure 7.3. Chronic cortical lesions. There are obsolescent sclerotic glomeruli and a hypoperfused glomerulus with a wide Bowman's space and retracted capillaries. On one of its sides there is a small arteriole with a recanalized thrombus and two lumina. On the other side there are two completely occluded arterioles showing thrombosis, recanalization, and refibrosis. A tortuous arteriole with slightly cellular subendothelial fibrosis is also seen (PAS).

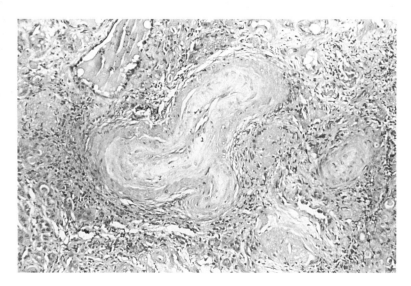

Figure 7.4. Typical histology of an interlobular arteriole which is almost occluded by a slightly cellular mucoid material. The lumen is distorted and the muscular media is partially destroyed and fibrotic. There is interstitial fibrosis with a moderate inflammatory infiltration. A dilated tubule containing hyaline material is seen (Masson).

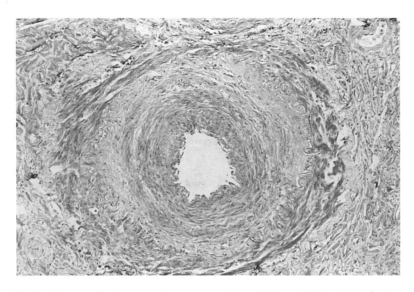

Figure 7.5. Chronic stage of an intraparenchymatous renal artery. Slight medial hyperplasia, fractures of the internal elastica, severe subendothelial fibrosis, myofibroblastic proliferation, and a drastic reduction of the lumen (Masson).

nephropathy. A non-inflammatory vasculopathy with or without thrombosis (the "APS vasculopathy") is a common finding in larger vessels. Of course, TMA is not pathognomonic of PAPS, as there is a wide range of conditions that present the same histologic appearance (Table 7.3). Nochy et al [31] have confirmed our initial observations on glomerular and interlobular arteriolar lesions, and, in addition, have emphasized the common presence of focal cortical atrophy (Fig. 7.6).

Finally, isolated cases of glomerulonephritis [32] and vasculitis [33] associated with aPL but without SLE, have also been published. These associations are hard to explain according to the current knowledge of aPL.

Table 7.3. Some conditions that associate with TMA.

Thrombotic thrombocytopenic purpura
Hemolytic uremic syndrome
Postpartum renal failure
Pre-eclampsia
Scleroderma
Malignant arterial hypertension
Oral contraceptives
Renal transplantation/allograft rejection
Cyclosporin A toxicity
Chemotherapy

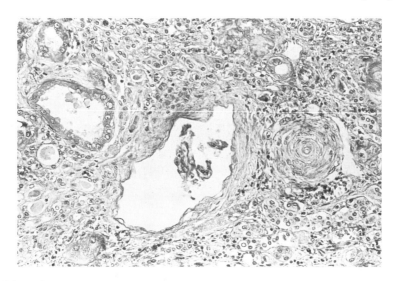

Figure 7.6. Focal cortical atrophy. There are ischemic glomeruli, an arteriole with "onion skin" hyperplasia of the media and a "pin-point" lumen, generalized tubular atrophy with early dilation in one, and interstitial fibrosis (Masson).

Cortical Renal Ischemia

Occlusion of small isolated parenchymatous renal vessels gives rise to small foci of cortical necrosis. These are generally asymptomatic; however, if they are multiple or generalized they may lead to patchy or diffuse cortical necrosis as described in the catastrophic APS [34]. These cases feature oligo/anuria, severe hypertension, and frequently have a fatal outcome. Some cases, eventually recover leaving a variable degree of renal impairment expressing cortical ischemia. Isolated cases and series of patients with cortical renal ischemia and aPL have been published [14, 31, 35, 36]. One of the first reported cases [35] was a 27-year-old man with coronary occlusion, arterial hypertension, thrombophlebitis, atrial thrombus, and positive aPL. An abdominal computerized tomography (CT) scan revealed cortex hypodensity in both kidneys. Renal biopsy showed diffuse interstitial fibrosis, mononuclear infiltration, sclerotic and ischemic glomeruli, and negative immunofluorescence studies. These findings suggested cortical sclerosis and atrophy as sequelae from old cortical necrosis. In this patient, aside from arterial hypertension, there was no additional clinical evidence of renal damage.

Cacoub's series of five cases [14] included patients with sudden presentation of malignant hypertension. While large renal vessels were patent on angiography, renal biopsy revealed glomerular ischemia, interstitial fibrosis, tubular atrophy, and vascular sclerosis with thrombosis. There was no vasculitis and immunofluorescence studies were negative. Four of these patients did well and one died, probably as a result of a catastrophic syndrome.

Pérez et al [36] reported on a man with PAPS and multiorgan arterial and venous thrombosis, seemingly a catastrophic syndrome. This patient had a 2-cm renal cortical infarction and multiple petechiae in the renal cortex. At autopsy, an organizing interlobular vein thrombus plus microthrombi in the microvasculature of the medulla were found. This case exemplifies medium and small vessel thrombosis affecting the intra- and extrarenal vasculature.

From the above observations, it may be concluded that cortical renal ischemia (Fig. 7.6) is a well-defined clinicopathologic entity in patients with APS. The lesion may recover ad integrum or it may leave a variable impairment of renal function.

An additional presentation of renal cortical ischemia was described by Leaker et al [37]. This is an insidious, slowly progressive nephropathy that causes renal failure in the long term. Clinically, patients have arterial hypertension, mild proteinuria, and a slowly progressive renal failure.

In a recent multicenter study, Nochy et al [31] reported 16 patients with PAPS followed for at least 5 years, all of whom had renal biopsy. In all patients there were small vessel vaso-occlusive lesions and focal cortical atrophy was present in 10.

Renal Vein Thrombosis

The main renal vein as well as minor veins may thrombose in APS. Hughes and his team [38] first described the association between aPL and renal vein thrombosis in two cases of SLE with proliferative nephritis and nephrotic syndrome. An interesting study by Glueck et al [17] demonstrated renal vein thrombosis in three of 18 SLE patients with LA, compared with none in the 59 patients without. Liano et al [39] described a man with SLE, LA, and end-stage renal disease who received a renal transplant. Nineteen months after transplantation, thrombosis of the graft's renal vein occurred and autopsy showed membranous glomerulonephritis.

Isolated cases of renal vein thrombosis have been reported in patients with PAPS [40] including one case with bilateral renal vein thrombosis in the postpartum period [41].

End-stage Renal Disease (ESRD)

A poorly studied issue is the occasional presence of aPL in patients with ESRD [42]. The information at hand about this interesting finding is incomplete and little more can be said about it. Similar considerations apply to the high titers of aCL and positive LA found in patients undergoing hemodialysis, a setting in which vascular access thrombosis is very common [43]. Recently, in a study of 97 hemodialysis patients, Brunet et al [44] found a prevalence of 31 % of aPL (LA in 16.5% and aCL in 15.5%). The presence of aPL was independent of age, time on dialysis, gender, type of dialytic membrane used, drugs used, or presence of hepatitis B or C. There was a higher prevalence of aPL when the cause of the ESRD could not be determined. Analyzing the association between vascular access thrombosis and aPL, they found a striking correlation with the presence of LA (62% versus 26% $P = 0.01$) but not with aCL.

Renal Transplantation

Very few studies have addressed the impact of aPL on renal transplantation. Reports of aPL-related morbidity among SLE transplant patients are limited by the relatively small number of subjects available for study at any given center. In the UCSF study, 15.4% of allograft failures were attributed to aPL-associated events [45].

Radhakrishnan et al [46] in a retrospective study of SLE, compared eight patients with aCL to five patients without, transplanted during the same period. Thrombotic episodes occurred in three patients in the aCL-positive group but none in the a CL-negative group. Neither of the two groups differed in the number of rejection episodes, rate of graft loss or renal function at follow-up. The authors concluded that patients with SLE and aCL can be succesfully transplanted.

Findings have been quite different in PAPS. Mondragón-Ramírez et al [47], reported two cases of PAPS with renal thrombotic microangiopathy who underwent renal transplantation and in whom despite intensive anticoagulant therapy the disease relapsed in the graft. Massive thrombosis in the graft in one case (Figs 7.7 and 7.8) and thrombotic microangiopathy in the other suggested recurrence of the disease. We postulated that the surgical procedure plus endothelial damage, a common feature of allograft rejection, may act synergistically in amplifying the hypercoagulable state. Both patients also had thrombosis in the vascular access used for hemodialysis as has been reported by others [43, 44].

In an interesting report by Knight et al [48], a woman with aCL lost a renal allo-graft in the immediate postoperative period due to renal artery thrombosis. Six months later she underwent successful retransplantation under full anticoagulation despite the presence of postoperative bleeding.

Recently, Vaidya et al [49] confirmed that patients with APS are at high risk for post-transplant renal thrombosis. Within a group of 78 patients who received renal transplant, six had APS. Each of these six patients thrombosed their renal allografts within a week of the transplant. In contrast, the remaining 72 patients were all

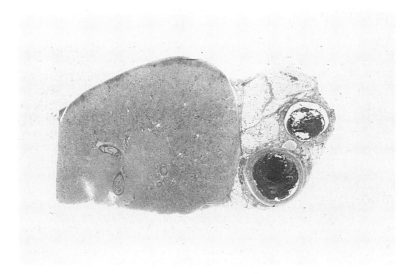

Figure 7.7. Fragment of the transplanted kidney in a female patient with PAPS. The whole vascular tree (from the intraparenchymatous vessels to the main intrarenal artery and vein) shows recent thrombotic occlusion (hematoxylin/eosin).

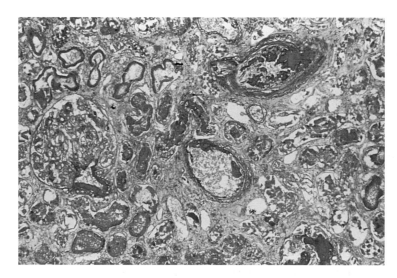

Figure 7.8. This micrograph belongs to the same kidney showed in Fig. 7.7. There is generalized thrombosis of the microvasculature including glomerular capillaries, afferent arterioles, and interlobular arteries. Generalized necrosis without inflammatory cell infiltration is also observed (Masson).

doing well 1 year post-transplant. With these data one should question whether patients with APS should be transplanted at all, and if so, which therapeutic intervention(s) could be used to avoid a catastrophic outcome.

Closing Comments

In agreement with Nochy et al [31] we believe thrombotic microangiopathy to be the characteristic nephropathy of PAPS. The lesion may have an abrupt or an insidious onset and may vary in severity and exent. All vascular structures of the kidney may be affected including glomeruli, arterioles, and parenchymatous arteries. Acute lesions as they heal give way to reparative fibrosis and focal atrophy. They are worsened by recurrent acute damage. In other cases, the lesion is insidious and slowly progressive, causing however, similar focal reparative fibrosis and tissue atrophy, arterial hypertension, and in some instances ESRD.

References

1. Piette JC, Cacoub P, Wechsler B. Renal manifestations of the antiphospholipid syndrome. Semin Arth Rheum 1994;23:357–366.
2. Harris EN, Gharavi AE, Boey C et al. Anticardiolipin antibodies: detection by radioimmunoassay and association with thrombosis in systemic lupus erythematosus. Lancet 1983;2:1211–1214.
3. Alarcón-Segovia D, Cardiel MH, Reyes E.Antiphospholipid arterial vasculopathy. J Rheumatol 1989;16:762–767.
4. Ostuni PA, Lazzarin P, Pengo V, Ruffarti A, Schiavon F, Gambari P. Renal artey thrombosis and hypertension in a 13 year-old girl with antiphospholipid syndrome. Ann Rheum Dis 1990;49:184–187.

5. Hernández D, Domínguez ML, Díaz F, Fernández ML, Lorenzo V, Rodríguez A et al. Renal infarction in a severely hypertensive patient with lupus erythematosus and antiphospholipid antibodies. Nephron 1996;72:298–301.
6. Asherson RA, Noble GE, Hughes GRV. Hypertension, renal artery stenosis and "primary "antiphospholipid syndrome. J Rheumatol 1991;18:1413–1415.
7. Ames PRJ, Cianciaruso B, Vellizzi V, Balletta M, Lubrano E, Scarpa R, Brancaccio V. Bilateral renal artery occlusion in a patient with primary antiphospholipid antibody syndrome: thrombosis, vasculitis or both? J Rheumatol 1992;19:1802–1806.
8. Rossi E, Sani C, Zini M, Casoli MC, Restori G. Anticardiolipin antibodies and renovascular hypertension. Ann Rheum Dis 1992;51:1180–1181.
9. Mandreoli M, Zuccala A, Zucchelli P. Fibromuscular dysplasia of the renal arteries associated with antiphospholipid auotantibodies: two case reports. Am J Kidney Dis 1992;20:500–503.
10. Mandreoli M, Zucchelli P. Renal vascular disease in patients with primary antiphospholipid antibodies. Nephrol Dial Transplant 1993;8:1277–1280.
11. Poux JM, Boudet R, Lacroix P, Jauberteau MO, Plouin PF, Aldigier JC et al. Renal infarction and thrombosis of the infrarenal aorta in a 35 year-old man with primary antiphospholipid syndrome. Am J Kidney Dis 1996;27:721–725.
12. Sonpal GM, Sharma A, Miller A. Primary antiphospholipid antibody syndrome, renal infarction and hypertension. J Rheumatol 1993;20:1221–1223.
13. Peribasekar S, Chawla K, Rosner F, Depestre M. Complete recovery from renal infarcts in a patient with mixed connective tissue disease. Am J Kidney Dis 1995;26:649–653.
14. Cacoub P, Wechsler B, Piette JC et al. Malignant hypertension in antiphospholipid syndrome without overt lupus nephritis. Clin Exper Rheumatol 1993;11:479–485.
15. Hughes GRV, Harris EN, Gharavi AE. The anticardiolipin syndrome. J Rheumatol 1987;13:486–489.
16. Kant KS, PollaK VE, Weiss MA, Glueck HI, Miller MA, Hess EV. Glomerular thrombosis in systemic lupus erythematosus: Prevalence and significance. Medicine 1981;60:71–86.
17. Glueck HI, Kant KS, Weiss MA, Pollak VE, Miller MA, Coots M. Thrombosis in systemic lupus erythematosus. Relation to the presence of circulating anticoagulants. Arch Intern Med 1985;145:1389–1395.
18. Leaker B, Cairley KF, Dowling J, Kincaid-Smith P. Lupus nephritis: clinical and pathological correlation. Quart J Med 1987;238:163–179.
19. Cervera, R, Khamashta MA, Font J et al. Systemic lupus erythematosus: clinical and immunologic patterns of disease expression in a cohort of 1000 patients. Medicine 1993;72:113–124.
20. Miranda JM, García-Torres R, Jara LJ, Medina F, Cervera H, Fraga A. Renal biopsy in systemic lupus erythematosus: significance of glomerular thrombosis. Analysis of 108 cases. Lupus 1994;3:25–29.
21. Bhathena DB, Sobel BJ, Migdal SD. Non-inflammatory renal microangiopathy of systemic lupus erythematosus ("lupus vaculitis"). Am J Nephrol 1981;1:144–159 .
22. Baldwin DS, Gluck MC, Lowenstein J, Gallo GR. Lupus nephritis: clinical course as related to morphological forms and their transitions. Am J Med 1977;62:12–30.
23. Kleinknecht D, Bobrie G, Meyer O, Noel LH, Callard P, Ramdane M. Recurrent thrombosis and renal vascular disease in patients with a lupus anticoagulant. Nephrol Dial Transplant 1989;4:854–858.
24. Kincaid-Smith P, Fairley KF, Kloss M. Lupus anticoagulant associated with renal thrombotic microangiopathy and pregnancy-related renal failure. Quart J Med 1988;69:795–815.
25. Becquemont L, Thervet E, Rondeau E, Lacave R, Mougenot B, Sraer JD. Systemic and renal fibrinolytic activity in a patient with anticardiolipin syndrome and renal thrombotic microangiopathy. Am J Nephrol 1990;10:254–258.
26. D'Agati V, Kunis C, Williams G, Appel GB. Anti-cardiolipin antibody and renal disease: a report of three cases. J Am Soc Nephrol 1990;1:777–784.
27. Amigo MC, García-Torres R, Robles M, Bochiccio T, Reyes PA. Renal involvement in Primary Antiphospholipid Syndrome. J Rheumatol 1992;19:1181.
28. Hughson MD, Nadasdy T, McCarty GA, Sholer C, Min K-W, Silva F. Renal thrombotic microangiopathy in patients with systemic lupus erythematosus and the antiphospholipid syndrome. Am J Kidney Dis 1992;20:150–158.
29. Lacueva J, Enríquez R, Cabezuelo JB, Arenas MD,Teruel A, González C. Acute renal failure as first clinical manifestation of the primary antiphospholipid syndrome. Nephron 1993;64:479–480.
30. Domrongkitchaiporn S, Cameron EC, Jetha N, Kassen BO, Sutton RAL. Renal microangiopathy in the primary antiphospholipid syndrome: a case report with literature review. Nephron 1994;68:128–132.
31. Nochy D, Daugas E, Droz D et al. The intrarenal vascular lesions associated with primary antiphospholipid syndrome. J Am Soc Nephrol 1999;10: 507–518.
32. Wilkowski M, Arroyo R, McCabe K. Glomerulonephritis in a patient with anticardiolipin antibody. Am J Kidney Dis 1990;15:184–186.

33. Almeshari K, Alfurayh O, Akhtar M. Primary antiphospholipid syndrome and self-limited renal vasculitis during pregnancy: case report and review of the literature. Am J Kidney Dis 1994;24:505–508.
34. Asherson RA. The catastrophic antiphospholipid syndrome. J Rheumatol 1992;19:508–512.
35. Ramdane M, Gryman R, Bacques P, Callard P, Kleinknecht D. Ischémie rénale corticale, thrombose auriculaire droite et occlusion coronaire au cours d'un syndrome des anticorps antiphospholipides. Néphrologie 1989;10:189–193.
36. Pérez RE, McClendon JR, Lie JT. Primary antiphospholipid syndrome with multiorgan arterial and venous thromboses. J Rheumatol 1992;19:1289–1292.
37. Leaker B, Mc Gregor AO, Griffiths M, Snaiyh A, Neild GH, Isenberg D. Insidious loss of renal function in patients with anticardiolipin antibodies and absence of overt nephritis. Br J Haematol 1991;30:422–425.
38. Asherson RA, Lanham JG, Hull RG, Boey ML, Gharavi AE, Hughes GR. Renal vein thrombosis in systemic lupus associated with the lupus anticoagulant. Clin Exp Rheumatol 1984;2:47–51.
39. Liano F, Mampaso F, García Martín F. Allograft membranous glomerulonephritis and renal vein thrombosis in a patient with a lupus anticoagulant factor. Nephrol Dial Transplant 1988;3:684–689.
40. Morgan RJ, Feneley CL. Renal vein thrombosis caused by primary antiphospholipid syndrome. Br J Urol 1994;74:807–808.
41. Asherson RA, Buchanan N, Baguley E, Hughes GRV. Postpartum bilateral renal vein thrombosis in the primary antiphospholipid syndrome. J Rheumatol 1993;20:874–876.
42. García-Martín F, De Arriba G, Carrascosa T et al. Anticardiolipin antibodies and lupus anticoagulant in end stage renal disease. Nephrol Dial Transplant 1991;6:543–547.
43. Nied Prieto L, Suki NW. Frequent hemodyalisis graft thrombosis: association with antiphospholipid antibodies. Am J Kidney Dis 1994;23:587–590.
44. Brunet P, Aillaud MF, SanMarco M et al. Antiphospholipids in hemodialysis patients: relationship between lupus anticoagulant and thrombosis. Kidney Int 1995;48:794–800.
45. Stone J, Amend W, Criswell L. Outcome of renal transplantation in SLE: 97 cyclosporine-era patients and matched controls. Arthritis Rheum 1997;27:17–26.
46. Radhakrishnan J, Williams GS, Appel GB, Cohen DJ. Renal transplantation in anticardiolipin antibody-positive lupus erythematosus patients. Am J Kidney Dis 1994;23:286–289.
47. Mondragón-Ramírez G, Bochicchio T, García-Torres R et al. Recurrent renal thrombotic angiopathy after kidney transplantation in two patients with primary antiphospholipid syndrome (PAPS). Clin Transplant 1994;8:93–96.
48. Knight RJ, Schanzer H, Rand JH, Burrows L. Renal allograft thrombosis associated with the antiphospholipid antibody syndrome. Transplantation 1995;60:614–615.
49. Vaidya S, Wang CC, Gugliuzza C, Fish JC. Relative risk of post-transplant renal thrombosis in patients with antiphospholipid antibodies. Clin Transplant 1998;12:439–444.

8 The Ear and Antiphospholipid Syndrome

E. Toubi, A. Kessel, J. Ben-David and T. D. Golan

Introduction

Evidence now exists that inner-ear pathology is frequently associated with immune dysfunction, including the presence of anti-cardiolipin antibodies (aCL) in the sera of such patients.

The pathogenesis of sensorineural hearing loss (SNHL) is still considered idiopathic, in most cases. Sudden deafness ((SD), severe hearing loss of acute onset) is usually unilateral but may occur bilaterally as well. Patients with progressive SNHL, develop bilateral progressive hearing loss over a course of a few days to 1–2 months, although as many as 20% initially present a unilateral loss. Both disabilities occur in previously healthy subjects, with equal preponderance among males and females.

In addition to auditory symptoms, these patients may also present vestibular complaints, such as true vertigo, light-headedness or ataxia. Tinnitus and aural pressure are also frequent symptoms, and may happen in one-half and one-third of patients, respectively.

The potential role of autoimmunity in the pathogenesis of SNHL was first described by MaCabe in 1979 [1], who demonstrated in 25% of these patients a positive lymphocyte inhibition test to cochlear antigens. Later, additional support followed. Both cellular and humoral elements of the immune system can normally be identified in inner-ear tissue; Animal models demonstrate inner-ear damage after immunization with inner-ear tissue extracts; Such an injury is transferable with sensitized T cells; human SNHL can occur in the context of systemic immunological diseases; SNHL can be treated by immunosuppressive therapy; Patients with SNHL demonstrate enhanced immune response to inner-ear antigens [2–5]. However, the definite proof of an autoimmune etiology is still lacking, since the exact nature of the immunizing antigenic epitope(s) has not yet been identified in most studies.

The Association of SNHL with Autoimmune Diseases

During the last decade many reports described the association of SNHL with various autoimmune disorders such as: systemic lupus erythematosus, Sjögren's syndrome, chronic ulcerative colitis, rheumatoid arthritis, polyarteritis nodosa, polymyositis, Hashimoto's thyroiditis and Cogan's syndrome [6–8]. The beneficial effect of immunosuppressive therapy observed in some of these patients supports the immune-mediated etiology. It was stressed that immediate treatment with cortico-steroids or other immunosuppressive agents is essential, since delay may lead to irreversible hearing loss [9]. In a recent study, the benefits of plasmapheresis given during the active phase of disease was evaluated: improved hearing was observed in 8/16 (50%) patients and only 25% of patients required in addition immunosuppres-sive maintenance therapy [10].

Otolaryngologists treating patients with unexplained sudden, fluctuating, or rapidly progressive hearing loss often consider SLE as the primary cause. In 1986, Bowman et al [11], prospectively tested the hearing status of 30 patients hospital-ized during SLE flares and observed an 8% incidence of substantial, previously undetected hearing loss. In the same year Caldarelli et al [12] reported profound SNHL of the right ear in a 51-year-old woman, followed 3 weeks later by similar finding in her left ear. This was concomitant with symptoms of her newly diagnosed SLE. In 1992, Kobayashi et al [13], described bilateral SNHL in a 32-year-old woman that improved dramatically after plasmapheresis, 2 years before the diagnosis of SLE was established. They suggested that circulating immune complexes or antiphospholipid antibodies might play a pathological role in the hearing impair-ment in SLE patients. In 1995, Kataoka et al [14], documented another case of inter-mittent bilateral SNHL in conjunction with SLE. In the same year Andonopoulos et al [15], reported an association between SNHL and SLE, without correlation to SLE disease activity, concluding that factors other than inflammation may be involved in the pathogenesis of this disorder. In a more recent study by Sperling et al, out of 84 SLE patients, 31% were reported to suffer from aural symptoms, such as tinnitus and hearing loss, suggesting that these findings are also related to the immune complex nature of the disease [16].

In yet another study, 38% of 37 unselected systemic sclerosis (SSC) patients the symptoms of SNHL were observed, suggesting that SSC may be included among the autoimmune diseases which may cause audiovestibular disturbances [17].

The association between Behçet's disease and SNHL was also reported in one patient, who had fluctuating hearing loss, tinnitus and dizziness, proposing a causative relationship between autoimmune vasculitis and endolymphatic hydrops [18].

Animal Models for Immune-mediated SNHL

To help in the investigation of SNHL, several animal models were introduced. In 1983, Yoo et al [19] immunized rats with native bovine type II collagen, a major structural element of the inner-ear, and induced SNHL in these animals. A recent study by Ruckenstein et al [20] proposed the MRL-lpr/lpr mouse strain as a poten-tial model of autoimmune inner-ear pathology, (a strain known to develop an SLE-like disease at the age of 4–5 months), in which the authors observed cochlear pathology in 6/11 animals of this age. Based on the above, Iwai et al [21] demon-strated in severe combined immunodeficient (SCID) mice infused with MRL-lpr/lpr derived spleen cells, the induction of cochlear damage which normally would not develop in such animals. However, a similar study by Inouey et al. [22] was not supportive of this data.

Immunological Profile in Sensorineural Hearing Disorders

Laboratory studies of peripheral blood lymphocytes from patients suffering from SNHL and serological assays of antigen-specific immune responses to sonicated inner-ear antigen preparations, have provided evidence that the disease may have an autoimmune etiology: both by enzyme-linked immunoabsorbent assay (ELISA) and indirect immunofluorescence the presence of circulating autoantibodies directed against inner-ear antigens was demonstrated in sera of such patients [23, 24].

In 1993, Mayot et al [25], reported in 57 individuals with SD ($n = 17$; group 1) or progressive SNHL ($n = 40$; group 2) an abnormality of the T-cell subgroups in peripheral blood: reduced presence of CD3+ and CD4+ cells was observed in group 1, and a marked decrease of CD8+ cells in both groups. In addition, antinuclear and antithyroid antibodies were detected frequently in sera of group 2 patients (75%), whereas anticochlear and anticartilage antibodies were present in both groups in similar frequency (71%).

Harris and Sharp used two-dimensional gel electrophoresis and immunoblot analysis to define, at the molecular level, the inner-ear autoantigens recognized by autoantibodies in sera of patients suffering from inner-ear diseases [26]. They found that 19/54 sera, derived from such patients, selectively bound an antigen migrating as a single or double band at 68 kDa, whereas only 1/14 sera derived from healthy human volunteers bound this antigen.

A more recent immunoblot study by Shin et al [27] suggested that approximately 40% of patients with rapidly progressive SNHL have antibodies to 68 kDa (heat-shock protein-70; hsp-70) inner-ear antigen. Such immunoblot testing provides 58% sensitivity and 98% specificity for hsp-70 antibodies.

In a different study, sera from patients with various inner-ear diseases, especially Meniere's disease, were investigated by western blot against guinea-pig inner-ear proteins. Out of 45 patients, 24 (53%) with various inner-ear diseases had antibodies against inner-ear proteins compared with 0/10 in control subjects without inner-ear diseases. Of the 10 proteins that showed a positive reaction with patient's sera, the 28-kDa band was unique in that it appeared only in the membranous fraction of the inner-ear proteins and was highly positive (28%) in reaction with Meniere's disease patient's sera. These results suggest that the antibody to the 28-kDa protein may be a candidate for detecting autoimmune inner-ear disease [28].

In another study, 16/18 SLE patients had antibodies to guinea-pig inner-ear antigens (detected by immunoblotting), whereas none were detected in the sera of the 11 normal subjects. This suggested that the inner ear might be one of the targets involved in SLE [29].

A more recent study demonstrated immunological abnormalities in 25/50 patients with SNHL: High immunoglobulin titers were observed in 18/50. Six patients were seropositive for antinuclear antibody and rheumatoid factor, whereas 2/50 revealed high anti-DNA titers [30]. In addition, abnormal low serum complement levels were detected in six cases.

In summary, based on all of the above, sensorineural hearing loss is associated with immunological dysregulation.

Sensorineural Hearing Loss and APS

Since the internal auditory artery is an end artery, disturbed circulation of the inner ear has long been suggested as the cause of sudden SNHL. In 1944 de Kleyn postulated a central vascular lesion in many SNHL cases [31]. Later, some authors have attributed these symptoms to a deficient hemostasis, often in conjunction with additional risk factors for vascular disease, such as arteriosclerosis and high blood viscosity. Others have postulated a viral cause, having a detrimental effect on the rheologic properties of blood.

Primary APS and SNHL

Because microthrombosis associated with antiphospholipid antibodies is known to affect both dermal or retinal vasculature, a similar involvement of the cochlear vessels could be envisioned, causing sudden SNHL.

In 1996, Hisashii et al. [32], reported three female patients with sudden SNHL to have elevated levels of aCL in their sera: 1/3 had IgM aCL only; 2/3 had IgG aCL. Corticosteroid therapy was effective only in the first patient, whereas in the third case, hearing loss improved after adding to the corticosteroids prostaglandin E and ticlopidine. The authors concluded that corticosteroids as well as prostaglandin E and ticlopidine therapy might be effective in patients with SNHL with anticardiolipin antibody.

In 1997 we reported our results on the presence of aCL in sera of patients with SNHL [32]. Thirty consecutive patients fulfilling the diagnostic criteria of either SD in 11 or progressive SNHL in 19 patients were included,. None of the patients recalled a recent clinical history of systemic disease, previous thromboembolic events or viral infections. Low to moderate positive aCL to one or both IgG/IgM isotypes (range 18–35 units) were found in 8/30 (27%) patients, whereas none were detected in healthy controls ($P < 0.02$).

The eight aCL-positive patients were followed for one year: two SD patients who retained reactivity relapsed, whereas no relapse was recorded in those who turned aCL seronegative. In contrast, fluctuations were observed in the follow-up of progressive SNHL patients, regardless of aCL positivity. Since fluctuations of aCL serum titers on follow-up evaluations are frequently reported (including their disappearance), it is not surprising that in our series 6 patients turned seronegative on re-examination.

Screening for antiviral antibodies was performed in sera of aCL-positive patients, which revealed antihepatitis B antibodies to both surface and core antigens in 4/8 of these patients. The finding of antihepatitis B antibodies in our patients is consistent with their prevalence in Israel in general and thus could be independent of aCL seropositivity. However, this does not exclude the possibility that the aCL antibodies presence is secondary to infection. Although the association of SNHL with hemostatic defects was studied by others, this report was the first to show in a relatively large group of patients the association between aCL and this disorder.

Recently, another study supported the notion that primary APS is associated with the development of SNHL. In the sera of 55 patients with SD and 80 with progressive SNHL, aCL were present in 49 and in 50% of these patients, respectively [34].

Secondary APS and progressive SNHL

In the past SNHL has been reported to be one of the symptoms complicating auto-immune diseases, but only recently its association with aCL seropositive data was reported. In 1993 Hisashi et al [35], reported the occurrence of SNHL in a patient with SLE who was also seropositive for IgG aCL. In 1995, Casoli and Tumiati [36] reported, in a 55-year-old woman with Sjögren's syndrome and aCL, seropositivity of IgG and IgM isotypes, who developed a sudden SNHL in association with vertigo, suggesting the presence of atypical Cogan's syndrome.

In a different study [37], 30 women suffering from Sjögren's syndrome were evaluated for audiovestibular disorders, in comparison with 40 healthy age-matched female controls. In 14/30 patients (46%), SNHL was found, compared to only one control subject (2.5%). Nine of the above 14 patients (64%) tested seropositive for aCL compared with 3/40 controls. This study suggested that SNHL in Sjögren's syndrome is correlated with aCL presence.

Recently, Naarendrop and Spiera [38] reported six SLE patients who developed SD in association with moderate to high levels of aCL and/or a positive lupus anti-coagulant test. Many studies evaluated the association between autoimmune SNHL and various viral infections, such as parvovirus B19, measles, mumps and influenza [39, 40], suggesting that these viruses may be of possible etiology in this inner-ear disease. On the other hand, the finding of positive aCL was also related frequently to such viruses, but without clear evidence that aCL may be the cause of recurrent thrombosis. Therefore, it is important to analyze the possible relationship between SNHL, aCL and various viral infections. If such a positive association can be established, the use of anticoagulant therapy should be its logical consequence.

Concluding Remarks

The goal of the current review is to focus on the reported association between APS, SNHL and the presence of aCL. However, a well-defined cause–effect correlation is still lacking for the following reasons:

1. Most of the current available information is based on small series of patients, or on case reports, both of which are of limited statistical value.
2. The requirement for a definite positive aCL test is based on at least two consecutive seropositive aCL results. This information is often missing.
3. Not all-seropositive aCL data are based on identical laboratory procedures as required by the consensus workshops on aCL analysis, and thus could be misleading.
4. A broad-spectrum infections screening of sera to rule out a post-infectious aCL immune response is not always performed, thus allowing for the inclusion of possible false-positive aCL data.

References

1. MaCabe BF. Autoimmune sensorineural hearing loss. Ann Otol 1979:88:585–589.
2. Hughes GB, Kinney SE, Hamid MA, Barna BP, Calabrese LH. Autoimmune vestibular dysfunction. Laryngoscope 1984;95:758–766.

3. Harris JP. Experimental autoimmune sensorineural hearing loss. Laryngoscope 1987;97:63–76.
4. Kanzaki J, Ouchi T. Steroid-responsive bilateral sensorineural hearing loss and immune complexes. Arch Otorhinolaryngol 1981;230:5–9.
5. Veldman JE. The immune system in hearing disorders. Acta Otolaryngol (Suppl) (Stockh) 1988;458:67–75.
6. Kumar BN, Walsh RM, Wilson PS, Carlin WV. Sensorineural hearing loss and ulcerative colitis. J Laryngol Otol 1997:111:277–278.
7. Wolf M, Kronenberg MD, Engelberg S et al. Rapidly progressive hearing loss as a symptom of polyarteritis nodosa. Am J Otolaryngol 1987;8:105–108.
8. Haynes BF, Kaiser-Kupfer MI, Mason P et al. Cogan's syndrome: studies in thirteen patients, long-term follow-up, and a review of the literature. Medicine 1980;56:426–441.
9. Saracaydin A, Katircioglu S, Katircioglu S, Karatay MC. Azathioprine in combination with steroids in the treatment of autoimmune inner-ear disease. J Intern Med Res 1993;21:192–196.
10. Luetje CM, Berliner KI. Plasmapheresis in autoimmune ear disease: long-term follow-up. Am J Otol 1997;18:572–576.
11. Bowman CA, Linthicum FH Jr, Nelson RA, Mikami K, Quismorio F. Sensorineural hearing loss associated with systemic lupus erythematosus. Otolaryngol Head Neck Surg 1986;94:197–204.
12. Caldarelli DD, Rejowski JE, Corey JP. Sensorineural hearing loss in lupus erythematosus. Am J Otol ;7:210–213.
13. Kobayashi S, Fujishiro N, Sugiyama K. Systemic lupus erythematosus with sensorineural hearing loss and improvement after plasmapheresis using the double filtration method. Intern Med 1992;31:778–781.
14. Kataoka H, Takeda T, Nakatani H, Saito H. Sensorineural hearing loss of suspected autoimmune ethiology: a report of three cases. Auris Nasus Larynx 1995;22:53–58.
15. Andonopoulos AP, Naxakis S, Goumas P, Lygatsikas C. Sensorineural hearing disorders in systemic lupus erythematosus. A controlled study. Clin Exp Rheumatol 1995;13:137–141.
16. Sperling NM, Tehrani K, Liebling A, Ginzler E. Aural symptoms and hearing loss in patients with lupus. Otolaryngol Head Neck Surg 1998;118:762–765.
17. Berrettini S, Ferri C, Pitaro N, Bruschini P, Latorraca A, Sellari-Franceschini S et al. Audiovestibular involvement in systemic sclerosis. ORL J Otorhinolaryngol Relat Spec 1994;56:195–198.
18. Igarashi Y, Watanabe Y, Aso S. Case of Behcet's disease with otologic symptoms. ORL J Otorhinolaryngol Relat Spec 1994;56:295–298.
19. Yoo TJ, Tomoda K, Stuart JM, Cremer MA, Townes AS, Kang AH. Type II collagen-induced autoimmune SNHL and vestibular dysfunction in rats. Ann Otol Rhinol Laryngol 1983;92:267–271.
20. Rukemstein MJ, Mount RJ, Harrison RV. The MRL-*lpr/lpr* mouse: a potential model of autoimmune inner-ear disease. Acta Oto-Laryngologica 1993;113:160–165.
21. Iwai H, Tomoda K, Hosaka N et al. Induction of immune-mediated hearing loss in SCID mice by injection of MRL/lpr mouse spleen cells. Hearing Res 1998;117:173–177.
22. Inoue Y, Kanzaki J, Ogawa K, Hashiguchi K, Masuda M. Hearing in the MRL/*lpr* mouse as a possible model of immune-mediated sensorineural hearing loss. Eur Arch Otorhinolaryngol 1998;255:240–243.
23. Hughes GB, Kinney SE, Barna BP, Calabrese LH. Practical versus theoretical Management of autoimmune inner-ear disease. Laryngoscope 1984;94:758–766.
24. Harris JP, Sharp PA. Inner-ear autoantibodies in patients with rapidly progressive sensorineural hearing loss. Laryngoscope 1990;100:516–524.
25. Mayot D, Bene MC, Dron K, Perrin C, Faure GC. Immunologic alterations in patients with sensorineural hearing disorders. Clin Immunol Immunopathol 1993;68:41–45.
26. Harris PJ, Sharp PA. Inner-ear autoantibodies in patients with rapidly progressive SNHL. Laryngoscope 1990; 100:516–524.
27. Shin S, Billings P, Keithley EM, Harris PJ. Comparison of anti-heat shock protein-70 (anti hsp-70) and anti 68-kDa inner-ear protein in the sera of patients with Meniere's disease. Laryngoscope 1997; 107:222–227.
28. Suzuki M, Krug MS, Cheng KC, Yazawa Y, Bernstein J, Yoo TJ. Antibodies against inner-ear proteins in the sera of patients with inner-ear diseases. ORL J Otorhinolaryngol Relat Spec 1997;59:10–17.
29. Xiao H, Wang J. Western blot analysis of serum autoantibodies against inner-ear antigens in patients with systemic lupus erythematosus. Chung Hau Erh Pi Yen Hou Ko Chih 1995;30:236–238.
30. Takahashi M, Sakata A, Unno T, Hokunan K, Shigyo H. Immunological abnormalities in patients with etiology unknown sensorineural hearing loss. Nipon Jibiinkoka Gakkai Kaiho 1998;101:1260–1265.
31. de Kleyn A. Sudden complete or partial loss of function of the octavus-system in apparently normal persons. Acta Otolaryngol (Stockh) 1944;32:407–429.
32. Hisashi K, Komune S, Komiyama S, Nakamura K. Sudden sensorineural hearing loss associated with anticardiolipin antibody. Nippon Jibiinkoka Gakkai Kaiho 1996;99:1157–1161.

33. Toubi E, Ben-David J, Kessel A, Podoshin L, Golan TD. Autoimmune aberation in sudden sen-sorineural hearing loss: association with anti-cardiololipin antibodies. Lupus 1997;6:540–542.
34. Heller U, Becker EW, Zenner HP, Berg PA. Incidence and clinical relevance to phospholipids, sero-tonin and ganglioside in patients with sudden deafness and progressive inner-ear hearing loss. HNO 1998;46:583–586.
35. Hisashi K, Komune S, Taira T, Uemura T, Sadoshima S, Tsuda H. Anticardiolipin antibody-induced sudden profound sensorineural hearing loss. Am J Otolaryngol 1993;14:275–277.
36. Casoli P, Tumiati B. Cogan's syndrome: a new possible complication of antiphospholipid antibodies? Clin Rheumatol 1995;14:197–198.
37. Tumiata B, Casoli P, Parmeggiani A. Hearing loss in the Sjögren syndrome. Ann Intern Med 1997;15:450–453.
38. Naarendorp M, Spiera H. Sudden sensorineural hearing loss in patients with systemic lupus erythe-matosus or lupus-like syndrome and antiphospholipid antibodies. J Rheumatol 1998;25:589–592.
39. Cotter CS, Singleton GT, Corman LC. Immune-mediated inner era disease and parvovirus B19. Laryngoscope 1994:104:1235–1239.
40. Casani A, Fattori B, Berrettini S, De Ciccio M, Vannucci G, Ghilardi PL. Delayed endolymphophatic hydrops: an analysis of 12 cases. Acto Otorhinolaryngol Ital 1993:13:297–303.

9   The Eye in the Primary Antiphospholipid Syndrome (Hughes Syndrome)

C. Castañon, and P. A. Reyes

Clinical associations of antiphospholipid antibodies include venous and arterial thrombosis, recurrent fetal loss, blood cytopenias, and mostly thrombocytopenia and multi-organ compromise [1–13]. Vessel occlusion is a hallmark of this association, it may occur within the context of several diseases, mainly autoimmune disorders such as systemic lupus erythematosus, or it may be present without any recognizable disease, the so called primary antiphospholipid syndrome or Hughes syndrome [14].

The eye is frequently involved in the primary antiphospholipid syndrome and serious ocular damage may occur. This is because the eye is a good mirror for blood vessels, especially micro-vessels at arteriolar, capillary and venous level and considered an extension of the central nervous system. A systematic fundus eye examination is usually used to evaluate the vessel architecture in different diseases that involve occlusive, proliferative or destructive wall changes caused by thrombosis or emboli.

In the past there were isolated reports describing optic neuritis and ocular vaso-occlusive disease in patients with Hughes syndrome. [15–17] This association was challenged by Merry et al [18] based on the absence of antiphospholipid antibodies in a group of patients with ocular vaso-occlusive disease, however, Asherson et al [19] found that the presence of ocular vaso-occlusive disease in patients with systemic lupus erythematosus was definitely related to the presence of antiphospholipid autoantibodies and several studies agree on a high prevalence of vasculopathic eye disease in subjects with Hughes syndrome [20–25]. Maybe the different appreciation reflects both a selection bias (the presence of ocular disease was the inclusion criterion in some studies) and a low prevalence of Hughes syndrome among patients with ocular vaso-occlusive disease of miscellaneous origin.

Clinical Study

We performed and reported a cross-sectional ophthalmology study [26] on 28 consecutive patients (18 women, 10 men; median ages, 30.5 and 40 years, respectively) with Hughes syndrome; all of them were seen at the Instituto Nacional de Cardiología Ignacio Chávez, Mexico City from 1987 to 1996. Irrespective of visual symptoms, 27 patients were evaluated prospectively by the ophthalmologist. One patient had visual symptoms, and primary antiphospholipid antibody syndrome was subsequently identified. The diagnosis was based on proposed clinical criteria [5]. Systemic lupus erythematosus was ruled out clinically and serologically over a 48-month follow up. Anticardiolipin antibodies were detected by enzyme-linked immunosorbent assay according to Gharavi et al [27], with some modifications by the authors [28]. Tests for serum lipid profile, fluorescent antinuclear antibodies, rheumatoid factors, syphilis (VDRL), fluorescent treponemal absorbed antibody, and a clotting profile, were performed in every patient using standard laboratory techniques.

The eye examination included a survey of ocular symptoms; tests for visual acuity, ocular movements, and intraocular pressure; and slit-lamp biomicroscopy to evaluate the anterior segment and the fundus. Twenty-four patients agreed to a standard retinal fluorangiography [29].

All patients (Table 9.1) had high-titer (>5 standard deviations above the mean) IgG anticardiolipin antibodies in at least two determinations. No other non-organ-specific antibodies nor lipid abnormalities were detected. In 14 out of 17 patients, a prolonged phospholipid-dependent clotting assay (partial thromboplastin time; PTT) was identified. In the remaining 11 patients, the test was not performed because the patients were receiving anticoagulant drugs. A false-positive VDRL test was present in 11 patients. Nine patients had thrombocytopenia, one more case had persistent leukopenia. Four out of nine patients in whom the test was done presented a positive lupus anticoagulant test.

Table 9.1. Primary antiphospholipid syndrome: clinical and laboratory findings.

Clinical findings	No.	Laboratory findings	No.
Ocular disease	24/28	IgG anticardiolipin	28/28*
Recurrent fetal loss	8/10[†]	PTT > 10 min	14/17
Venous thrombosis	16/28	False-positive results of VDRL	11/28
Arterial occlusion[‡]	10/28	Lupus anticoagulant	4/9[†]
Migraine	11/28	Cytopenia	10/28[§]
Livedo reticularis	7/28	FANA (low titer)	3/28
Leg ulcers	3/28		
Chorea	1/28		

PTT = partial thromboplastin time; FANA = fluorescent antinuclear antibodies.
* More than 5 standard deviations above the mean value.
[§] Thrombocytopenia; 9, leukopenia; 1.
[†] Subjects at risk or those in whom the test was done.
[‡] Seven of these ten patients had brain infarction demonstrated by computed tomography.

Ocular Findings

As shown in Table 9.2; 19 (68%) patients had visual symptoms. Transient visual disturbance (transient blurred vision or amaurosis fugax) was present in 16 eyes (eight patients), decreased vision in seven (four patients), transient diplopia in eight (four patients), and transient field loss associated with headache and photopsy in eight (four patients). Visual acuity with or without correction was 20/20 to 20/40 in 46 eyes, 20/60 to 20/100 in three eyes, and 20/400 or worse in seven eyes (four patients). All patients had normal intraocular pressures (12–18 mmHg), except for a case with

Table 9.2. Ocular vaso-occlusive disease in primary antiphospholipid syndrome.

																													Case No.	
	1	2	3	4	5	6	7	8	9	10	11	12	13	14	15	16	17	18	19	20	21	22	23	24	25	26	27	28	Total No. Eyes
Ocular findings – visual symptoms (18/28)																													
Decreased vision	R/L											L	R/L											R/L					7
Transient blurring						R/L	R/L						R/L						R/L	R/L	R/L			R/L		R/L			16
Transient diplopia			R/L						R/L												R/L				R/L				8
Transient field loss											R/L						R/L			R/L	R/L						R/L		8
Photopsy																R/L	R/L											R/L	6
Ocular findings – anterior segment (9/28)																													
Conjunctival telangiectases										R/L				R/L	R/L				R/L	R/L					R/L				12
Conjunctival microaneurysms										R/L				R/L	R/L				R/L	R/L					R/L				12
Simple episcleritis				R/L																									2
Limbal keratitis																R													1
Corneal opacity									R																				1
Ocular findings – eye fundi (24/28)																													
Vitreous hemorrhage	R											L												L					3
Preretinal hemorrhage													R/L																2
Swelling optic disk	R											L	R											R					4
Venous tortuosity	R/L		R/L		R/L	R/L	R/L	R/L		R/L	R/L	R/L	R/L	R/L	R/L	R/L	R/L		R/L			R/L	R/L		R/L		R/L		38
Vascular sheathing	R/L*		R/L*					L*	L*											R/L*				L		R			10
Rarefaction and rectification																		R/L											2
Pigment abnormalities			R/L				R/L			R/L		L														R/L			9
Flame-shaped hemorrhages					R/L				L	R/L			R/L																7
Cotton-wool spots	R												R																2
Microaneurysms								L	L				L											L					4
Macular serous detachment								L																					1
IRMAs													L																1
Peripheral drusen				R/L																								R/L	4

R = right eye; L = left eye; IRMAs = intraretinal microvascular abnormalities
* Peripheral vessels.

cerebrovascular disease and 20-mmHg intraocular pressure in both eyes who had an inferior temporal quadrantanopia, due to an obstruction of a branch of retinal artery.

Anterior segment abnormalities were mild and relatively uncommon: conjunctival telangiectases or microaneurysms were present in 12 eyes (six patients), simple episcleritis in two (one patient), and limbal keratitis in one. The latter two abnormalities resolved with local corticosteroid treatment. One patient had a monocular post-traumatic superficial corneal opacity since childhood.

Posterior segment abnormalities were found in 24 patients (86%) (Table 9.2). Tortuosity of first-order venous vessels or peripheral terminals in 38 eyes (19 patients) was the most common finding. Swelling of the optic disk was found in four eyes (cases 1, 12, 13, 24). Vitreous hemorrhage occurred in three eyes (cases 1, 12, 24); vitreous bands adherent to the optic disk subsequently developed in two of these eyes (case 12, 24) after the hemorrhage. One of these cases (case 1) fully recovered under treatment. Serous detachment at the macula with preretinal hemorrhage was observed in one eye (case 13). Other patient had segmental dilatation of capillary vessels, microaneurysms, and intraretinal microvascular abnormalities in one eye (case 8). There were cotton-wool spots in two eyes (cases 1, 13), flame-shaped hemorrhages in eight eyes (cases 1, 8, 9, 12, 13, 24), microaneurysms in three eyes (cases 8, 9, 14); sheathing of first-order veins in two eyes (case 1), arterial sheathing in one additional patient (case 25). Equatorial and peripheral hypopigmentation was noted in two eyes (case 3), and reticular pigment clumps around the temporal vascular arcade of both eyes, associated with widespread areas of atrophy, were seen in case 10. Two eyes (case 26) presented grayish lines extended radially on temporal retina from the optic disk, with a hypertrophic scar in the temporal aspect of the macula in the right eye. One eye had minor irregular clumps of pigment near superior temporal vessels (case 28).

Retinal fluorescein angiography was performed in 24 patients (Table 9.3) and was abnormal in 18 eyes (12 patients, 50%). Although in general the procedure confirmed the fundoscopic findings, it showed unsuspected occlusion of the perimacular arteriole in one eye (case 9), focal late hyperfluorescence and leakage of retinal capillaries superior in one eye (case 20), pigment epithelial window defects considered to be secondary to choriocapillary vessels obstruction in two eyes (case 3). In case 10, early hyperfluorescence of atrophic areas around pigment clumps created a window effect, which was interpreted as reticular degeneration of the pigmentary epithelium. Two eyes (case 26) showed fluorescence in the arterial phase which persisted after the dye had disappeared from retinal veins; these angioid streaks did occur in the absence of systemic evidence of pseudoxanthoma elasticum. This patient also had vessel occlusion inferior to the macula and a hypertrophic scar in the right eye. Case 24 had hyperfluorescence and poor arterial filling because of retinal central artery occlusion in the right eye with vitreous hemorrhage and vaso-occlusive retinopathy in the left eye. A generalized vaso-occlusive retinopathy with fluorescein leakage and areas of hypoperfusion was noted in five eyes (cases 1, 12, 25). In another patient, a macular serous detachment was present (case 13). Of particular interest were the angiographic findings in one eye (case 8), including focal occlusion of temporal arterioles and venules near the macula, areas of capillary hypoperfusion, fluorescein leakage, and retinal neovascularization. Emergency photocoagulation treatment was used on this patient; 4 years later recurrence in these vessels required further treatment.

Table 9.3. Ocular vaso-occlusive-disease in primary antiphospholipid syndrome.*

Abnormalities	(12/24)	Case No.												
		1	3	8	9	10	12	13	20	24	25	26	28	Total No. Eyes
Vitreous	Hemorrhage	R						L		L				3
Choroidal	Blocked fluorescence					R/L			L			R	R	5
	Window defects		R/L		L	R/L						R/L		7
Vascular	Tortuosity	R/L	R/L	R/L	R/L		R/L	R/L		L	L			14
	Microaneurysms			R/L	L			R/L						5
	Capillary ectasis	R/L		L				R/L		L				6
	Leakage	R/L		L					L	L				5
	Non-capillary perfusion	R/L		L	L		L	L		R/L	L			9
	Obstruction (*)	R/L		L	L			L		R/L	L	R		9
	Neoformation			L										1
Retinal	Hemorrhages	R/L		L	L			R/L						6
	Cotton-wool spots	R						R						2
Optic disk	Leakage	R						R		R				3

R right; L left.
* Ocular findings – retinal fluorescein angiography (12/24)

Follow-up

Six patients were lost, two of them died and four left the hospital. Ophthalmologic follow up from 5 to 9 years has been completed in eight patients, 11 more were followed from 1 to 3 years, and three for less than a year. All cases were treated with long-term anticoagulants, with international normalization ratio (INR) between 2 and 3, as well as chronic low dosage of acetylsalicylic acid, except case 19, who had an associated clotting defect, von Willebrand disease, which prevented the use of anticlotting measures.

Most patients recovered and stay visually asymptomatic for long periods, up to 9 years. Some of them required photocoagulation therapy, usually once, but one of them required a second treatment. A patient (case 13) with extensive bilateral arterial and venous ocular obstruction, developed a neovascular glaucoma and right-eye ptisis bulbi in a 2-year period; the left eye conserved a corrected 20/50 vision without further problems. Another patient, (case 18), developed retinal microaneurysms and hemorrhages in both eyes, which disappeared in a year.

In summary, ocular vaso-occlusive disease is a common finding in Hughes syndrome; it is easy to identify this complication by systematic eye examination. Prompt recognition and anticlotting therapy limits organ damage and usually achieves sustained improvement.

Discussion

Our study confirms a high prevalence of ocular disease in patients with primary antiphospholipid antibody syndrome. Because thrombosis is the hallmark of this syndrome, eye involvement would be expected to occur in this condition. Retinal vasculopathy has been described in patients with systemic lupus erythematosus associated with the antiphospholipid syndrome. According to Asherson et al [19], the prevalence of ocular vaso-occlusive disease in patients with lupus without antiphospholipid antibodies is less than 2%. When these antibodies are present its prevalence increases fourfold. In the case of Hughes syndrome this situation is definitively demonstrated.

Twenty-four of our 28 patients (86%) had ocular involvement at the posterior eye segment, although only 19 of these patients were symptomatic. Anterior eye segment findings were minor. In contrast, fundoscopic abnormalities were common and included vein tortuosity, swelling of the optic disease, vitreous and preretinal hemorrhage, microaneurysms and intra-retinal vascular abnormalities. Retinal fluorangiography demonstrated retinal vascular occlusive disease in eight patients. Three of them had a worsening or recurrent disease (cases 8, 9, 13), four remain stable (cases 12, 24, 25, 26) and one more (case 1) improved. Choroidal damage probably related to obstructive vascular disease also was observed. Of particular interest was a patient with a history of vascular headaches who suddenly had bilaterally decreased vision. This patient was referred with a probable diagnosis of Eales disease. On ocular examination, retinal venous vasculopathy was observed. The patient had high-titer IgG antiphospholipid antibodies as well as extensive myocardial perfusion abnormalities. Her condition responded dramatically including recovery of vision, to anticoagulation plus antiplatelet drugs.

Interestingly, of our 28 patients with primary antiphospholipid antibody syndrome, 7 had central nervous system vascular disease. Among these seven patients, four had ocular vaso-occlusive disease. These findings support the long-held view that a relationship exists between ocular and central nervous system vascular disease.

In conclusion, a high prevalence of vasculopathic eye disease involving retinal and choroidal vessels was demonstrated in our patients with Hughes syndrome. Retinal vascular obstruction occurred in 33% of our cases; it involves both; venous and arterial vessels (Table 9.4) even in the same eye and its evolution is not predictable independently of treatment. A complete eye examination including retinal fluorescein angiography appears warranted in evaluating patients with this interesting syndrome.

Table 9.4. Retinal vascular obstruction 12/56 eyes.

Case No.	CRA	RA branch	CRV
1	–	–	R/L
8	–	–	L
9	–	L	–
12	–	–	L
13	R	–	R/L
24	R	–	L
25	–	L	–
26	–	L	–

CRA = Central retinal artery, RA branch = retinal artery branch, CRV = central retinal vein.

References

1. Shapiro SS, Thiagarajan P. Lupus anticoagulants. Progr Hemost Thromb 1982;6:263–85.
2. Harris EN, Gharavi AE, Hughes GRV. Antiphospholipid antibodies. Clin Rheum Dis 1985;11:591–609.
3. Triplett DA, Brandt JT, Musgrave KA, Orr CA. The relationship between lupus anticoagulants and antibodies to phospholipid. JAMA 1988;259:550–554.
4. Mackworth-Young CG, Loizou S, Walport MJ. Primary antiphospholipid syndrome: features of patients with raised anticardiolipin antibodies and no other disorder. Ann Rheum Dis 1989;48:362–367.
5. Alarcón-Segovia D, Sanchez-Guerrero J. Primary antiphospholipid syndrome. J Rheumatol 1989;16:482–8
6. Asherson RA, Khamashta MA, Ordi-Ros J et al. The "primary" antiphospholipid syndrome: major clinical and serological features. Medicine 1989;68:366–374.
7. Sammaritano LR, Gharavi AE, Lockshin MD. Antiphospholipid antibody syndrome: immunologic and clinical aspects. Sermin Arthritis Rheum 1990;20:81–96.
8. Khamashta MA, Cervera R, Asherson RA et al. Association of antibodies against phospholipids with heart valve disease in systemic lupus erythematosus. Lancet 1990;335:1541–1543.
9. Reyes López PA, Casanova JM, Amigo MC. The anticardiolipin syndrome – a clinical study. In: Ring J, Pryzbilla B, editors. New trends in allergy III. Berlin: Springer-Verlag, 1991;382–394.
10. Amigo M-C, Garcia-Torres R, Robles M et al. Renal involvement in primary antiphospholipid syndrome. J Rheumatol 1992;19:1181–1185.
11. Hachulla E, Leys D, Deleume JF, Pruvo JP, Devulder B. Manifestations neurologiques associees aux anticorps antiphospholipides. Ou que reste-t-il du neurolupus?. Rev Med Interne 1995;16: 121–130.
12. Badui E, Soloni S, Martinez E et al. The heart in the primary antiphospholipid syndrome. Arch Med Res 1995;26:115–120.
13. Cervera R, Asherson RA, Lie JT. Clinicopathologic correlation of the antiphospholipid syndrome. Semin Arthritis Rheum 1995;24: 262–272.
14. Hughes GRV, Harris EN, Gharavi AE. The anticardiolipin syndrome. J Rheumatol 1986;13: 486–489.
15. Levin SR, Crofts JW, Lesser GR, Floberg J, Welch KMA. Visual symptoms associated with the presence of a lupus anticoagulant. Ophthalmology 1988;95:686–692.
16. Kleiner RC, Najarian LV, Schatten S et al. Vaso-occlusive retinopathy associated with antiphospholipid antibodies (lupus anticoagulant retinopathy). Ophthalmology 1989;96:896–904.
17. Gerber SL, Cantor LB. Progressive optic atrophy and the primary antiphospholipid syndrome [letter]. Am J Ophthalmol 1990;110:443–444.
18. Merry P, Acheson JF, Asherson RA, Hughes GR. Management of retinal vein occlusion [letter]. Br Med J 1988;296:294.
19. Asherson RA, Merry P, Acheson JF et al. Antiphospholipid antibodies: a risk factor for occlusive ocular vascular disease in systemic lupus erythematosus and the "primary" antiphospholipid syndrome. Ann Rheum Dis 1989;48:358–361.
20. Dunn JP, Noorily SW, Petri M, Finkelstein D, Rosenbaum JT, Jabs DA. Antiphospholipid antibodies and retinal vascular disease. Lupus 1996;5:313–322.
21. Wiechens B, Schroder JO, Potzsch B, Rochels R. Primary antiphospholipid antibody syndrome and retinal occlusive vasculopathy. Am J Ophthalmol 1997;123:848–850.
22. Susuki A, Okamoto N, Watanabe M, Kiritoshi H, Motokura M, Fakuda M. The time course of white retinal arterioles in two cases of antiphospholipid antibody syndrome. Nippon Ganka Gakkai Zasshi 1998;102:455–461.
23. Inhara M, Tanaka H, Nishimura Y. Primary antiphospholipid syndrome with recurrent transient ischemic attacks: report of a case and its successful treatment. Intern Med 1998;37:704–707.
24. Leo-Kottler B, Klein R, Berg PA, Zrenner E. Ocular symptoms in association with antiphospholipid antibodies. Graefes Arch Clin Exp Ophthalmol 1998;236:658–668.
25. Dori D, Gelfand YA, Brenner B, Miller B. Cilioretinal artery occlusion: an ocular complication of primary antiphospholipid syndrome. Retina 1997;17:555–557.
26. Castañon C, Amigo MC, Bañales JL, Nava A, Reyes PA. Ocular vaso-occlusive disease in primary antiphospholipid syndrome. Ophthalmology 1995;102:256–262.
27. Gharavi AE, Harris EN, Asherson RA, Hughes GRV. Anticardiolipin antibodies: isotype distribution and phospholipid specificity. Ann Rheum Dis 1987;46:1–6.
28. Nava A, Bañales JL, Reyes PA. Effect of heat inactivation and sheep erythrocyte adsorption on the titer of anticardiolipin antibodies in primary antiphospholipid syndrome and healthy blood donor's sera. J Clin Lab Anal 1992;6:148–150.
29. Novotny HR, Alvis DL. A method of photographing fluorescence in circulating blood in the human retina. Circulation 1961;24:82–86.

10 Pulmonary Hypertension and Antiphospholipid Antibodies

J. -C. Piette and B. J. Hunt

Pulmonary hypertension (PH) is defined as a mean pulmonary artery pressure greater than 25 mmHg [1, 2]. After many years of debate, it is now agreed that PH can be classified according to three features: anatomical localization of vascular disorder, presence or not of any associated disease, and severity, with the magnitude of reduction of cardiac output as the best predictor survival (1, Table 10.1). The term primary pulmonary hypertension (PPH) has been used extensively in literature, leading to some confusion. PPH usually means that diverse mechanisms have been ruled out, especially chronic causes of hypoxia, left ventricular failure, and repeated pulmonary embolism, and that plexogenic arteriopathy can be found on histological lung examination. PPH is a rare but life-threatening condition, whose pathophysiology has remained mysterious for a while. Recent advances have suggested the importance of diverse factors, such as: imbalance in vasoactive agents – i.e. deficiency of nitric oxide and prostacyclin synthase versus overexpression of endothelin-1 -, vascular endothelial growth factor (VEGF) expression, K^+ channel anomalies, genetic susceptibility, and, last but not least, clonal expansion of endothelial cells in primary but not secondary PH [2–6]. Though PPH frequently remains "unexplained", several comorbid conditions have been identified as possible etiologies, with human immuno-deficiency virus (HIV) infection, prior use of anorectic agents, and connec-

Table 10.1. Classification of pulmonary hypertension.

Arterial pulmonary hypertension (changes in precapillary arteries)
  "Primary" arterial PH
  Secondary arterial PH (scleroderma, MCTD and other CTD, congenital heart disease, portal hypertension, HIV, anorectic agents, cocaine, etc.)

Postcapillary pulmonary hypertension (changes in pulmonary veins)
  Left-sided heart failure
  Rarely: pulmonary veno-occlusive disease, pulmonary hemangiomatosis, chronic sclerosing mediastinitis, congenital pulmonary vein anomaly

Proximal pulmonary artery involvement
  Mainly: chronic thromboembolic PH
  Rarely: metastatic neoplasm, parasites, miscellaneous emboli

Extrinsic vascular compression

Secondary to all chronic causes of hypoxia

tive tissue diseases (CTD) as leaders [2, 7, Table 10.1]. Whatever the "cause", severe PH may be complicated by (a) superimposed in situ thromboses affecting distal pulmonary arteries [8] and, (b) the development of plexogenic lesions, both thought to occur as a consequence of chronic endothelial injury [1, 6].

This chapter will give a brief overview of PH within the antiphospholipid syndrome (APS), question the possible role of antiphospholipid antibodies (aPL) in the pathophysiology of "unexplained" PPH, and then discuss practical aspects of the management.

Pulmonary Hypertension and APS

APS mainly occurs either in association with systemic lupus erythematosus (SLE), or as a primary disorder named primary APS [9]. Within these two subsets, the prevalence of PH has been estimated 1.8 and 3.5%, respectively, in a multicenter study [10]. In two other large studies performed on SLE patients, the prevalence of PH was 2% [11], and 5% [12]. Within APS, PH may result from various causes listed in Table 10.2 [13, 14].

Pulmonary embolism is assumed to be the leading cause of PH in APS. Due to the frequent mixing of the terms pulmonary embolism with deep venous thrombosis in articles, its frequency cannot be precisely determined, but it ranged 17–33% in three non-purely obstetrical APS series [10, 15, 16], and seemed to be similar in SLE-related and in primary-APS: 21 versus 24%, respectively [10]. Though the "catastrophic" APS is characterized by widespread microvascular involvement, eight of 50 patients had multiple pulmonary emboli in a recent series [17]. Pulmonary embolism approximately occurs in one third of APS patients with deep venous thrombosis [18]. It may originate from nearly all sites, including inferior vena cava and/or renal vein thrombosis [19], tricuspid valve vegetations [20] or right-sided intracardiac thrombosis [21, 22]. The latter site underlines the need to systematically perform an echocardiography in all patients with APS and pulmonary embolism. The presence of anticardiolipin antibodies (aCL) has been shown to be associated with the further occurrence of deep venous thrombosis/pulmonary embolism in a cohort of healthy males [23]. Among patients with a first episode of

Table 10.2. Pulmonary hypertension within APS.

APS-related
    Pulmonary embolism (acute/chronic)
    Left-sided heart failure
        Heart valve dysfunction
        Myocardial infarction
        Myocardiopathy
    "Primary" pulmonary hypertension (?)
    Miscellaneous (rare)
        Portal hypertension
        Pulmonary veno-occlusive disease

Not directly APS-related
    Chest disorder leading to chronic hypoxia
        Mainly fibrosing alveolitis
    Coincidental

"idiopathic" venous thromboembolism, the presence of aCL [24] or of a lupus anti-coagulant (LA) [25] was significantly associated with recurrences. Permanent PH may be found in patients with SLE-related or primary APS and pulmonary embolism [12, 26–28], sometimes as the presenting manifestation [29], but its occurrence has not yet been quantified by prospective studies. It is probably higher than the estimated 0.1% prevalence seen after acute pulmonary embolism in the general population [27]. Fatalities may result from embolic recurrences [16, 26, 30], and pulmonary embolism was responsible for 4% of 222 deaths in a collaborative study on SLE [31].

The diverse causes of left-sided heart failure leading to PH being discussed in another part of this book, they will be briefly summarized. Heart valve dysfunction is a frequent feature of SLE-related and primary APS [32–34]. It mainly affects the mitral, then the aortic valve, and features as valve incompetence or incompetence plus stenosis, rarely as stenosis alone. Echocardiogram usually shows diffuse valve thickening and rigidity, whereas nodular masses are less frequent. These valve lesions may lead over years to significant hemodynamic intolerance [35], and though frank improvement has been reported in some cases under steroid treatment [36], surgical replacement or repair may be necessary [35, 37]. Despite the recent finding of sub-endothelial aCL deposits [34], the pathophysiology of these valve lesions remains poorly understood. Myocardial infarction is a well-established manifestation of the APS [38], and the presence of antiphospholipid antibodies (aPL) must be looked for, especially when it occurs in patients aged less than 50 years. Diffuse myocardiopathy thought to result from distal microthromboses may occur, especially within "cata-strophic" APS [17, 39, 40]. Myocardial dysfunction may also be the consequence of systemic hypertension resulting from thrombosis affecting renal vessels.

Other mechanisms leading to PH, such as portal hypertension [41] or pulmonary veno-occlusive disease [42], are ocasionally encountered within APS.

"Primary" Pulmonary Hypertension and aPL

Data concerning the "heart of the topic" remain scarce. PH is known for years to occur in association with CTD, mainly mixed connective tissue disease (MCTD) and scleroderma, especially in the Calcinosis, Raynaud's, esophageal dysmotility, sclero-dactyly, telangiectasia (CREST) variety [2]. Within this setting, PH may complicate the course of chronic interstitial lung disease leading to pulmonary fibrosis or occur in its absence, then featuring as "primary" PH. aCL are frequently found in these diverse CTD [43], but interestingly it has been recently shown that the only auto-antibodies that were specifically associated with PH-related deaths in a long-term study of patients with MCTD were IgG aCL [44]. None of these aCL-positive patients had thromboembolic manifestations. However, in this study, pulmonary involvement was statistically associated with PH, though the four autopsied patients had little or no interstitial fibrosis [44].

Concerning SLE, the relationship between PH and aPL was first suspected as early as 1983 [45]. The same group reported in 1990 an extended study on 24 patients with PH, of whom 22 had SLE [12]. Two had thromboembolic PH, and one with SLE–scleroderma overlap had pulmonary fibrosis. In the others, PH was said to resemble PPH, i.e., "with clear lung fields and no overt clinical evidence of pul-monary thromboembolism," and it was prudently suggested that the higher than expected prevalence of aPL (68%) observed in the whole group might be relevant to the pathogenesis of SLE-related PH [12]. Raynaud's phenomenon was also highly prevalent among these 24 patients. However, due to the absence of systematically performed pulmonary angiograms/nuclear perfusion scans, this study carries several limitations concerning the classification of PH as "primary" in most of patients. Subsequent data came from the Mexican group directed by Alarcon-Segovia. In a prospective analysis of 500 consecutive patients with SLE, these authors reported that PH was statistically associated with the presence of IgA aCL above 2 SD, whereas results were neither significant for higher IgA titers nor for IgG, IgM, or any aCL isotype [46]. An extended study performed on 667 SLE patients confirmed the association of PH with aPL, but the criteria used were not precisely defined [11]. Subsequently, Alarcon-Segovia proposed to delete PH and transverse myelitis from criteria for "definite" APS, due to their rare occurrence [47]. Sturfelt et al also found an increased frequency of aCL in SLE patients with mild HT [48]. On the other hand, Petri et al found no association between aPL and PH in a short series of 60 patients with SLE [49], and Miyata et al were unable to correlate aCL titer and the mean pulmonary artery pressure in 10 SLE patients whereas a significant correlation was present in 12 patients with MCTD [50]. PH has also been reported in patients with aPL and either Sjögren' syndrome [51] or anticentromere antibodies [52], but in both cases, it was probably due to thromboembolism.

Several cases of PPH complicating primary APS have been described or mentioned [15, 53–55]. Despite the anatomical demonstration of plexogenic lesions [53], the diagnosis of PPH has been debated in the patient reported by Luchi et al, due to the coexistence of a large thrombus in the right main pulmonary artery [27]. In a multicenter study of 70 patients with primary APS, PH was present in two, thromboembolic in one and suggestive of PPH in the other, to compare with 18 patients in the series who had pulmonary embolism [15].

The alternative way to investigate the potential role of aPL in PPH is to study aPL prevalence in large series of consecutive patients with "unexplained" PPH. Similar studies have shown that diverse autoantibodies, namely antinuclear [56] and anti-Ku antibodies [57] are frequently found in this setting. In the group of 30 patients with idiopathic (without SLE) PPH studied by Asherson et al, four had aPL, i.e., LA in two and low IgG aCL in three [12]. None of the 31 patients with PPH reported by Isern et al had aCL above mean + 5 SD [57]. Martinuzzo et al recently studied 54 consecutive patients with PH: 23 with primary PH, 20 with secondary PH (mainly congenital heart diseases, CTD or pulmonary disorders), and 11 with chronic thromboembolic PH [58]. The latter group was characterized by a strikingly higher prevalence of LA and IgG antibodies directed to cardiolipin, β_2-glycoprotein I and prothrombin, whereas both primary and secondary PH patients usually had negative or low-positive tests. Similarly, in a recent study, high aPL were much more prevalent in thromboembolic PH compared to PPH [59]. Among 216 patients referred for a possible surgical treatment of chronic thromboembolic PH, Auger et al found positive LA in 10.6%, of whom none had SLE, but aCL were not determined [60]. Conversely, Karmochkine et al reported the presence of aPL in four of nine patients with "unexplained" PPH, but also in seven of 29 patients with precapillary PH secondary to diverse causes, whereas the eight patients with postcapillary PH were all aPL-negative [61]. This raises the central question of the true nature of aPL, i.e., cause or consequence? Keeping in mind that all forms of severe PH may be complicated by superimposed in situ thromboses [8], a risk exists to categorize as

Definite APS [62] some patients with PH due to other causes. This theoretical risk is illustrated by the example of PH associated with HIV infection, given that aCL of questionable pathogenic significance are frequently present in this condition [63].

Finally, the possible role of aPL in the pathophysiology of "unexplained" PPH remains unclear to date. Consideration of the mechanisms potentially involved are therefore highly speculative. It seems unlikely that the "classical" thrombogenic properties of aPL are initially involved in the diffuse process leading to PPH. Other explanations could imply a role for activated platelets or for an interaction between aPL and endothelial cells of pulmonary arteries, leading to vascular remodeling. Similar mechanisms may also be proposed to explain the development of aPL-associated heart valve thickening. The occurrence of these peculiar lesions in some but not all patients might result from a double heterogeneity, i.e., that of aPL and of endothelial cells. In vitro studies using aPL from patients with distinct vascular manifestations and focusing on the interaction of aPL with endothelial cells orig-inated from various sites might help to solve this question. Another point that deserves comment is the possible implication of endothelin-1, a peptide known to induce a strong vasoconstriction and to stimulate the proliferation of vascular muscle cells. High levels of endothelin-1 have been found on the one hand in both plasma and lung tissue of patients with PPH [64], and on the other hand, in plasma of APS patients with systemic arterial thrombosis [65]. It would then be interesting to study plasma endothelin-1 levels of patients with "unexplained" PPH, according to the presence, or not, of aPL. Beside aPL but in keeping with endothelin-1, antiendothelial cell antibodies might also be involved in the pathogenesis of SLE-associated non-thromboembolic PH [66, 67].

Practical Management

Evaluation includes careful personal and familial history, complete physical exam-ination, electrocardiogram, chest-X ray, transesophageal echocardiogram, pul-monary function tests with arterial blood gas tension and additional sleep studies when sleep apnea may be suspected, routine blood tests, liver function tests, com-plete autoantibody screening including aPL determination, HIV serology, and either pulmonary angiogram or helicoidal chest computerized tomography scan that should be prefered to ventilation–perfusion isotopic scan. It should be emphasized that chronic thromboembolic PH may masquerade as PPH until appropriate imaging studies, as attested by our experience of several patients referred for severe PPH and possible heart–lung transplantation, who in fact had thromboembolic PH. Within the peculiar setting of aPL-related manifestations, the need to look for malig-nancies needs to be underlined. Indeed, cancer may present not only as recurrent venous thromboembolic events [68] sometimes associated with aPL [69–71], but can also masquerade as PPH, the correct diagnosis of pulmonary tumour micro-embolism being only made at necropsy [72]. In this respect, de novo occurrence of aPL-related events should be regarded cautiously in patients aged 60 or more [73].

Treatment options are conditioned by the mechanism and cause of PH. However, chronic anticoagulation is needed in all cases, at least to prevent the development of superimposed thrombosis [3], and this seems especially true for patients with aPL.

When PH results from chronic thromboembolism, inferior vena cava filter may be recommended [60], and successful thromboendarterectomy has been performed in some patients with very severe disease [27, 28, 60]. Within this setting, Auger et al have reported a high incidence of thrombocytopenia induced by unfractionated heparin in LA-positive patients [60].

Concerning aPL-related PPH, given the absence of definite management guidelines, the following regimens are those used in "unexplained" or CTD-associated PPH. Beside chronic anticoagulation and oxygen administration, patients are given vasodilators according to the results of acute drug testing. Calcium channel blockers may be sufficient in moderate forms, whereas continuous intravenous prostacyclin infusion using a pump is needed in severe cases, where it frequently provides a substantial benefit but may require sustained upward dosage adjustement [3, 54, 74]. The initiation of this complex and costly procedure is restricted to experienced centers. Monthly cyclophosphamide infusions have been claimed to be beneficial in a few reports of CTD-associated PPH [75, 76]. Diverse surgical procedures are discussed in advanced forms refractory to medical regimens. Atrial septectomy is used by several teams [3]. Transplantation, either double-lung, single lung or heart–lung, may cure the disease [3, 12], but mortality remains high and donors scarce.

A better understanding of PPH pathophysiology and the development of new drugs are both needed to improve the prognosis of this rare disorder.

References

1. Gosney JR. Pulmonary hypertension. In: An introduction to vascular biology. Halliday, Hunt, Poston, Schachter Eds. Cambridge: Cambridge University Press, 1998;p100–111.
2. Galie N, Manes A, Uguccioni L, Serafini F, De Rosa M, Branzi A et al. Primary pulmonary hypertension: insights into pathogenesis from epidemiology. Chest 1998;114(3 Suppl):184S–194S.
3. Haworth SG. Primary pulmonary hypertension. J R Coll Physicians Lond 1998;32:187–190.
4. Lee SD, Shroyer KR, Markham NE, Cool CD, Voelkel NF, Tuder RM. Monoclonal endothelial cell proliferation is present in primary but not secondary pulmonary hypertension. J Clin Invest 1998;101:927–34.
5. Mecham RP. Conference summary: biology and pathobiology of the lung circulation. Chest 1998;114(3 Suppl):106S–111S.
6. Voelkel NF, Cool C, Lee SD, Wright L, Geraci MW, Tuder RM. Primary pulmonary hypertension between inflammation and cancer. Chest 1998;114(3 Suppl):225S–230S.
7. Fishman AP. Etiology and pathogenesis of primary pulmonary hypertension: a perspective. Chest 1998;114(3 Suppl):242S–247S.
8. Chaouat A, Weitzenblum E, Higenbottam T. The role of thrombosis in severe pulmonary hypertension. Eur Respir J 1996;9:356–63.
9. Piette JC. 1996 diagnostic and classification criteria for the antiphospholipid/cofactors syndrome: a "mission impossible"? Lupus 1996;5:354–363.
10. Vianna JL, Khamashta MA, Ordi-Ros J, Font J, Cervera R, Lopez-Soto A et al. Comparison of the primary and secondary antiphospholipid syndrome: a european multicenter study of 114 patients. Am J Med 1994;96:3–9.
11. Alarcon-Segovia D, Perez-Vazquez ME, Villa AR, Drenkard C, Cabiedes J. Preliminary classification criteria for the antiphospholipid syndrome within systemic lupus erythematosus. Semin Arthritis Rheum 1992;21:275–286.
12. Asherson RA, Higenbottam TW, Dinh Xuan AT, Khamashta MA, Hughes GRV. Pulmonary hypertension in a lupus clinic: experience with twenty-four patients. J Rheumatol 1990;17:1292–1298.
13. Koike T, Tsutsumi A. Pulmonary hypertension and the antiphospholipid syndrome. Intern Med 1995;34:938.
14. Kunieda T. Antiphospholipid syndrome and pulmonary hypertension. Intern Med 1996;35:842–843.
15. Asherson RA, Khamashta MA, Ordi-Ros J , Derksen RHW, Machin SJ, Barquinero J et al. The "primary" antiphospholipid syndrome: major clinical and serological features. Medicine (Baltimore) 1989;68:366–374.

16. Font J, Lopez-Soto A, Cervera R, Balasch J, Pallares L, Navarro M et al. The "primary" antiphospho-
    lipid syndrome: antiphospholipid antibody pattern and clinical features of a series of 23 patients.
    Autoimmunity 1991;9:69–75.
17. Asherson RA, Cervera R, Piette JC, Font J, Lie JT, Burcoglu A et al. "Catastrophic" antiphospholipid
    syndrome: clinical and laboratory features of 50 patients. Medicine (Baltimore) 1998;77:195–207.
18. Cervera R, Garcia-Carrasco M, Asherson RA. Pulmonary manifestations in the antiphospholipid
    syndrome. In: The antiphospholipid syndrome, Asherson RA, Cervera R, Piette JC, Shoenfeld Y,
    editors. Boca Raton: CRC Press, 1996;161–167.
19. Mintz G, Acevedo-Vazquez E, Guttierrez-Espinosa G, Avelar-Garnica F. Renal vein thrombosis and
    inferior vena cava thrombosis in systemic lupus erythematosus. Arthritis Rheum 1984;27:539–544.
20. Brucato A, Baudo F, Barberis M, Redaelli R, Casadei G, Allegri F et al. Pulmonary hypertension sec-
    ondary to thrombosis of the pulmonary vessels in a patient with the primary antiphospholipid syn-
    drome. J Rheumatol 1994;21:942–944.
21. Day SM, Rosenzweig BP, Kronzon I. Transesophageal echocardiographic diagnosis of right atrial
    thrombi associated with the antiphospholipid syndrome. J Am Soc Echocardiogr 1995;8:937–940.
22. O'Hickey S, Skinner C, Beattie J. Life-threatening right ventricular thrombosis in association with
    phospholipid antibodies. Br Heart J 1993;70:279–281.
23. Ginsburg KS, Liang MH, Newcomer L, Goldhaber SZ, Schur PH, Hennekens CH et al. Anticardiolipin
    antibodies and the risk for ischemic stroke and venous thrombosis. Ann Intern Med 1992;117:997–1002.
24. Schulman S, Svenungsson E, Granqvist S and the Duration of Anticoagulation Study Group.
    Anticardiolipin antibodies predict early recurrence of thromboembolism and death among patients
    with venous thromboembolism following anticoagulant therapy. Am J Med 1998;104:332–338.
25. Kearon C, Gent M, Hirsh J, Weitz J, Kovacs Mj, Anderson Dr et al. A Comparison of three months of
    anticoagulation with extended anticoagulation for a first episode of idiopathic venous thromboem-
    bolism. N Engl J Med 1999;340:901–7
26. Anderson NE, Ali MR. The lupus anticoagulant, pulmonary thromboembolism, and fatal pulmonary
    hypertension. Ann Rheum Dis 1984;43:760–763.
27. Sandoval J, Amigo MC, Barragan R, Izaguirre R, Reyes PA, Martinez-Guerra ML et al. Primary
    antiphospholipid syndrome presenting as chronic thromboembolic pulmonary hypertension.
    Treatment with thromboendarterectomy. J Rheumatol 1996;23:772–775.
28. Ando M, Takamoto S, Okita Y, Matsukawa R, Nakanishi N, Kyotani S, Satoh T. Operation for
    chronic pulmonary thromboembolism accompanied by thrombophilia in 8 patients. Ann Thorac
    Surg 1998;66:1919–1924.
29. Miyashita Y, Koike H, Misawa A, Shimizu H, Yoshida K, Yasutomi T. Asymptomatic pulmonary
    hypertension complicated with antiphospholipid syndrome case. Intern Med 1996;35:912–915.
30. Jeffrey PJ, Asherson RA, Rees PJ. Recurrent deep vein thrombosis, thromboembolic pulmonary
    hypertension and the "primary" antiphospholipid syndrome. Clin Exp Rheumatol 1989;7:567–569.
31. Rosner S, Ginzler EM, Diamond HS, Weiner M, Schlesinger M, Fries JF, et al. A multicenter study of
    outcome in systemic lupus erythematosus. II. Causes of death. Arthritis Rheum 1982;25:612–617.
32. Khamashta MA, Cervera R, Asherson RA, Font J, Gil A, Coltart DJ et al. Association of anti-
    bodies against phospholipids with heart valve disease in systemic lupus erythematosus. Lancet
    1990;335:1541–1544.
33. Cervera R, Khamashta MA, Font J, Reyes PA, Vianna JL, Lopez-Soto A et al. High prevalence of
    significant heart valve lesions in patients with the "primary" antiphospholipid syndrome. Lupus
    1991;1:43–47.
34. Hojnik M, George J, Ziporen L, Shoenfeld Y. Heart valve involvement (Libman–Sacks endocarditis)
    in the antiphospholipid syndrome. Circulation 1996;93:1579–1587.
35. Roldan CA, Shively BK, Crawford MH. An echocardiographic study of valvular heart disease associ-
    ated with systemic lupus erythematosus. N Engl J Med 1996;335:1424–1430.
36. Nesher G, Ilany J, Rosenmann D, Abraham AS. Valvular dysfunction in antiphospholipid syndrome:
    prevalence, clinical features, and treatment. Semin Arthritis Rheum 1997;27:27–35.
37. Piette JC, Amoura Z, Papo T. Valvular heart disease and systemic lupus erythematosus (letter).
    N Engl J Med 1997;336:1324.
38. Asherson RA, Khamashta MA, Baguley E, Oakley CM, Rowell NR, Hughes GRV. Myocardial infarc-
    tion and antiphospholipid antibodies in SLE and related disorders. Q J Med 1989;73:1103–1115.
39. Kattwinkel N, Villanueva AG, Labib SB et al. Myocardial infarction caused by cardiac microvasculo-
    pathy in a patient with the primary antiphospholipid syndrome. Ann Intern Med 1992;116:974–976.
40. Nihoyannopoulos P, Gomez PM, Joshi J, Loizou S, Walport MJ, Oakley CM. Cardiac abnormalities in
    systemic lupus erythematosus: association with raised anticardiolipin antibodies. Circulation
    1990;82:369–375.

41. De Clerck LS, Michielsen PP, Ramael MR, Janssens E, Van Maercke YM, Van Marck EA et al. Portal and pulmonary vessel thrombosis associated with systemic lupus erythematosus and anticardiolipin antibodies. J Rheumatol 1991;18:1919–1921.
42. Hussein A, Trowitzsch E, Brockmann M. Pulmonary veno-occlusive disease, antiphospholipid antibody and pulmonary hypertension in an adolescent. Klin Padiatr 1999;211:92–95.
43. Merkel PA, Chang YC, Pierangeli SS, Convery K, Harris EN, Polisson RP. The prevalence and clinical associations of anticardiolipin antibodies in a large inception cohort of patients with connective tissue diseases. Am J Med 1996;101:576–583.
44. Burdt MA, Hoffman RW, Deutscher SL, Wang GS, Johnson JC, Sharp GC. Long-term outcome in mixed connective tissue disease: longitudinal clinical and serologic findings. Arthritis Rheum 1999;42:899–909.
45. Asherson RA, Mackworth-Young CG, Boey ML, Hull RG, Saunders A, Gharavi AE et al. Pulmonary hypertension in systemic lupus erythematosus. Br Med J 1983;287:1024–1025.
46. Alarcon-Segovia D, Deleze M, Oria CV, Sanchez-Guerrero J, Gomez-Pacheco L, Cabiedes J et al. Antiphospholipid antibodies and the antiphospholipid syndrome in systemic lupus erythematosus. A prospective analysis of 500 consecutive patients. Medicine (Baltimore) 1989;68:353–365.
47. Alarcon-Segovia D. Clinical manifestations of the antiphospholipid syndrome. J Rheumatol 1992;19:1778–1781.
48. Sturfelt G, Eskilsson J, Nived O, Truedsson L, Valind S. Cardiovascular disease in systemic lupus erythematosus. A study of 75 patients from a defined population. Medicine (Baltimore) 1992;71:216–223.
49. Petri M, Rheinschmidt M, Whiting-O'Keefe Q, Hellmann D, Corash L. The frequency of lupus anti-coagulant in systemic lupus erythematosus. A study of sixty consecutive patients by activated partial thromboplastin time, Russell viper venom time, and anticardiolipin antibody level. Ann Intern Med 1987;106:524–531.
50. Miyata M, Suzuki K, Sakuma F, Watanabe H, Kaise S, Nishimaki T et al. Anticardiolipin antibodies are associated with pulmonary hypertension in patients with mixed connective tissue disease or systemic lupus erythematosus. Int Arch Allergy Immunol 1993;100:351–354.
51. Biyajima S, Osada T, Daidoji H, Hisaoka T, Sakakibara Y, Tajima J et al. Pulmonary hypertension and antiphospholipid antibody in a patient with Sjögren's syndrome. Intern Med 1994;33:768–772.
52. Tilley S, Newman J, Thomas A. Antiphospholipid and anticentromere antibodies occurring together in a patient with pulmonary hypertension. Tenn Med 1996;89:166–168.
53. Luchi ME, Asherson RA, Lahita RG. Primary idiopathic pulmonary hypertension complicated by pulmonary arterial thrombosis. Association with antiphospholipid antibodies. Arthritis Rheum 1992;35:700–705.
54. De la Mata J, Gomez-Sanchez MA, Aranzana M, Gomez-Reino JJ. Long-term iloprost infusion therapy for severe pulmonary hypertension in patients with connective tissue diseases. Arthritis Rheum 1994;37:1528–1533.
55. Nagai H, Yasuma K, Katsuki T, Shimakura A, Usuda K, Nakamura Y et al. Primary antiphospholipid syndrome and pulmonary hypertension with prolonged survival. A case report. Angiology 1997;48:183–187.
56. Rich S, Kieras K, Hart K, Groves BM, Stobo JD, Brundage BH. Antinuclear antibodies in primary pulmonary hypertension. J Am Coll Cardiol 1986;8:1307–1311.
57. Isern RA, Yaneva M, Weiner E, Parke A, Rothfield N, Dantzker D et al. Autoantibodies in patients with primary pulmonary hypertension: association with anti-Ku. Am J Med 1992;93:307–312.
58. Martinuzzo ME, Pombo G, Forastiero RR, Cerrato GS, Colorio CC, Carreras LO. Lupus anticoagulant, high levels of anticardiolipin, and anti-beta2-glycoprotein I antibodies are associated with chronic thromboembolic pulmonary hypertension. J Rheumatol 1998;25:1313–1319.
59. Wolf M, Boyer-Neumann C, Parent F, Eschwege V, Jaillet H, Meyer D, Simonneau G. Thrombotic risk factors in pulmonary hypertension. Eur Respir J In press.
60. Auger WR, Permpikul P, Moser KM. Lupus anticoagulant, heparin use, and thrombocytopenia in patients with chronic thromboembolic pulmonary hypertension: a preliminary report. Am J Med 1995;99:392–396.
61. Karmochkine M, Cacoub P, Dorent R, Laroche P, Nataf P, Piette JC et al. High prevalence of antiphospholipid antibodies in precapillary pulmonary hypertension. J Rheumatol 1996;23:286–290.
62. Wilson WA, Gharavi AE, Koike T, Lockshin MD, Branch DW, Piette JC et al. International consensus statement on preliminary classification criteria for definite antiphospholipid syndrome: report of an international workshop. Arthritis Rheum 1999;42:1309–1311.
63. Opravil M, Pechere M, Speich R, Joller-Jemelka HI, Jenni R, Russi EW et al. HIV-associated primary pulmonary hypertension. A case control study. Swiss HIV Cohort Study. Am J Respir Crit Care Med 1997;155:990–995.

64. Cacoub P, Dorent R, Nataf P, Carayon A, Riquet M, Noe E et al. Endothelin-1 in the lungs of patients with pulmonary hypertension. Cardiovasc Res 1997;33:196–200.
65. Atsumi T, Khamashta MA, Haworth RS, Brooks G, Amengual O, Ichikawa K et al. Arterial disease and thrombosis in the antiphospholipid syndrome: a pathogenic role for endothelin 1. Arthritis Rheum 1998;41:800–807.
66. Yoshio T, Masuyama J, Sumiya M, Minota S, Kano S. Antiendothelial cell antibodies and their relation to pulmonary hypertension in systemic lupus erythematosus. J Rheumatol 1994;21:2058–2063.
67. Yoshio T, Masuyama J, Mimori A, Takeda A, Minota S, Kano S. Endothelin-1 release from cultured endothelial cells induced by sera from patients with systemic lupus erythematosus. Ann Rheum Dis 1995;54:361–365.
68. Prandoni P, Lensing Awa, Büller HR, Cogo A, Prins MH, Cattelan AM et al. Deep-vein thrombosis and the incidence of subsequent symptomatic cancer. N Engl J Med 1992;327:1128–1133.
69. Zuckerman E, Toubi E, Golan TD, Rosenvald-Zuckerman T, Sabo E, Shmuel Z, Yeshurun D. Increased thromboembolic incidence in anti-cardiolipin-positive patients with malignancy. Br J Cancer 1995;72:447–451.
70. Ruffatti A, Aversa S, Del Ross T, Tonetto S, Fiorentino M, Todesco S. Antiphospholipid antibody syndrome associated with ovarian cancer. A new paraneoplastic syndrome? J Rheumatol 1994;21:2162–2163.
71. Papagiannis A, Cooper A, Banks J. Pulmonary embolism and lupus anticoagulant in a woman with renal cell carcinoma. J Urol 1994;152:941–942.
72. Hibbert M, Braude S. Tumour microembolism presenting as "primary pulmonary hypertension". Thorax 1997;52:1016–1017.
73. Piette JC, Cacoub P. Antiphospholipid syndrome in the elderly: caution (editorial). Circulation 1998;97:2195–2196.
74. Humbert M, Sanchez O, Fartoukh M, Jagot JL, Sitbon O, Simonneau G. Treatment of severe pulmonary hypertension secondary to connective tissue diseases with continuous IV epoprostenol (prostacyclin). Chest 1998;114:80S–82S.
75. Groen H, Bootsma H, Postma DS, Kallenberg CGM. Primary pulmonary hypertension in a patient with systemic lupus erythematosus: partial improvement with cyclophosphamide. J Rheumatol 1993;20:1055–1057.
76. Tam LS, Li EK. Successful treatment with immunosuppression, anticoagulation and vasodilator therapy of pulmonary hypertension in SLE associated with secondary antiphospholipid syndrome. Lupus 1998;7:495–497.

11　Off the Beaten Track: A Clinician's View

G. R. V. Hughes

Introduction

The original title of this chapter was to have been "other organs". I thought that this would be an ideal opportunity to track through the body, touching on selected, lesser known features of the syndrome. This approach will, I hope, allow me to focus on aspects of the syndrome which seem to me to be clinically relevant, but which, in some instances, have yet to be verified.

Dr Munther Khamashta has previously used the sobriquet "eminence-based medicine" as an antidote to "evidence-based medicine". This author is a clinician, not an eminence. I hope that some of the points discussed in this tour of the body will stimulate clinical discussion.

Brain

Memory Loss ("Alzheimer's")

Although strokes are the pre-eminent feature of the antiphospholipid syndrome (APS), for me, the more subtle (and sometimes not-so-subtle) neuropsychiatric and cognitive disorders are the most haunting aspect.

Few studies have systematically addressed the frequency and severity of memory impairment in APS. Often, the degree of impairment is only brought out after more searching history taking. The degree can vary from: "I thought it was just early old age"; to more gross examples – the woman who forgot to pick her children up from school; the patient who couldn't remember which exit to take from the traffic circle on her way home.

In clinical practice, these patients seem to have so much in common. The worst cases – patients whose diagnosis has remained elusive and whose job and normal life have long since gone – are heartbreaking. How many such patients are there in the community with this potentially preventable disorder?

Two practical questions still await answers. First, would lifelong (and possibly aggressive) anticoagulation help these patients? (My feeling is "yes".) Second, can we improve on the magnetic resonance imaging (MRI) – often normal or equivocal in such cases?

Migraine

Some years ago, we carried out a survey that did not show migraine as a major feature of APS [1]. I do not believe our study. Migraine, or even "atypical" migraine is a recurring feature in our patients. Ask the 35-year-old with APS-associated transient ischemic attacks (TIA) – did you suffer recurrent migraine as a teenager? Yes. Having asserted this association (non-evidence-based medicine), a number of clinical questions arise. Is the known association of teenage migraine with TIA and cerebrovascular disease associated in part with APS? Are there cases of the syndrome where severe recurrent migraine is worth treating with anticoagulation. In my own anecdotal experience, there have been dramatic responses to coumadin/warfarin treatment. However, this observation will undoubtedly be answered in time by appropriate studies. It will take a brave physician to argue that some migraine patients need anticoagulants.

Seizures

Our original reports in the early 1980s included seizures – as might be expected. All forms of electrical abnormalities have been seen in APS patients. As with migraine (and with chorea) there have been cases where a recurrent seizure tendency has been stopped when anticoagulation has been introduced. It is difficult to explain this observation other than as a reversal of cerebral small vessel "sludging".

Strokes

This subject will be discussed in more detail elsewhere in this volume. From the first description of the syndrome, it was clear that strokes of every type were a major complication – a feature which immediately distinguishes APS from almost all other forms of coagulopathy. Much has been made in recent times of the economic, as well as social impact of strokes on Western medicine.

In the UK alone there are over 120 000 strokes per annum [2]. Even if the most conservative estimate of 5% of strokes being associated with APS is taken, this constitutes some 6000 potentially preventable strokes per annum.

Other forms of cerebral thrombotic disease, which we and others have seen in APS, are saggital sinus thrombosis and benign intracranial hypertension.

Spinal Cord

Transverse myelopathy was described in our original publications in the early 1980s, and was the reason I became involved in studies of antiphospholipid antibodies (aPL) in 1975 [3]. In a later large lupus study, an association between aPL and transverse myelopathy was noted [4]. The association has not been confirmed by others. The topic is of immense importance. In a sick lupus patient with acute transverse myelopathy, does one add in immediate and urgent anticoagulation, or treat with pulse cyclophosphamide? Important light on the subject has been shed by Gharavi and his colleagues in their mouse model. Some APS mice develop myelopathy, the pathology of which is clearly seen to be spinal cord vessel thrombosis [5].

Eyes and Ears

Acute ischemia of the eye (often monocular) is a major feature of APS. Careful screening of fields is vital. Quadrantanopia or hemianopia in a sick lupus patient is a strong pointer to APS, and the need for anticoagulation, rather than more "conventional" CNS lupus treatment.

The ear, nose and throat surgeon will also see APS patients. *Acute vertigo* has been described [6] and has certainly been a major feature in a number of our patients. We are currently studying our APS patients more thoroughly for more subtle middle ear disease. The vascular supply of the middle ear is precarious and it is not surprising that ischemia here presents itself in APS. One recent case report described acute ischemia and swelling of the skin of the earlobes in APS ("Hughes ears") [7].

Skin

There is a comprehensive review of skin manifestations of APS in this book. Here I touch briefly on two aspects – nailfold infarcts and livedo.

Nailfold infarcts or splinter hemorrhages are prominent in a small number of APS patients [8]. We have often wondered whether they represent a subset, e.g., associated with heart-valve vegetations, but to date have not found any such association. It is notable that in some women, the nailfold splinters occur premenstrually each month.

Livedo poses one of the interesting questions concerning APS. It was a feature described in my earliest descriptions of the antiphospholipid syndrome [9]. Most studies of Sneddon's' syndrome show only a minority with aPL. The reason for the absence of these antibodies in the majority of patients still remains poorly explained, though Piette and his group in Paris have made important contributions to the clinical description of subsets of livedo types.

In terms of treatment, it was traditional practice to treat Sneddon's syndrome mainly with aspirin. Maybe this policy needs radical overhaul.

Genitalia

Impotence, not surprisingly, has been a development in a number of APS patients with peripheral vascular disease. Not yet reported in the literature, it is a feature that may be common, and one for which there is now some treatment. Infarction of the tissue of the penis, and of the skin of the scrotum have been seen. Surprisingly, perhaps, testicular and epididymal infarction appear to be a less common complication than in, say, polyarteritis.

Thymus

A number of cases of "late onset lupus" have been described in patients who have undergone thymectomy [10]. One of our patients, a woman in her 60s, developed polyarthritis, high-titer anti-DNA, high levels of IgM and IgG aPL and clinical thrombosis, 5 years following thymectomy for benign thymic tumour. This is indirect support for APS being another autoimmune disease.

Blood

The three clinical aspects I choose to discuss here are difficulties in anticoagulation, the problem of borderline platelet counts, and the management of Evans' syndrome.

A number of patients with APS prove very resistant to conventional doses of warfarin, some requiring doses well over 20 mg daily. Although this is a therapeutic problem well recognized in anticoagulation clinics, it is still uncertain whether APS present particular difficulties in this regard.

Platelet counts of 70 000–90 000 are common in APS patients. Normal clinical practice is to treat conservatively, but as yet there has been no major audit of these patients to see, for example, whether they are more at risk from severe thrombocytopenic attacks, especially during infection. The inter-relationships of aPL, other antiplatelet antibodies, antiprothrombin antibodies, and thrombocytopenia are complex, and are given detailed discussion by Galli and Barbui elsewhere in this book (Chapter 41).

It has been suggested that hemolytic anemia may be more associated with IgM aCL [11]. Certainly, autoimmune hemolytic anemia, sometimes associated with thrombocytopenia (Evans' syndrome) is a difficult therapeutic problem in some APS patients, often proving very resistant to conventional steroid treatment.

Finally, the bone marrow, as an organ, is no more immune from the thrombotic complications of APS and marrow infarction has been described [12].

Vascular Disease

In addition to the known risks of venous and arterial thrombosis, other practical therapeutic problems in some APS patients include difficulties with venous access and cannulation (thrombosis) and skin ulceration.

The tendency to accelerated arterial disease in a number of APS patients is a major clinical discovery, and is discussed elsewhere in this book. Lupus is a known risk factor for atherosclerosis. The known risks include hypercholesterolemia, inflammation, nephrotic syndrome, steroids and hypertension. APS patients with accelerated arterial disease have, in many cases, none of these risks. It seems likely that aPL are a direct risk factor for atheroma [13].

Liver

The liver is rarely involved in lupus. Abormal liver function tests (LFTs) in lupus are usually due to aspirin, azathioprine, or a second diagnosis. To the list should now be added APS. APS is a major cause of liver thrombosis including Budd–Chiari syndrome [14]. It is important for the clinician to realize that less extreme forms of hepatic thrombosis, with abnormal LFTs, are common in APS.

Heart

One of the major differences of the heart valve disease seen in APS and rheumatic fever is that atrial fibrillation is rare in APS [15]. The relationship between APS and heart valve disease is clinically complex. We have seen, for example, a valve thrombus the size of a table-tennis ball removed from a lupus patient negative at the time for aPL, who has, several years later, become aPL antibody strongly positive.

The association with coronary artery thrombosis is now well described, and discussed elsewhere in this book.

Endocrine System

Adrenal infarction is now recognized as a severe complication of APS. It is probably a significant cause of Addison's disease [16]. The importance of adrenal insufficiency in patients with the catastrophic APS has yet to be evaluated. Pituitary infarction in APS patients is, to my knowledge, not described. But I am sure that some cases of Sheehan's syndrome – pituitary infarction after pregnancy delivery – must be caused by APS.

Kidneys

The degree to which renal thrombosis plays a part in the pathology of APS is unresolved [17]. Renal biopsies from APS patients in our practice have shown a number to have considerable interstitial ischemia – this is still an area for more detailed clinical analysis.

Renal artery stenosis has been a major finding in a number of our patients, and warrants consideration in any APS patient with hypertension.

Finally, some of our primary APS patients have developed membranous nephritis (without lupus). We are not sure if there is a connection.

Joints

Our paper suggesting an association with avascular necrosis (AVN) was stimulated by a case of multiple AVN in a man with APS who had never received steroids. In a collaborative study with colleagues in Paris, we found the incidence of AVN in lupus patients with aPL to be twice that of lupus patients without – despite the same steroid background [18]. Others have not confirmed this link and the jury is still out.

Therapeutic Considerations

The presence of aPL is an important risk factor for both venous and arterial (especially strokes) thrombosis. Our own retrospective analysis over 10 years suggested that one half of asymptomatic individuals carrying aPL would go on to develop thrombosis [19]. We are therefore embarking on a national study of prophylactic antithrombotic regimes (aspirin versus low-dose warfarin/coumadin) in aPL positive individuals.

We also need further observation on the additional dangers of other prothrombotic risks in these patients. How dangerous is flying? – or climbing? – a 20-year-old aPL positive student developed saggital sinus thrombosis whilst climbing in the Andes. How dangerous is infection? – or organ transplantation? – aPL probably increases the risk of postoperative failure of renal transplantation in lupus patients. What are the future dangers for women found in pregnancy to have aPL? – possibly the largest group of individuals to be routinely screened.

These are all questions which *can* be answered by careful clinical practice.

References

1. Montalban J, Cervera R, Font J, Ordi J, Vianna J, Haga HJ et al. Lack of association between anti-cardiolipin antibodies and migraine in systemic lupus erythematosus. Neurology 1992;42:681–682.
2. Potter JF. What should we do about blood pressure and stroke? Quart J Med 1999;92:63–66.
3. Wilson WA, Hughes GRV. Aetiology of Jamaican neuropathy. Lancet 1975;i:240.
4. Alarcon-Segovia D, Deleze M, Oria CV, Sanchez-Guerrero J, Gomez-Pacheco L, Cabiedes J et al. Antiphospholipid antibodies and the antiphospholipid syndrome in systemic lupus erythematosus: a prospective study of 500 consecutive patients. Medicine (Baltimore) 1989;68:353–365.
5. Garcia CO, Kanbour-Shakir A, Tang H, Molina JF, Espinoza LR, Gharavi AE. Induction of experimental antiphospholipid antibody syndrome in PL/J mice following immunization with β_2-GPI. Am J Reprod Immunol 1997;37:118–124.
6. Toubi E, Ben-David J, Kessel A, Podoshin L, Golan TD. Autoimmune aberration in sudden sensorineural hearing loss: association with anticardiolipin antibodies. Lupus 1997;6: 540–542.
7. O'Gradaigh D, Scott DGI, Levell N. Hughes' ears: an unusual presentation of antiphospholipid syndrome. Ann Rheum Dis 1999;58:65–66
8. Mujic F, Lloyd M, Cuadrado MJ, Khamashta MA, Hughes GRV. Prevalence and clinical significance of subungual splinter haemorrhages in patients with the antiphospholipid syndrome. Clin Exp Rheumatol 1995;13:327–331.
9. Hughes GRV. Connective tissue disease and the skin: the 1983 Prosser-White Oration. Clin Exp Dermatol 1984;9:535–544.
10. Mevorach D, Perrot S, Buchanan NMM, Khamashta M, Laoussadi S, Hughes GRV et al. Appearance of systemic lupus erythematosus after thymectomy: four case reports and review of the literature. Lupus 1995;4:33–37.
11. Deleze M, Alarcon-Segovia D, Oria CV, Sanchez-Guerrero J, Fernandez-Dominguez L et al. Hemocytopenia in systemic lupus erythematosus. Relationship to antiphospholipid antibodies. J Rheumatol 1989;16:926–930.
12. Bulvik S, Aronson I, Ress S, Jacobs P. Extensive bone marrow necrosis associated with antiphospholipid antibodies. Am J Med 1995;98:572–574.
13. George J, Shoenfeld Y. The antiphospholipid (Hughes) syndrome: a crossroads of autoimmunity and atherosclerosis. Lupus 1997;6:559–560.
14. Pelletier S, Landi B, Piette JC et al. Antiphospholipid syndrome is the second cause of non-tumorous Budd–Chiari syndrome. J Hepatol 1994;21:76–80.
15. Cuadrado MJ, Fofi C, Khamashta MA, Hughes GRV. Absence of atrial fibrillation in patients with heart valve disease associated with the antiphospholipid syndrome. Q J Med 200, in press.
16. Asherson RA, Hughes GRV. Addison's disease and primary antiphospholipid syndrome. Lancet 1989;ii:874.
17. Amigo MC, Garcia-Torres R, Robles M, Bochiccio T, Reyes PA. Renal involvement in the primary antiphospholipid syndrome. J Rheumatol 1992;19:1181–1185.
18. Asherson RA, Liote F, Bernard P, Meyer O, Buchanan N, Khamashta MA et al. Avascular necrosis of bone and antiphospholipid antibodies in systemic lupus erythematosus. J Rheumatol 1993;20:284–288.
19. Shah NM, Khamashta MA, Atsumi T, Hughes GRV. Outcome of patients with anticardiolipin antibodies: a 10 year follow-up of 52 patients. Lupus 1998;7:3–6.

12 The Primary Antiphospholipid Syndrome

T. Vincent and C. Mackworth-Young

Introduction

The emergence of the antiphospholipid syndrome (APS) over the last thirty-odd years has been one of the most striking developments in clinical autoimmunity. The identification of a pure or "primary" variant of the syndrome has been central to this story, not least in enabling us to establish the place of this remarkable condition in the wide spectrum of autoimmune disease.

Circulating antiphospholipid antibodies (aPL), as detected by the false positive biological test for syphilis, have been known for more than 40 years [1], and their ability to cause prolongation of the partial thromboplastin or kaolin clotting time generated the term "lupus anticoagulant" (LA) [2]. Although the phenomenon was initially described in a systemic lupus erythematosus (SLE) patient associated with a haemorrhagic disorder, by the 1960s it was apparent that the presence of the LA was paradoxically linked to the risk of thrombosis [3]. Following this, associations with thrombocytopenia [4], and recurrent miscarriage [5–7] were established. Not all of these patients had SLE – so the term "lupus anticoagulant" was thus misleading, not only because of its procoagulant associations in vivo, but also because some patients had no evidence of lupus.

In vitro studies showed that the LA activity was mediated by antibodies [8]. The association of false positive tests for syphilis led to the suggestion that these antibodies may bind to phospholipids. This was supported by an earlier study, which demonstrated that LA activity could be partially abolished by pre-absorption of test serum with cardiolipin [9].

Direct confirmation came in 1983 with the development of a sensitive immunoassay for anticardiolipin activity in serum [10]. Antibodies detected by this method were subsequently shown to exhibit LA activity [11]. Derivatives of this assay still perform a pivotal role in the diagnosis of the antiphospholipid syndrome.

Defining the APS

The direct detection of anticardiolipin antibodies (aCL) enabled Hughes and coworkers to make the first formal description of the APS [12, 13]. They recognized a group of patients with SLE who had raised levels of these antibodies and clinical features including recurrent venous thrombosis, central nervous system disease and

Table 12.1. Clinical and serological features of the primary antiphospholipid syndrome.

	Mackworth-Young et al [75]		Asherson et al [21]		Alarcon-Segovia et al [76]	
	Number	(%)	Number	(%)	Number	(%)
No. of patients	20		70		9	
M : F ratio	NS		26 : 44		1 : 8	
Age range	17–53		21–59		16–43	
aCL IgG	14/20	(70)	60/70	(86)	8/9	(89)
aCl IgM	12/20	(60)	27/70	(39)	5/9	(56)
LA	NS		60/70	(86)	5/5	(100)
Thrombosis						
Venous	7/20	(35)	38/70	(54)	6/9	(67)
Arterial	5/20	(25)	31/70	(44)	5/9	(56)
Pregnancy loss	12/15	(80)	24/70	(34)	4/4	(100)
Thrombocytopenia	6/20	(30)	32/70	(46)	4/9	(44)
Migraine	4/20	(20)	NS		NS	
Livedo reticularis	1/20	(5)	14/70	(20)	5/9	(56)

LA, lupus anticoagulant.
NS, not specified.

recurrent miscarriage. Serologically the majority of these patients demonstrated antiphospholipid antibodies. By 1985 it had become apparent that some of such patients exhibited few or no features of underlying connective tissue disease, and the concept emerged that this syndrome could exist as a separate entity [14–16].

In 1989 three units published clinical series establishing the primary antiphospholipid syndrome (PAPS) (Table 12.1). They described a group of patients in whom recurrent thrombosis, miscarriage and thrombocytopenia were associated with aCL. Although several patients were positive for anti-nuclear antibodies, none fulfilled classification criteria for the diagnosis of SLE.

APS as a Clinical Spectrum

From these early reports four categories of APS, or Hughes syndrome, could be defined:

1. antiphospholipid syndrome associated with underlying connective tissue disease, most usually SLE;
2. patients with antiphospholipid syndrome with no underlying features of connective tissue disease, the primary antiphospholipid syndrome;
3. patients with APS and "lupus like" disease who have features of connective tissue disease but who do not fulfill classification criteria for the diagnosis of SLE;
4. APS due to other causes, such as drugs, malignancy and infection. Many of these patients exhibit increased aCL in the absence of an overt clinical syndrome. When clinical disease is apparent it is usually mild and transient.

These are a heterogeneous group of patients and as such are likely to represent a spectrum of disease rather than discrete disease entities. This is supported by documented development of overt SLE in patients with an original diagnosis of PAPS. In a 5-year follow up by Asherson et al [17], 19 patients with APS (nine with associated SLE; seven with lupus like disease; and three with PAPS) were studied. During this interval three patients with lupus like disease progressed to a diagnosis of SLE, and one patient with PAPS developed lupus like disease.

In some instances this transition may take many years. The same unit [18] performed a retrospective study of 80 patients seen over a 10-year period with PAPS. Two cases developed SLE more than 10 years following the initial presentation of PAPS and one developed lupus like disease. Andrews et al [19] described two patients with PAPS developing SLE after 8 and 10 years. These findings and similar anecdotal experience mean that clinicians should be mindful of the long transition times from PAPS to SLE-associated APS, even though the studies would suggest that this is a relatively uncommon event.

Differentiation Between SLE-associated APS and PAPS

There are both clinical and serological features that help differentiate between these groups of patients. Vianna et al [20] conducted a multicenter study of primary and secondary APS. Of 114 patients, 56 had SLE-associated APS and 58 had PAPS. They found that both groups of patients had similar clinical presentations with the exception of endocardial valve disease, which occurred in 63% of lupus patients versus 37% of patients with PAPS ($P < 0.005$). Other more predictable differences included autoimmune hemolytic anemia (21 versus 7%, $P < 0.05$), neutropenia (11 versus 0%, $P < 0.01$), antinuclear antibodies (ANA) positivity (81 versus 41%), and low C4 levels, all of which were significantly more common in patients with SLE-associated APS. No patient with PAPS had antibodies to extractable nuclear antigens or dsDNA.

The female:male ratio in this study was 7 : 1 for SLE-associated APS and 4.2:1 for PAPS. Other studies have also documented this relatively low female : male ratio in PAPS compared to SLE where it is 9:1:Asherson et al [21], 2:1; and Font et al [22], 5:1. Given that fetal loss may result in more females presenting with APS than males, these findings suggest that female sex is considerably less of a predisposing factor for APS than for SLE.

Antibody Specificity

The past few years have seen major advances in our understanding of the antibodies present in APS, in particular their ligand-binding specificities. Indeed many so called "antiphospholipid" antibodies may not directly bind phospholipid at all, but associated plasma proteins. As with other autoimmune conditions, work in this field has major implications for our understanding of the pathogenesis. It also has the potential for improving the specificity and sensitivity of laboratory assays for both diagnosis and prognosis. Studies in this area have included patients with SLE-associated APS and with PAPS. At this stage it is too early to tell if there are significant differences between these two variants of the condition. The subject of ligand binding specificity is covered in detail elsewhere. The following summarizes some of the main findings.

Antibodies to Phospholipids

As in SLE-associated APS, the serum of patients with PAPS generally contains antibodies which have specificity for anionic phospholipids (such as cardiolipin and phosphatidylserine). Some cross-reactivity is sometimes seen with neutral phospholipids (such as phosphatidylcholine), but this is much less common than in patients who have raised aPL levels in the context of infections [23].

Antibodies to β_2-glycoprotein I

Initially aCL assays were performed in the presence of serum. Removal of serum factors resulted in a drop in detection of aCL suggesting that serum proteins might be involved in the binding of the antibodies to cardiolipin. Considerable interest was generated when β_2-glycoprotein I (β_2GPI) was identified as a cofactor for the binding of aCL [24], and was shown to potentiate the anticoagulant activity of aCL [25]. β_2GPI is a 50-kDa, heavily glycosylated protein that binds negatively charged molecules such as phospholipids. It is thought to act as a natural inhibitor of thrombosis, by inhibiting the conversion of prothrombin to thrombin, the activation of the intrinsic clotting cascade, and protein C activation [26].

Different populations of aCL exist. Although some bind phospholipid in the absence of β_2GPI, if high sensitivity microtiter plates are employed most aCL can be shown to bind to β_2GPI [27–29]. In addition, those antibodies which bind to cardiolipin in the absence of serum factors can have their binding disrupted by addition of human β_2GPI, suggesting competition at this phospholipid site [30].

Antibodies to Prothrombin

Bajaj et al initially demonstrated the presence of high-affinity autoantibodies to prothrombin in two patients with LA and hypoprothrombinemia [31]. Antiprothrombin antibodies have also been found in lupus patients without hypoprothrombinemia [32, 33]. Arvieux et al showed that in 139 patients with LA, 55% had antibodies to prothrombin [34]. In his study antibodies were present in 70% of LA-positive patients with lupus or APS but only 20% of LA-positive patients with associated infection or malignancy.

Antibodies to Platelets

There have been two studies of platelet antibodies which looked exclusively at patients with PAPS. They report conflicting results as to the relationship with thrombocytopenia. Godeau et al [35] studied 25 PAPS patients of whom 15 had thrombocytopenia and 10 had normal platelet counts. They found 73% of thrombocytopenic patients had serum platelet antibodies. The most common specificity was for the surface glycoprotein GpIIbIIIa. Only 10% of non-thrombocytopenic patients were platelet antibody positive.

In a study by Panzer et al [36], 22 patients with PAPS were examined for platelet antibodies. 15/22 had raised levels for such antibodies (mainly GPIIbIIIa) but they found no correlation with the presence of thrombocytopenia, LA activity or history of thromboembolic disease.

Others

Several other ligand binding specificities have been described in APS. These include antibodies to complement factor H which has high homology to β_2GPI [37], and antibodies to clotting factors X and V, which have LA activity. Some are not detectable in standard assays used in APS and include antibodies to a number of regulatory proteins of the coagulation pathway, e.g., protein C, protein S, thrombomodulin, annexin V, CD36, and kininogens [30].

Antibody Sensitivity and Specificity in PAPS

Diagnosis

To date, solid-phase assays for aCL have provided the main laboratory test in the diagnosis of SLE-associated APS and PAPS. More recently interest has grown in assays for cofactor antibodies, the detection of which appears to improve diagnostic accuracy. Cabiedes et al [38] studied the prevalence of anti-β_2GPI antibodies in patients with SLE. Thirty-five out of 39 patients with associated APS had antibodies to β_2GPI, compared to only two out of 55 SLE patients with no evidence of APS ($P < 0.0001$). Najmey et al in 1997 [39] conducted a meta-analysis on the use of anti-β_2GPI antibodies in the diagnosis of APS. They selected studies where anti-β_2GPI antibodies had been measured and where clinical details of patients were available. Studies included patients with both SLE and PAPS. Out of a total of 90 individuals, 65 had two or more clinical manifestations of APS. Anti-β_2GPI antibodies were present in 89% of APS patients compared to 44% of those who failed to fulfill criteria for the syndrome. No significant difference was found in levels of anti-β_2GPI antibodies between PAPS and SLE-associated APS.

These observations of the diagnostic specificities of β_2GPI antibodies in the diagnosis of APS have been mirrored by two studies in PAPS. Cabral et al [40], studied 15 patients with PAPS, 13 aCL-positive syphilis controls and 76 healthy controls. They found antibodies to β_2GPI in 12 out of 15 patients with PAPS compared to none in the syphilis or healthy control groups ($P < 0.0001$). Day et al [41] studied the prevalence of these antibodies in patients with PAPS or SLE-associated APS. They demonstrated a high prevalence of IgG anti-β_2GPI antibodies in PAPS (58%) compared to SLE-associated APS (33% $P = 0.008$). They suggested that using a combination of anti-β_2GPI antibodies, aCL, and the LA test would improve diagnostic accuracy.

Clinical Disease Prediction

It has long been known that aCL titer, isotype and ligand specificity predict clinical sequelae in APS in the context of SLE. For instance, fetal loss is associated with high aCL titers [42] and the presence of IgG, but not IgM or IgA aCL, have good diagnostic accuracy in identifying a preceding history of thrombosis [43]. Viard et al [44] have demonstrated a higher level of thrombosis in those with anti-β_2GPI antibodies compared to aCL, and Lopez-Sotol et al [45] showed that IgM aCL is more often associated with hemolytic anemia at presentation, whereas raised IgG antibodies are more likely to be associated with thrombosis, thrombocytopenia and pregnancy loss.

Most clinicians in the field feel that a similar pattern of association holds true for PAPS. However there are relatively few data. Levine et al [46] showed that high aCL titers were associated with a shorter time to recurrence of cerebral ischemia compared to low titers. Prothrombin antibodies have been shown to be predictive of risk of myocardial infarct in middle-aged men without SLE [47].

Classification Criteria for PAPS

Classification criteria for APS were first suggested by Harris et al [15] in 1987. They initially included:

1. thrombosis (venous or arterial); or
2. miscarriage (at least two); and
3. LA or aCL (>20 units, IgG or IgM), identified on two occasions more than 8 weeks apart.

Following this, Alarcon-Segovia et al [48] proposed more detailed criteria which took into consideration of both the number of aCL-related manifestations and aCL titres. (Table 12.2).

These criteria do not take into account the presence of antibodies of other relevant specificities, such as β_2GPI and prothrombin antibodies. Such criteria may

Table 12.2. Preliminary classification criteria for APS in patients with SLE.

Clinical manifestations associated with aPL
    Livedo reticularis
    Thrombocytopenia
    Recurrent fetal loss
    Venous thrombosis
    Haemolytic anaemia
    Arterial occlusion
    Leg ulcer
    Pulmonary hypertension
    Transverse myelitis

Classification groups and APS categories

aCL level	Number of clinical manifestations		
	2	1	0
High (>5SD)	definite	probable	doubtful
Low (>2 <5SD)	probable	doubtful	negative
Negative (<2SD)	doubtful	negative	negative

Reproduced from Alarcon-Segovia D 1992 [48].

therefore fail to recognize small but significant groups of patients. Indeed, there are clearly documented cases in the literature of patients with the clinical features of APS who have raised levels of β_2GPI antibodies but no detectable levels of aCL by standard aPL assays [49, 50]. It is therefore likely that in the future such antibodies will be included in the classification criteria.

It is generally accepted that criteria for the diagnosis of PAPS should include:

1. fulfillment of criteria for APS; and
2. exclusion of the diagnosis of an underlying connective tissue disease, in particular SLE.

In practice this can be difficult. Several of the clinical criteria for the classification of SLE are shared by the APS. For example thrombocytopenia and pleuritic chest pain are clinical manifestations of both SLE and APS even though the underlying pathology may be different [51]. This led Piette et al [52] to propose specific exclusion criteria for primary APS (Table 12.3). The presence of any of the listed clinical features would exclude the diagnosis of PAPS. They stipulate that a follow up of longer than 5 years after the first clinical manifestation is necessary to rule out the subsequent emergence of SLE. This is of course an arbitrary period. In practice it seems sensible to make a diagnosis of PAPS in patients with appropriate criteria, while accepting that an associated connective tissue disease, such as SLE, may present in time.

Stringent adherence to these guidelines will necessarily identify a large group of patients who have neither SLE nor PAPS, and whose condition can be viewed as falling into the category of "lupus like" APS. In a proportion of such individuals – as in those with true primary APS – a definitive diagnosis of SLE may emerge at a later date.

Table 12.3. Exclusion criteria for diagnosis of PAPS.

The presence of any of these criteria excludes the diagnosis of primary antiphospholipid syndrome.

Malar rash
Discoid rash
Oral or pharyngeal ulceration, excluding nasal septum ulceration or perforation
Arthritis
Pleuritis, in the absence of pulmonary embolism or left-sided heart failure
Pericarditis, in the absence of myocardial infarction or uraemia
Persistent proteinuria greater than 0.5 g per day, due to biopsy-proven immune complex-related glomerulonephritis
Lymphopenia $< 1.0 \times 10^9$/l
Antibodies to native DNA (detected by radio-immunoassay or Crithidia fluorescence)
Antibodies to "extractable nuclear antigens"
Antinuclear antibodies $> 1 : 320$
Treatment with drugs known to induce aPL.

A follow-up longer than 5 years after the first clinical manifestation is necessary to rule out the subsequent emergence of SLE.

Reproduced from Piette JC 1993 [52].

Clinical Presentation

The APS is largely a non-inflammatory autoimmune disorder. For the most part, thrombosis is the most important underlying pathological process and accounts for many of the clinical features of all forms of APS. The way in which it presents is similar in PAPS and SLE-associated APS, although in the former the syndrome is often not defined until a clinically apparent thrombosis has occurred. With patients who already have SLE there is usually a heightened awareness of the possibility that features of APS may develop. There have been a large number of studies and case reports documenting clinical features in patients with PAPS. Allowing for differences in the selection and reporting of cases, there is no reason to suppose that the spectrum of clinical features in PAPS is significantly different from that seen in SLE-associated APS. All of the standard features of APS – such as venous or arterial thrombosis, fetal loss, thrombocytopenia, neurological disease, migraine and livedo reticularis – are well described in PAPS. Some of these areas are worth considering in more detail.

Thrombosis

In most other prothrombotic diseases, for example, proteins C and S deficiency, homocysteinuria and antithrombin III deficiency, thromboses are usually restricted to the venous or to the arterial vasculature. APS is unusual because both systems may be affected. In any given patient, however, one arterial event is likely to predispose to another arterial event; the same is true for venous thrombosis. These observations apply to PAPS as well as to SLE-associated APS. Histologically, these are generally bland thromboses with no evidence of vascular endothelial damage, or vasculitis [53] although vasculitis has been reported in some patients, especially with lupus-associated APS [54].

Arterial and venous thromboses have been described in virtually every organ system. Some examples of these occurring in PAPS are summarized in Table 12.4.

Table 12.4. Thrombotic manifestations reported in primary antiphospholipid syndrome.

Organ	No. of patients	Clinical manifestations	Author
Liver	10	Budd–Chiari syndrome	Asherson 1991 [77]
			Pomeroy 1984 [78]
	1	Hepatic artery occlusion	Mor 1989 [79]
	1	Portal hypertension	Lee 1997 [80]
	1	Inferior vena cava thrombosis	Tatrai 1996 [81]
Kidney	1	Hypertension, Renal artery thrombosis	Asherson 1991 [82]
	1	Renal infarction and hypertension	Sonpal 1992 [83]
Adrenal	1	Hypoadrenalism	Grottolo 1988 [84]
	1	Bilateral infarction	Marie I 1997 [85]
Heart	1	Large vessel occlusion	Takeuchi 1998 [86]
Lungs	3	Primary pulmonary hypertension	Nagai 1997 [87]
			Sandoval 1996 [88]
CNS	40	CVA Amaurosis fugax Ischemic optic neuropathy Retinal artery occlusion	Levine 1990 [89]
	1	Arterial and venous thrombosis	Keller 1996 [90]
	2	Superior saggital sinus thrombosis	Nagai 1998 [87]
			Khoo 1995 [91]

Although large and small vessel thrombosis can account for many of the organ restricted clinical presentations, some organ-specific features are less well characterized. Some of these will be considered further.

Cardiovascular System

One of the most striking lesions seen in APS is the aseptic vegetation on cardiac valves. Such vegetations, which are partly thrombotic, probably account for most cases of Libman–Sacks endocarditis seen in SLE. The advent of sensitive echocardiography has increased the frequency of diagnosis of such lesions. They have been well described in PAPS. As in SLE, they are usually asymptomatic. Badui et al [55] found them in 13 out of 20 women with PAPS. Most of these (10 patients) were mitral, and all caused regurgitation. They authors also found electrocardiograph (ECG) abnormalities in 12 patients, and a raised pulmonary artery pressure in one. Other cardiac abnormalities have been described by Coudray et al [56]. They studied 18 patients with PAPS who were asymptomatic for cardiac disease but who demonstrated abnormal relaxation and impaired filling dynamics of the left ventricle on pulsed Doppler echocardiography. It may well be that such cardiac pathology is due in part to coronary ischemia, but this has not yet been established. One retrospective study found 21% of patients under 45 years with acute myocardial infarction had raised aCL levels [57]. These findings have been the subject of some controversy, but raise the possibility that a significant proportion of young patients with myocardial infarction may have a form of PAPS.

Central Nervous System

Neurological involvement is an important cause of morbidity and mortality in PAPS. A wide range of clinical syndromes in the CNS have been described. Some, such as stroke and chorea, are clearly associated with raised aCL whilst others are less well established, e.g., migraine and Guillain–Barré syndrome. In some instances it is likely that in situ thrombosis is responsible for the clinical manifestations, whereas in others embolic phenomena are likely to be important. The 1990 Antiphospholipid Antibodies in Stroke Study Group (APASS) study [58] reported 16 of 72 patients with cerebral ischemia who also had predominantly left-sided cardiac valve lesions.

Several CNS syndromes have been associated with raised levels of aCL even though by current guidelines many of these patients fail to fulfill classification criteria for PAPS. In patients with cerebral ischemia, an increased prevalence of aPL – 6.8% – has been found in unselected patients with stroke [59], and this figure rises to 46% if the patients less than 50 years of age are selected [60]. The 1993 APASS study [61] evaluated 255 consecutive first ischemic stroke patients and 255 matched controls for the presence of aCL as an independent risk factor for stroke. The prevalence of aCL in the stroke group was 9.7% compared with 4.3% in controls. They determined an odds ratio of 2.3 after adjustment for other known risk factors for ischemic events. None of these patients had SLE.

A study by Verrot et al [62] looked at 163 patients with idiopathic epilepsy. They found 19% positive for IgG aCL, but none fulfilled clinical criteria for APS. The absence of any ischemic damage on magnetic resonance imaging (MRI) scan suggested that thromboembolism was an unlikely cause of the epilepsy. This view is not shared by Inzelberg et al [63] who claim that within an SLE population most patients with seizures have evidence of ischemic injury on MRI.

Sneddon first described the clinical association of cerebrovascular lesions and livedo reticularis in 1965[64]. Patients with this syndrome exhibit a range of neurological manifestations from headache, dizziness and focal neurological deficits to progressive cognitive defects and dementia. Kalashnikova et al [65] recognized the association between aPL and the syndrome. Although not all patients express these antibodies, those that do can be considered to have a subset of PAPS.

Chorea is usually a transient clinical manifestation that can occur in the presence of aPL. Both SLE-associated and PAPS-associated disease is recognized [16]. In patients with raised aPL levels, these movement disorders may be induced by estrogens, for example the oral contraceptive pill [66], or by pregnancy [67].

Recurrent Abortion

Ten to 15% of all recognized pregnancies result in abortion. By far the majority of these occur in the pre-embryonic (less than 5 weeks post-menstrual date) or early embryonic (between 5 and 10 weeks post-menstrual) periods. Thereafter, fetal loss is rare. In a study by Goldstein [68], 232 women with apparently normal early pregnancies were examined, 13.4% had pregnancy loss, of which 87% occurred in the pre-embryonic or embryonic periods.

Several studies have examined the frequency of raised aCL in such individuals who have recurrent miscarriages but who are otherwise healthy (Table 12.5). The reported prevalence of aCL in this population varies from 7 to 42%. By far the majority of these patients with raised aCL levels may be considered to have PAPS rather than SLE-associated APS. The broad range of results is likely to reflect inconsistent aCL and LA tests, variability in the clinical criteria used in assessment of recurrent miscarriages, and differences in patient selection. What is clear, however, is that a significant population of these women do have raised aCL levels.

These studies also failed to delineate accurately the stage of pregnancy loss. Oshiro et al [69] have shown that 50% of pregnancy losses in aCL or LA positive

Table 12.5. The prevalence of aCL-positivity in "healthy" women with recurrent abortions.

Author	Patients		Type of aPL	No. of abortions	SLE
	Total number	%			
Lockwood et al 1986 [92]	55	27%	IgG aCL	≥ 2 or IUGR or stillbirth	ND
Cowchock et al 1986 [93]	61	13.1%	IgG or IgM aCL	≥ 2	3*
Unander et al 1987 [94]	99	42% 10%	IgG or IgM aCL (high titre IgG)	≥ 3	1
Petri et al 1987 [95]	44	11%	IgG aCL	≥ 3	ND
Granger et al 1997 [96]	387	16%	IgG aCL or LA	≥ 2	4

IUGR, Intrauterine growth retardation.
ND, not determined.
* Serology suggestive of SLE.

recurrent miscarriers ($n = 76$) were fetal deaths (>10 weeks) compared to only 15% in aCL negative recurrent miscarriers ($n = 290$). In other words, aCL is more strongly associated with late abortion (sensitivity of 76%) compared to early losses (sensitivity of 6%). This is not to say that aCL antibodies are not also associated with early losses, but more common causes of early loss such as genetic, hormonal and anatomical are numerically more important. Low titer IgG and IgM antibodies do not confer a greater miscarriage risk compared to normal controls in some studies [70], whereas in others a significantly greater proportion of recurrent miscarriage has been found [71].

Comparison of pregnancy loss in PAPS and SLE- associated APS is difficult because of increased losses in lupus per se due to features such as renal impairment. Furthermore, there is likely to be considerable selection bias against patients with connective tissue diseases in recurrent miscarriage clinics in which most of these studies have been performed. It is likely that most aCL-associated recurrent miscarriage falls into the PAPS group. However, it is not an uncommon finding for recurrent miscarriage to predate the diagnosis of SLE, suggesting that at least some of these patients show an evolution from PAPS into SLE-associated APS [72]. Other pregnancy complications such as intrauterine growth retardation, premature delivery and pre-eclampsia are seen in PAPS, as in SLE-associated APS.

Thrombocytopenia

Thrombocytopenia is a common manifestation of both SLE-associated APS and PAPS but is generally mild. In a patient with lupus it is often difficult to determine whether thrombocytopenia is APS related, since low platelet counts are a frequent manifestation of SLE itself. Both platelet autoantibodies and platelet activation have been implicated in the pathogenesis of thrombocytopenia in APS, and platelet activation may also play a role in the development of thrombosis. Fanelli et al [73] have found high levels of CD62 and CD63 (markers of platelet activation) on platelets in patients with PAPS. Emmi et al [74] have confirmed these high levels of CD62-positive platelets in 16 patients with PAPS. They found that the level of CD62-positivity in patients with neurological disease was significantly higher than in PAPS patients without neurological manifestations. They also showed a linear relationship in all patients between the aCL IgG level and the CD62-positive platelet percentage. In PAPS – as in SLE-associated APS – thrombocytopenia is usually mild (platelet counts are rarely lower than $80 \times 10^9/l$), and not usually of clinical importance.

The Catastrophic APS

This syndrome has been described in PAPS as well as SLE-associated APS and is considered further elsewhere in this book.

Treatment in PAPS

The principles of managing patients with PAPS are broadly similar to those for patients with SLE-associated APS. They are covered elsewhere in this book.

Conclusion

The primary antiphospholipid syndrome has emerged as an important disease entity. Depending on the organ systems involved, it can produce a highly variable clinical picture, with severity ranging from mild asymptomatic disease (often undiagnosed) to major life-threatening events. It may be regarded as the "pure" form of a condition which is also frequently seen in the context of other autoimmune diseases. In particular it is intricately linked to APS seen in the context of SLE; and these two variants of the condition appear to behave in a similar fashion. Defining PAPS provides us with the opportunity to study the disease in the absence of other comorbid conditions such as SLE. Advances in our understanding of the pathogenesis of PAPS should facilitate the development of improved treatment and outlook for patients with all forms of the antiphospholipid syndrome.

References

1. Moore JE, Mohr CF. Biologically false positive serologic tests for syphilis, type incidence and cause. JAMA 1952;150:467–473.
2. Feinstein DI, Rapaport SI. Acquired inhibitors of blood coagulation. [Review] [95 refs]. Prog Hemost Thromb 1972;1:75–95.
3. Bowie WEJ, Thompson JH, Pascuzzi CA, Owen CA. Thrombosis in SLE despite circulation anticoagulant. J Clin Invest 1963;62:413–430.
4. Margolius A, Jackson DP, Ratnoff OD. Circulation anticoagulants: a study of 40 cases and a review of the literature. Medicine (Baltimore) 1961;40:145–202.
5. Nilsson IM, Astedt B, Hedner U, Berezin D. Intrauterine death and circulating anticoagulant ("antithromboplastin"). Acta Med Scand 1975;197(3):153–159.
6. Firkin BG, Howard MA, Radford N. Possible relationship between lupus inhibitor and recurrent abortion in young women [letter]. Lancet 1980;2(8190):366.
7. Carreras LO, Defreyn G, Machin SJ, Vermylen J, Deman R, Spitz B et al. Arterial thrombosis, intrauterine death and "lupus" anticoagulant: detection of immunoglobulin interfering with prostacyclin formation. Lancet 1981;1(8214):244–246.
8. Yin ET, Gaston LW. Purification and kinetic studies on a circulating anticoagulant in a suspected case of lupus erythematosus. Thromb Diath Haemorrhag 1965;14:88–115.
9. Laurell AB, Nilsson IM. Hypergammaglobulinaemia, circulating anticoagulant and biologic false positive Wassermann reaction. J Lab Clin Med 1957;49:694–707.
10. Harris EN, Gharavi AE, Boey ML, Patel BM, Mackworth-Young CG, Loizou S et al. Anticardiolipin antibodies: detection by radioimmunoassay and association with thrombosis in systemic lupus erythematosus. Lancet 1983;2(8361):1211–1214.
11. Violi F, Valesini G, Ferro D, Tincani A, Balestrieri G, Balsano F. Anticoagulant activity of anticardiolipin antibodies. Thromb Res 1986;44(4):543–7.
12. Boey ML, Colaco CB, Gharavi AE, Elkon KB, Loizou S, Hughes GR. Thrombosis in systemic lupus erythematosus: striking association with the presence of circulating lupus anticoagulant. Br Med J 1983;287(6398):1021–1023.
13. Hughes GR. Thrombosis, abortion, cerebral disease, and the lupus anticoagulant. Br Med J 1983;287:1088–1089.
14. Hughes GR. The anticardiolipin syndrome [editorial]. Clin Exp Rheumatol 1985;3:285–286.
15. Harris EN, Baguley E, Asherson RA, Hughes GRV. Clinical and serological features of the "antiphospholipid syndrome" (APS). Br J Rheumatol 1987;26:19.
16. Asherson RA. A "primary" antiphospholipid syndrome? J Rheumatol 1988;15:1742–1746.
17. Asherson RA, Baguley E, Pal C, Hughes GR. Antiphospholipid syndrome: five year follow up. Ann Rheum Dis 1991;50:805–810.
18. Mujic F, Cuadrado MJ, Lloyd M, Khamashta MA, Page G, Hughes GR. Primary antiphospholipid syndrome evolving into systemic lupus erythematosus. J Rheumatol 1995;22:1589–1592.
19. Andrews PA, Frampton G, Cameron JS. Antiphospholipid syndrome and systemic lupus erythematosus [letter; comment]. Lancet 1993;342:988–989.

20. Vianna JL, Khamashta MA, Ordi-Ros J, Font J, Cervera R, Lopez-Soto A et al. Comparison of the primary and secondary antiphospholipid syndrome: a European Multicenter Study of 114 patients [see comments]. Am J Med 1994;96:3–9.

21. Asherson RA, Khamashta MA, Ordi-Ros J, Derksen RH, Machin SJ, Barquinero J et al. The "primary" antiphospholipid syndrome: major clinical and serological features. Medicine 1989;68:366–74.

22. Font J, Lopez-Soto A, Cervera R, Balasch J, Pallares L, Navarro M et al. The "primary" antiphospholipid syndrome: antiphospholipid antibody pattern and clinical features of a series of 23 patients. Autoimmunity 1991;9:69–75.

23. Loizou CG, Mackworth-Young C, Cofiner C, Walport MJ. Heterogeneity of binding reactivity to different phospholipids of antibodies from patients with systemic lupus erythematosus (SLE) and with syphilis. Clin Exp Immunol 1990;80:171–176.

24. Galli M, Comfurius P, Maassen C, Hemker HC, de Baets MH, van Breda-Vriesman PJ et al. Anticardiolipin antibodies (ACA) directed not to cardiolipin but to a plasma protein cofactor [see comments]. Lancet 1990;335:1544–1547.

25. McNeil HP, Simpson RJ, Chesterman CN, Krilis SA. Anti-phospholipid antibodies are directed against a complex antigen that includes a lipid-binding inhibitor of coagulation: beta 2-glycoprotein I (apolipoprotein H). Proc Natl Acad Sci USA 1990;87:4120–4124.

26. Harris EN, Pierangeli S. Anticardiolipin antibodies: specificity and function. [Review] [58 refs]. Lupus 1994;3:217–222.

27. Matsuura E, Igarashi Y, Yasuda T, Triplett DA, Koike T. Anticardiolipin antibodies recognize beta 2-glycoprotein I structure altered by interacting with an oxygen modified solid phase surface. J Exp Med 1994;179:457–462.

28. Roubey RA, Eisenberg RA, Harper MF, Winfield JB. "Anticardiolipin" autoantibodies recognize beta 2-glycoprotein I in the absence of phospholipid. Importance of Ag density and bivalent binding. J Immunol 1995;154:954–960.

29. Arvieux J, Roussel B, Jacob MC, Colomb MG. Measurement of anti-phospholipid antibodies by ELISA using beta 2-glycoprotein I as an antigen. J Immunol Methods 1991;143:223–229.

30. Roubey RA. Immunology of the antiphospholipid antibody syndrome. [Review] [116 refs]. Arthritis Rheum 1996;39:1444–1454.

31. Bajaj SP, Rapaport SI, Fierer DS, Herbst KD, Schwartz DB. A mechanism for the hypoprothrombinemia of the acquired hypoprothrombinemia-lupus anticoagulant syndrome. Blood 1983;61:684–692.

32. Edson JR, Vogt JM, Hasegawa DK. Abnormal prothrombin crossed-immunoelectrophoresis in patients with lupus inhibitors. Blood 1984;64:807–816.

33. Fleck RA, Rapaport SI, Rao LV. Anti-prothrombin antibodies and the lupus anticoagulant. Blood 1988;72:512–9.

34. Arvieux J, Darnige L, Caron C, Reber G, Bensa JC, Colomb MG. Development of an ELISA for autoantibodies to prothrombin showing their prevalence in patients with lupus anticoagulants. Thromb Haemost 1995;74:1120–1125.

35. Godeau B, Piette JC, Fromont P, Intrator L, Schaeffer A, Bierling P. Specific antiplatelet glycoprotein autoantibodies are associated with the thrombocytopenia of primary antiphospholipid syndrome. Br J Haematol 1997;98:873–879.

36. Panzer S, Gschwandtner ME, Hutter D, Spitzauer S, Pabinger I. Specificities of platelet autoantibodies in patients with lupus anticoagulants in primary antiphospholipid syndrome. Ann Hematol 1997;74:239–242.

37. Kertesz Z, Yu BB, Steinkasserer A, Haupt H, Benham A, Sim RB. Characterization of binding of human beta 2-glycoprotein I to cardiolipin. Biochem J 1995;310:315–321.

38. Cabiedes J, Cabral AR, Alarcon-Segovia D. Clinical manifestations of the antiphospholipid syndrome in patients with systemic lupus erythematosus associate more strongly with anti-beta 2-glycoprotein-I than with antiphospholipid antibodies. J Rheumatol 1995;22:1899–1906.

39. Najmey SS, Keil LB, Adib DY, DeBari VA. The association of antibodies to beta 2 glycoprotein I with the antiphospholipid syndrome: a meta-analysis. Ann Clin Lab Sci 1997;27:41–46.

40. Cabral AR, Cabiedes J, Alarcon-Segovia D. Antibodies to phospholipid-free beta 2-glycoprotein-I in patients with primary antiphospholipid syndrome. J Rheumatol 1995;22:1894–1898.

41. Day HM, Thiagarajan P, Ahn C, Reveille JD, Tinker KF, Arnett FC. Autoantibodies to beta 2-glycoprotein I in systemic lupus erythematosus and primary antiphospholipid antibody syndrome: clinical correlations in comparison with other antiphospholipid antibody tests. J Rheumatol 1998;25:667–674.

42. Loizou S, Byron MA, Englert HJ, David J, Hughes GR, Walport MJ. Association of quantitative anticardiolipin antibody levels with fetal loss and time of loss in systemic lupus erythematosus. Quart J Med 1988;68:525–531.

43. Escalante A, Brey RL, Mitchell BD, Jr., Dreiner U. Accuracy of anticardiolipin antibodies in identifying a history of thrombosis among patients with systemic lupus erythematosus. Am J Med 1995;98:559–565.

44. Viard JP, Amoura Z, Bach JF. Association of anti-beta 2 glycoprotein I antibodies with lupus-type circulating anticoagulant and thrombosis in systemic lupus erythematosus [see comments]. Am J Med 1992;93:181–186.
45. Lopez-Soto A, Cervera R, Font J, Bove A, Reverter JC, Munoz FJ et al. Isotype distribution and clinical significance of antibodies to cardiolipin, phosphatidic acid, phosphatidylinositol and phosphatidylserine in systemic lupus erythematosus: prospective analysis of a series of 92 patients. Clin Exp Rheumatol 1997;15:143–149.
46. Levine SR, Brey RL, Sawaya KL, Salowich-Palm L, Kokkinos J, Kostrzema B et al. Recurrent stroke and thrombo-occlusive events in the antiphospholipid syndrome. Ann Neurol 1995;38:119–124.
47. Vaarala O, Puurunen M, Manttari M, Manninen V, Aho K, Palosuo T. Antibodies to prothrombin imply a risk of myocardial infarction in middle-aged men. Thromb Haemost 1996;75:456–459.
48. Alarcon-Segovia D, Perez-Vazquez ME, Villa AR, Drenkard C, Cabiedes J. Preliminary classification criteria for the antiphospholipid syndrome within systemic lupus erythematosus. Semin Arthritis Rheum 1992;21:275–286.
49. Cabral AR, Amigo MC, Cabiedes J, Alarcon-Segovia D. The antiphospholipid/cofactor syndromes: a primary variant with antibodies to beta 2-glycoprotein-I but no antibodies detectable in standard antiphospholipid assays. Am J Med 1996;101:472–481.
50. Alarcon-Segovia D, Mestanza M, Cabiedes J, Cabral AR. The antiphospholipid/cofactor syndromes. II. A variant in patients with systemic lupus erythematosus with antibodies to β_2-glycoprotein I but no antibodies detectable in standard antiphospholipid assays. J Rheumatol 1997;24:1545–1551.
51. Piette JC, Wechsler B, Francis C, Godeau P. Systemic lupus erythematosus and the antiphospholipid syndrome: reflections about the relevance of ARA criteria [editorial] [see comments]. J Rheumatol 1992;19:1835–1837.
52. Piette JC, Wechsler B, Frances C, Papo T, Godeau P. Exclusion criteria for primary antiphospholipid syndrome [letter]. J Rheumatol 1993;20:1802–1804.
53. Johannsson EA, Niemi KM, Mustakillio KK. A peripheral vascular syndrome overlapping with SLE: recurrent venous thrombosis and hemorrhagic capillary proliferation with circulating anticoagulants and false-positive reactions for syphilis. Dermatologica 1977;15:257–267.
54. Alegre VA, Gastineau DA, Winkelmann RK. Skin lesions associated with circulating lupus anticoagulant. Br J Dermatol 1989;120:419–429.
55. Badui E, Solorio S, Martinez E, Bravo G, Enciso R, Barile L et al. The heart in the primary antiphospholipid syndrome. Arch Med Res 1995;26:115–120.
56. Coudray N, de Zuttere D, Bletry O, Piette JC, Wechsler B, Godeau P et al. M mode and Doppler echocardiographic assessment of left ventricular diastolic function in primary antiphospholipid syndrome. Br Heart J 1995;74:531–535.
57. Hamsten A, Norberg R, Bjorkholm M, de Faire U, Holm G. Antibodies to cardiolipin in young survivors of myocardial infarction: an association with recurrent cardiovascular events. Lancet 1986;1:113–116.
58. APASS. The Antiphospholipid Antibodies in Stroke Study Group. Clinical and laboratory findings in patients with antiphospholipid antibodies and cerebral ischaemia. Stroke 1990;21:1268–1273.
59. Montalban J, Codina A, Ordi J, Vilardell M, Khamashta MA, Hughes GR. Antiphospholipid antibodies in cerebral ischemia. Stroke 1991;22:750–753.
60. Brey RL, Hart RG, Sherman DG, Tegeler CH. Antiphospholipid antibodies and cerebral ischemia in young people. Neurology 1990;40:1190–1196.
61. APASS. The Antiphospholipid Antibodies in Stroke Study Group. Anticardiolipin antibodies are an independent risk factor for first ischemic stroke. Neurology 1993;43:2069–2073.
62. Verrot D, San-Marco M, Dravet C, Genton P, Disdier P, Bolla G et al. Prevalence and signification of antinuclear and anticardiolipin antibodies in patients with epilepsy. Am J Med 1997;103:33–37.
63. Inzelberg R, Korczyn AD. Lupus anticoagulant and late onset seizures [see comments]. Acta Neurol Scand 1989;79:114–118.
64. Sneddon IB. Cerebral vascular lesion in livedo reticularis. Br J Dermatol 1965;77:180–185.
65. Kalashnikova LA, Nasonov EL, Kushekbaeva AE, Gracheva LA. Anticardiolipin antibodies in Sneddon's syndrome. Neurology 1990;40:464–467.
66. Asherson RA, Harris NE, Gharavi AE, Hughes GR. Systemic lupus erythematosus, antiphospholipid antibodies, chorea, and oral contraceptives [letter]. Arthritis Rheum 1986;29:1535–1536.
67. Lubbe WF, Walker EB. Chorea gravidarum associated with circulating lupus anticoagulant: successful outcome of pregnancy with prednisone and aspirin therapy. Case report. Br J Obstet Gynaecol 1983;90:487–490.
68. Goldstein SR. Embryonic death in early pregnancy: a new look at the first trimester. Obstet Gynecol 1994;84:294–297.

69. Oshiro BT, Silver RM, Scott JR, Yu H, Branch DW. Antiphospholipid antibodies and fetal death. Obstet Gynecol 1996;87:489–493.

70. Silver RM, Porter TF, van Leeuween I, Jeng G, Scott JR, Branch DW. Anticardiolipin antibodies: clinical consequences of "low titers". Obstet Gynecol 1996;87:494–500.

71. Aoki K, Hayashi Y, Hirao Y, Yagami Y. Specific antiphospholipid antibodies as a predictive variable in patients with recurrent pregnancy loss. Am J Reprod Immunol 1993;29:82–87.

72. Derue G, Englert HJ, Harris EN et al. Foetal loss in systemic lupus: association with anticardiolipin antibodies. J Obstet Gynaecol 1985;5:207–209.

73. Fanelli A, Bergamini C, Rapi S, Caldini A, Spinelli A, Buggiani A et al. Flow cytometric detection of circulating activated platelets in primary antiphospholipid syndrome. Correlation with thrombocytopenia and anticardiolipin antibodies. Lupus 1997;6:261–267.

74. Emmi L, Bergamini C, Spinelli A, Liotta F, Marchione T, Caldini A et al. Possible pathogenetic role of activated platelets in the primary antiphospholipid syndrome involving the central nervous system. Ann N Y Acad Sci 1997;823:188–200.

75. Mackworth-Young CG, Loizou S, Walport MJ. Primary antiphospholipid syndrome: features of patients with raised anticardiolipin antibodies and no other disorder. Ann Rheum Dis 1989;48:362–367.

76. Alarcon-Segovia D, Sanchez-Guerrero J. Primary antiphospholipid syndrome [published erratum appears in J Rheumatol 1989 Jul;16(7):1014]. J Rheumatol 1989;16:482–488.

77. Asherson RA, Khamashta MA, Hughes GR. The hepatic complications of the antiphospholipid antibodies [editorial]. Clin Exp Rheumatol 1991;9:341–344.

78. Pomeroy C, Knodell RG, Swaim WR, Arneson P, Mahowald ML. Budd–Chiari syndrome in a patient with the lupus anticoagulant. Gastroenterology 1984;86:158–161.

79. Mor F, Beigel Y, Inbal A, Goren M, Wysenbeek AJ. Hepatic infarction in a patient with the lupus anticoagulant. Arthritis Rheum 1989;32:491–495.

80. Lee HJ, Park JW, Chang JC. Mesenteric and portal venous obstruction associated with primary antiphospholipid antibody syndrome [see comments]. J Gastroenterol Hepatol 1997;12:822–826.

81. Tatrai T, Kiss G, Sevcic K. Inferior vena cava thrombosis developing in primary antiphospholipid syndrome [Hungarian]. Orv Hetil 1996;137:135–137.

82. Asherson RA, George EN, Hughes GRV. Hypertension, renal artery stenosis and the "primary" antiphospholipid syndrome. J Rheumatol 1991;18:1413–1415.

83. Sonpal GM, Sharma A, Miller A. Primary antiphospholipid antibody syndrome, renal infarction and hypertension. J Rheumatol 1993;20:1221–1223.

84. Grottolo A, Ferrari V, Mariano M, Zambruni A, Tincani A, Del Bono R. Primary adrenal insufficiency, circulating lupus anticoagulant and anticardiolipin antibodies in a patient with multiple abortions and recurrent thrombotic episodes. Haematologica 1988;73:517–519.

85. Marie I, Levesque H, Heron F, Cailleux N, Borg JY, Courtois H. Acute adrenal failure secondary to bilateral infarction of the adrenal glands as the first manifestation of primary antiphospholipid antibody syndrome [letter]. Ann Rheum Dis 1997;56:567–568.

86. Takeuchi S, Obayashi T, Toyama J. Primary antiphospholipid syndrome with acute myocardial infarction recanalised by PTCA. Heart 1998;79:96–98.

87. Nagai S, Horie Y, Akai T, Takeda S, Takaku A. Superior sagittal sinus thrombosis associated with primary antiphospholipid syndrome – case report [Review] [23 refs]. Neurol Med Chir 1998;38:34–39.

88. Sandoval J, Amigo MC, Barragan R, Izaguirre R, Reyes PA, Martinez-Guerra ML et al. Primary antiphospholipid syndrome presenting as chronic thromboembolic pulmonary hypertension. Treatment with thromboendarterectomy. J Rheumatol 1996;23:772–775.

89. Levine SR, Deegan MJ, Futrell N, Welch KM. Cerebrovascular and neurologic disease associated with antiphospholipid antibodies: 48 cases. Neurology 1990;40:1181–1189.

90. Keller E, Sommer T, Lutterbey G, Schild HH. Coincident arterial and venous cerebral thrombosis in primary antiphospholipid syndrome [German]. Rofo Fortschr Geb Rontgenstr Neuen Bildgeb Verfahr 1996;165:300–302.

91. Khoo KB, Long FL, Tuck RR, Allen RJ, Tymms KE. Cerebral venous sinus thrombosis associated with the primary antiphospholipid syndrome. Resolution with local thrombolytic therapy. [Review] [14 refs]. Med J Aust 1995;162:30–32.

92. Lockwood CJ, Reece EA, Romero R, Hobbins JC. Anti-phospholipid antibody and pregnancy wastage [letter]. Lancet 1986;2:742–743.

93. Cowchock S, Smith JB, Gocial B. Antibodies to phospholipids and nuclear antigens in patients with repeated abortions. Am J Obstet Gynecol 1986;155:1002–1010.

94. Unander AM, Norberg R, Hahn L, Arfors L. Anticardiolipin antibodies and complement in ninety-nine women with habitual abortion. Am J Obstet Gynecol 1987;156:114–119.

95. Petri M, Golbus M, Anderson R, Whiting OKQ, Corash L, Hellmann D. Antinuclear antibody, lupus anticoagulant, and anticardiolipin antibody in women with idiopathic habitual abortion. A controlled, prospective study of forty-four women. Arthritis Rheum 1987;30:601–606.
96. Granger KA, Farquharson RG. Obstetric outcome in antiphospholipid syndrome. Lupus 1997;6;509–513.

13   Catastrophic Antiphospholipid Syndrome

H. M. Belmont

Introduction

The syndrome of multiple vascular occlusions associated with high titer anti-phospholipid antibodies (aPL) is known as the catastrophic antiphospholipid syndrome (APS). Although APS is typically characterized by thrombotic events that either occur singly or, when recurrent, are seen many months or even years apart, some patients with this syndrome may develop widespread, non-inflammatory vascular occlusions. The prevalence and incidence of this condition both in the general population, as well as those with SLE or antiphospholipid antibodies, is unknown. However, expanding numbers of patients fulfilling criteria for catastrophic APS are now reported which reflects increasing familiarity with the disorder.

The first reports of patients with multiple non-inflammatory vascular occlusions appeared in 1974 by Dosekun [1] and in 1987 by Ingram [2]. However, it was not until Greisman reported in 1991 on two patients with "acute, catastrophic, widespread non-inflammatory visceral vascular occlusions associated with high titer antiphospholipid antibodies" that the full spectrum of clinical features associated with antiphospholipid antibodies (aPL) became appreciated [3]. This spectrum was outlined in an editorial by Harris and Bos that accompanied the Greissman report [4]. The authors described two additional patients with "acute disseminated coagulopathy–vasculopathy associated with antiphospholipid syndrome" and identified three cohorts of patients with these antibodies. They recognized that aPL may be "asymptomatic" and observed in patients free of thrombosis or associated with one or two episodes of thrombosis typically involving only one artery or vein at a time with long periods (months to years) free of occlusive events. Alternatively, aPL may confer a risk for an ominous disorder characterized by multiple, typically three or more, widespread thrombotic occlusions often with marked ischemic changes in the extremities, livido reticularis, as well as renal, cerebral, myocardial, pulmonary and other visceral organ thrombotic vasculopathy. Asherson, describing 10 such patients in an article published in 1992, first proposed the term catastrophic APS [5]. This chapter will describe the clinical, therapeutic, and pathogenic aspects of this condition.

Clinical Aspects

Our appreciation of the clinical features of catastrophic APS is immeasurably assisted by a review of the subject ably completed by Asherson and published in a

1998 issue of *Medicine* [6]. The authors performed a comprehensive computer-assisted search of medical literature to identify all cases of catastrophic APS published between 1992 and 1996. After reviewing 56 references they summarized the data. I identified seven additional references since 1996 to generate a total of 57 reported patients with catastrophic APS [7–14].

Patients with catastrophic APS can be broadly categorized into those with SLE, "lupus-like" illness satisfying two to three of the modified ACR criteria, primary APS, or secondary to an another autoimmune, connective tissue disease such as rheumatoid arthritis [6], scleroderma [14] or primary, systemic nercotizing vasculitis [12].

Demographic Characteristics

Amongst 57 patients with catastrophic APS, 37 (66%) were females and 20 (34%) males (2:1 female:male ratio) with an age range of 9 to 74 years and an average of 36 years. Five (7%) patients developed the clinical picture before the age of 15 and 13 (23%) after the age of 50. Thirty-one (55%) who developed acute, multi-organ involvement suffered from primary APS, 15 (30%) from SLE, 6 (12%) from "lupus-like" illness, and 3 (3%) from other connective tissue disease.

Preceding Thrombotic History

The majority of the patients did not have a prior history of thrombophilia and thrombotic event. However, a total of 20 (37%) of the 57 patients had a history of venous occlusions. Deep venous thrombophlebitis (DVT) were reported in 17 (33%) patients, and in 7 (14%) were accompanied or followed by pulmonary embolism. Two patients had prior superior vena cava thrombosis and one each inferior vena cava and Budd–Chiari syndrome (hepatic vein thrombosis).

In addition to venous events, major arterial occlusions occurred in 12 (23%) of the 57 patients. Femoral, popliteal, and digital artery peripheral arterial occlusions were reported in four patients, myocardial infarctions in four, cerebral events as either transient ischemic attacks or completed cerebral vascular accidents in three, adrenal infarction in two, renal infarction in two, and mesenteric and splenic artery thrombosis in one. Spontaneous fetal losses had occurred in only eight (23%) of the 37 female patients and thrombocytopenia in five (8%). One patient 31 years before developing catastrophic APS had experienced an atypical pre-eclampsia – eclampsia presentation known as the HELLP syndrome (hemolysis, elevated liver enzymes, and low platelets) [15]. Other potential thrombotic manifestations of pre-existing hypercoagulability include non-healing cutaneous ulcers of the lower extremities in 7 (13%) patients.

Potential Precipitating Factors

In 11 (21%) of the 57 patients precipitating factors may have contributed to the development of catastrophic APS. These included infections in three patients (upper respiratory tract, intestinal, and undefined), ingestion of drugs in three (thiazide, captropril, and oral contraceptive), minor surgical procedures in three (dental extraction, endoscopic retrograde cholangiopancreatography, and uterine dilatation and curettage), anticoagulation withdrawal in two, and major surgical procedure in one (hysterectomy). Catastrophic APS occurred in the postpartum period in three patients, including in two after fetal losses. The biological significance of these risks is uncertain. As this summary data was culled from numerous investigator's published reports it may contain biases. The likelihood that the authors ascertained potential risks and chose to include the information can not be certain. Only a prospective study which is designed to audit all identified, hypothetical risk factors could reveal which are significantly associated with developing catastrophic APS.

Clinical Presentation

Presentation of the catastrophic APS is often complex as it involves multiple organs concurrently over a short period of time, typically days to weeks. Figure 13.1 shows the clinical manifestations attributed to thrombotic events at the time of catastrophic APS in the 57 reviewed patients.

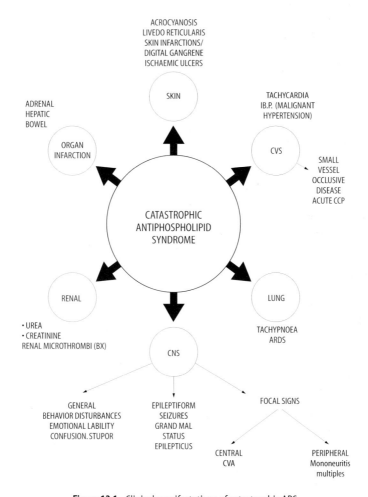

Figure 13.1. Clinical manifestations of catastrophic APS.

In catastrophic APS the most characteristic involvement is of renal, pulmonary, cerebral, gastrointestinal and cerebral vessels. In contrast to the non-catastrophic APS, DVT is uncommon. However, atypical occlusive events such as of adrenal, pancreatic, splenic, testicular and cutaneous vessels typify catastrophic APS.

In the 57 patients, 43 (80%) had renal involvement usually accompanied by hypertension. Pathological material revealed renal microangiopathy with small vessel occlusive disease.

Pulmonary involvement occurred in 36 (67%) of the patients. Symptoms included severe dyspnea but frank adult respiratory distress syndrome (ARDS) developed in 18. Eight suffered multiple pulmonary emboli, in 7 interstitial infiltrates predominated and three experienced intraalveolar hemorrhage.

The central nervous system was involved in 30 (57%) of patients although only nine demonstrated major cerebral infarctions on computerized tomography (CT) or magnetic resonance imaging (MRI) scans and one patient had a cerebral sinus thrombosis. However, the finding of microthrombi and microinfarctions in the pathological material from 13 patients suggests that the thrombophilia that characterizes the catastrophic APS results in thrombotic events involving the microcirculation.

Cardiac manifestations were described in 25 (48%) patients although typical myocardial infarction occurred in only a few patients while diffuse myocardial involvement was present in 18. Again, pathological material revealed multiple myocardial microthrombi.

Twenty patients had gastrointestinal involvement. Vascular occlusions of mesenteric, portal and inferior vena cava were common and arterial occlusions were accompanied by gangrene of the bowels and splenic infarctions. Hepatic involvement occurred in 17 (33%), splenic in 10 (19%), and 6 (5%) demonstrated pancreatitis. Microthrombi characterized the organs examined at autopsy.

Adrenal thrombosis was present in 14 (26%) patients. Three patients experienced testicular infarction and another patient necrosis of the prostate gland. Another characteristic feature was skin involvement with 25 (49%) demonstrating livedo reticularis, ulcerations, gangrene, purpura, acrocyanosis or digital ischemia.

Laboratory Findings

Thrombocytopenia (<100 000/mm) was reported in 36 (69%) patients, hemolytic anemia in 13 (25%), findings consistent with disseminated intravascular coagulation (DIC) (prolonged coagulation tests with increased fibrinogen degradation factors and hypofibrinogenemia) in 14 (27%), and evidence of microangiopathy with schistocytes (fragmented erythrocytes) reported in peripheral blood smears in 7 (13%) patients. Lupus anticoagulant was detected in 46 of the 49 (95%) patients and anticardiolipin antibodies (aCL) was positive in 50 of 53 (95%) patients. The ANA was positive in 28 of 48 (57%) patients, usually in low titer. On the other hand, in the SLE patients with catastrophic APS anti-dsDNA antibodies were found in 13 of 15 (87%) patients.

Outcome

Death occurred in 27 of the 57 (49%) patients and most commonly from cardiac events, predominately from myocardial microthrombi producing cardiac failure, or less often acute myocardial infarction. Respiratory failure especially with ARDS or diffuse alveolar hemorrhage, was often a complicating feature in fatal cases. Cerebrovascular involvement was a less common cause of death although coma, large vessel strokes, multiple small vessel strokes, seizures, and cerebral hemorrhage contributed to significant morbidity. Renal involvement although a common clinical features was not a usual cause of death. Death occurred from gastrointestinal involvement in two patients: esophageal perforation in one and bowel infarction in another.

Therapeutic Aspects

In the absence of randomized controlled trials, optimal therapy for patients with catastrophic APS is uncertain. In contrast to the experience with APS where Khamashta [16] reviewed retrospectively, in 147 patients, the efficacy of warfarin, low-dose aspirin, or both in the secondary prevention of thrombosis; no single center, large series of patients with catastrophic APS exists. Treatment is therefore empiric. Since catastrophic APS is a thrombophilic disorder characterized by widespread microvasculopathy the rationale of treatment is to prevent thrombosis by anticoagulation, to prevent the production and circulation of mediators (i.e. aPL, cytokines, complement degradation products, anti-endothelial cell antibodies, etc.) which generate the hypercoagulable state, or to prevent both. In other words, treatment may consist of anticoagulation, immunosuppressives, such as corticosteroids or cytotoxics, or plasmapheresis. The role of antiplatelet agents, intravenous immunoglobulin and fibrinolytic treatment is less certain.

Patients treated with the combination of anticoagulation in addition to steroids plus a therapy which can achieve a prompt reduction in aPL titer, either plasmapheresis or intravenous gammaglobulin [17], had the highest survival rate of almost 70% [6]. A role for cyclophosphamide is suggested by its use in many of the most severe cases and knowledge it prevents the rebound production of pathogenic autoantibodies by autoaggresive lymphocytes. Patients have received ancrod, purified fraction of Malayan snake pit viper venom, as well as defibrotide [6] and fibrinolytics such as streptokinase [18] with uncertain benefit.

Pathogenic Aspects

Catastrophic APS occurs in a minority of patients with aPL, is characterized by acute, vascular occlusions involving multiple organs, and is an example of a non-inflammatory thrombotic microvasculopathy. The pathogenesis of microvacsulopathy in autoimmune disease includes: (1) classic leukocytoclastic vasculitis secondary to subendothelial immune complex deposition in vessel walls; (2) leukothrombosis secondary to intravascular activation of complement, neutrophils, and endothelium in the absence of local immune complex deposition; or (3) thrombosis of vessels secondary to a non-inflammatory vasculopathy [19–21].

Besides APS, other thrombotic microangiopathic syndromes include thrombotic thrombocytopenia purpura (TTP), hemolytic uremic syndrome (HUS), DIC, and HELLP syndrome. The latter is an uncommon complication of pregnancy and, interestingly, Neuwelt described a woman who developed catastrophic APS 31 years after a pregnancy accompanied by HELLP suggesting a unifying pathophysiologic mechanism [15]. On the other hand, evidence suggests that an inhibitor of von Willebrand factor-cleaving protease causes the thrombotic microangiopathic hemolytic anemia that characterizes autoimmune associated TTP [22]. The uncatabolized von Willebrand multimers promote disseminated intravascular platelet aggregation.

The diffuse and multiorgan, yet episodic, nature of catastrophic APS occurring in only a minority of patients with likely long-standing circulating aPL is consistent with the hypothesis that an additional biological factor is required for the widespread microvasculopathy. A candidate target for activation that would then be permissive for the development of APS is endothelial cells [19, 23]. There are groups of immune stimuli that activate endothelial cells and likely contribute to providing preparatory signals for catastrophic APS. These stimuli include cytokines, complement components and autoantibodies.

Cytokines are likely to be important mediators of endothelial cell activation required for the development of catastrophic APS. Tumor necrosis factor-α (TNF-α), interferon-γ (INF-γ, and interleukin-1 (IL-1) each stimulate endothelial cells [24]. Several products of the activated complement system (e.g. C3b, iC3b, and C5a) are known to activate the endothelium [24]. Additionally, assembly of the membrane attack complex (MAC), consisting of C5b-9, on endothelial cells results in the upregulation of adhesion molecules [25]. Specifically, MAC has been shown to participate in the upregulation of endothelial cell tissue factor activity and this expression of tissue factor by the endothelium promotes a procoagulant state that is likely to contribute to the vascular injury typical of catastrophic APS [25]. There is also evidence that C1q is a cofactor required for immune complexes to stimulate endothelial cells [26]. Finally, autoantibodies including aPL, anti-endothelial cell and anti-dsDNA have each been demonstrated to react with endothelial cells in vitro, provide a stimulatory signal, and upregulate adhesion molecules or tissue factor [27, 28]. Simanitov showed that IgG from patients with aPL is able to enhance endothelial cell adhesion molecule expression and monocyte adherence [29]. This capacity of aPL to activate endothelial cells may be required in catastrophic APS before aPL interacts with platelets or coagulation proteins to mediate diffuse thrombotic microvasculopathy.

The activation of endothelial cells and accompanying upregulation of adhesion molecules and tissue factor is likely pivotal to the development of catastrophic APS. It is the collaboration of cytokines, activated complement components and autoantibodies that act on endothelial cells to increase its adhesiveness and procoagulant activity that provides the preparatory signals for aPL in catastrophic APS. These same mediators can act on leukocytes and platelets to increase their adhesion to vascular endothelium and to promote microthrombosis and the local release of toxic mediators, including proteases and oxygen-derived free radicals [19, 21]. This interaction between activated endothelial cells, neutrophils and platelets in the presence of aPL generates the diffuse microvasculopathy that characterizes catastrophic APS. This widespread, thrombotic microvasculopathy is responsible for the clinical features of catastrophic APS by producing tissue injury, which can include pulmonary capillary leak or ARDS, brain capillary leak or "acute cerebral distress syndrome", myocardial dysfunction and potentially systemic inflammatory response syndrome (SIRS) with multi-organ failure [19–21].

It is now recognized that SIRS may arise both from sepsis and from noninfectious causes, such as immune-mediated organ injury [30]. SIRS is a reaction characterized by widespread inflammation primarily affecting vascular endothelium, however, the same cascade of mediators have been invoked in catastrophic APS [31]. The main endogenous mediators of both include TNF-α and IL-1 with a prominent role for platelet-activating factor, vasodilator prostaglandins, complement activation, and upregulation of adhesion molecules on leukocytes, platelets, and endothelial cells [32]. Catastrophic APS and SIRS share similar clinical consequences with multiorgan failure and manifestations, which include impaired renal function, ARDS, cerebral dysfunction, decreased myocardial contractility, and catecholamine unresponsive hypotension.

Summary

Catastrophic APS develops in a minority of patients with aPL and is characterized by acute, vascular occlusion involving three or more organs. The disorder is characterized by a diffuse thrombotic microvasculopathy with a predilection for kidney, lung, brain, heart, skin, and gastrointestinal tract. Treatment is empiric and, although mortality may approach 50%, outcomes appear best for patients that receive combinations of heparin anticoagulation, steroids, plasmapheresis, intravenous gammaglobulin and cyclophosphamide. The etiology of catastrophic APS awaits clarification but likely involves the activation of vascular endothelium to express surface adhesion molecules and possibly tissue factor that interact with circulating cellular inflammatory cells, elements of the phospholipid-dependent coagulation factors and platelets in the presence of aPL. Improved therapy awaits better understanding of the underlying immunologic, coagulation, and vascular pathology.

References

1. Dosekun AK, Pollak VE, Glas-Greenwalt P, et al. Ancrod in systemic lupus erythematosus with thrombosis. Clinical and firbrinolytic effects. Arch Intern Med 1984;144:37–42.
2. Ingram SB, Goodnight SH , Bennett RH. An unusual syndrome of a devastating non-inflammatory vasculopathy associated with anticardiolipin antibodies. Arthritis Rheum, 1987;30:1167–1171.
3. Greisman SG, Thayaparan R-S, Godwin TA, Lockshin MD. Occlusive vasculopathy in systemic lupus erythematosus-Association with anticardiolipin antibody. Arch Intern Med 1991;151:389–392.
4. Harris EN and K Bos. An acute disseminated coagulopathy–vasculopathy associated with the antiphospholipid syndrome. Arch Intern Med 1991;151:231–232.
5. Asherson RA. The catastrophic antiphospholipid syndrome. J. Rheumatol 1992;19:508–512.
6. Asherson RA, Cervera R, Piette J-C, Font J, Lie JT, Burcoglu A, et al. Catastrophic antiphospholipid syndrome: Clinical and laboratory features of 50 patients. Medicine 1998;77:195–207.
7. Le Loet X, Vittecoq O, Joen-Beades F, Tron F. Catastrophic antiphospholipid syndrome. Presse Medicale 1997;26:131–134.
8. Petras T, Rudolph B, Filler G, Zimmering M, Ditscherlein G, Loening SA. An adolescent with acute renal failure, thrombocytopenia and femoral vein thrombosis. Nephrology, Dialysis, Transplantation 1998;13:480–483.
9. Falcini F, Taccetti G, Ermini M, Trapani S, Matucci Cerinic M. Catastrophic antiphospholipid antibody syndrome in pediatric systemic lupus erythematosus. J Rheumatol 1997;24:389–392.
10. Provenzale JM, Spritzer CE, RC Nelson, TL Ortel. Disseminated thrombosis in primary antiphospholipid syndrome: MR findings. Eur J of Radiol 1998;26:244–247.
11. Argento A, DiBenedetto RJ. ARDS and adrenal insufficiency associated with the antiphospholipid antibody syndrome. Chest 1998;113:1136–1138.
12. Dasgupta B, Almond MK, Tanqueray A. Polyarteritis nodosa and the antiphospholipid syndrome. Br J Rheumatol 1997;36:1210–1212.

13. Chinnery PF, Shaw PJ, Ince PG, Jackson GH, Bishop RI. Fulminant encephalopathy due to the catastrophic primary antiphospholipid syndrome (letter). J Neurol Neurosurg Psych 1997;62:300–301.
14. Kane D, McSweeney F, Swan N, Bresnihan B. Catastrophic antiphospholipid antibody syndrome in primary systemic sclerosis. J Rheumatol 1998;25:810–812.
15. Neuwelt CM, Daikh DI, Linfoot JA, Pfister DA, Young RG, Webb RL, et al. Catastrophic antiphospholipid syndrome. Response to repeated plasmapheresis over three years. Arthritis Rheum 1997;40:1534–1539.
16. Khamashta MA, Cuadrado MJ, Mujic F, Taub NA, Hunt BJ, Hughes GRV. The management of thrombosis in the antiphospholipid-antibody syndrome. N Engl J Med 1995;332:993–997.
17. Yu Z, Lennon VA. Clinical implications of basic research: mechanism of intravenous immune globulin therapy in antibody-mediated autoimmune diseases. N Engl J Med 1999;340:227–228.
18. Kitchens C. Thrombotic storm. Am J Med 1998;164:381.
19. Belmont HM, Abramson SB, Lie JT. Pathology and pathogenesis of vascular injury in systemic lupus erythematosus. Interactions of inflammatory cells and activated endothelium. Arthritis Rheum 1996;39:9–22.
20. Golden BD, Belmont HM. The role of microvasculopathy in the catastrophic antiphospholipid syndrome: comment on the article by Neuwelt et al (letter). Arthritis Rheum 1997;40:1534–1539.
21. Abramson SA, Belmont HM. SLE: mechanisms of vascular injury. Hospital Practice 1998;33:107–127.
22. Tsai H-M, Lian EC-Y. Antibodies to von Willebrand factor-cleaving protease in acute thrombotic thrombocytopenic purpura. N Engl J Med 1998;339:1585–1594.
23. Cockwell P, Tse WY, Savage CO. Activation of endothelial cells in thrombosis and vasculitis. Scan J Rheumatol 1997;26:145–150.
24. Arnaout MA, Colten HR. Complement C3 receptors: structure and function. Molec. Immun. 1984;21:1191–1199.
25. Kilgore KS, Shen JP, Miller BF, Ward PA, Warren JS. Enhancement by the complement membrane attack complex of tumor necrosis factor-alpha-induced endothelial cell expression of E-selectin and ICAM-1. J Immunol 1995;155:1434.
26. Lozada C, Levin RI, Huie M, Hirschhorn R, Naime D, Whitlow M, et al. Identification of C1q as the heat-labile serum cofactor required for immune complexes to stimulate endothelial expression of the adhesion molecules E-selectin and intercellular and vascular cell adhesion molecules. Proc Natl Acad Sci USA 1995;92:8378–8382.
27. Neng Lai LK, Leung JC, Bil Lai K, Li PK, Lai CK. Anti-DNA autoantibodies stimulate the release of interleukin-1 and interleukin-6 from human endothelial cells. J Pathol 1996;178:451–458.
28. Lai KN, Leung JC, Lai KB, Wong KC, Lai CK. Upregulation of adhesion molecule expression on endothelial cells by anti-DNA autoantibodies in systemic lupus erythematosus. Clin Immunol Immunopathol 1996;81:229–238.
29. Simantov R, LaSala J, Lo SK, Gharavi A, Sammaritano LR, Salmon JE, et al. Activation of cultured vascular endothelial cells by antiphospholipid antibodies. J Clin Invest 1995;96:2211–2219.
30. Bone RC. Why new definitions of sepsis and organ failure are needed. Am J Med 1993;95:348.
31. Nogare D. Septic shock. Am J Med Sci 1991;302:50–65.
32. Waage A, Brandtzaeg P, Espevik T, Halstensen A. Current understanding of the pathogenesis of gram-negative shock. Infect Dis Clin North Am 1991;5:781–789.

14 Infections and Antiphospholipid Antibodies

A. E. Gharavi and S. S. Pierangeli

Historical Background: Serological Test for Syphilis (STS)

Antiphospholipid antibodies (aPL) were detected for the first time in sera from patients with syphilis. Wassermann et al [1] in 1906 used saline extract of liver and spleen of fetus with congenital syphilis as an antigen in a complement fixation test and demonstrated positive reaction with syphilitic sera. The antibody was called Wassermann reagin and the test was introduced as a serological test for syphilis (STS). Although these investigators first believed that in this test, sera reacted with specific antigens derived from *Treponema palladium,* within a year it was shown that extract of normal human or animal tissues reacted similarly with syphilitic sera [2]. The antigenic component of this test was isolated and identified from bovine heart extracts as cardiolipin by Pangborn [3] in 1941. Later, a flocculation test using suspension of liposomes containing cardiolipin, lecithin and cholesterol was adopted

Table 14.1. Antiphospholipid antibodies in infectious diseases.

	References
Viral infections	
Human immunodeficiency virus	Canoso et al [66] (1987); Gris et al [67] (1996); Silvestris et al [68] (1996)
Cytomegalovirus	Cheng et al [69] (1997)
Hepatitis C Virus	Matsuuda et al [70] (1995); Prieto et al [58] (1996); Sanmarco et al [71] (1997); Leroy et al [50] (1998); Giordano et al [72] (1998)
Epstein–Barr Virus	Yamazaki et al [73] (1991)
Varicella zoster virus	Manco-Johnson et al [28] (1996)
Parvovirus B	Gratacos et al [74] (1995)
Bacterial infections	
Syphilis	Santiago et al [22] (1990); Forastiero et al [49] (1996)
Q fever	Galvez et al [25] (1990); Ordi Ros et al [75] (1994)
Lyme disease	Mackworth-Young et al [20] (1988); Garcia Monco et al [76] (1993); Oteo et al [77] (1993)
Mediterranean spotted fever	Chaumentin et al [26] (1997)
Tuberculosis	Adebajo et al [78] (1993)
Mycoplasma	Snowden et al [79] (1990); Catteau et al [21] (1995)
Leprosy	Hojnik et al [52] (1994); Fiallo et al [23] (1998)
Legionnaires' disease	Durupt et al [80] (1996)

as a serodiagnostic test for syphilis referred to as the VDRL (Venereal Disease Research Laboratory) test [4].

False Positive STS Using the Complement Fixation Test for Syphilis and VDRL

The presence of aPL detected as Wassermann reagin in conditions other than syphilis was reported as early as 1907 [2]. Detection of Wassermann reagin in the serum of a person who did not have syphilis was called "biological false-positive serological test for syphilis" (BFP-STS) and in a retrospective study of false-positive reactors, Moore and Mohr identified two distinct groups of patients with acute and chronic reactions [5]. Acute reactions are transient and are seen during non-syphilis infections such as viral pneumonia, viral hepatitis, measles, varicella, and scarlet fever [6]. Vaccination against smallpox may also cause BFP-STS [7]. The chronic BFP-STS reactors whose BFP test persisted for a period of 6 months or more, had a high prevalence of autoimmune disorders such as SLE, Sjögren's syndrome, autoimmune hemolytic anemia, Hashimoto's thyroiditis, and rheumatoid arthritis [5, 8–9]. In 1957, Laurell and Nilsson found that the so-called lupus coagulation inhibitor (or "lupus anticoagulant", LA) was frequently associated with BFP-STS [10] and Lee and Saunders [11] showed that these were aPL, and this observation was confirmed by later studies using monoclonal antibodies [12]. In clinical studies, Bowie et al reported that the lupus anticoagulant was associated paradoxically with thrombotic episodes [13].

Solid Phase Immunoassays for aCL

In 1983 Harris, et al designed a radioimmunoassay using cardiolipin as antigen [14] to detect antibodies to cardiolipin in SLE patients with a positive lupus anticoagulant (LA) test. LA tests detect the ability of aPL antibodies to prolong phospholipid-dependent clotting reactions (such as the activated partial thromboplastin time) in vitro. This assay that was later converted to an enzyme-linked immunoassay (ELISA) [15], was subsequently standardized in several International Workshops [16] and gave a new dimension to the field of aPL antibodies. The anticardiolipin (aCL) ELISA was first thought to be just a more sensitive test for detecting aPL antibodies than STS. However, it was recognized soon that the two tests detected somewhat different antibody populations and not all sera with positive STS were always positive in solid-phase assay for cardiolipin [17]. In fact, the aCL ELISA did not help diagnosing more patients with syphilis, but it resulted in the recognition of a new syndrome characterized by thrombosis, recurrent abortion, and thrombocytopenia associated with aPL antibodies, the antiphospholipid syndrome (APS) [18]. The aCL ELISA is now commonly used to detect autoimmune aCL antibodies, present in APS.

This assay also detected aPL antibodies in patients with other infections [19] such as Lyme disease [20], mycoplasma [21], tuberculosis [22], leprosy [23], Legionnaires disease [24], Q fever [25], Mediterranean spotted fever [26], etc. Furthermore, aPL antibodies in viral infections have also been reported. These include: cytomegalovirus [27], varicella zoster virus [28], human immunodeficiency virus (HIV) [29], hepatitis C [30]. Furthermore, transient LA activity has been reported in patients with Epstein–Barr virus infections [31].

Differentiation of Autoimmune and Infectious-induced aPL: β_2-glycoprotein- I

The association of the aPL detected by solid-phase assays with serious clinical complications such as venous and arterial thrombosis, recurrent spontaneous abortion, stroke and myocardial infarction [18] underlined the importance of differentiating the infection-induced aPL antibodies that seemed not to be associated with these clinical complications, from aPL associated with autoimmune conditions that are closely associated with these life-threatening complications [32]. Several groups studied these two types of aPL antibodies with respect to: the differences in binding to CL and other individual PL [33] or phospholipid mixtures [34], the differences in IgG sub-classes, in light chain distribution and in their affinity [35]. However, most of these findings remained controversial among different investigators [36].

The important observation that the autoimmune aPL antibodies required a lipid binding normal plasma protein which is an inhibitor of coagulation: β_2-glycoprotein I (β_2GPI) by three groups simultaneously in 1990 [37–39] shed a new light on this issue. Matsuura et al reported that binding of aPL in sera from autoimmune diseases (SLE) to CL-coated plates is enhanced by β_2GPI and called these autoimmune aPL "β_2GPI-dependent aPL" [37]. In contrast, the binding of aPL from syphilis sera (infection) is inhibited by β_2GPI, and these infection-associated aPL antibodies were called "β_2GPI-independent aPL" . It is generally believed that β_2GPI-dependent antibodies are associated with clinical features of APS, such as thrombosis and pregnancy losses, and the β_2GPI-independent aPL antibodies are not. These findings were confirmed by other investigators. We purified IgG and IgM aPL antibodies from sera of patients with syphilis, HIV infection, SLE and chlorpromazine-induced aPL and demonstrated that the binding of autoimmune and drug-induced aPL was enhanced by β_2GPI, but the binding of syphilis and HIV induced aPL was significantly inhibited by β_2GPI [40]. Hunt et al used purified IgG, IgA and IgM aPL from patients with infectious or autoimmune diseases and had similar findings [41]. In an elegant study, Celli et al recently studied the interaction of aPL antibodies from two different populations (autoimmune and infectious) with CL arranged in a defined bilayer. In this system, β_2GPI increased, the binding of autoimmune aPL to CL and induced the leakage of the fluorescent probe, carboxyfluorescein (CF), entrapped in the vesicles. In contrast, β_2GPI inhibited the binding of syphilitic aPL to CL-containing vesicles [42]. The authors concluded that CL-β_2GPI complex is the most likely epitope for autoimmune aPL, and in syphilis β_2GPI is not likely to be part of the epitope.

Some studies have shown that syphilis and autoimmune aPL antibodies differ not only in specificity or β_2GPI requirement, but also in functional effects. Campbell et al studied the effects of affinity purified aCL antibodies from APS patients and syphilis on platelet activation and aggregation [43]. These investigators showed that in the presence of low concentrations of platelet activators (thrombin, ADP or collagen), all APS samples ($n = 6$), but none of the syphilis ($n = 5$) samples induced platelet aggregation and activation [43]. In another study, affinity purified aPL antibodies from APS patients and not from syphilis were shown to inhibit the conversion of prothrombin into thrombin (prothrombinase reaction) when liposomes composed of phosphatidylserine and phosphatidylcholine were used to support the enzymatic reaction [44].

Several investigators have reported that autoimmune aPL may bind to β_2GPI coated on irradiated, high-binding or oxidized polystyrene plates [45, 46], and the anti-β_2GPI antibodies that are detected by this method in the sera of APS and SLE patients would represent only the autoimmune ("pathogenic") aPL antibodies [47, 48]. In a recent study, Forastiero et al showed that 29 out of 35 APS samples, and only one out of 37 syphilis sera (that were aCL positive), bound to β_2GPI coated on irradiated ELISA plates, concluding that performing both ELISA (aCL and anti-β_2GPI) makes it possible to distinguish between APS and syphilitic sera [49]. In another recent study, Leroy et al examined the prevalence of aPL, anti-β_2GPI and antiprothrombin antibodies in chronic hepatitis C patients. Twenty-four percent of the patients had low to moderate levels of aCL antibodies, compared with 3.5 % in the control population. In contrast the prevalence of anti-β_2GPI and antiprothrombin antibodies was not different from the control [50]. The presence of aCL antibodies in hepatitis C patients did not correlate with thrombosis or pregnancy losses, indicating that in the absence of associated anti-β_2GPI antibodies aPL is not associated with the clinical complications of APS [50].

In a study involving 58 HIV positive patients, Constans et al showed that 3–4% of the patients were anti-β_2GPI positive, whereas the frequency of aCL antibodies was 41% [51].

β_2GPI-dependent aPL and anti-β_2GPI Antibodies Associated with Infections

Recently, the widely believed dogma that the infection-associated aPL antibodies are β_2GPI independent, do not bind β_2GPI in the absence of phospholipids, and are not associated with thrombosis has been challenged by several reports. (Table 14.2)

In a study, aCL antibodies present in leprosy patients were shown to be heterogeneous with respect to their β_2GPI requirement: in 10 of 31 leprosy sera, the aCL were β_2GPI-dependent and 16 of 31 did not require β_2GPI for binding to CL [52]. These observations were confirmed by other investigators who indicated that these β_2GPI-dependent aPL were associated with thrombosis in leprosy [23].

In another study, parvovirus B19 associated aCL antibodies were shown to be β_2GPI dependent and behaved in a similar fashion as the autoimmune aPL [53]. Furthermore, some cases of viral hepatitis C-associated aPL have been reported to be complicated with thrombosis [54]. (Table 14.2)

Anti-β_2GPI antibodies without aPL were detected in patients with human T lymphotrophic virus-1 (HTLV-1) infections associated with tropical spastic paraparesis (TSP) [55]. TSP, which is also called Jamaican neuropathy, is believed to be an autoimmune condition that complicates the HTLV-1 infection only in a small proportion of patients (about 5%).

In a series of experiments by our group, in 184 samples from non-APS patients who had syphilis or other autoimmune disorders, 18 out of 184 samples were positive for anti-β_2GPI antibodies, yielding a specificity of 82% [56].

Table 14.2. β_2GPI-dependent antiphospholipid antibodies and anti-β_2GPI antibodies associated with clinical features of APS in infectious diseases.

Disease	Clinical complications	References
Parvovirus B 19	n/d	Loizou et al [53] (1997)
Leprosy	Thrombosis	Hojnik et al [52] (1994); Fiallo et al [23] (1998)
Hepatitis C virus	Thrombosis	Prieto et al [58] (1996); Violi et al [81] (1997)
Human immunodeficiency virus	Endothelial cell activation, thrombosis, protein S deficiency, stroke.	Keeling et al [82] (1990); Hassell et al [83] (1994); Narayanan et al [84] (1998);
Epstein–Barr virus	LA and protein S deficiency	Yamazaki et al [73] (1991); Manco Johnson et al [28] (1996)
Adenovirus	LA and hypoprothrombinemia	Jaeger et al [59] (1993)
Cytomegalovirus	Thrombosis	Labarca et al [27] (1997)
Varicella zoster virus	Thrombosis	Manco-Johnson et al [28] (1996); Peyton et al [74] (1998)

The approach of using an anti-β_2GPI assay to diagnose APS and distinguish autoimmune aPL from infection associated aPL seems to have two major problems: (a) the assay is not sensitive enough and many autoimmune aPL may be not detected; (b) some sera with infection-induced aPL (syphilis, leprosy, parvo virus, etc.) may be positive for anti-β_2GPI antibodies.

The clinical significance of finding β_2GPI-dependent and anti-β_2GPI antibodies in infectious diseases sera, remains unknown. It is possible that these anti-β_2GPI antibodies be transient and disappear within two or three months or may raise the question of whether infections may be a *trigger* for the development of aPL antibodies in autoimmune diseases [57], particularly in susceptible individuals.

Do Infections Induce Autoimmune aPL?
Viral Peptide Induced aPL

There are several reports of aPL and/or LA associated with thrombosis in patients with Epstein–Barr virus [28], leprosy [23], cytomegalovirus [27] and HIV infection [51], hepatitis C [30, 58] and adenovirus [59]. These observations may suggest that certain infections in genetically predisposed individuals may induce autoimmunity. This hypothesis is further supported by our recent experiments: following induction of aPL antibodies [60, 61], associated with recurrent fetal death and thrombosis [62] in laboratory animals by immunization with β_2GPI, we induced aPL in mice by immunization with a 15-amino acid peptide representing the PL-binding region of the β_2GPI [63]. These aPL antibodies had properties similar to autoimmune aPL: they were shown to be thrombogenic in an in vivo model of thrombosis and to activate endothelial cells in vivo in an animal model of microcirculation [64]. Then, we identified PL-binding peptides that had structural similarity to the PL-binding site of β_2GPI with viral and bacterial origin that induced aPL and anti-β_2GPI antibodies with properties similar to autoimmune aPL in mice [65]. These findings suggest that incidental immunization, during a subclinical infection, with these viral and bacterial proteins, may trigger aPL antibody production.

References

1. Wassermann A, Neisser A, Bruck C. Eine serodiagnostiche Reaction bei Syphilis. Dtsch Med Wochenschr 1906;32:475–489.

2. Lansdteiner K, Muller R, Potzl O. Zur Frage der Komplementbindungsreaktion bei Syphilis. Wein Klin Wochenschr 1907;20: 565–1569.

3. Pangborn MC. A new serologically active phospholipid from beef heart. Proc Soc Exp Biol Med 1941;48:484–486.

4. Harris A, Rosenberg AA, Riedel L. A microflocculation test for syphilis using cardiolipin antigen. Preliminary report. J Vener Dis Inf 1946;27:169–174.

5. Moore JE, Mohr CF. Biologically false-positive test for syphilis: type, incidence, and cause. JAMA. 1952;150:467–473.

6. Putkonen T. Biologic false-positive seroreactions for syphilis: type, incidence, and cause. JAMA 1952;150:467–473.

7. Lynch FW, Boynton RE, Kimball AC. False positive serologic reactions for syphilis due to smallpox vaccination (vaccinia) JAMA 1941;115:591–595.

8. Moore JE, Lutz WB. Natural history of SLE: approach to its study through chronic biologic false positive reactions. J Chron Dis 1949;1:297–316.

9. Harvey AM, Shulman LE. Systemic lupus erythematosus and chronic biological false-positive test for syphilis. In: Dubouis E, edition. Lupus erythematosus , 4th edn. Los Angeles: University of California Press, 1974;196–209.

10. Laurell AB, Nilsson IM. Hypergammaglobulinemia and biological false positive Wassermann reaction: a study of two cases. J Lab Clin Med 1957;49:694–707.

11. Lee SL, Saunders M. A disorder of blood coagulaiton in SLE. J Clin Invest 1955;34:1814–1822.

12. Thiagarajan P, Shapiro SS, DeMarco L. Monoclonal immunoglobulin M lambda coagulation inhibitor with phospholipid specificity: mechanism of lupus anticoagulant. J Clin Invest 1980;66:397–407.

13. Bowie EJ, Thompson JH Jr, Pascuzzi CA, Owen CA Jr. Thrombosis in SLE despite cirulating anticoagulants. J Lab Clin Med 1963;62:416–420.

14. Harris EN, Gharavi AE, Boey M, Patel BM, Macworth-Young CG, Loizou S et al. Anticardiolipin antibodies: detection by radioimmunoassay and association with thrombosis in systemic lupus erythematosus. Lancet 1983;ii:1211–1214.

15. Gharavi AE, Harris EN, Asherson RA, Hughes GRV. Antiphospholipid antibodies: isotype distribution and phospholipid specificity. Ann Rheum Dis 1987;46:1–6.

16. Harris EN, Gharavi AE, Patel BM, Hughes GRV. Evaluation of the anticardiolipin antibody test: report of an international workshop held April 4 1986. Clin Exp Immunol l; 1987;68:215–222.

17. Harris EN, Gharavi AE, Loizou S, Derue G, Chan JKH, Patel BM et al. Cross-reactivity of antiphospholipid antibodies. J Clin Lab Immunol 1985;16:1–6.

18. Wilson WA, Gharavi AE Hughes syndrome: perspectives on thrombosis and antiphospholipid antibody. Am J Med 1996;101:574–576.

19. Vaarala O, Kleemola M, Palosuo T, Aho K. Anticardiolipin in response in acute infections. Clin Immunol Immunopathol 1986;41:8–15.

20. Mackworth-Young CG, Harris EN, Steere AC, Malawista SE, Hughes GRV, Gharavi AE. Anticardiolipin antibodies in Lyme disease. Arthritis Rheum 1988;31:1052–1057.

21. Catteau B, Delaporte E, Hachulla E, Piette F, Bergoend H. Mycoplasma infection with Stevens–Johnson syndrome and antiphospholipid antibodies: apropos of 2 cases. Rev Med Interne. 1995;16:10–14.

22. Santiago MB, Cossemelli W, Tuma MF, Oliveira RM. Anticardiolipin antibodies in infectious diseases. Clin Rheumatol 1989;8:23–28.

23. Fiallo P, Ninzi. β_2-glycoprotein I-dependent anticardiolipin antibodies as a risk factor for reactions in borderline leprosy patients. Int J Lepr Other Mycobact Dis 1998;66:387–388.

24. Durupt S, Rosselli S, Manchon J, Lopez M. Presence of antiphospholipid antibodies in "Legionnaires disease". Presse Med 1996;25:1649.

25. Galvez J, Martin I, Medino D, Pujol E. Thrombophlebitis in a patient with abute Q fever and anticardiolipin antibodies. Med Clin (Barc) 1997;108:396–397.

26. Chaumentin G, Zenone T, Bibollet C, Denoyel GA, Boibieux A, Biron F et al. Malignant boutonneuse fever and polymyalgia rheumatica: a coincidental association? Infection 1997;25:320–322.

27. Labarca JA, Rabaggliatti RM, Radrigan FJ, Rojas PP, Perez CM, Ferres MV, et al. Antiphospholipid syndrome associated with cytomegalovirus infection: case report and review. Clin Infect Dis 1997;24:197–200.

28. Manco-Johnson MJ, Nuss R, Key N, Moertel C, Jacobson K, Meech S et al. Lupus anticoagulant and protein S deficiency in children with postvaricella purpura fulminans or thrombosis. J Pediatr 1996;128:319–323.

29. Intrator L, Oksenhendler E, Desforgs L. Anticardiolipin antibodies in HIV infected patients with or without autoimmune thrombocytopenia purpura. Br J Haematol 1988;67:269–270.

30. Herzenberg Am, Telford JJ, De Luca LG, Holden JK, Magil AB. Thrombotic microangiopathy associated with cryoglobulinemic membranoproliferative glomerulonephritis and hepatitis C. Am J Kidney Dis 1998;31:521–526.

31. Poux JM, Jauberteau MO, Boudet R, Leroux-Robert C, Loizou F. Transient lupus anticoagulant induced by Epstein–Barr virus infections. Blood Coagul Fibrinolysis.1991;2:771–774.

32. Sammaritano, LR, Gharavi, AE, Lockshin MD. Antiphospholipid antibody: immunologic and clinical aspects. Semin Arthritis Rheum 1990;20:81–96.

33. Harris EN, Gharavi AE, Wasley GD, Hughes GRV. Use of an enzyme-linked immunosorbent assay and of inhibition stduies to distinguish betwen antibodies to cardiolkipin from patients with syphilis or autoimmune disorders. J Infect Dis 1988;157:23–31.

34. Harris EN, Pierangeli SS. A more ELISA assay for the detection of antiphospholipid antibodies. Clin Immunol Newslett. 1995;15:26–28.

35. Levy RA, Gharavi AE, Sammaritano LR, Habina L, Qamar T, Lockshin MD. Characteristics of IgG antiphospholipid antibodies in patients with systemic lupus erythematosus and syphilis. J Immunol 1990;17:1036–1041.

36. Costello PB, Green FA. Reactivity patterns of human anticardiolipin and other antiphospholipid antibodies in syphilitic sera. Infect Immun 1986;51:771–775.

37. Matsuura H, Igarashi T, Fujimoto M, Ichikawa K, Koike T. Anticardiolipin cofactor(s) and differential diagnosis of autoimmune disease (Letter). Lancet 1990;336:177–178.

38. Galli M, Comfurius P, Hemker HC, Debaets MH, van Breda-Vreisman PJC, Barbui T et al. Anticardiolipin antibodies (ACA) directed not to cardiolipin but to a plasma protein cofactor. Lancet 1990;335:1544–1547.

39. McNeil HP, Simpson RJ, Chesterman CJ, Krilis SA. Antiphospholipid antibodies are directed against a complex antigen that includes lipid binding inhibitor of coagulation: B$_2$ glycoprotein I (apolipoprotein H). Proc Natl Acad Sci USA 1990;87:4120–4124.

40. Gharavi AE, Sammaritano LR, Wen J, Miyakawi N, Morse JH, Zarrabi MH et al. Characteristics of HIV and chlorpromazine induced antiphospholipid antibodies: effect of β_2-glycoprotein I on binding to phospholipid. J Rheum 1984;21:94–99.

41. Hunt J and Krilis S. A phospholipid-β_2-glycoprotein I complex is an antigen for anticardiolipin antibodies occurring in autoimmune disease but not with infection. Lupus 1992;1:75–81.

42. Celli M, Gharavi AE, Chaimovich H. Opposite β_2-glycoprotein I requirement for the binding of infectious and autoimmune antiphospholipid antibodies to cardiolipin liposomes is associated with antibody avidity. Biochim Biophys Acta 1999;12:1416:225–238.

43. Campbell AL, Pierangeli SS, Wellhausen S, Harris EN. Comparison of the effects of anticardiolipin antibodies from patients with the antiphospholipid syndrome and with syphilis on platelet aggregation. Thromb Haemost 1995;73:529–534.

44. Pierangeli SS, Goldsmith GH, Krnic S, Harris EN. Differences in functional activity of anticardiolipin antibodies from patients with syphilis and the antiphospholipid syndrome,. Infect Immun 1994;62:4081–4084.

45. Matsuura E, Igarashi M, Yasuda T, Koike T, Triplett DA. Anticardiolipin antibodies recognize β_2-glycoprotein I structure altered by interacting with in oxygen modified solid phase surface. J Exp Med. 1994;179:457–462.

46. Roubey RAS. Autoantibodies to phospholipid-binding plasma proteins: a new view of lupus anticoagulantas and other "antiphospholipid" autoantibodies. Blood 1994;84:2854–2867.

47. Tsutsumi A, Matsuura E, Ichikawa K, Fujisake A, Mukai M, Kobayashi S et al. Antibodies to β_2-glycoprotein I and clinical manifestations in patients with systemic lupus erythematosus. Arthritis Rheum 1996;39:1466–1474.

48. Roubey RA. Comparison of an enzyme-linked immunosorbent assay for antibodies to β_2-glycoprotein I and a conventional anticardiolipin immunoassay. Arthritis Rheum 1996;39:1606–1607.

49. Forastiero RR, Martinuzzo ME, Kordich LC, Carreras LO. Reactivity to β_2-glycoprotein 1 clearly differentiates anticardiolipin antibodies from antiphospholipid syndrome and syphilis. Thromb Haemost 1996;75:717–720.

50. Leroy V, Arvieux J, Jacob MC, Maynard M, Baud M, Zarski JP. Prevalence and significance of anticardiolipin, antiβ_2-Glycoprotein I and anti-prothrombin antibodies in chronic hepatitis C. Br J Haematol 1998;101:468–474.

51. Constans J, Guerin V, Couchouron A, Seigneur M, Ryman A, Blann AD et al. Autoantibodies directed against phospholipids or human β_2-glycoprotein I in HIV-seropositive patients: relationship with endothelial activation and antimalonic dialdehyde antibodies. Eur J Clin Invest 1998;28:115–122.

52. Hojnik M, Gilburd B, Ziporen L, Blank M, Tomer Y, Scheinberg MA et al. Anticardiolipin antibodies in infections are heterogenous in their dependency on β_2-glycoprotein I: analysis of anticardiolipin antibodies in leprosy. Lupus 1994;3:515–521.

53. Loizou S, Cazabon JK, Walport MJ, Tait D, So AK. (1997). Similarities of specificity and cofactor dependence in serum antiphospholipid antibodies from patients with human parvovirus B19 infection and from those with systemic lupus erythematosus. Arthritis Rheum 1997;40:103–108.

54. Giordano P, Galli M, Del Vecchio GC, Altomare M, Norbis F, Ruggeru L et al. Lupus anticoagulant, anticardiolipin antibodies and hepatitis C virus infection in thalassaemia. Br J Haematol 1998;102:903–906.

55. Wilson WA, Morgan Ost C, Barton EN, Smikle M, Hanchard B, lattner WA et al. IgA antiphospholipid antibodies in HTLV-1 associated tropical spastic paraparesis. Lupus 1995;4:138-141.

56. Abreu I, Pierangeli SS, Harris EN. Comparison of threee assays for the detection of antiphospholipid and anti-β_2-glycoprotein I antibodies. Lupus 1998;7:S211.

57. Gharavi AE, Pierangeli SS. Origin of antiphospholipid antibodies: induction of aPL by viral peptides. Lupus 1998;7:S52-S54.

58. Prieto P, Yuste JR, Beloqui O, Civeira MP, Riez JI, Aguirre B et al. Anticardiolipin antibodies in chronic hepatitis C: implication of hepatitis C virus as the cause of antiphospholipid syndrome. Hepatology 1997;23:199–204.

59. Jaeger U, Kapiotis S, Pabinger I, Puchhammer E, Kyrle PA, Lechner K. Transient lupus anticoagulant associated with hypoprothrombinemia and factor XII deficiency following adenovirus infection. Ann Hematol 1993;67:95–99.

60. Gharavi AE, Sammaritano LR, Wen J, Elkon KB. Induction of antiphospholipid autoantibodies by immunization with β_2-glycoprotein I (apolipoprotein H). J Clin Invest 1992;90:1105–1109.

61. Pierangeli SS, Harris EN. Induction of phospholipid-binding antibodies in mice and rabbits by immunization with human β_2-glycoprotein I or anticardiolipin antibodies alone. Clin Exp Immunol 1993;78:233–238.

62. Garcia CO, Kanbour-Shakir A, Tang H, Molina JF, Espinoza LR, Gharavi AE. Induction of experimental antiphospholipid syndrome in PL/J mice following immunization with β_2-GPI. Am J Reprod Immunol 1997;37:118–124.

63. Gharavi AE, Tang H, Gharavi E, Wilson WA, Espinoza LR. Induction of aPL by immunization with a 15 amino acid peptide. Arthritis Rheum 1995;39:S296.

64. Pierangeli SS, Liu Xwei, Harris EN, Gharavi AE. Murine monoclonal antibodies against the phospholipid binding site of human β_2-glycoprotein 1 are thrombogenic and activate endothelial cells. Arthritis Rheum 1997;40:S103.

65. Gharavi EE, Chaimovich H, Cucurull E, Celli C, Tang H. Wilson W, Gharavi AE. Induction of antiphospholipid antibodies by immunization with synthetic viral and bacterial peptides. Lupus 1999;8:449–455.

66. Canoso RT. Anticardiolipin antibodies associated with HTLV-III infection. Br J Haematol 1987;65(4):495–498.

67. Gris JC. The relationship between plasma microparticles, protein S and anticardiolipin antibodies in patients with human immunodeficiency virus infection. Thromb Haemost 1996;76(1):38–45.

68. Silvestris F, Frassanito MA, Cafforio P, Potenza D, Diloreto M, Tucci M, Grizzuti MA, Nico B, Dammacco F. Antiphosphatidylserine antibodies in human immunodeficiency virus-1 patients with evidence of T-cell apoptosis and mediate antibody-dependent cellular cytotoxicity. Blood 1996;87(2):5185–5195.

69. Cheng HM, Khairullah NS. Induction of antiphospholipid autoantibody during cytomegalovirus infection. Clin Infect Dis 1997;25(6):1493–1494.

70. Matsuda J, Saitoh N, Gotoh M, Gohchi K, Tsukamoto M, Syoji S, Mijake K, Yamanaka M. High prevalance of anti-phospholipid antibodies and anti-thyroglobulin antibody in patients with hepatitis C virus infection treated with interferon-α. Am J Gastroenterol 1995;90(7):1131–1141.

71. Sanmarco M, Soler C, Christides C, Raoult D, Weiller PJ, Gerolami V, Bernard D. Prevalence and clinical significance of IgG isotype and anti-$\beta_2$glycoprotein I antibodies in antiphospholipid syndrome: a comparative study with anticardiolipin antibodies. J Lab Clin Med 1997;129(5):499–506.

72. Giordano P, Galli M, Del Vecchio GC, Altomare M, Norbis F, Ruggeri L, et al. Lupus anticoagulant, anticardio;ipin antibodies and hepatitis C virus infection in thalassemia. Br J Haematol 1998;102(4):903–906.

73. Yamazaki M, Asakura H, Kawamura Y, Ohka T, Endo M, Matsuda T. Blood coagul Fibrinolysis 1991;2(6):771–774.

74. Gratacos E, Torres PJ, Vidal J, Font J, Antolin E, Cararach V, Fortuny A. Prevalence and clinical significance of anticardiolipin antibodies in pregnancies comlicated by parvovirus B19 infection. Prenat Diagn 1995;15(2):1109–1113.

75. Ordi-Ros J, Selva-O'Callaghan A, Monegal F, Monasterio-Aspiri Y, Juste-Sanchez C, Vilardell-Torres M. Prevalence, significance, and specificity of antibodies to phospholipids in Q fever. Clin Infect Dis 1994;18(2):213–218.

76. Garcia Monco JC, Wheeler CM, Benach JL, Furie RA, Lukehart SA, Stanek G, et al. Reactivity of neuroborreliosis patients (Lyme disease) to cardiolipin and gangliosides. J Neurol Sci 1993;117(1–2):206–214

77. Oteo Revuelta JA, Elias Calvo C, Martinez de Artola V, Perez Surribas D. Infection by Borrelia burgdorferi in patients with the human immunodeficiency virus. A diagnostic problem. Med Clin (Barc) 1993;101(6):207–209.

78. Adebajo AO, Charles P, Maini RN, Hazleman BL. Autoantibodies in malaria, tuberculosis and hepatitis B in a west African population. Clin Exp Immunol 1993;92(1):73–76.

79. Snowden N, Wilson PB, Longson M, Pumphrey RS. Antiphospholipid antibodies and Mycoplasma pneumoniae infection. Postgrad Med J 1990;66(775):356–362.

80. Durupt S, Rosselli S, Manchon J, Lopez M. Presence of antiphospholipid antibodies in Legionnaires' disease. Presse Med 1996;25(34):1649.

81. Violi F, Ferri D, Basili S. Hepatitis C virus, antiphospholipid antibodies, and thrombosis. Hepatology 1997;25(3):782.

82. Keeling DM, Birley H, Machin SJ. Multiple transient ischemic attacks and a mild thrombotic stroke in a HIV-positive patient with anticardiolipin antibodies. Blood Coagul Fibrinolysis 1990;1(3):333–335.

83. Hassell KL, Kressin DC, Neumann A, Ellison R, Marlar RA. Correlation of antiphospholipid antibodies and protein S deficiency with thrombosis in HIV-infected men. Blood Coagul Fibrinolysis 1994;5(4):455–462.

84. Narayanan TS, Narawane NM, Phadke AY, Abraham P. Multiple abdominal venous thrombosis in HIV-seropositive patient. Indian J Gastroenterol 1998;17(3):105–106.

15   Drug-induced Antiphospholipid Antibodies

L. R. Sammaritano

Autoimmune antiphospholipid antibodies (aPL) have been extensively described, and remain the subject of considerable debate and scrutiny [1, 2]. Pathogenicity of these antibodies has been well documented, including the prospective identification of IgG anticardiolipin antibody (aCL) as a risk factor for deep venous thrombosis and pulmonary embolism in a large cohort of healthy males [3]. The etiology and mechanism of action of these antibodies are becoming clearer as newly adapted molecular biology techniques define epitopes on phospholipid binding proteins [4].

A distinction is made between the autoimmune aPL associated with both systemic lupus erythematosus (SLE) and the primary antiphospholipid antibody syndrome (PAPS), and those aPL secondarily induced by infection or medication. These "non-autoimmune" aPL are common, accounting for up to 50% of lupus anticoagulant (LA) detected in routine coagulation assays [5]. Infection-induced aPL are clearly different from the autoimmune antibodies in both antibody characteristics and potential pathogenicity: they are not associated with thrombotic complications [6]. Analysis of drug-induced aPL yields a more ambiguous picture: pathogenicity of these antibodies is variable, and is closely related to the identity of the specific drug involved. In general, phenothiazine-induced aPL are considered fairly benign [7], while procainamide and other drug-induced aPL are more frequently associated with thrombosis [8]. Drug-induced aPL have long been acknowledged as a significant proportion of non-SLE associated lupus anticoagulants (LA) (5). Lupus syndromes caused by medications have also drawn attention to the presence of drug related aPL antibodies, both as LA and as aCL [9, 10].

Drug-induced Lupus Erythematosus

The induction of autoantibodies in drug-induced SLE has the potential to provide insight into idiopathic autoimmune antibody production. Over 25 drugs have been implicated in producing a lupus-like syndrome [11–13]. Hydralazine and procainamide are the most closely associated drugs [13]; other commonly used medications include isoniazid, phenytoin, and propylthiouracil [14]. Antinuclear antibodies (ANA) develop in at least one-half of patients receiving procainamide [13]. While similar proportions of patients receiving phenothiazines also have a positive antinuclear antibody (ANA), phenothiazines are rarely associated with drug-induced SLE [7]. Criteria for the diagnosis of drug-induced lupus match those for clinical SLE, but, in addition, the drug must have been administered before the onset of SLE symptoms, and the disease process must reverse upon cessation of the drug. Clinical signs and symptoms typically clear within days, although serologic findings, including aPL, may persist for months or years [14, 15]. Drug-induced lupus differs from classic SLE in the characteristics of the populations affected, the specific clinical manifestations, and the autoantibody profile. Occurring in an older age group, the female to male ratio is low and clinical features are milder. Central nervous system (CNS) and renal involvement are rare in the drug-induced disorder [13, 14, 16]. Patients have a characteristic antibody profile with antibodies to single-stranded DNA (ssDNA) and to histones H2A/2B [13, 14, 17–20]. The presence of a genetically determined slow acetylator phenotype for the hepatic enzyme N-acetyl transferase reduces drug metabolism and is a risk factor for drug-induced SLE in patients taking hydralazine, procainamide, and quinidine. The slow acetylator phenotype may predispose to drug-induced aPL as well [13, 14, 16, 19–22].

Drug-induced aPL

Analysis of multiple series of LA-positive patients suggests a 12% prevalence of drug-induced LA [23, 24]. Non-SLE aPL patients (including aPL induced by drug, infection, or malignancy) develop fewer complications than do patients with aPL associated with SLE. No significant association has been found between presence of non-SLE aPL and thrombotic complications or recurrent fetal loss. Rates of thrombosis in patients with drug-induced LA or aCL vary from 0% (with phenothiazines) to 56% (with procainamide). Drugs implicated in both LA and aCL production include chlorpromazine and other phenothiazines, procainamide, quinidine, hydralazine, and phenytoin [24, 25]: with the notable exception of phenothiazines, these are, not surprisingly, drugs which also induce clinical SLE.

Chlorpromazine-induced aPL

Development of a lupus syndrome in chlorpromazine (CPZ)-treated patients is rare, despite the presence of a positive ANA in a majority of these patients [26, 27]. A distinct clinical syndrome secondary to CPZ has been described, however: in addition to the development of ANA and aPL antibodies, up to 50% of treated patients manifest elevated serum levels of IgM and splenomegaly [28, 29]. Prevalence of any aPL (LA or aCL) in schizophrenic patients treated with CPZ varies from 38 to 89% (Table 15.1). Development of a positive aPL is linked to dose and duration of drug therapy [27–30]: there is a positive correlation between both serum IgM level and activated partial thromboplastin time (aPTT) prolongation with either CPZ dose or duration of therapy [28, 30]. Patients are rarely reported to develop thromboses [26–31].

Whether phenothiazines other than CPZ induce aPL is controversial: if so, there is clearly a much lower likelihood of aPL induction. Absolute distinctions are difficult to make since medications are often changed, and patients on newer phenothiazines may have been treated with CPZ in the past [27, 30–32]. Early studies did not reveal an association of autoantibodies with other phenothiazines [28, 33]. A recent evaluation of autoantibody prevalence in 185 patients on long-term neuroleptic therapy does, however, suggest a low but measurable rate of aPL with non-CPZ neuroleptic

Table 15.1. Large series of psychiatric patients evaluated for chlorpromazine-induced aPL.

Author	Medication	n	LA	aCL	IgG aCL	IgM aCL	Comments
Zarrabi, et al 1979 [28]	CPZ ± PTZ	47	42/47				(1)
	CPZ ≤ 2.5 years	28	0/28				
Canoso et al 1982 [29]	CPZ	30	11/30				
	CPZ + PTZ	13	5/13				
	controls	53	0/53				(2)
Canoso et al 1988 [7]	CPZ + LA	54	54/54		3/54	37/54	
	CPZ − LA	42	0/42		0/42	8/42	(3)
Lillicrap et al 1990 [27]	CPZ ± PTZ	71	21/71			23/71 IgM aCL/aPS	
	Non- CPZ PTZ	26	[Total with LA and aCL : 7/26]				
Canoso et al 1990 [31]	CPZ	64	29/64		21/64		
	Non-CPZ PTZ	53	7/53		8/53		
	Non-PTZ						
	Neuroleptics	67	9/67		11/67		
	Controls	35	0/35		0/35		
Metzer et al 1994 [30]	Neuroleptics	27	nr	10/27	7/27	5/27	(4)

nr not reported.
CPZ, chlorpromazine;
PTZ, phenothiazine.

Comments:
(1) 20/42 patients with splenomegaly on nuclear scan.
(2) Controls had no psychiatric disease.
(3) One patient with +LA developed DVT; two patients with low titer IgM aCL developed (1)DVT and (1)DVT/PE.
(4) CVA in patient with (−) aCL; no report of LA status; excluded patients with known cardiovascular disease.

drugs [31]. Patients treated with CPZ alone (minimum of 100 mg/day for at least 1 year), non-CPZ phenothiazines in comparable dosage for at least 1 year, or non-phenothiazine neuroleptics were compared. Forty-five percent of CPZ-treated patients were positive for LA, 34% for aCL, 39% for ANA, and 50% for rheumatoid factor (RF). Small numbers (13–17%) of patients in the non-CPZ treatment groups had positive tests for LA and aCL. Interestingly, all patients had an increased incidence of RF (41–61%), making it unclear whether its presence reflects an association with the drug therapy or with an underlying psychiatric disease. In contrast, the low incidence of aPL in the non-CPZ treated patients suggests that antigenic stimulation and aPL antibody response vary among different antipsychotic medications regardless of underlying diagnosis [31].

Most CPZ-induced aCL are IgM in isotype; the IgG isotype is generally observed in less than 10% of patients [7, 31], although there are exceptions [33]. Like autoimmune aPL, drug-induced LA and aCL are concordant only part of the time [7, 27, 31]. A detailed evaluation of phospholipid-binding specificities of plasmas from phenothiazine-treated psychiatric patients confirmed a discordance in results for LA versus aCL, showing differences in aPL reactivity with the anionic phospholipids phosphatidylserine, phosphatidylinositol, and cardiolipin in enzyme-linked immunosorbent assay (ELISA) [27]. Varying results in activated partial thromboplastin and kaolin clotting times have also been noted. About one-third of

Table 15.2. Reported cases of thrombosis due to phenothiazine-related antiphospholipid antibodies.

Author	Sex	Age	Type of thrombosis	Drug
El-Mallakh et al [38]	F	35	Lacunar infarcts	Perphenazine
Kelley et al [35]	M	52	TIA	Fluphenazine
Mueh et al [36]	F	37	PE	Fluphenazine
	M	66	MCA CVA, DVT	"Phenothiazine"
	M	37	DVT	Haloperidol
Walker et al [37]	M	69	Thrombosis, CABG	Chlorpromazine
	M	55	DVT	Chlorpromazine
Triplett et al [8]	M	–	"complication"	Chlorpromazine
Canosa et al [7]	nr	nr	DVT	Chlorpromazine
	nr	nr	DVT	Chlorpromazine*
	nr	nr	DVT / PE	Chlorpromazine*

*Low level of IgM aCL with negative LA; all other patients LA positive.
DVT, deep venous thrombosis; MCA, middle cerebral artery; CVA, cerebrovascular accident; CABG, coronary artery bypass graft; TIA, transient ischemic attack.

phenothiazine-treated patients have a heterogeneous pattern of antibody reactivity against negatively charged phospholipids. A single study suggests that the majority of IgG aPL reactivity is directed towards phosphatidylserine and cardiolipin but not phosphatidylinositol, in contrast to the more uniform pattern of anionic phospholipid reactivity described for autoimmune aPL [32]. No difference in clinical characteristics between IgG and IgM patients has been noted [33].

The rarity of thrombosis in patients with CPZ – induced aPL is striking [7, 26, 27, 34, 35]. Over a 5-year period only three of 96 prospectively followed CPZ-treated patients developed thromboses [7]. In this series, a single patient with LA developed a deep venous thrombosis (DVT), and two patients with low titer IgM aCL developed DVT (one with subsequent pulmonary embolus) [7]. Table 15.2 presents the cases of phenothiazine-induced aPL with thromboses, taken from six series of several hundred psychiatric patients [7, 8, 35–38].

Procainamide-induced aPL

Procainamide is the medication most closely associated with drug-induced SLE. Unlike phenothiazine-induced aPL, procainamide-induced aPL are often identified as part of a drug-induced autoimmune syndrome [10, 13, 18, 22, 39–42]. The immunoglobulin nature of drug-induced LA was first recognized by Davis et al using column chromatography to purify an "inhibitor" from the plasma of a 59-year-old man with procainamide-induced SLE. LA activity was limited to the IgG fraction [40]. As with idiopathic aPL, most drug-related aPL complications are deep vein thromboses (DVTs) or ischemic strokes [1]. Other thromboses have been reported as well, including a patient with procainamide-induced SLE, IgM aCL and multiple pulmonary emboli [10], and a case of severe retinal vaso-occlusive disease secondary to procainamide-induced lupus with a LA [42].

Procainamide-induced LA may also occur as an isolated finding in the absence of SLE [37, 43–46]. Up to 21% of asymptomatic cardiac patients on procainamide are

Table 15.3. Case reports of procainamide-induced antiphospholipid antibodies.

Author	Sex	Age	aPL	Thrombosis	SLE
Bell et al [22]	M	69	circ.anticoag.	–	+
Davis et al [41]	M	59	circ. anticoag.	–	+
Edwards et al [9]	–	–	LA	–	+
Asherson et al [10]	M	67	IgM aCL	Multiple PE	+
Nichols et al [42]	M	66	LA	Bilateral vaso-occlusive retinopathy	+
Freeman et al [40]	M	68	LA	– *	+
Li et al [45]	M	69	LA	DVT	–
O'Brien et al [44]	F	80	LA	DVT	–
Heyman et al [46]	M	68	LA	–	–
	F	66	LA	–	–
Metzdorff et al [48]	M	75	LA	–	–
List et al [47]	M	63	LA	(L) CVA	–
	M	67	LA	DVT / PE	–
Gastineau et al [25]	[10 patients]		LA	–	+
Walker et al [37]	F	73	LA	CVA/angina	–
Triplett et al [8]	[15 patients]		LA	thrombosis/CVA [n = 11]	–
Derkson et al [23]	[5 patients]		LA	–	–

*Thrombocytopenia (platelet count 8000).
DVT, deep venous thrombosis; CVA, cerebrovascular accident; PE, pulmonary embolus; (L), left.

positive for aCL in a moderate to high titer [43]. As expected, most patients with procainamide-induced aPL are older (mean age 68 years), with a 1:1 female:male sex ratio [25]. As with idiopathic autoimmune aPL, thrombotic complications secondary to drug-induced aPL occur independently of the presence or activity of underlying SLE. The spectrum of clinical complications attributed to procainamide-induced aPL is summarized in Table 15.3, including one case of severe thrombocytopenia [40]. A therapeutic dilemma common in autoimmune LA-positive patients has been reported for a procainamide-treated preoperative patient: anticoagulation parameters for coronary artery bypass surgery were altered by LA-induced prolongation of the activated partial thromboplastin time (aPTT), and frequent intraoperative heparin levels were necessary to monitor anticoagulation (48).

aPL Induced by Other Drugs

Other medications have been reported to induce aPL [8, 23, 25, 37], although this is rare. Drugs other than chlorpromazine or procainamide that have been implicated include hydralazine, quinidine, phenytoin and streptomycin. Chlorpromazine is by far the most common medication associated with drug-induced aPL, although it is not clear whether this reflects, in part, a screening bias due to the accessibility of phenothiazine-treated patients, who are often in hospital. A review of over 650 LA-positive patients in 25 separate studies revealed 78 patients to have drug-induced antibodies; most were attributed to phenothiazines ($n = 69$) or procainamide ($n = 5$), but four patients had aPL induced by hydralazine ($n = 3$), and phenytoin ($n = 1$) [23].

A single series of drug-induced aPL implicated hydralazine ($n = 1$), quinidine ($n = 2$), diphenylhydantoin ($n = 1$) and propranolol ($n = 1$). The single patient on quinidine developed pulmonary emboli, and the patient on diphenylhydantoin had a DVT and arterial occlusive disease. Hydralazine induced splenomegaly without evidence of thrombosis, and the single propranolol-treated patient was asymptomatic [37]. Finally, drugs implicated in the series of 34 drug-induced LA from Triplett et al included quinidine ($n = 7$) and phenytoin [4] in addition to a single case each of valproic acid, amoxycillin, hydralazine, and propranolol. As expected, CPZ and procainamide accounted for a large proportion of positive tests. In this series of LA-positive patients identified by routine coagulation tests, procainamide accounted for 15 cases and CPZ only four cases, again likely influenced by the nature of the population evaluated. Complications, which were defined as thrombosis, abortion, cerebrovascular accident (CVA) and seizures, occurred in 10 of the 34 patients [8].

Therapy

Therapy of drug-induced aPL requires prompt discontinuation of the offending drug. While drug-induced SLE symptoms, if present, resolve within days, serologic abnormalities such as aPL may take months or years to resolve [16, 22, 26, 42, 44]. As with idiopathic autoimmune aPL, therapy involves anticoagulation rather than immunosuppression. Duration of therapy need not be for life, given that the antibody generally disappears over time. There has been a single attempt to use plasmapheresis to eradicate a chlorpromazine-induced aCL in an asymptomatic schizophrenic patient. The therapy was ineffective in reducing the serum aCL level [49].

Genetics

Risk of various drug-related complications has been linked to specific human leukocyte antigen (HLA) genotypes. There is an increased chance of gold-induced proteinuria, for example, in rheumatoid arthritis patients who are DR3 positive [50]. Risk of developing chlorpromazine-induced aPL has been demonstrated to be higher in patients with the HLA alleles Bw44 and DR7 [51–53]. The relative risk of exhibiting a positive aPL or ANA for HLA Bw44-positive patients treated with CPZ is 3.5 [51]. Incidence of DR7 is elevated in idiopathic aPL-positive patients (whether SLE or APS) [54]; this provides a further link between drug-induced aPL and the naturally occurring autoantibodies [52–54].

The increased predisposition to autoantibody formation in schizophrenic patients has been suggested to relate at least partly to the nature of the underlying disease itself [33]. The presence of autoantibodies (including ANA and aCL), underlying psychiatric diagnosis and pharmacological therapy have been analyzed and compared in patients with various chronic mental illnesses [33]. Prevalence of a positive ANA was 40% and correlated with age > 55 years old, female sex, diagnosis of schizophrenia, and CPZ therapy. Chronic administration of CPZ was associated with presence of both ANA and aCL (IgM in particular). The diagnosis of schizophrenia alone was associated with presence of an ANA. IgG and IgM aCL may also be elevated in association with the diagnosis of schizophrenia in untreated patients and has been reported to be elevated in first-degree family members free of disease [55].

Genetic predisposition may be important in susceptibility to other CPZ- related side effects. Tardive dyskinesia is a movement disorder closely associated with CPZ administration. Overall the presence of tardive dyskinesia in neuroleptic-treated patients is about 30%. Ninety-four percent of HLA Bw44 positive patients treated with chlorpromazine, however, show evidence of moderate to severe tardive dyskinesia. The comparable proportion for the HLA Bw44 negative group without immunologic abnormalities is 30% [56].

HLA typing of patients with LA induced by medications other than the phenothiazines has not been extensively evaluated. The presence of the genetically determined slow-acetylator phenotype for the hepatic enzyme N-acetyl transferase is present in most, if not all, patients on procainamide who develop evidence of drug-induced autoimmunity, including LA.

Immunology and Pathogenesis

Understanding the process that leads to autoantibody formation as a response to drug therapy may lend insight into the induction of spontaneous autoantibodies [31, 57, 58]. Chlorpromazine increases cell membrane fluidity, and may impair resealing of large membrane pores. This has been proposed to lead to shedding of membrane antigens, leakage of nuclear immunogens, and possible production of autoantibodies [31]. CPZ itself may react in the presence of ultraviolet light to become antigenic [57], and procainamide has been reported to bind DNA to form an antigenic complex [14, 16]. Wide occurrence of natural anti-procainamide antibodies [58] may also increase occurrence of autoantibody formation because of predisposition or antibody cross-reactivity.

Early studies of circulating inhibitors in procainamide-induced lupus described more than one antibody population within a given sample, although not all circulating anticoagulants behaved as LA. Two separate antibody populations have been described in at least three different drug-induced LA-positive plasmas, with different in vitro mechanisms of action [9, 22, 41]. These have included antibodies directed against factor XII, prothrombin, the prothrombin–thrombin activator complex and factor XI. Isotypes may be IgG or IgM [9]. The multiple epitopes described in drug-induced lupus anticoagulant sera mirror the more recent identification of multiple phospholipid-binding protein epitopes in idiopathic LA.

Antiprothrombin antibodies with reactivity in ELISA have been identified in 55% of LA-positive sera overall, and in 80% of drug-induced cases of LA. An IgG2 predominant pattern is found on subclass analysis [59]. This IgG subclass skewing, also found in autoimmune (but not infection-induced) aCL [60] and in antibodies reactive in the anti β_2-GPI ELISA [61], has been proposed as an important factor in antibody pathogenicity [62]. IgG subclasses have not been reported in CPZ-induced aPL, presumably since most of these antibodies are IgM in isotype.

β_2-glycoprotein I-dependent binding is characteristic of autoimmune aCL, and may be a more specific indicator of thrombosis risk than aCL as measured in the traditional cardiolipin assay [60]. Prevalence of anti β_2-GPI antibody in drug-induced LA is only 40%, considerably lower than that seen in autoimmune aPL [59]. Provocative data regarding epitope specificity in drug-induced aCL, however, documents β_2GPI-dependent binding for CPZ-induced IgM aCL, similar to that seen with autoimmune but not human immunodeficiency virus (HIV)- or syphilis-induced IgG aCL [63, 64]. The dependence of CPZ-induced IgM aCL binding on β_2GPI suggests an epitope specificity similar to that of autoimmune aCL despite the paucity of reported thrombotic complications. While procainamide-induced aCL are predominantly IgG in isotype, subclass distribution has not been reported. Anti-β_2GPI antibodies have been identified, however, in 21% of sera from patients taking procainamide [43], and it is likely that the procainamide-induced pathogenic antibodies are also IgG2 predominant.

Chlorpromazine may provide its own compensatory anticoagulant effect to reduce risk of aPL-related thrombosis. Phenothiazines are cationic amphipathic drugs that inhibit calmodulin and stabilize membranes, which may exert a protective effect against thrombosis at the endothelial cell level [7]. CPZ action on platelet membranes inhibits the aggregation response to physiologic agonists such as adenosine diphosphate (ADP) and may also, in part, explain the lack of thrombotic complications encountered in the CPZ-induced aPL syndromes [27, 64]. As thrombosis is more closely associated with IgG aCL, the IgM isotype reported for most CPZ-induced aCL may reduce relative risk as well. It should be noted, however, that in series of CPZ-induced aCL with a high proportion of IgG antibodies there is not an increased rate of thrombosis [30]. Alternatively, subtle differences in phospholipid epitope specificities may distinguish the CPZ-induced aCL from those associated with SLE or PAPS, and even from other drug-induced (e.g., procainamide-induced) aCL. This is possible given the lack of drug-induced SLE and may relate to the presence of the other immunological abnormalities described with CPZ [7].

Not surprisingly, the IgG isotype predominance of procainamide-induced aCL has been suggested as a possible explanation for the greater pathogenicity of procainamide as opposed to CPZ-induced antibodies. Autoimmune IgM aCL are associated with complications, however, although the risk is lower than that associated with IgG. This may be true for procainamide-induced aCL as well: although primarily IgG in isotype, it is clear that drug-induced IgM aCL may be implicated in thrombosis [10]. It is also possible that procainamide-treated patients may be at increased risk of thrombosis due to the presence of established cardiovascular disease [8, 46].

Summary

The advent of newer neuroleptics with less tardive dyskinesia and fewer other side effects has dramatically decreased the use of chlorpromazine. At present, when chlorpromazine is prescribed, it is usually in an episodic fashion, often for migraine or antiemesis therapy [65, 66]. Procainamide may be less commonly used than in the past as newer antiarrythmics with fewer side effects become available. Drug-induced aPL do not, however, represent a closed chapter in the evolving text of antiphospholipid antibodies. Other medications in common use such as isoniazid and phenytoin may induce aPL, and awareness of drug-induced antibody is still critical. Perhaps more importantly, drug-induced aPL have the potential to serve as a model of idiopathic antibody induction, given that they are similar to autoimmune aPL in phospholipid-binding protein dependence, and may similarly promote thrombosis. Given the appropriate genetic setting, particular medications, in contrast to infections, have the ability to induce antibodies that are closely related to the naturally produced antibodies. Drug-induced aPL present one path of exploration towards understanding idiopathic aPL production and pathogenesis, and may serve as a clue to possible therapeutic intervention: unlike naturally occurring aPL, these pathogenic antibodies have the potential to simply disappear.

References

1. Harris EN, Gharavi AE, Hughes GRV. Anti-phospholipid antibodies. Clin Rheum Dis 1985;11:591–609.
2. Finazzi G, Brancaccio V, Moia M et al. Natural history and risk factors for thrombosis in 360 patients with antiphospholipid antibodies: four year prospective study from the Italian Registry. Am J Med 1996;100:530–536.
3. Ginsberg KS, Liang MH, Newcomer L et al. ACL and the risk for ischemic stroke and venous thrombosis. Ann Intern Med 1992;117:997–1002.
4. Koike T, Ichikawa K, Kasahara H, Atsumi T, Tsutsumi A, Matsuura. Epitopes on β_2GPI recognized by anticardiolipin antibodies. Lupus 1998;7:S14–S17.
5. Schleider MA, Nachman RL, Jaffe EA, Coleman M. A clinical study of the lupus anticoagulant. Blood 1976;48:499–509.
6. Canoso RT, Zon LI, Groopman JE. Anticardiolipin antibodies associated with HTLV-III infection. Br J Haematol 1987;65:495–498.
7. Canoso RT, deOliveira RM. Chlorpromazine-induced anticardiolipin antibodies and lupus anticoagulant: absence of thrombosis. Am J Hematol 1988;27:272–275.
8. Triplett DA, Brandt JT, Musgrave KA, Orr CA. The relationship between lupus anticoagulants and antibodies to phospholipid. JAMA 1988;259:550–554.
9. Edwards RL, Rick ME, Wakem CJ. Studies on a circulating anticoagulant in procainamide-induced lupus erythematosus. Arch Intern Med 1989;141:1688–1690.
10. Asherson RA, Zulman J, Hughes GRV. Pulmonary thromboembolism associated with procainamide induced lupus syndrome and anticardiolipin antibodies. Ann Rheum Dis 1989;48:232–235.
11. Dustan HP, Taylor RD, Corcoran AC, Page IH. Rheumatic and febrile syndrome during prolonged hydralazine therapy. JAMA 1954;154:23–29.
12. Ladd AT. Procainamide-induced lupus erythematosus. N Engl J Med 1962;267:1357–1358.
13. Harmon CE, Portonova JP. Drug-induced lupus: clinical and serological studies. Clin Rheum Dis 1982;8:121–135.
14. Lee SL, Chase PH. Drug-induced systemic lupus erythematosus: a critical review. Semin Arthritis Rheum 1975;5:83–102.
15. Irias JJ. Hydralazine-induced lupus erythematosus-like syndrome. Am J Dis Child 1975;129:862–864.
16. Blomgren SE, Condemi JJ, Vaughn JH. Procainamide-induced lupus erythematosus. Am J Med 1972;52:338–343.
17. Blomgren SE, Condemi JJ, Bignall MC, Vaughn JH. Antinuclear antibody induced by procainamide: a prospective study. N Engl J Med 1969;281:64–66.
18. Mongey AB, Donovan-Brand R, Thomas TJ, Adams LE, Hess EV. Serologic evaluation of patients receiving procainamide. Arthritis Rheum 1992;35:219–223.
19. Hughes GRV, Rynes RI, Gharavi AE, Ryan PFJ, Sewell, Mansilla R. The heterogeneity of serologic findings and predisposing host factors in drug-induced lupus erythematosus. Arthritis Rheum 1981;24:1070–1076.
20. Reidenberg MM. Aromatic amines and the pathogenesis of lupus erythematosus. Am J Med 1983;75:1037–1042.
21. Blumenkrantz N, Christiansen AH, Ullman S, Asboe-Hansen. Hydralazine-induced lupoid syndrome. Acta Med Scand 1974;195:443–449.
22. Bell WR, Boss GR, Wolfson JS. Circulating anticoagulant in the procainamide-induced lupus syndrome. Arch Intern Med 1977;137:1471–1473.
23. Derkson RHWM, Kator L. Lupus anticoagulant: revival of an old phenomenon. Clin Exp Rheum 1985;3:349–357.
24. Love PE, Santoro SA. Antiphospholipid antibodies: anticardiolipin antibodies and the lupus anticoagulant in systemic lupus erythematosus and non-systemic lupus erythematosus disorders. Ann Intern Med 1990;112:682–698.

25. Gastineau DA, Kazmier FJ, Nichols WL, Bowie EJW. Lupus anticoagulant: an analysis of the clinical and laboratory features of 219 cases. Am J Hematol 1985;19:265–275.
26. Canoso RT, Hutton RA. A chlorpromazine-induced inhibitor of blood coagulation. Am J Hematol 1977;2:183–191.
27. Lillicrap DP, Pinto M, Benford K, Ford PM, Ford S. Heterogeneity of laboratory test results for antiphospholipid antibodies in patients treated with chlorpromazine and other phenothiazines. Am J Clin Pathol 1990;93:771–775.
28. Zarrabi MH, Zucker S, Miller F et al. Immunologic and coagulation disorders in chlorpromazine treated patients. Ann Intern Med 1979;91:194–199.
29. Canoso RT, Sise HS. Chlorpromazine-induced lupus anticoagulant and associated immunologic abnormalities. Am J Hematol 1982;13:121–129.
30. Metzer WS, Canoso RT, Newton JEO. Anticardiolipin antibodies in a sample of chronic schizophrenics receiving neuroleptic therapy. Southern Med J 1994;87:190–192.
31 .Canoso RT, deOliviera RM, Nixon RA. Neuroleptic-associated autoantibodies: a prevalence study. Biol Psychiatry 1990;27:863–870.
32. Levy RA, Gharavi AE, Sammaritano LR et al. Characteristics of IgG antiphospholipid antibodies in patients with systemic lupus erythematosus and syphilis. J Rheumatol 1990;17:1036–1041.
33. Yannitsi SG, Manoussakis MN, Mavridis AK et al. Factors related to the presence of autoantibodies in patients with chronic mental disorders. Biol Psychiatry 1990;27:747–756.
34. Kaslow K, Rosse RB, Zeller JA, Nagy JA, Deutsch SI. Phenothiazine-induced lupus anticoagulant. J Clin Psychiatry 1992;53:103–104.
35. Kelley RE, Gilman PB, Kovacs AG. Cerebral ischemia in the presence of lupus anticoagulant. Arch Neurol 1984;41:521–523.
36. Mueh JR, Herbst KD, Rapaport SI. Thrombosis in patients with the lupus anticoagulant. Ann Intern Med 1980;92:156–159.
37. Walker TS, Triplett DA, Javed N, Musgrave K. Evaluation of lupus anticoagulants: antiphospholipid antibodies, endothelium associated immunoglobulin, endothelial prostacyclin secretion, and antigenic protein S levels. Thromb Res 1988;51:267–281.
38. El-Mallakh RS, O'Donaldson JO, Kranzler HR, Racy A. Phenothiazine-associated lupus anticoagulant and thrombotic disease. Psychosomatics 1988;29:104–113.
39. Meisner DJ, Carlson RJ, Gottlieg AJ. Thrombocytopenia following sustained release procainamide. Arch Intern Med 1985;145:700–702.
40. Freeman NJ, Fajardo L, Carvalho A. Simultaneous procainamide-induced immune thrombocytopenia and lupus anticoagulant. Am J Hematol 1995;48:133–134.
41. Davis S, Furie BC, Griffin JH, Furie B. Circulating inhibitors of blood coagulation associated with procainamide-induced lupus erythematosus. Am J Hematol 1978;4:401–407.
42. Nichols CJ, Mieler WF. Severe retinal vaso-occlusive disease secondary to procainamide-induced lupus. Ophthalmology 1989;96:1535–1540.
43. Merrill JT, Shen C, Gugnani M, Lahita RG, Mongey AB. High prevalence of antiphospholipid antibodies in patients taking procainamide. J Rheumatol 1997;24:1083–1088.
44. O'Brien DC, Shimomura SK. DIAS Rounds: drug information analysis service: Procainamide and the lupus anticoagulant. Drug Intell Clin Pharm 1984;18:971
45. Li GC, Greenberg CS, Curric MS. Procainamide-induced lupus anticoagulants and thrombosis. Southern Med J 1988;81:262–264.
46. Heyman MR, Flores RH, Edelman BB, Carliner NH. Procainamide-induced lupus anticoagulant. Southern Med J 1988;81:934–936
47. List AF, Doll DC. Thrombosis associated with procainamide-induced lupus anticoagulant. Acta Haematol 1989;82:50–52.
48. Metzdorff MT, Hansen KS, Wright GL, Fried SJ. Interference with anticoagulation monitoring by procainamide-induced lupus anticoagulant. Ann Thorac Surg 1996;61:994–995.
49. Matsukawa Y, Satoh M, Itoh T et al. Plasmapheresis for a schizophrenic patient with drug-induced lupus anticoagulant. J Int Med Res 1996;24:147–150.
50. Woody PH, Griffin J, Panayi GS et al. HLA-DR antigens and toxic reaction to sodium aurothiomalate and D-penicillamine in patients with rheumatoid arthritis. N Engl J Med 1980;303:300–308.
51. Canoso RT, Lewis ME, Yunis EJ. Association of HLA Bw44 with chlorpromazine-induced autoantibodies. Clin Immunol Immunopathol 1982;25:278–282.
52. Vargas-Alarcon G, Yamamoto-Furusho JK, Zuniga J, Canoso RT, Granados J. HLA DR7 in association with chlorpromazine-induced lupus anticoagulant. J Autoimmunity 1997;10:579–583.
53. Tincani A, Carella G, Balestrieri G, Cattaneo R. Antiphospholipid antibodies and HLA. Clin Exp Rheumatol 1986;4:294–295.

54. Sammaritano LR. Pediatric and familial antiphospholipid syndromes. In: The Antiphospholipid Syndrome. RA Asherson, R Cervera, JC Piette, Y Shoenfeld, editors. Boca Raton: CRC Press, 1996;259–266.

55. Firer M, Sirota P, Schild K, Elizur A, Slor H. Anticardiolipin antibodies are elevated in drug-free, multiply affected families with schizophrenia. J Clin Immunol 1994;14:73–78

56. Canoso TR, Romero JA, Yunis EJ. Immunogenetic markers in chlorpromazine-induced tardive dyskinesia. J Neuroimmunol 1986;12:247–252.

57. Kahn G, Davis BP. In vitro studies on long wave ultraviolet light-dependent reactions of the skin photosensitize chlorpromazine with nucleic acids, purines, and pyrimidines. J Invest Dermatol 1970;55:47–52.

58. Russell AS, Ziff M. Natural antibodies to procainamide. Clin Exp Immunol 1968;3:901–909.

59. Arvieux J, Darnigl L, Caron C, Bensa JC, Colomb MG. Development of an ELISA for autoantibodies to prothrombin showing their prevalence in patients with lupus anticoagulants. Thromb Haemost 1995;74:1120–1125.

60. Gharavi AE, Harris EN, Lockshin MD, Hughes GRV, Elkon KB. IgG subclass and light chain distribution of anticardiolipin and anti-DNA antibodies in systemic lupus erythematosus. Ann Rheum Dis 1988;47:286–290.

61. Arvieux J, Roussel B, Ponard D, Colomb MG. IgG2 restriction of anti-β_2 glycoprotein I antibodies in autoimmune patients. Clin Exp Immunol 1994;95:310–315.

62. Gharavi AE, Sammaritano LR, Wen J et al. Characteristics of human immunodeficiency virus and chlorpromazine-induced antiphospholipid antibodies: effect of β_2-glycoprotein I on binding to phospholipid. J Rheumatol 1994;21:94–99.

63. Matsuura E, Igarashi Y, Fujimoto M, Ichikawa K, Koike T. Anticardiolipin cofactor(s) and differential diagnosis of autoimmune disease. Lancet 1990;336:177–178.

64. Mills DCB, Roberts GCK. Membrane active drugs and the aggregation of human platelets. Nature 1967;213:35–38.

65. Owens DG. Adverse effects of antipsychotic agents. Do newer agents offer advantages? Drugs 1996;51:895–930.

66. Cameron JD, Lane PL, Speechley M. Intravenous chlorpromazine versus intravenous metoclopramide in acute migraine headache. Acad Emerg Med 1995;2:597–602.

16 Antiphospholipid Antibodies and Antiphospholipid Syndromes in Children

L. B. Tucker

Introduction

The scientific and clinical understanding of the phenomenon of antiphospholipid antibodies (aPL) has grown enormously since the first descriptions of an inhibitor of in vitro clotting tests in the serum of some patients with systemic lupus erythematosus (SLE) by Conley and Hartman [1], and the subsequent connection of these inhibitors to the occurrence of thromboses [2]. The lupus anticoagulant described in these early studies was found to be an antibody directed against phospholipid [3]. Extensive studies of adult populations has further identified the primary clinical associations of aPL; recurrent venous and arterial thromboses, thrombocytopenia, and recurrent fetal losses [4, 5]. Other less common or minor clinical findings described in adults with aPL include valvular heart disease, early myocardial infarction, pulmonary hypertension, renovascular microthrombotic disease, hemolytic anemia, transverse myelitis, chorea, and livedo reticularis [6].

In comparison to the enormous amount of information concerning aPL in adults, there has been relatively less research in the area of aPL in pediatrics [7–10]. The presence of aPLs and associated clinical events have been well described in some children with SLE but occurs in those without SLE as well. In children, the most common reported clinical problem associated with aPL is that of cerebral ischemic stroke, in general a relatively rare occurrence in childhood. The less common thrombotic events in children found to have aPL have mainly been the subject of individual case reports.

This chapter will review the current state of knowledge of aPL in pediatrics. The focus of the chapter will be clinical; to date, there is no information to suggest that aPL in children are immunochemically different from those found in adults.

Clinical Associations of aPL in Childhood

Although the first description of aPL was in patients with SLE, it is well known that aPL can be found in a number of other conditions. Infections, certain medications, and other autoimmune conditions can be associated with the development of aPL, although not all may be associated with clinical events. The incidence of aPL in healthy populations is generally low, if the testing is done in a reliable laboratory [5]. The incidence of aPL in a healthy pediatric population has not been determined in a large and reliable study. A study done by Kontiainin et al in Finland reported a surprisingly high incidence of positive IgG anticardiolipin antibodies (aCL) (82%) in healthy children compared with 27% of adults positive [11]. The significance of such a high percentage of well children testing positive for aCL is unknown, particularly since these results are very different from those found in other studies. Few other studies of children with aPL have included healthy control children; these are listed in Table 16.1 [12–15]. As shown, the incidence of aPL in healthy children in all of these studies appears to be well under 10%. Larger population-based studies with different ethnic groups need to be done to provide more accurate data.

aPL have been described in adult patients with a broad range of infections, including acute common viral infections [16]. Infection-related aPL differ immunochemically from those seen in patients with autoimmune disease and have not been associated with the typical clinical features of aPL. Kratz et al [15] studied a group of 88 children with primarily upper airway infections and found 30% were positive for aPL. The majority of the aPL identified were IgM isotype as would be expected in an acute infection. In the same study, 22% of a group of 20 children with inherited metabolic conditions and 25% of children with a variety of conditions including malignancies (excluding autoimmune diseases) were also positive for aPL. None of the children with positive aPL and infection, metabolic disease, or other conditions in this study developed thrombosis, consistent with findings in adult populations. Therefore, it is important for clinicians to remember that aPL can be found incidentally in children after any common viral infection. Since most children suffer from frequent viral infections, all positive aPL titers should be verified on at least two occasions, preferably at a time when the child has not had a recent infection.

In one study of children with human immunodeficiency virus (HIV) infection, 82% of the patients were found to have IgG aCL [17]; these results are similar to those described in adults with HIV as well.

There has been controversy concerning a possible association of aPL and clinical findings in acute rheumatic fever (ARF). Figueroa et al reported that 80% of their patients with active ARF had aCL compared with 40% of those with inactive ARF [18]. The control subjects in this study, however, were adults. No correlation could be established between the presence of chorea and aCL positivity. The authors reported a correlation of carditis and IgM aCL; however, this conclusion was based on the results from only six children with carditis (100% positive for IgM aCL) compared with eight children without carditis (37% of whom were positive for IgM aCL). A second study of

Table 16.1. Incidence of antiphospholipid antibodies in healthy children.

Reference	No. patients	% + aPL (IgG: IgM if available)
Caporali et al [12]	42	IgG 0%; IgM 5%
Shergy et al [13]	15*	7%
Singer et al [14]	20	IgG 10%
Kratz et al [15]	20	IgG 0; IgM 5%
Kontiainen et al [11]	173	IgG 82%

* Patients had asthma.

children with ARF [19] could not substantiate elevated aCL levels in children with ARF compared with healthy children as controls, and there was no correlation of aCL with disease activity.

The presence of aPL has been examined in several small groups of children with tic disorders who do not have autoimmune disease. Although one study [20] suggested the presence of lupus anticoagulant and aCL in 4/9 children with Tourette's syndrome, a larger study done by Singer et al [14] did not show a significant increase in prevalence of aPL in 21 children tested, compared with healthy age-matched control subjects.

The presence of IgG aCL has been shown in 24% of a group of 29 children and adolescents with insulin-dependent diabetes mellitus (type 1 diabetes) [21]. Patients with aCL antibodies had a shorter disease duration than those without aCL; however, there were no other autoantibodies or specific clinical associations among these patients.

The prevalence of aPL among children with juvenile chronic arthritis (JCA) has ranged from 8–53% in a small number of studies [12, 22, 23]. However, there has not been any association of thrombosis or other aPL-related clinical events in aPL+ children with JCA, nor does there appear to be any association with JCA subtype or other characteristics of the disease. There is only one reported case of a child with JCA who developed a deep vein thrombosis (DVT) and was found to be positive for lupus anticoagulant (LA); however, this child was also immobilized due to a lower limb fracture and therefore had an additional risk factor for development of DVT [24]. Therefore, aPL in children with JCA may be an incidental finding.

The clinical significance of positive aPL or LA discovered incidentally in children is unknown, and a matter of concern. A recent study examined and followed 95 children found to have LA, identified in a single pediatric tertiary care center over a 27-year time period [25]. Eighty-four percent of these children had a LA diagnosed incidentally, in most cases during preoperative screening tests. One of these patients was found to have SLE. However, in follow-up, none of these asymptomatic children developed bleeding, thrombosis, or autoimmune disease. This study provides evidence that most children with a LA discovered incidentally during laboratory screening will not have any clinical manifestations of antiphospholipid syndrome (APS), both at the time of diagnosis and in further follow-up.

aPL in Childhood-onset SLE

aPLs have been reported present in a high frequency of adult patients with SLE. Adult patients with SLE and associated aPLs have a high risk of thromboembolic events of all types, cardiac valvular disease, thrombocytopenia and other autoimmune cytopenias. Similarly, studies examining children with SLE have reported finding aPLs in 19–87% of patients (Table 16.2) [8, 13, 22, 26–30]. In some cases, a thrombosis associated with aPL was the presenting sign for the diagnosis of SLE [31]. These studies of small populations of pediatric patients with SLE are somewhat limited by small numbers of patients included (average of 30 subjects per study) and variation in laboratory testing methods for aPLs.

Investigators have attempted to show whether the presence of a positive aPL in children with SLE is associated with specific clinical events with varying results. In looking at thrombosis in pediatric patients with SLE, studies show a wide variation

Table 16.2. Antiphospholipid antibodies in pediatric systemic lupus erythematosus (case series).

Reference	No. patient	% aPL +	% aCL/% LA
Molta et al [30]	37	38	19/11
Montes de Oca et al [29]	120	19	ND/19
Shergy et al [13]	32	50	50/ND
Gattorno et al [22]	19	90	79/42
Ravelli et al [27]	30	87	87/20
Berube et al [32]	59	–	19/24
Massengill et al [26]	36	67	50/6
Seaman et al [28]	29	65	66/62

in incidence, ranging from 7/29 (24%) [28] to 1/30 (3%) [27]. In most studies, there appears to be a clear association of aPL with thrombotic events. Several studies suggest that the presence of a LA confers a higher risk for thrombosis than aCL antibodies alone [22, 28, 32]. Berube et al [32] showed a significant relationship of a positive LA test to thrombotic events, with a less significant trend of relationship of a positive aCL to thrombosis. However, Ravelli et al [27] did not find an association of thrombotic events with aPL positivity in a group of 30 children with SLE, 87% of whom were positive for at least one aPL. In a recent study, Massengill et al [26] studied a group of 36 children with lupus nephritis, finding 67% positive for aPL and 22% having had a thrombotic event; however, aPL positivity was not significantly increased among the patients who suffered thrombosis.

The types of thrombotic events reported in these studies, and in case reports [13, 22, 26, 28–30, 32–36], include DVTs, ischemic stroke, retinal artery occlusion, renal artery thrombosis, pulmonary embolism, transverse myelitis and superior vena cava (SVC) thrombosis. These reports should alert clinicians caring for children with SLE to investigate all patients who present with these clinical findings for the presence of aPL, particularly since therapeutic management will be affected if the child is aPL positive. The implication of finding a positive aPL in a child with SLE who has not developed any clinical problem which could be related to the aPL is less clear. Many clinicians are treating such patients with low- aspirin but are reluctant to give oral anticoagulation unless a documented thrombosis has occurred.

Some studies have examined the association of aPL in pediatric SLE patients and central nervous system (CNS) disease of SLE. Shergy et al [13] reported that the highest titers of aCL seen among a group of 32 children with SLE were found in those with CNS disease, although overall there was no significant difference in the prevalence of aCL in patients with CNS disease and those without. Ravelli et al commented that of nine patients who developed increasing high titers of IgG aCL during follow-up, six had neuropsychiatric manifestations [27]. Although these data are suggestive that children with SLE and aPL, particularly those with high titer aPL, may be at higher risk of developing aPL-related CNS disease, larger prospective studies are needed to determine the level of risk.

Two studies [27, 28] have reported a trend towards positive aCL in children with SLE who have autoimmune cytopenias. In several studies, aPL titers were determined in serial samples over time and attempts were made to correlate disease activity or treatment with aPL titers. In every instance, aPL titers were found to fluctuate widely over time in the same patient [13, 22, 26, 28]. It was unclear from these small studies whether increases of aPL accompanied active disease. Some patients with aPL who were treated aggressively with cyclophosphamide for their disease activity were found to have decreased or negative aPL titers after their treatment course [22, 28].

aPL-associated Clinical Events

The major clinical events associated with aPL are arterial or venous thrombosis, thrombocytopenia, and recurrent fetal loss. Minor, or less common, clinical events also associated with aPL include livedo reticularis, migraine, chorea, transverse myelitis, cardiac valvular abnormalities, Coomb's positivity, and hemolytic anemia. Most of these clinical findings have been described in children (excluding recurrent fetal loss which will not be addressed in this review), although some are quite rare. aPL-associated events have been described in children of all ages, even some as young as a few months of age.

Thrombosis

Thrombosis, either of arterial or venous vessels, is a central pathogenic phenomenon leading to a long list of clinical problems that have been related to the presence of aPL. In contrast to adults, thrombosis in general is a very uncommon clinical problem in pediatrics. Therefore, the finding of elevated aPL in many children with thrombotic conditions reported in an ever increasing number of studies suggests that the presence of aPL is one of the most common precipitating factors for this clinical problem when it occurs in children. Venous and arterial thromboses have been reported in children. The range of clinical problems that may result from thrombosis associated with aPL is shown in Table 16.3. The specific types of thrombotic and neurologic problems reported in the literature in children with aPL are shown in Table 16.4.

Venous occlusions due to aPL can occur in any blood vessel. Deep vein thrombosis is the most common venous thrombotic condition reported in children associated with aPL. In some cases the DVT was accompanied by pulmonary embolism [29, 31, 37], suggesting that clinicians evaluating a child with DVT should carefully evaluate the patient for other concomitant thrombosis. Pulmonary hypertension related to microthromboembolic phenomenon is rare but reported in children [38], and therefore APS should be included in the differential of a child presenting with idiopathic

Table 16.3. Clinical conditions resulting from thrombosis associated with aPL in children.

Deep vein thrombosis	Cerebral ischemic stroke
Pulmonary embolism	Chorea
Pulmonary hypertension	Transverse myelitis
Budd–Chiari syndrome	Myocardial infarction
Addison's disease	Renal arterial thrombosis
Cerebral sinus thrombosis	Renal thrombotic microangiopathic disease
Renal vein thrombosis	

Table 16.4. Antiphospholipid-associated clinical events in children (not associated with SLE)

Reference	No. patients	Neurologic events	Thrombotic events	Additional comments
Bernstein et al [39]	2		Iliac vein, DVT, partial Budd–Chiari	
Sheridan-Pereira et al [63]	1		Neonatal aortic thrombosis	Mother aCL +
Falcini et al [42]	1	Chorea	Myocardial infarction	Thrombocytopenia, livedo reticularis
Vlachoyiannopoulous [71]	1	Chorea	DVT	
Roddy and Giang [70]	1	Infantile stroke		
Ravelli et al [72]	1		SVC thrombosis	
Silver et al [63]	2	Fetal stroke		Mothers aCL +
Hasegawa et al [50]	1	Spinal cord infarction		
Schoning et al [47]	8	Ischemic stroke		
Toren et al [55]	19	Ischemic stroke (1) Tourettes (3)	DVT (3)	Thrombocytopenia (10) IgA nephritis (1) Vasculitis (1)
Angelini et al [43]	10	Cerebral ischemia		
Olson et al [46]	2	Ischemic stroke		Family + for primary APS
Manco-Johnson and Nuss [31]	14	Ischemic stroke	Pulmonary embolism, central venous, arterial	
Di Nucci et al [45]	1	Ischemic stroke		
Baca et al [69]	10	Ischemic stroke		
Von Scheven et al [38]	5	Ischemic stroke, chorea	Pulmonary embolism	Digital ischemia, Addison disease
Brady et al [40]	1		Portal vein thrombosis	
Nuss et al [37]	3		Pulmonary embolism DVT	
Ohtomo et al [52]	1			Renal thrombotic microangiopathy
Male et al [25]	5	TIA (1)	DVT (4)	

pulmonary hypertension. aPL is likely a primary precipitant of Budd–Chiari syndrome, the thrombotic occlusion of the inferior vena cava and hepatic veins. There are a number of reports of children with Budd–Chiari syndrome who have elevated aPL [39] and it is likely that other children with this syndrome may have associated aPL but have not yet been tested. One case of isolated portal vein thrombosis has been reported secondary to APS [40]. Addison's disease and hypoadrenalism are also known to be caused by infarction of the adrenal glands due to aPL [41]; this has also been reported in children [38]. Myocardial infarction at a young age should prompt the clinician to search for aPL, as there have been rare reports of this relationship in children [42].

Cerebral ischemic stroke is the most common neurologic event reported in association with aPL, and the most common arterial thrombotic condition. Increasingly, it is becoming clear that a significant proportion of children who suffer idiopathic stroke, at any age, have elevated aPL [43–46]. Angelini and colleagues reported that among an unselected group of 13 children with idiopathic cerebral ischemia, 76% had moderate- to high-titer aPL [43]. Of great interest is the finding that 50% of these children had multiple ischemic events. A study by Schoning et al confirms these findings [47]. These data suggest that aPL in children may rarely be associated with a condition similar to multi-infarct dementia in adults [48, 49].

There are other less-common arterial thrombotic conditions reported in children with aPL, in association with SLE or not. Renal artery thrombosis, retinal artery thrombosis, and myocardial infarction have been reported in rare situations in children with high titers of aPL. Transverse myelitis, seen rarely in children with SLE, appears to be a thrombotic complication of aPL in nearly all cases [50]. Renal thrombotic microangiopathy, a rare finding in adults with APS [51], has been also described in an adolescent with primary APS who presented with severe hypertension, renal impairment, and a history of Raynaud's phenomenon [52].

Thrombocytopenia

Thrombocytopenia is one of the major clinical associations of aPL reported in adults, and is one of the criteria for diagnosis of the APS. Patients with SLE and thrombocytopenia have a very high incidence of APL [5], as do those with Evans' syndrome (hemolytic anemia and thrombocytopenia) [53]. APL were found as well in 30% of patients with chronic idiopathic thrombocytopenic purpura (ITP) [54]. Thrombocytopenia has been reported in children with primary APS and in two-thirds of children with SLE and aPL [28]. Toren et al reported thrombocytopenia present in 52% of the children they reviewed with primary APS [55]. Ura et al described a 3-year-old child with immune thrombocytopenic purpura and aPL who later developed clinical findings suggesting APS [56].

Other Clinical Features

Chorea has been reported in children with aPL, either in association with SLE or not, similar to what is seen in adults [35, 57, 71]. Livedo reticularis is mentioned frequently in children with APS as a concomitant clinical finding.

Hematologic abnormalities other than thrombocytopenia may occur with some frequency in patients who have aPL. Patients with autoimmune hemolytic anemia and Evans syndrome have been reported to have a high frequency of associated aPL. In one report of 12 SLE patients with aPL and Evans' syndrome, two of the patients had childhood-onset SLE [53]. Gattorno et al reported two adolescent girls presenting with autoimmune hemolytic anemia who later developed thrombosis and were found to have aCL and/or LA [22].

Neonatal Effects of aPL

One of the more interesting questions concerning aPLs is whether transplacentally transferred aPL can cause clinical problems in human infants. Investigators have shown that pregnant mice injected with human monoclonal aPL exhibit an increase in fetal wastage related to placental insufficiency and thrombosis [58]. However, the issue is not as clear when one looks at human mothers and infants.

Three studies have examined a total of 129 newborns born to women with aPL detected during or before pregnancy [59–61]. No significant aPL-related clinical pathology was detected in these studies. In one study [61], mothers were treated with calcium heparin during the pregnancy, and although there was an increased rate of prematurity, no other problems were seen in these infants. In a study by Botet et al [60], 33 pregnancies were studied. All the women were treated with low-dose aspirin and again, a higher than expected rate of prematurity was found but no other problems.

Despite these encouraging studies, there is an increasing number of case reports of infants suffering neonatal stroke or thrombosis who were found to have aPL, and whose mothers were then identified as having aPL as well. Contractor et al [62] described a neonate with renal vein and vena caval thrombosis. The infant and mother were both positive for IgG aCL, with antibodies disappearing in the infant after 4 months of age, supporting the suggestion of a transplacental transfer of aCL in this case. Silver et al described two infants with cerebral infarctions at ages 6 and 7 months of age whose mothers were positive for aCL [63], and Sheridan-Pereira et al described an infant with aortic thrombus whose mother had a positive LAC [64]. Hage et al described an infant with hydrops fetalis and a fetal renal vein thrombosis whose mother had aPL detected postpartum [65]. Although these are obviously rare occurrences described in case reports, they suggest that not all transplacentally trans-ferred aPL is benign. All infants with thromboses, and their mothers, should be inves-tigated for the presence of aPL. The important question remains however; what is the risk to an infant born to a mother with known aPL? Further large studies are required to answer this question, which will provide information in deciding whether treat-ment of pregnant women with aPL is necessary for protection of the fetus from harm.

Primary APS in Children

Primary APS is a disorder, described by Hughes and colleagues [6, 66], in which patients have documented aPL (IgG or IgM aCL or LA) with one or more major clinical manifestations of aPL (thrombosis, recurrent fetal loss, or thrombocyto-penia). These patients do not have the diagnosis of SLE or any other underlying autoimmune condition. The actual prevalence of APS in pediatrics is not known although many of the children reported in the literature with aPL-related clinical problems would fulfill these criteria for the diagnosis of APS (Table 16.4). Primary APS may be less common in childhood than in adults, as most major pediatric rheumatology center may only follow one or two such patients. However, it could be suggested that the criteria for diagnosing APS may not be appropriate for chil-dren since recurrent fetal loss is not a pediatric problem. If cerebral ischemic stroke was added to the clinical criteria for pediatric APS, the sensitivity for diagnosing children with APS might be greatly enhanced.

Treatment of APS and aPL-related Events in Children

The treatment of children with APS or aPL-related events in children has been similar to adults with these problems; however, there are not standard recommendations for therapy based on long term observation of the outcome of APS in children. In adults, the standard recommendations are [6, 67, 68]:

1. No therapy in asymptomatic individuals who are identified with aPL or LA and who have no evidence of autoimmune disease.
2. Long-term intensive oral anticoagulation with warfarin for individuals who have had a thrombosis associated with positive aPL or LA (whether or not the individual has SLE or any other autoimmune disease).

Ravelli and Martini, in a review of aPL in pediatrics, recommend no therapy of a child who has aPL but is asymptomatic [8]. The study by Male et al would substantiate this approach, as all asymptomatic patients identified with LA in their study remained well on follow-up [25]. Antithrombotic therapy is recommended for children who present with thrombosis and have aPL and/or LA; however, the duration and intensity of this therapy is a question. Several sources [8] have suggested "intermediate intensity anticoagulation therapy" for such patients. The effectiveness of such therapy and the length of treatment required are unknown. Ravelli's previous review of this subject suggested the need for anticoagulation for children who experienced a thrombotic event and had a persisting aPL. Many clinicians are hesitant to recommend long-term aggressive anticoagulation of children given that the potential risks for hemorrhage in active children may exceed the risk of recurring thrombosis. The report of Baca et al [69] describing 10 children with cerebral infarctions in association with aPL provides a picture of the current state of confusion and lack of consistency in treating such patients. In their study, one child had a "lupus-like" disease and was treated with intravenous methylprednisolone and cyclophosphamide. All aCL positive patients were treated with low-dose aspirin and no recurrences of cerebral infarctions or other thromboses were seen over a 15-month follow-up. No patient underwent oral anticoagulation with warfarin. Until large-scale, multicenter studies are undertaken to determine the natural history of children who have had a thrombosis or clinical problem due to aPL, the necessity for treatment is unknown and certainly the type and duration of treatment can not be rationally determined.

References

1. Conley CL, Hartman RC. A hemorrhagic disorder caused by circulating anticoagulant in patients with disseminated lupus erythematosus. J Clin Invest 1952;31:621–622.
2. Bowie EJ, Thompson JH, Pascuzzi CA, Owen CA. Thrombosis in systemic lupus erythematosus despite circulating anticoagulants. J Lab Clin Med 1963;62:416–430.
3. Harris EN, Gharavi AE, Boey ML. Anticardiolipin antibodies: detection by radioimmunoassay and association with thrombosis in systemic lupus erythematosus. Lancet 1983;2:1211–1214.
4. Alarcon-Segovia D. Clinical manifestations of the antiphospholipid syndrome. J Rheumatol 1992;19:1778–1781.
5. Sammaritano LR, Gharavi AE, Lockshin MD. Antiphospholipid antibody syndrome: immunologic and clinical aspects. Semin Arthritis Rheum 1990;20:81–96.
6. Ames PRJ, Khamashta MA, Hughes GRV. Clinical and therapeutic aspects of the antiphospholipid syndrome. Lupus 1995;4:S23–S25
7. Tucker LB. Antiphospholipid syndrome in childhood: the great unknown. Lupus 1994;3:367–369.
8. Ravelli A, Martini A. Antiphospholipid antibody syndrome in pediatric patients. Rheum Dis Clin North Am 1997;23:657–676.
9. Ravelli A, Martini A, Burgio GR. Antiphospholipid antibodies in paediatrics. Eur J Pediatr 1994;153:472–479.

10. Szer IS. Clinical development in the management of lupus in the neonate, child, and adolescent. Curr Opin Rheumatol 1998;10:431–434.

11. Kontiainen S, Miettinen A, Seppala I, Verkasalo M, Maenpaa J. Antiphospholipid antibodies in children. Acta Paediatr 1996;85:614–615.

12. Caporali R, Ravelli A, De Gennaro F, Neirotti G, Montecucco C, Martini A. Prevalence of anticardiolipin antibodies in juvenile chronic arthritis. Ann Rheum Dis 1991;50:599–601.

13. Shergy WJ, Kredich DW, Pisetsky DS. The relationship of anticardiolipin antibodies to disease manifestations in pediatric systemic lupus erythematosus. J Rheumatol 1988;15:1389–1394.

14. Singer HS, Krumholz A, Giuliano J, Kiessling LS. Antiphospholipid antibodies: An epiphenomenon in Tourette syndrome. Movement Disorders 1997;12:738–742.

15. Kratz C, Mauz-Korholz C, Kruck H, Korholz D, Gobel U. Detection of antiphospholipid antibodies in children and adolescents. Pediatr Hematol Oncol 1998;15:325–332.

16. Vaarala O, Palosuo T, Kleemola M. Anticardiolipin responses in acute infections. Clin Immunol Immunopathol 1986;41:8–15.

17. Carreno L, Monteagudo I, Lopez-Longo FJ. Anticardiolipin antibodies in pediatric patients with human immunodeficiency virus. J Rheumatol 1994;21:1344

18. Figueroa F, Berrios X, Gutierrez M, Carrion F, Goycolea JP, Riedel I et al. Anticardiolipin antibodies in acute rheumatic fever. J Rheumatol 1992;19:1175–1180.

19. Narin N, Kutukculer N, Narin F, Keser G, Doganavsargil E. Anticardiolipin antibodies in acute rheumatic fever and chronic rheumatic heart disease: is there a signficant association? Clin Exp Rheumatol 1996;14:567–569.

20. Toren P, Toren A, Weizman A, Mozes T, Eldar S, Magor A et al. Tourette's disorder: is there an association with the antiphospholipid syndrome? Biol Psychiatry 1994;35:495–498.

21. Lorini R, d'Annunzio G, Montecucco C, Caporali R, Vitali L, Pessino P et al. Anticardiolipin antibodies in children and adolescents with insulin-dependent diabetes mellitus. Eur J Pediatr 1995;154:105–108.

22. Gattorno M, Buoncompagni A, Molinari AC, Barbano GC, Morreale B, Stalla F et al. Antiphospholipid antibodies in paediatric systemic lupus erythematosus, juvenile chronic arthritis, and overlap syndromes: SLE patients with both lupus anticoagulant and high-titre anticardiolipid antibodies are at risk for clinical manifestations related to the antiphospholipid syndrome. Br J Rheumatol 1995;34:873–881.

23. Leak AM, Colaco CB, Isenberg DA. Anticardiolipin and anti-ss DNA antibodies in antinuclear positive juvenile chronic arthritis and other childhood onset rheumatic diseases. Clin Exp Rheumatol 1987;5:18

24. Caporali R, Ravelli A, Ramenghi B, Montecucco C, Martini A. Antiphospholipid antibody associated with thrombosis in juvenile chronic arthritis. Arch Dis Child 1992;67:1384–1386.

25. Male C, Lechner K, Eichinger S, Kyrle PA, Kapiotis S, Wank H et al. Clinical significance of lupus anticoagulants in children. J Pediatr 1999;134:199–205.

26. Massengill SF, Hedrick C, Ayoub EM, Sleasman JW, Kao KJ. Antiphospholipid antibodies in pediatric lupus nephritis. Am J Kid Dis 1997;29:355–361.

27. Ravelli A, Caporali R, Di Fuccia G. Anticardiolipin antibodies in pediatric systemic lupus erythematosus. Arch Pediatr Adolesc Med 1994;148:398

28. Seaman DE, Londino V, Kent Kwoh C, Medsger TA, Manzi S. Antiphospholipid antibodies in pediatric systemic lupus erythematosus. Pediatrics 1995;96:1040–1045.

29. Montes de Oca MA, Babron MC, Bletry O, Broyer M, Courtecuisse V, Fontaine JL et al. Thrombosis in systemic lupus erythematosus: a French collaborative study. Arch Dis Child 1991;66:713–717.

30. Molta C, Meyer O, Dosquet C. Childhood-onset systemic lupus erythematosus: Antiphospholipid antibodies in 37 patients and their first degree relatives. Pediatrics 1993;92:849

31. Manco-Johnson M, Nuss R. Lupus anticoagulant in children with thrombosis. Am J Hematol 1995;48:240–243.

32. Berube C, Mitchell L, Silverman E, David M, Saint Cyr C, Laxer R et al. The relationship of antiphospholipid antibodies to thromboembolic events in pediatric patients with systemic lupus erythematosus. Pediatr Res 1998;44:351–356.

33. Dungan DD, Jay MS. Stroke in an early adolescent with systemic lupus erythematosus and coexistent antiphospholipid antibodies. Pediatrics 1992;90:96–98.

34. Kwong T, Leonidas JC, Ilowite NT. Asymptomatic superior vena cava thrombosis and pulmonary embolism in an adolescent with SLE and antiphospholipid antibodies. Clin Exp Rheumatol 1994;12:215–217.

35. Besbas N, Damarguc I, Ozen S, Aysun S, Saatci U. Association of antiphospholipid antibodies with systemic lupus erythematosus in a child presenting with chorea: a case report. Eur J Pediatr 1994;153:891–893.

36. Baca V, Sanchez-Vaca G, Martinez-Muniz I, Ramirez-Lacayo M, Lavalle C. Successful treatment of transverse myelitis in a child with systemic lupus erythematosus. Neuropediatrics 1996;27:42–44.

37. Nuss R, Hays T, Chudgar U, Manco-Johnson M. Antiphospholipid antibodies and coagulation regulatory protein abnormalities in children with pulmonary emboli. J Pediatr Hematol Oncol 1997;19:202–207.

38. von Scheven E, Athreya B, Rose CD, Goldsmith DP, Morton L. Clinical characteristics of antiphospholipid antibody syndrome in children. J Pediatr 1996;129:339–345.

39. Bernstein ML, Salusinsky-Sternbach M, Bellefleur M, Esseltine DW. Thrombotic and hemorrhagic complications in children with the lupus anticoagulant. Am J Dis Child 1984;138:1132–1135.

40. Brady L, Magilavy D, Black DD. Portal vein thrombosis associated with antiphospholipid antibodies in a child. J Pediatr Gastroenterol Nutr 1996;23:470–473.

41. Asherson RA, Hughes GRV. Hypoadrenalism, Addison's disease, and antiphospholipid antibodies. J Rheumatol 1991;18:1.

42. Falcini F, Taccetti G, Trapani S, Tafi L, Petralli S, Mattuci-Cerinic M. Primary antiphospholipid syndrome: a report of two cases. J Rheumatol 1991;18:1085–1087.

43. Angelini L, Ravelli A, Caporali R, Rumi V, Nardocci N, Martini A. High prevalence of antiphospholipid antibodies in children with idiopathic cerebral ischemia. Pediatrics 1994;94:500–503.

44. Takanashi J, Sugita K, Miyazato S et al. Antiphospholipid antibody syndrome in childhood strokes. Pediatr Neurol 1995;13:323

45. Di Nucci GD, Mariani G, Arcieri P, Cerbo R, Tarani L, Bruni L et al. Antiphospholipid syndrome in young patients. Two cases of cerebral ischemic accidents. Eur J Pediatr 1995;154:334

46. Olson JC, Konkol RJ, Gill JC, Dobyns WB, Coull BM. Childhood stroke and lupus anticoagulant. Pediatr Neurol 1994;10:54–57.

47. Schoning M, Klein R, Krageloh-Mann I, Falck M, Berg PA, Michaelis R. Antiphospholipid antibodies and cerebrovascular ischemia and stroke in childhood. Neuropediatrics 1993;25:8–14.

48. Pope JM, Canny CHL, Bell DA. Cerebral ischemic events associated with endocarditis, retinal vascular disease, and lupus anticoagulant. Am J Med 1991;90:299–309.

49. Coull BM, Bourdette DN, Goddnight SH Jr et al. Multiple cerebral infarctions associated with antiphospholipid antibodies. Stroke 1987;18:1107–1112.

50. Hasegawa M, Yamashita J, Yamashima T, Ikeda K, Fujishima Y, Yamazaki M. Spinal cord infarction associated with primary antiphospholipid syndrome in a young child. J Neurosurg 1993;79:446–450.

51. Amigo M-C, Garcia-Torres R, Robles M, Bochicchio T, Reyes P. Renal involvement in primary antiphospholipid syndrome. J Rheumatol 1992;19:1181–1185.

52. Ohtomo Y, Matsubara T, Nishizawa K, Unno A, Motohashi T, Yamashiro Y. Nephropathy and hypertension as manifestations in a 13-year-old girl with primary antiphospholipid syndrome. Acta Paediatr 1998;87:903–907.

53. Deleze M, Oria CV, Alarcon-Segovia D. Occurrence of both hemolytic anemia and thrombocytopenic purpura (Evan's Syndrome) in systemic lupus erythematosus. Relationship to antiphospholipid antibodies. J Rheumatol 1988;15:611–615.

54. Harris EN, Gharavi AE, Hegde U, Derue G, Morgan SH, Englert H et al. Anticardiolipin antibodies in autoimmune thrombocytopenic purpura. Br J Haematol 1985;59:231–234.

55. Toren A, Toren P, Many A, Mandel M, Mester R, Neumann Y et al. Spectrum of clinical manifestations of antiphospholipid antibodies in childhood and adolescence. Pediatr Hematol Oncol 1993;10:311–315.

56. Ura Y, Hara T , Mori Y, Matsuo M, Fujioka Y, Kuno T et al. Development of Perthes' disease in a 3-year-old boy with idiopathic thrombocytopenic purpura and antiphospholipid antibodies. Pediatr Hematol Oncol 1992;9:77–80.

57. Cervera R, Asherson RA, Font J, Tikly M, Pallares L, Chamorro A et al. Chorea in the antiphospholipid syndrome. Clinical, radiologic, and immunologic characteristics of 50 patients from our clinics and the recent literature. Medicine 1997;76:203–212.

58. Ziporen L, Blank M, Schoenfeld Y. Animal models for antiphospholipid syndrome in pregnancy. Rheum Dis Clin North Am 1997;23:99–117.

59. Zurgil N, Bakimer R, Tincani A, Faden D, Cohen J, Lorber M et al. Detection of anti-phospholipid and anti-DNA antibodies and their idiotypes in newborns of mothers with anti-phospholipid syndrome and SLE. Lupus 1993;2:233–237.

60. Botet F, Romera G, Montagut P, Figueras J, Carmona F, Balasch J. Neonatal outcome in women treated for the antiphospholipid syndrome during prenancy. J Perinat Med 1997;25:192–196.

61. Ruffati A, Dalla Barba B, Del Ross T, Vettorato F, Rapizzi E, Tonello M et al. Outcome of fifty-five newborns of antiphospholipid antibody-positive mothers treated with calcium heparin during pregnancy. Clin Exp Rheumatol 1998;16:605–610.

62. Contractor S, Hiatt M, Kosmin M, Kim HC. Neonatal thrombosis with anticardiolipin antibody in baby and mother. Am J Perinatol 1992;9:409–410.
63. Silver RK, MacGregor SN, Paternak JF, Neely SE. Fetal stroke associated with elevated maternal anticardiolipin antibodies. Obstet Gynecol 1992;80:497–499.
64. Sheridan-Pereira M, Porreco RP, Hays T, Shannon Burke M. Neonatal aortic thrombosis associated with the lupus anticoagulant. Obstet Gynecol 1988;71:1016–1018.
65. Hage ML, Liu R, Marcheschi DG, Bowie JD, Allen NB, Macik BG. Fetal renal vein thrombosis, hydrops fetalis, and maternal lupus anticoagulant. A case report. Prenat Diagn 1994; 14:873–877.
66. Asherson RA, Khamashta MA, Ordi-Ros J, Derksen RHWM, Machin SJ, Barquinero J et al. The "primary" antiphospholipid syndrome: major clinical and serological features. Medicine 1989;68:366–374.
67. Khamashta MA, Wallington T. Management of the antiphospholipid syndrome. Ann Rheum Dis 1991;50:959–962.
68. Khamashta MA, Cuadrado M, Mujic F, Taub N, Hunt B, Hughes GRV. The management of thrombosis in the antiphospholipid-antibody syndrome. N Engl J Med 1995;332:993–997.
69. Baca V, Garcia-Ramirez R, Ramirez-Lacayo M, Marquez-Enriquez L, Martinez I, Lavalle C. Cerebral infarction and antiphospholipid syndrome in children. J Rheumatol 1996;23:1428–1431.
70. Roddy SM, Giang DW. Antiphospholipid antibodies and stroke in an infant. Pediatrics 1991;87:933–935.
71. Vlachoyiannopoulos PG, Dimou G, Siamopoulou-Mavirdou A. Chorea as a manifestation of the antiphospholipid syndrome in childhood. Clin ExpRheumatol 1991;9:303–305.
72. Ravelli A, Caporali R, Montecucco C, Martini A. Superior vena cava thrombosis in a child with antiphospholipid syndrome. J Rheumatol 1992;19:502–503.

17 Antiphospholipid Antibodies as a Risk Factor for Atherosclerosis

R. G. Lahita

Etiologic Factors and Atherosclerosis

There is no greater contribution that our understanding of the antiphospholipid syndrome (APS; Hughes syndrome) might give us than the etiopathogenesis of atherosclerosis, the most common cause of death in the world. Although the etiology remains unknown, It is a multifactorial disease. What we do know is that it is dependent on a number of variables. Some factors known to be associated with the progression of atherosclerosis include hypercholesterolemia and modified lipids, high homocysteine levels [1], hypertension, and infection. Perhaps the latter might seem surprising, but there is solid evidence that infection – suspected for many years – might be at the heart of atherosclerosis [2].

One of the most interesting ideas regarding the cause of this chronic disease is the suspicion that the immune system is involved in its etiology [3]. First is evidence that the complement system is directly involved in plaque formation. This is not surprising since complement is a complex of enzymes and regulators which has multiple biological effects in circulation and in tissues inducing opsonization, the chemoattraction of leukocytes, cell lysis, and finally apoptosis [4–6]. Immune complexes also deposit in the affected arterial wall, specifically in the intima and the media, and as a result there is local activation of the complement system. Immunoglobulins like IgG, IgM, and IgA are also found in the areas of intimal thickening and in the fibrous plaques. The membrane attack complex of complement, C5b-9 is also present in the human atherosclerotic samples. Finally, interleukin-6, -8, and tumor necrosis factor-α are also found in the lesions [7]. Chemokines may be responsible for the chemotaxis and the accumulation of macrophages in the fatty streak. Mice that lack apolipoprotein E are naturally hypercholesterolemic [8, 9], and have constitutive expression of intercellular adhesion molecule-1 at lesion prone sites in the vasculature. Mice deficient in this adhesion molecule have no atheromata development, indicating its importance in the etiology. Not only are smooth muscle cells important in the development of the atherosclerotic plaque, but the migration of monocyte-derived macrophages and T cells is also important [10]. The macrophages produce cytokines, proteolytic enzymes (like the metalloproteinases) and other growth factors.

Activated macrophages at the vascular wall express class II human leukocyte antigen (HLA) antigens like HLA-DR that allow the presentation of antigens to lymphocytes. Cell-mediated immune reactions that are important aspects of the development of the atherosclerotic plaque depend on this mechanism [10]. Moreover, T cells of both CD4 and CD8 classes are present in the plaque. The cytokine profile of the atherosclerotic immune reaction was clearly identified as a T helper 2 (Th2) profile [11] in recent work. This gives more validity to its accelerated development in Th2 diseases like systemic lupus erythematosus (SLE).

The antigens for the immune response might be oxidized low-density lipoprotein (LDL), produced by macrophages or heat-shock protein-60 known to prevent, among other things, the local breakdown of denatured protein [12–15].

Atherosclerosis in Lupus

There is no doubt that premature atherosclerosis occurs in SLE and is a major cause of death in that disease [16]. In fact, the cause of death in most patients with lupus is early myocardial infarction [17, 18]. The early observation of atherosclerosis development in crossed inbred lupus mice indicated that this aspect of the disease was both important and could have relevance to the pathogenic process for human atherosclerosis [19].

Arteritis may also be a component of the coronary vascular disease found in lupus patients [20]. It is also known that immune complexes from lupus sera increase the uptake of cholesterol by smooth muscle cells [21].

There are other risk factors in SLE and these include hypertension more prevalent in those patients with renal disease and hyperlipidemia because of medications like the corticosteroids. Petri et al found that only three coronary artery disease (CAD) risk factors were found in her Hopkins' cohort of SLE patients: weight, mean cholesterol and mean arterial pressure. Interestingly, all of the above mentioned risk factors are exacerbated by corticosteroid therapy [22, 23].

Phospholipid Antibodies and Atherosclerosis

The antiphospholipid syndrome (Hughes syndrome) is characterized by a predisposition for thromboembolic events, Thrombocytopenia, recurrent fetal loss and systemic phenomena like accelerated atherosclerosis.

An attractive explanation for this accelerated atherosclerosis is the presence of antiphospholipid antibodies (aPL). Compared with a control group, SLE patients had significantly more pericardial abnormalities, valvular disease, left ventricular hypertrophy, left atrial enlargement, left ventricular dysfunction and verrucous valvular thickening. There are data to explain some of the observations and associate the phospholipid antibodies with certain of these pathologic features. The presence of aPL is associated with isolated left ventricular (global or segmental dysfunction), verrucous valvular disease, and consequently global valvular dysfunction in the heart [24]. Some mechanisms come from observations. First is the purported cross-reactivity of aPL with oxidized LDL antibodies [25]. It was suggested that the one-third of patients with SLE who have aPL might be those with accelerated atherosclerosis. Moreover, this cross-reactivity might enhance the uptake of such oxidized LDL by macrophages. The binding of oxidized LDL by macrophages was significantly increased by the simultaneous addition of anticardiolipin antibody and the antigenic target "cofactor" β_2-glycoprotein I (apolipoprotein H) [26]. A second observation indicates that immunization of mice with β_2-glycoprotein I results in the induction of early atherosclerosis. These experiments which involved control of diet and other variables are very provocative.

In another observation, we reported low total plasma cholesterol levels and low high-density lipoproteins (HDL) in patients with high levels of anticardiolipin IgG [27]. In further research, we found by enzyme-linked immunosorbent assay (ELISA) an antibody against apolipoprotein A1, the major component of HDL. These data were obtained using gamma-irradiated ELISA plates [28]. Therefore, apolipoprotein A1 can be an immunogenic epitope at times as steric changes alter structure. A gene identified as that for apolipoprotein A1 was isolated from a mouse cDNA library using the serum of a patient who suffered from severe atherosclerosis and had a cerebrovascular accident. The overall significance of this antibody in the development of atherosclerosis is unknown. Although antibody to apolipoprotein A1 was found in 32.5% of patients with SLE and 22.9% of patients with primary APS. It is apparent that several cofactors exist with phospholipid which themselves can become the principal target of antibody. It is logical to assume that most apolipoprotein molecules could become cofactors to negatively charged phospholipid and thus with steric change become antigenic.

Other Considerations

Atherosclerosis is common in the hypoestrogenic state and in procoagulant states. However, lupus is not a condition where estrogenic metabolites are absent. Rather, it is a condition where hyperestrogenicity is the norm and metabolism of estrone is distinctly directed towards very feminizing compounds. One would therefore expect protection against the development of atherosclerosis [29] in SLE. However, aPL result in a procoagulant state that can have many effects on a developing atheroma and these antibodies as well as immune functions are stimulated by estrogen. Taken together, the hyperestrogenic state [30, 31] together with the presence of procoagulation might enhance the development of the atherosclerotic plaque. While it is certainly true that hormones by themselves cannot explain the accelerated atheroma of the lupus patient, hormones in the context of a "stimulated" immune system can contribute to the formation of the atheroma, if as we suppose, the atheroma is an immune lesion like the pannus of the rheumatoid arthritic patient.

Several other factors might enhance the progression of the plaque, among them the association between free protein S levels and aPL. The homology between protein S and sex hormone binding globulin could mean that estrogen might lower protein S levels and enhance coagulability in this manner [32]. Additionally protein S might also be lowered via binding to C4BP a suppressor of the complement system. It is apparent therefore that atherosclerosis is likely to be directly related to the presence of aPL. The exact mechanism awaits elucidation.

References

1. Tsai J-C, Perrella MA, Yoshizumi M. Promotion of vascular smooth muscle cell growth by homocysteine: a link to atherosclerosis. Proc Natl Acad Sci USA 1994;91:6369.
2. Folsom AR. Antibiotics for prevention of myocardial infarction? Not yet! JAMA 1999;281:461–462.
3. Bittner V. Atherosclerosis and the immune system. Arch Int Med 1998;158:1395–1396.
4. Rus HG, Niculescu F, Constantinescu E, Cristea A, Vlaicu R. Immunoelectron microscopic localization of the terminal C5b-9 complement complex in human atherosclerotic vascular lesions. Atherosclerosis 1986;61:35–42.
5. Shin ML, Rus HG, Niculescu FI. Membrane attack by complement: assembly and biology of terminal complement complexes.In: AK Lee, editor. Biomembranes. Greenwich, CT: JAI Press, 1996;123.
6. Vlaicu R, Rus HG, Niculescu F, Cristea A. Immunoglobulins and complement components in human aortic atherosclerotic intima. Atherosclerosis 1985;55:50.
7. Niculescu F, Rus H. Atherosclerosis and the immune system. Arch Int Med 1999;159:315.
8. Tam S-P, Archer TK, Deeley RG. Biphasic effects of estrogen on apolipoprotein synthesis in human hepatoma cells: mechanism of antagonism by testosterone. Proc Natl Acad Sci USA 1986;83:3111–3115.
9. Zuckerman SH, Bryan-Poole N. Estrogen-induced alterations in lipoprotein metabolism in autoimmune MRL/lpr mice. Arterioscler ThrombVasc Biol 1995;15:1556–1562.
10. Hansson GK. Cell mediated immunity in atherosclerosis. Curr Opin Lipidol 1997;8:301–311.
11. Zhou X, Paulsson G, Stemme S, Hansson GK. Hypercholesterolemia is associated with a T helper (Th)1/Th2 switch of the autoimmune resonse in atheroslcerotic apoE-knockout mice. J.Clin Invest 1998;101:1717–1725.
12. Assmann G, Funke H. HDL metabolism and atherosclerosis. J Cardiovasc.Pharmacol 1990;16 (Suppl 9):S15–S20.
13. George J, Afek A, Gilburd B, Blamk M, Levy Y, Aron-Maor A et al. Induction of early atherosclerosis in LDL-receptor deficient mice immunized with β_2-glycoprotein I. Circulation 1998;98:1108–1115.
14. Palinski W, Rosenfield ME, Yla-Herttuala S. Low density lipoprotein undergoes oxidative modification in vivo. Proc Natl Acad Sci USA 1989;86:1372.
15. Salonen JT, Yla-Herttuala S, Yamamoto R, Butler S, Korpela H, Salonen R et al. Autoantibody against oxidised LDL and progression of carotid atherosclerosis. Lancet 1992;339:883–887.
16. Doherty NE, Siegel RJ. Cardiovascular manifestations of systemic lupus erythematosus. Am Heart J 1985;110:1257.
17. Urowitz MB, Bookman AM, Koehler BE, Gordon DA, Smythe HA, Ogryzlo MA. The bimodal mortality pattern of SLE. Am J Med 1976;60:221–225.
18. Asherson R, Cervera R. The antiphospholipid syndrome: a syndrome in evolution. Ann Rheum Dis 1992;51:147–150.
19. Hang LM, Izui S, Dixon FJ. (NZWBXSB) F1 hybrid: a model of acute lupus and coronary vascular disease with myocardial infarction. J Exp Med 1981;154:216.
20. Juvonen T, Juvonen J, Savolainen MJ. Is vasculitis a significant component of atherosclerosis? Curr Opin Rheumatol 1999;11:3–10.
21. Kabakov AE, Tertov VV, Saenko VA, Poverenny AM, Orekhov AN. The atherogenic effect of lupus sera: systemic lupus erythematosus-derived immune complexes stimulate the accumulation of cholesterol in cultured smooth muscle cells from human aorta. Clin Immunol Immunopathol 1992;63:214.
22. Petri M, Perez-Gutthann S, Spence D, Hochberg MC. Risk factors for coronary artery disease in patients with systemic lupus erythematosus. Am J Med 1992;93:513–519.
23. Petri M, Spence D, Bone LR, Hochberg MC. Coronary artery disease risk factors in the Hopkins lupus cohort; prevalence, patient recognition, and preventive practices. Medicine 1992;71:291.
24. Leung W-H, Wong K-L, Lau C-P, Wong C-K, Liu H-W. Association between antiphospholipid antibodies and cardiac abnormalities in patients with systemic lupus erythematosus. Am J Med 1990;89:411–418.
25. Vaarala O, Alfthan G, Jauhainen M. Crossreaction between antibodies to oxidized low-density lipoprotein and to cardiolipin in systemic lupus erythematosus. Lancet 1993;341:923.
26. Hasunuma Y, Matsuura E, Makita Z. Involvement of β_2-glycoprotein I and anticardiolipin antiobdies in oxidatively modified low-density lipoprotein uptake by macrophages. Clin Exp Immunol 1997;107:569.
27. Lahita RG, Rivkin E, Cavanagh I, Romano P. Low levels of total cholesterol, high-density lipoprotein, and apolipoprotein A1 in association with anticardiolipin antibodies in patients with systemic lupus erythematosus. Arthritis Rheum 1993;36:1566–1574.

28. Dinu AR, Merrill JT, Shen C, Antonov IV, Myones BL, Lahita RG. Frequency of antibodies to the cholesterol transport protein apolipoprotein A1 in patients with SLE. Lupus 1998;7:1–7.
29. Nathan L, Chaudhuri G. Estrogens and atherosclerosis. Annu Rev Pharmacol Toxicol 1999;37:477–515.
30. Bucala R, Lahita RG, Fishman J, Cerami A. Nonenzymatic modification of red cell and lymphocyte membrane proteins by 16-alpha hydroxyestrone in patients with systemic lupus erythematosus. Arthritis Rheum 1984;27:s40 (Abstract).
31. Lahita RG, Bradlow HL, Kunkel HG, Fishman J. Increased 16 alpha hydroxylation of estradiol in systemic lupus erythematosus. J Clin Endocrinol Metab 1981;53:174–178.
32. Ginsberg JS, Demers C, Brill-Edwards P, Bona R, Jofnston M, Wong A, Denburg J. Aquired free protein S deficiency is associated with antiphospholipid antibodies and increased thrombin generation in patients with systemic lupus erythematosus. Am J Med 1995;98:379–383.

18 Accelerated Atherosclerosis in Antiphospholipid Syndrome

O. Vaarala

Introduction

Atherosclerosis can be considered as a systemic arterial disease characterized by narrowing arteries with endothelial dysfunction, impaired vascular relaxation and hemostatic imbalance. The basic feature in the atherosclerotic vessel is the accumulation of lipids, lipoproteins and inflammatory cells, such as macrophages and T lymphocytes, in the arterial intima and the proliferation of the smooth muscle cells [1]. Inflammatory reaction in the atheroma can be seen already in early atherosclerotic lesions and is an important determinant for the development of the clinical complications of atherosclerotic disease, such as atherothrombosis.

The "oxidative-modification hypothesis" in the pathogenesis of atherosclerosis is based on the oxidative modification of low-density lipoprotein (LDL) which takes place in the arterial wall and leads to lipid accumulation due to the enhanced uptake of oxidized LDL by scavenger receptors of macrophages [2]. Elevated levels of autoantibodies to oxidized LDL are associated with atherosclerosis and have been reported to imply an active atherosclerotic process [3, 4]. Antibodies to oxidized LDL occur frequently also in the patients with systemic lupus erythematosus (SLE) [5] in whom premature atherosclerosis is a considerable clinical problem [6–8]. According to Manzi and co-workers, women with SLE in the 35–44 years age group had over 50 times higher rate ratio of cardiovascular events than healthy women of similar age [7]. Classic risk factors for atherosclerosis, such as the prolonged treatment with prednisone, high blood pressure and high levels of LDL cholesterol also contribute to the atherosclerosis in SLE, but do not wholly explain this clinical peculiarity. Accumulating evidence indicates that antiphospholipid antibodies aPL (including antibodies binding to cardiolipin–β_2-glycoprotein I complex and antibodies to oxidized LDL) may be involved in the pathogenesis of atherosclerosis in SLE extending the clinical picture of antiphospholipid syndrome (APS; Hughes syndrome) to include accelerated atherosclerosis [9].

aPL in Atherosclerosis

Antibodies to oxidized LDL comprise a heterogenous groups of antibodies as regard to their specificity. A subpopulation of these antibodies binds to oxidized lipids in

LDL molecule and are likely responsible for cross-reactivity with phospholipids such as cardiolipin [10, 11]. A subpopulation of antibodies to oxidized LDL recognizes oxidized apolipoprotein B of LDL, which is modified during oxidation [12]. Antibodies to β_2-glycoprotein I may show binding to oxidized LDL [13] because small amounts of plasma β_2-glycoprotein I is bound to LDL molecule in circulation. However, studies on SLE sera-derived autoantibodies have not been able to demonstrate a true cross-reactivity between the antibodies to oxidized LDL and β_2-glycoprotein I [14, 15]. Since antibodies to oxidized LDL cross-react with antiphospholipid antibodies (aPL) they are considered as members of the family of aPL [5, 10, 11, 16]. The major population of the cross-reactive antibodies react likely with oxidized phospholipids (e.g., cardiolipin). Despite the overlapping specificities described above a separate population of antibodies to oxidized LDL with no cross-reactivity to cardiolipin can be eluted from SLE sera [10]. Also, clinical associations of the antibodies to oxidized LDL differ from those of antibodies binding to cardiolipin–β_2-glycoprotein I complex [17–19]. The antibodies to cardiolipin–β_2-glycoprotein I complex are associated with both arterial and venous thrombosis in SLE, but antibodies to oxidized LDL do not show association with venous thrombosis. Instead, these antibodies are associated with arterial thrombosis in APS [18, 19]. The question of the direct involvement of antibodies to oxidized LDL in the development of atherothrombosis is open but several studies indicate that these antibodies serve as markers of pathogenic determinants of atherosclerosis, such as oxidation of LDL, endothelial dysfunction and arterial inflammation. The frequent occurrence of antibodies to oxidized LDL in SLE and APS may be associated with enhanced oxidative stress and atherosclerotic process in SLE.

Studies in subjects without SLE on the role of aPL in atherosclerotic complications have a special importance since the diverse clinical problems and immunological abnormalities in patients with SLE do not interfere with the results. However, when evaluating the role of aPL in atherosclerosis the major problem is how to define atherosclerosis. Myocardial infarction is considered as a clinical manifestation of atherosclerosis in coronary arteries. Two prospective studies in non-SLE subjects have shown that antibodies to oxidized LDL are predictive for myocardial infarction [4, 20]. In addition, the levels of antibodies to oxidized LDL represented an independent determinant of impaired endothelium-dependent and endothelium-independent vasodilatation, which was detected in the forearm vasculature by strain-gauge plethysmography in a series of patients with coronary heart disease (Sinisalo et al, unpublished work). These findings suggest that antibodies to oxidized LDL may be closely associated with the atherosclerotic process in the vessel wall.

Elevated levels of antibodies binding to cardiolipin have been associated with myocardial infarction. Also, prospective studies have shown that elevated levels of cardiolipin-binding antibodies in non-SLE populations imply an increased risk for the development of myocardial infarction [20, 21–23]. Some evidence supports the view that cardiolipin-binding antibodies are a risk for myocardial infarction especially in young individuals [22, 23]. All prospective studies have not confirmed the association of cardiolipin antibodies with myocardial infarction [24, 25]. Cardiolipin-binding antibodies are a frequent finding in SLE and it is thus possible that the clinical significance of these antibodies in the development of myocardial infarction in SLE populations may indeed be more pronounced. However, prospective studies in SLE patients are not published yet.

The role of antibodies to β_2-glycoprotein I is unclear in human atherosclerosis. These antibodies were not associated with the development of myocardial infarction in a study including non-SLE patients [26]. However, both in vitro studies [27] and experimental studies in animal models suggest that these antibodies may be involved with the development of atherosclerosis [28]. This possibility is discussed later in this chapter.

Antibodies to prothrombin have been associated with myocardial infarction in a prospective follow-up of healthy dyslipidemic men. A twofold risk of myocardial infarction was found in middle-aged men with antibody levels to prothrombin in the highest tertile when compared to the men with antibody levels in the lowest tertile [26]. This risk was multiplied by an additive manner when the joint effect with other risk factors for myocardial infarction was accounted, such as high levels of antibodies to oxidized LDL, smoking and high Lp(a) levels.

Altogether it seems that several subspecificities of aPL may occur in the patients with atherosclerosis and some evidence suggests that these antibodies may contribute to the development of atherosclerosis. It is possible that aPL are initiated as a consequence of the underlying systemic arterial inflammatory disease and reflect the spreading of the autoimmune response against several antigens modified in the atherosclerotic vessel wall.

The Putative Mechanisms of Accelerated Atherosclerosis in APS

In vitro studies suggest that aPL may contribute to the development of atherosclerotic process in APS by enhancing of the lipid accumulation and inflammation in the arterial vessel wall. Antibodies to β_2-glycoprotein I have been shown to enhance the accumulation of oxidized LDL into macrophages [27]. The binding of antibodies to β_2-glycoprotein I–LDL complex may be the mechanism how these antibodies increase LDL uptake by Fc-receptors. This mechanism may be important in the development of premature atherosclerosis in patients with antiphospholipid syndrome who frequently have high levels of antibodies to β_2-glycoprotein I. Also animal studies indicate that immunity to β_2-glycoprotein I plays a role in the development of atherosclerosis. When LDL-receptor deficient or apolipoprotein E deficient mice were immunized with human β_2-glycoprotein I acceleration of early atherosclerosis was observed [28, 29]. Immunization with anticardiolipin antibodies (aCL) has also been reported to result in accelerated atherosclerosis in an animal model [30]. The mechanisms are not known but these studies indicate an involvement of β_2-glycoprotein I in the atherosclerotic process. The recent finding of the presence of β_2-glycoprotein I in the atherosclerotic plaque is of great interest and emphasized the role of antibodies to β_2-glycoprotein I in atherosclerosis [31].

Enhanced inflammation response in the atherosclerotic plaques, characterized by accumulation of macrophages and activated T lymphocytes, seems to be a crucial factor predisposing to plaque rupture. Atherosclerosis is converted to an acute clinical event by the induction of plaque rupture, which in turn leads to thrombosis. The risk of plaque rupture depends more on the structure of the plaque than on its size (i.e., the degree of stenosis) [32]. Vascular inflammatory process accompanying with multiple immunological abnormalities is a basic feature of SLE. The antibodies directed against the antigenic structures present in the atherosclerotic plaques may enhance the local inflammatory process and contribute to the atherosclerotic process. On the other hand high oxidative capacity in the arterial wall leads to oxidation of proteins trapped in the subendothelial space. Antibody responses to oxidized plasma proteins, such as oxidized LDL, β_2-glycoprotein I or prothrombin, may reflect the degree of the focal inflammatory reaction and thus be a markers for inflammation in atherosclerosis.

The pathogenic role of antibodies to oxidized LDL have been suggested by studies showing that in vitro these antibodies enhance the LDL accumulation into macrophages [2]. However, in vivo immunization with oxidized LDL has been shown to protect from atherosclerosis in ApoE deficient mice [33] and in LDL-receptor-deficient mice [34]. This effect seems not to be dependent on the generation of antibodies to oxidized LDL [34]. It must be pointed out that due to the absence of LDL receptor in these mice the mechanisms and the effect of immunization may differ from those observed in normal animals.

aPL may also contribute to the clinical manifestations of atherosclerosis due to their interference with blood coagulation. The occurrence of aPL in atherosclerosis may independently influence on the development of atherothrombosis by changing the hemostatic balance towards hypercoagulation. In Hughes syndrome, underlying vascular inflammation and the occurrence of aPL may essentially increase the risk of clinical manifestations of atherosclerosis as thrombosis. Several case reports on the occurrence of coronary occlusion with minimal atherosclerotic changes in association of antiphospholipid antibodis have been published [35, 36]. Besides the possible direct effect of aPL on blood coagulation, their occurrence has been associated with high Lp(a) levels which is a hemostatic risk factor for atherothrombosis [37, 38]. Thus, it is possible that already early atherosclerotic changes in Hughes syndrome may lead to the development of atherothrombosis (Fig. 18.1).

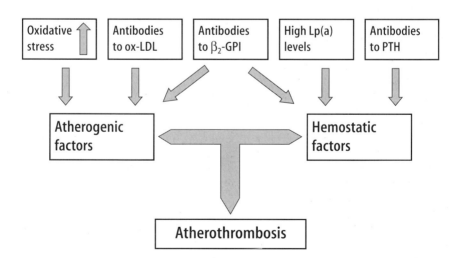

Figure 18.1. Factors contributing to development of atherothrombosis in APS.

Conclusions

In the Hopkins lupus cohort, the majority of the prospectively-followed thrombotic events were arterial thrombosis, such as myocardial infarction and stroke [39]. Venous thrombosis were clustered early in the history of the disease and arterial events occurred late pointing the poor therapeutical efficiency in prevention atherothrombosis in SLE. Several studies clearly indicate that accelerated atherosclerosis is a clinical challenge in the treatment of patients with SLE [6–8, 40]. The studies showing an association of aPL with clinical manifestations of atherosclerosis suggest that especially the patients with antiphosholipid syndrome are at an increased risk of atherosclerosis (Table 18.1). Markers of enhanced lipid peroxidation have been associated with aPL indicating an increased oxidative stress in APS [41, 42] and suggesting the use of antioxidants as a therapeutic choice in APS. The current knowledge on the pathogenesis of atherosclerosis emphasizes the importance of the intensive treatment of the classic risk factors of atherosclerosis, such as high blood pressure and LDL-cholesterol, while waiting for a specific treatment of the immunological atherogenic factors in patients with APS.

Table 18.1. Evidence linking atherosclerosis and antiphospholipid syndrome.

Antibodies to oxidized LDL occur in APS and crossreact with aCL [5, 18, 19]

aPL are associated with atherosclerotic complications in non-SLE population [20–23, 26]

Markers of enhanced lipid peroxidation are reported in APS [41, 42]

Antibodies to β_2-glycoprotein I increase the uptake of oxidized LDL [27]

Immunization with β_2-glycoprotein I or aCL resulted in accelerated atherosclerosis in LDL-receptor deficient mice [28–30]

References

1. Jonasson L, Holm J, Skalli O, Bondjers G, Hansson GK. Regional accumulations of T cells, macrophages, and smooth muscle cells in the human ahterosclerotic plaque. Arteriosclerosis 1986;6:131–138.
2. Witztum JL. The oxidation hypothesis of atherosclerosis . Lancet 1994;344:793–795.
3. Salonen JT, Ylä-Herttuala S, Yamamoto R, Butler S, Korpela H, Salonen R et al. Autoantibody against oxidized LDL and progression of carotid atherosclerosis. Lancet 1992;339:883–887.
4. Puurunen M, Mänttäri M, Manninen V, Tenkanen L, Alfthan G, Ehnholm C et al. Antibody against oxidized low-density lipoprotein predicting myocardial infarction. Arch Intern Med 1994;154:2605–2609.
5. Vaarala O, Alfthan G, Jauhiainen M, Leirisalo-Repo M, Aho K, Palosuo T. Crossreaction between antibodies to oxidized lipoprotein and to cardiolipin in systemic lupus erythematosus. Lancet 1993;341:923–925.
6. Urowitz MB, Bookman AAM, Koehler BE, Gordon DA, Smythe HA, Ogryzlo MA. The bimodal mortality pattern of systemic lupus eryhtematosus. Am J Med 1976;69:221–225.
7. Manzi S, Meilahn EN, Rairie JE, Conte CG, Medsger TA, Jansen-McWilliams L et al. Age-specific incidence rates of myocardial infarction and angina in women with systemic lupus erythematosus: comparison with the Framingham Study. Am J Epidemiol 1997;145:408–415.
8. Ward MM. Premature morbidity from cardiovascular and cerebrovascular diseases in women with systemic lupus erythematosus. Arthritis Rheum 1999;42:338–346
9. Vaarala O. Atherosclerosis in SLE and Hughes syndrome [editorial]. Lupus 1997;:489–490.
10. Vaarala O, Puurunen M, Lukka M, Alfthan G, Leirisalo-Repo M, Aho K et al. Affinity-purified cardiolipin-binding antibodies show heterogeneity in their binding to oxidized low-density lipoprotein. Clin Exp Immunol 1996;104:269–274.

11. Hörkkö S, Miller E, Dudl E, Reaven P, Curtiss LK, Zvaifler NJ et al. APL are directed against epitopes of oxidized phospholipids. J Clin Invest 1996;98:815–825.
12. Palinski W, Yla-Herttuala S, Rosenfeld ME, Butler SW, Socher SA, Parthasarathy S et al. Antisera and monoclonal antibodies specific for epitopes generated during oxidative modification of low density lipoprotein. Arteriosclerosis 1990;10:325–335.
13. Matsuura E, Katahira T, Igarashi Y, Koike T. β_2-glycoprotein I bound to oxidatively modified lipoproteins could be targeted by anticardiolipin antibodies. Lupus 1994;3:314.
14. Matsuda J, Gotoh M, Kawasugi K, Gohchi K, Tsukamoto M, Saitoh N. Negligible synergistic effect of beta2-glycoprotein I on the reactivity of antioxidized low-density lipoprotein antibody to oxidized low-density lipoprotein. Am J Hematol 1996;52:114–116.
15. Tinahones FJ, Cuadrado MJ, Khamashta MA, Mujic F, Gomez-Zumaquero JM, Collantes E et al. Lack of cross-reaction between antibodies to beta2-glycoprotein-I and oxidized low-density lipoprotein in patients with antiphospholipid syndrome. Br J Rheumatol 1998;37:746–749.
16. Mizutani H, Kurata Y, Kosugi S, Shiraga M, Kashiwagi H, Tomiyama Y et al. Monoclonal anti-cardiolipin autoantibodies established from the (New Zealand White BXSB)F1 mouse model of antiphospholipid syndrome cross-react with oxidized low-denstiy lipoprotein. Arhtritis Rheum 1995;38:1382–1388.
17. Aho K, Vaarala O, Tenkanen L, Julkunen H, Jouhikainen T, Alfthan G et al. Antibodies binding to anionic phospholipids but not to oxidized low-density lipoprotein are associated with thrombosis in patients with systemic lupus erythematosus. Clin Exp Rheumatol 1996;14:499–506.
18. Amengual O, Atsumi T, Khamashta MA, Tinahones F, Hughes GR. Autoantibodies against oxidized low-density lipoprotein in antiphospholipid syndrome. Br J Rheumatol 1997;36:964–968.
19. Cuadrado MJ, Tinahones F, Camps MT, de Ramon E, Gomez-Zumaquero JM, Mujic F et al. Antiphospholipid, anti-beta 2-glycoprotein I and anti-oxidized-low-density antibodies in antiphospholipid syndrome. Quart J Med 1998;91:619–626.
20. Wu R, Nityanand S, Berglund L, Lithell H, Holm G, Lefvert AK. Antibodies against cardiolipin and oxidatively modified LDL in 50-year-old men predict myocardial infarction. Arterioscler Thromb Vasc Biol 1997;17:3159–3163.
21. Vaarala O, Mänttäri M, Manninen V, Tenkanen L, Puurunen M, Aho K et al. Anti-cardiolipin antibodies and risk of myocardial infarction in a prospective cohort of middle-aged men. Circulation 1995;91:23–27.
22. Zuckerman E, Toubi E, Shiran A, Sabo E, Shmuel Z, Golan TD et al. Anticardiolipin antibodies and acute myocardial infarction in non-systemic lupus erythematosus: a controlled prospective study. Am J Med 1996;101:381–386.
23. Levine SR, Salowich-Palm L, Sawaya KL, Perry M. Spencer HJ, Winkler HJ et al. IgG anticardiolipin antibody titer > 40 GPL and the risk of subsequent thrombo-occlusive events and death. A prospective cohort study. Stroke 1997;28:1660–1665.
24. Sletnes KE, Smith P, Abdelnoor M, Arnesen H, Wisloff F. APL after myocardial infarction and their relation to mortality, reinfarction, and non-haemorrhagic stroke. Lancet 1992;339:451–453.
25. Tsakiris DA, Marbet GA, Burkat F, Duckert F. Anticardiolipin antibodies and coronary heart disease. Eur Heart J 1992;13:1645–1648.
26. Vaarala O, Puurunen M, Mänttäri M, Manninen V, Áho K, Palosuo T. Antibodies to prothrombin imply a risk of myocardial infarction in middle-aged men. Thromb Haemost 1996;75:456–459.
27. Hasunuma Y, Matsuura E, Makita Z, Katahira T, Nishi S, Koike T. Involvement of b2-glycoprotein I and anticardiolipin antibodies in oxidatively modified low-density lipoprotein uptake by macrophages. Clin Exp Immunol 1997;107:569–573.
28. George J, Afek A, Gilburd B, Blank M, Levy Y, Aron-Maor A et al. Induction of early atherosclerosis in LDL-receptor-deficient mice immunized with beta2-glycoprotein I. Circulation 1998;98:1108–1115.
29. Afek A, George J, Shoenfeld Y, Gilburd B, Levy Y, Shaish A et al. Enhancement of atherosclerosis in beta-2-glycoprotein I-immunized apolipoprotein E-deficient mice. Pathobiology 1999;67:19–25.
30. George J, Afek A, Gilburd B, Levy Y, Blank M, Kopolovic J et al. Atherosclerosis in LDL-receptor knockout mice is accelerated by immunization with anticardiolipin antibodies. Lupus 1997;6:723–729.
31. George J, Harats D, Gilburd B, Afek A, Levy Y, Schneiderman J et al. Immunolocalization of β_2-glycoprotein I (apolipoprotein H) to human atherosclerotic plaques. Potential implications for lesion progression. Circulation 1999;99:2227–2230.
32. Libby P. Molecular bases of the acute coronary syndromes. Circulation 1995;91:2844–2850.
33. George J, Afek A, Gilburd B, Levkovitz H, Shaish A, Goldberg I et al. Hyperimmunization of apo-E-deficient mice with homologous malondialdehyde low-density lipoprotein suppresses early atherogenesis. Atherosclerosis 1998;138:147–152.

34. Freigang S, Horkko S, Miller E, Witztum JL, Palinski W. Immunization of LDL receptor-deficient mice with homologous malondialdehyde-modified and native LDL reduces progression of atherosclerosis by mechanisms other than induction of high titers of antibodies to oxidative neoepitopes. Arterioscler Thromb Vasc Biol 1998;18:1972–1982.
35. Asherson RA, Mackay JR, Harris EN. Myocardial infarction in a young man with systemic lupus erythematosus, deep vein trhombosis, and antibodies to phospholipid. Br Heart J 1986;56:190–193.
36. Maaravi Y, Raz E, Gilon D, Rubinow A. Cerebrovascular accident and myocardial infarction associated with anticardiolipin antibodies in a young woman with systemic lupus erythematosus. Ann Rheum Dis 1989;48:853–855.
37. Yamazaki M, Asakura H, Jokaji H, Saito M, Uotani C, Kumabashiri I et al. Plasma levels of lipoprotein(a) are elevated in patients with the antiphospholipid antibody syndrome. Thromb Haemost 1994;71:424–427.
38. Atsumi R, Khamashta MA, Andujar C, Leandro MJ, Amengual O, Ames PR et al. Elevated plasma lipoprotein(a) level and its association with impaired fibrinolysis in patients with antiphospholipid syndrome. J Rheumatol 1998;25:69–73.
39. Petri M. Thrombosis and systemic lupus erythematosus: the Hopkins Lupus Cohort perspective. Scand J Rheumatol 1995;25:191–193.
40. Manzi S, Selzer F, Sutton-Tyrrell K, Fitzgerald SG, Rairie JE, Tracy RP et al. Prevalence and risk factors of carotid plaque in women with systemic lupus erythematosus. Arthritis Rheum 1999;42:51–60.
41. Iuliano L, Pratico D, Ferro D, Pittoni V, Valesini G, Lawson J et al. Enhanced lipid peroxidation in patients positive for aPL. Blood 1997;90:3931–3935.
42. Ames PR, Nourooz-Zadeh J, Tommasino C, Alves J, Brancaccio V, Anggard EE. Oxidative stress in primary antiphospholipid syndrome. Thromb Haemost 1998;79:447–449.

19 Pregnancy Loss and Antiphospholipid Antibodies

T. Flint Porter, R. M. Silver and D. Ware Branch

Introduction

Clinicians recognized that pregnancy loss was associated with antiphospholipid antibodies (aPL) nearly 20 years ago, and by the mid-1980s, rheumatologists had formalized this clinical feature as one criterion of the antiphospholipid syndrome (APS). Harris listed "fetal loss" as the pregnancy loss criterion for APS in his 1987 proposal entitled *The Syndrome of the Black Swan* [1], implying that embryonic loss or neonatal death, would not qualify. The last decade has seen considerable debate regarding the nature of pregnancy loss associated with or attributable to aPL. The 1999 criteria proposed at the International Antiphospholipid Symposium in Sapporo, Japan probably reflect the best current consensus. These criteria include any of the following three different types of pregnancy loss as a clinical criterion for APS: (1) one or more unexplained deaths of a morphologically-normal fetus at or beyond the 10th week of gestation with normal fetal morphology documented by ultrasound or direct examination of the fetus, (2) one or more premature births of a morphologically-normal neonate at or before the 34th week of gestation because of severe pre-eclampsia or placental insufficiency, (3) three or more consecutive spontaneous abortions before the 10th week of gestation with maternal anatomic, hormonal abnormalities, and paternal and maternal chromosomal causes excluded [2]. In addition to clinical pregnancy loss, a number of investigators have found that infertility is associated with aPL. However, the clinical implications of this association are uncertain. The purpose of this chapter is to critically analyze the relationship between aPL and these obstetric problems, as well as to outline appropriate management plans when aPL are found in association with pregnancy loss.

An Overview of Pregnancy Loss

Nomenclature and Classification

For an understanding of the relationship between aPL and pregnancy loss, it is important to clarify the nomenclature of pregnancy loss. Obstetricians traditionally have grouped all pregnancy losses prior to 20 weeks' gestation (menstrual dates) together as "abortions" and the death of the fetus thereafter as a stillbirth. While this term has been pragmatic, it is arbitrary and makes no sense in terms of what is now known about developmental biology and the nature of pregnancy loss. The *pre-embryonic period* lasts from conception through the 3rd or 4th week from the first day of the last menstrual period (1 or 2 weeks since conception). During this period, the early trophoblast differentiates from the tissue destined to become the embryo (the inner cell mass) and accomplishes implantation into the maternal endo-metrium (days 6–7 after fertilization). The pre-embryo develops into a bilaminar and then trilaminar disk of cells and microscopically observable alterations of the cell disk define the cranial end central neural axis of the pre-embryo. Oxygen and nutrient needs are met by diffusion across maternal tissues. From the 4th or 5th week of gestation through the 8th or 9th week of gestation encompasses the *embryonic period*, with the exact beginning and end of the period debated by authorities according to developmental criteria used. During the *embryonic period*, the trilaminar disk folds to become cylindrical, the head and tail regions become recognizable as cranial and caudal folds, definite segmentation is seen, the heart forms, circulation is established through the umbilical cord and placenta, and all organs form (organogenesis). The *fetal period* begins at the 9th or 10th week of gestation and extends through pregnancy until delivery. This period is characterized by relatively little organogenesis, but with substantial growth and differentiation of previously formed structures.

The classification of pregnancy loss is often made difficult because of its clinical presentation. The demise of the conceptus usually precedes the symptoms of miscarriage, typically uterine bleeding and cramping, by at least several days, and often by a week or more. For example, the onset of bleeding at 10 to 12 weeks' gestation represents pre-embryonic or embryonic losses in the vast majority of cases. Furthermore, fetal death may not always precede miscarriage as in cases of cervical incompetence where the fetus is usually alive at the time of presentation. Finally, the death of a live-born infant after 20 weeks' gestation usually is recorded as a "neonatal loss" or "neonatal death."

Epidemiology

Human reproduction is inefficient, with an estimated 50% of conceptions failing [3]. The majority are unrecognized, occurring prior to or with the expected next menses [4]. The clinical problem of pregnancy loss encompasses recognized pregnancies that progress beyond the expected next menses. Approximately 10–12% of these end in spontaneous abortions prior to 12–14 weeks' gestation (from last menses), most of which are pre-embryonic or embryonic in nature. In a study of 232 women with apparently normal early pregnancies, Goldstein and colleagues [5] showed that 13.4% had pregnancy loss. Fully 87% of these occurred in the pre-embryonic or embryonic periods, representing 12% of all pregnancies. Approximately 2% of pregnancies were lost as fetal deaths from 14 to 20 weeks' gestation. The period from 8.5–14 weeks' gestation appeared to be a period of infrequent embryonic or fetal loss with no embryos alive at 8.5 weeks' gestation dying before 14 weeks' gestation, suggesting that pregnancy loss is somewhat biphasic in its distribution. Including both fetal deaths and early neonatal deaths, approximately 5% of all pregnancies end in pregnancy loss from 14 weeks' gestation through term [6–8].

Table 19.1. Common causes of recurrent pre-embryonic and embryonic pregnancy loss.

Genetic abnormalities
    Parental structural chromosome abnormalities
    Numeric chromosome abnormalities of the conceptus
    Molecular genetic abnormalities of the conceptus or placenta

Hormonal and metabolic disorders
    Luteal phase defects
    Hypersecretion of luteinizing hormone

Uterine anatomic abnormalities
    Congenital uterine malformations
    Uterine synechiae
    Fibroids
    Cervical incompetence

APS

Thrombophilia
    Factor V resistance to activated protein C
    Deficiencies of antithrombin III, protein C, or protein S

The vast majority of pregnancy losses are sporadic in nature, i.e., they occur as an isolated event in a woman whose other pregnancies are successful. Recurrent pregnancy loss, traditionally defined as the loss of three or more consecutive pregnancies, occurs in an estimated 0.5 to 1% of women. In most cases of recurrent pregnancy loss, the losses are all pre-embryonic or embryonic in nature; recurrent fetal death is much less common. Commonly accepted causes of recurrent pre-embryonic or embryonic loss are listed in Table 19.1. Taken together, women with two successive pre-embryonic or embryonic losses have a recurrence risk similar to that of women with three previous losses (24–30%) [9–11]. Some investigators have found that the risk of pre-embryonic or embryonic losses in a next pregnancy increases after four or more successive miscarriages [12].

The risk of recurrent fetal death is less well understood. However, when one fetal death has occurred, the risk increases substantially [13, 14]. In one study of over 350 000 women in Norway, investigators found that one previous fetal death between 16–27 weeks increased the risk of recurrence 20-fold [13]. Fetal death at greater than 28 weeks' gestation was associated with a 5 fold increase in recurrence. Samueloff [14] reported that the risk fetal death increased 10 fold in patients with a fetal death after 20 weeks' gestation. The commonly accepted causes of fetal death are listed in Table 19.2.

Evaluation of the Patient with Pregnancy Loss

From the standpoint of determining the cause of pregnancy loss, fetal loss is fundamentally different than pre-embryonic or embryonic loss. In cases of fetal loss, the fetus itself may be examined. In addition, a wide variety of structural malformations and precursors to fetal death (such as hydrops fetalis) may be seen by sonographic examination of the fetus in utero. The finding of a morphologically-normal fetus (postmortem changes aside) excludes a chromosomal abnormality in over 95% of cases [10]. In any case, chromosomal abnormalities are relatively infrequent causes of fetal death, especially beyond 15–20 weeks' gestation. In contrast, chromosomal abnormalities are common causes of pre-embryonic or embryonic loss, even

Table 19.2. Common causes of recurrent fetal death.

Uterine anatomic abnormalities
    Congenital uterine malformations
    Uterine synechiae
    Fibroids
    Cervical incompetence
Autoimmune causes
    APS
    Other conditions
Factor V Leiden mutation resistance to activated protein C
Alloimmunization to Rh D antigen and other blood group antigens
Poorly controlled diabetes mellitus
Maternal hypertension

in cases of recurrent pre-embryonic and embryonic loss [15]. The clinical utility of pathologic evaluation of pre-embryonic and embryonic products of conception is questionable because specimens usually contain only decidual and placental tissue which demonstrate non-specific histological features that provide little insight into the cause of pregnancy loss, cannot be used to distinguish between sporadic and recurrent abortion, and provide no prognostic significance [16]. Early pregnancy sonographic examination of the embryo is unlikely to identify malformations, especially when performed with anything less than state-of-the art equipment and experienced personnel with a special interest in the morphology of the embryo.

The placenta from a fetal death case is likely to be retrieved with intact sections that can be examined. The finding of spiral artery vasculopathy and villus abnormalities consistent with chronic hypoxia, though somewhat non-specific, would be consistent with APS-related fetal death [17] In contrast, the placental material from the average pre-embryonic and embryonic pregnancy loss is disrupted, often has undergone substantial postmortem change, and typically demonstrates placental abnormalities that are non-specific [16, 18].

Finally, the evaluation of non-genetic known or suspected causes of fetal death is more satisfying than the evaluation of pre-embryonic and embryonic loss. Fetomaternal hemorrhage may be evaluated by obtaining a Kleihauer–Betke stain of maternal blood and the presence of anti-erythrocyte antibodies causing hemolytic disease of the fetus may be evaluated by standard antibody screening techniques. The possibility of a viral infection causing fetal death may be evaluated by culture standard molecular biology techniques, and by searching for specific histopathological features in appropriate fetal tissues. Bacterial infection as a cause may be sought by maternal evaluation, appropriate cultures, and by histopathological examination of appropriate fetal tissues and the chorioamnion. In both fetal loss and pre-embryonic and embryonic loss, the possibility of a uterine septum or other uterine abnormality can be evaluated easily by hysterosalpingography or hysteroscopy. In addition, the presence of aPL should be investigated. However, the certainty with which one might ascribe APS as the cause of fetal death is often, if not usually, greater than in cases of pre-embryonic or embryonic loss. Recommendations for routine evaluation of patients with recurrent pregnancy loss are presented in Table 19.3.

Neonatal death may be due to a large number of causes – the majority are due to infection (e.g., neonatal group B *Streptococcus* infection) or complications of premature birth due to preterm premature rupture of membranes or preterm labor.

Table 19.3. Suggested routine evaluation for recurrent pregnancy loss.

History
1. Pattern and trimester of pregnancy losses and whether a live embryo or fetus was present.
2. Exposure to environmental toxins or drugs
3. Known gynecologic or obstetric infections
4. Features associated with APS
5. Genetic relationship between reproductive partners (consanguinity)
6. Family history of recurrent miscarriage or syndrome associated with embryonic or fetal loss
7. Previous diagnostic tests and treatments

Physical
1. General physical examination
2. Examination of vagina, cervix, and uterus

Tests
1. Hysterosalpingogram or hysteroscopy
2. Luteal phase endometrial biopsy; repeat in next cycle if abnormal
3. Parental karyotypes
4. LA and aCL
5. Other laboratory tests suggested by history and physical examination

In a small proportion of cases, death results from complications of prematurity after severe pre-eclampsia or severe placental insufficiency mandates iatrogenic preterm birth.

Pregnancy Loss and aPL

Type of Pregnancy Loss

aPL are not associated with sporadic pregnancy loss <20 weeks' gestation [19]. A number of studies, however, indicate that positive tests for lupus anticoagualant (LA) or IgG or IgM anticardiolipin antibodies (aCL) may be found in up to 20% of women with "recurrent pregnancy loss" or "recurrent abortion" [20–27]. Unfortunately, recurrent pregnancy loss is defined variably in these studies as either two or more consecutive losses or three or more consecutive losses. Also, in most of these studies, the type of recurrent losses is not stated (i.e., recurrent pre-embryonic or embryonic losses versus recurrent fetal deaths versus a mixture of the two). Moreover, the rigor with which other common causes of recurrent pregnancy loss have been ruled out is unclear in many studies.

In one study of a highly-selected referral population of 366 women with two or more consecutive pregnancy losses, investigators compared the types of prior pregnancy losses in 76 women with and 290 women without LA or 20 G phospholipid units (GPL) aCL [28] and found that women with moderate-to-high levels of aPL had significantly different pregnancy loss histories compared to women without high levels of aPL. Both groups of women had similar rates of prior pregnancy loss (84%). But, 50% of the prior losses in women with aPL were fetal deaths, compared to less than 15% in women without aPL. More than 80% of women with aPL had at least one fetal death, compared with less than 25% of women without aPL ($P < 0.001$). Finally, the specificity of fetal death for the presence of aPL was 76% compared to only 6% for two or more pre-embryonic or embryonic losses without fetal death.

Isotype and Levels of aPL

In many studies of patients with recurrent pregnancy loss and aPL, a substantial proportion of the positives are low level IgG aCL or only IgM aCL isotype. The nature of the relationship between low positive IgG aCL antibodies or isolated IgM aCL antibodies is of uncertain [26] or questionable clinical significance. In one study [29], women with low positive IgG aCL or isolated IgM aCL had no greater risk for antiphospholipid-related events than women who tested negative [29]. In addition, their risk for APS-associated complications was markedly lower than the risk in women with LA or ≥20 GPL aCL antibodies. On the other hand, it is intriguing that two recent studies found a significant proportion of women with recurrent pregnancy loss (primarily pre-embryonic and embryonic losses) had normalized values indicating low levels of IgG aCL antibodies (defined as > 95th or 99th percentiles) [27, 30]. In one of these studies [27], those positive for low levels of IgG aCL antibodies did not have the clinical background typical of a population of women with well-characterized APS (e.g., lupus, thrombosis, etc.). It may be that low levels of aPL detected by immunoassay are associated with recurrent pre-embryonic and embryonic loss, but that women with LA and moderate-to-high levels of IgG aCL antibodies constitute a different population of patients. Similar contentions may be raised regarding IgM aCL in the absence of LA.

To fully understand the significance of low levels of IgG aCL, isolated IgM aCL, or phospholipid-binding autoantibodies other than LA and aCL, the individuals studied must be meticulously characterized from a clinical standpoint and their level of aPL carefully determined in a way that allows comparison between studies. The inclusion of appropriate controls is, of course, crucial.

Patient Selection in Studies of aPL and Pregnancy Loss

Nowhere is the degree of variability in patient selection more evident or more important than in treatment studies of women with aPL-related pregnancy loss. In two studies, all patients had bona fide APS, as defined by clinical and laboratory criteria [31, 33], and over 40% of prior pregnancies had ended in fetal death. In one study [32], over 80% of women had suffered at least one prior fetal death. Both studies found similarly high rates of hypertension in pregnancy, fetal growth impairment, fetal distress, and preterm delivery, even with treatment. The overall pregnancy success rates in these studies were 63 and 70%, respectively. In contrast, one-quarter or more of patients in three other studies of women with aPL and prior pregnancy loss did not meet criteria for APS and had only IgM aCL antibodies (without LA), or both [34–36]. No more than one-third of patients included in these studies had prior fetal deaths. Interestingly, treated pregnancy outcomes were better than in the studies including only patients with APS, with lower rates of complications (hypertension, fetal growth impairment, fetal distress, and preterm birth).

Other Complications of APS in Pregnancy

Apart from fetal loss, other obstetric complications seen in women with APS include pre-eclampsia, uteroplacental insufficiency, and preterm birth. Clinicians should realize that the reported rates of these conditions vary considerably between studies, most likely as a result of differences in patient selection [31] An unusually high rate of pre-eclampsia has been noted in several series of patients with well-characterized APS [31, 33, 37–39] and pre-eclampsia is a major contributor to the high rate of preterm delivery in this condition. Unfortunately, the rate of pre-eclampsia is not markedly diminished by treatment. In the two largest series of well-characterized APS pregnancies [31, 33] 18–48% of women developed pre-eclampsia. In contrast, Kutteh found that only 10% of less highly selected cases (women with IgG or IgM aCL antibodies and no LA) had pre-eclampsia [40].

Several studies attempted to determine the rate of aPL among patients with pre-eclampsia. Some investigators have no association with pre-eclampsia near term [41]. However, in four studies, 11.7% to 17% of pre-eclamptic patients had significant levels of aPL [42–45]. Two of these included only patients with early-onset, severe pre-eclampsia [42, 45]. A relationship between aPL and pre-eclampsia has been confirmed by two prospective studies of unselected obstetric patients [46, 47], but not by another [48]. The weight of evidence supports testing women with early onset (< 34 weeks' gestation), severe pre-eclampsia for aPL. However, routinely testing women with mild pre-eclampsia or pre-eclampsia near term is not justified.

Women with APS are at substantial risk for placental insufficiency as manifest by fetal growth impairment and fetal distress [31, 33, 38, 39]. The rate of fetal growth impairment is approximately 30% among women with well-characterized APS [31, 33]. Even in women with IgG or IgM aCL antibodies, but no LA, the rate of fetal growth impairment among live-born infants approaches 15% [36]. Whether all women with fetal growth impairment should be tested for aPL is another matter. One group of investigators found that 24% of mothers delivered of growth impaired infants had medium or high positive tests for aCL antibodies [49]. In the prospective study of Yasuda and colleagues, 12% of women testing positive for IgG aCL antibodies had small-for-gestational age infants compared to 2% of women testing negative [47]. However, in the two other prospective studies, investigators did not find a relationship between aPL and fetal growth impairment [46, 48]. Thus, testing women who deliver infants with idiopathic fetal growth impairment is not warranted unless other clinical features point to APS.

The diagnosis of fetal distress during labor is also relatively common in pregnancies complicated by APS [31, 33, 37–39]. In the two largest series of women with APS, half of all successful treated pregnancies were complicated by fetal distress requiring delivery [31, 33] However, as with fetal growth impairment, prospective studies have not confirmed this relationship in unselected patients.

Preterm delivery occurs in approximately one-third of treated APS pregnancies [31, 33] primarily because of fetal growth impairment and/or pre-eclampsia [31, 33, 37–39]. One investigator found preterm delivery in 13% of 31 women with either IgG or IgM aCL antibodies, but no LA [40] Another group found 12% of 60 women testing positive for IgG aCL were delivered early compared to 4% of those testing negative [47].

APS patients *without* a history of thrombosis appear to have a substantial risk (i.e., 1 to several percent) of thrombosis during pregnancy [31, 33], and some authorities have recommended thromboprophylaxis and even full anticoagulation [50, 51] If used, treatment should be continued during the postpartum period, probably for about 6–8 weeks. Warfarin may be substituted for heparin during the postpartum period to limit further risk of heparin induced osteoporosis and fracture.

Pathogenesis of Obstetric Problems in APS

The clinical problems of fetal death, growth impairment, pre-eclampsia, and abnormal fetal heart tracings are all consequences of abnormal placental function, probably resulting from thrombosis in the uteroplacental circulation. Indeed, several case reports and initial series reported extensive infarction, necrosis, and thrombosis in placentas from failed pregnancies in women with aPL [17, 38, 52–54]. A spiral arterial vasculopathy in decidual vessels also has been linked to aPL-related fetal loss [17, 53]. This decidual vasculopathy is characterized by acute atherosis, intimal thickening, fibrinoid necrosis, and an absence of the normal physiologic changes in the spiral arteries, and also has been associated with pre-eclampsia and fetal growth restriction [55]. A recent large case–control study confirmed these findings, reporting evidence of thrombosis or infarction in 82% of placentas from women with aPL and fetal death [21].

It must be said that the histologic abnormalities seen in APS cases are nonspecific [55]. Furthermore, they are not always present in gestational tissues of women with aPL [56]. It may be that other factors other than placental thrombosis are relevant to some cases of pregnancy loss associated with aPL.

Management of APS in Pregnancy

Preconceptional Counseling and Antenatal Surveillance

Patients with APS should undergo preconceptional assessment and counseling. A detailed medical and obstetrical history should be obtained, and the presence of significant levels of aPL (i.e., LA, medium-to-high levels of aCL antibodies, or both) should be confirmed. The patient should be informed of the potential maternal and obstetrical problems, including fetal loss, thrombosis or stroke, pre-eclampsia, fetal growth impairment, and preterm delivery. In those women who also have SLE, issues related to exacerbation of SLE also should be discussed. All patients with APS should be assessed for evidence of anemia and thrombocytopenia, since both may occur in association with APS. Assessment for underlying renal disease (urinanalysis, a serum creatinine, 24-hour urine for creatinine clearance and total protein) may be useful.

Once pregnant, the patient with APS should be seen frequently by a physician and instructed to notify the physician immediately if she develops signs or symptoms of thrombosis or thromboembolism, severe pre-eclampsia, or decreased fetal movement. Once the diagnosis of APS is made and confirmed, serial aPL determinations are not useful. A primary goal of the antenatal visits in APS patients after 20 weeks' gestation is the detection of hypertension and/or proteinuria. Because of the risk of uteroplacental insufficiency, fetal ultrasounds should be performed every 4–6 weeks starting at 18–20 weeks' gestation. In otherwise uncomplicated APS patients, standard antenatal surveillance for fetal compromise should be started at 30 to 32 weeks' gestation. Earlier and more frequent ultrasound and fetal testing is indicated in patients with poor obstetric histories, evidence of pre-eclampsia, or evidence of fetal growth impairment. In selected cases, fetal surveillance may be justified as early as 24–25 weeks' gestation [57].

Heparin and Other Therapies During Pregnancy

A number of medications and treatment regimens have been used to treat pregnant women in an attempt to improve pregnancy outcomes in women with APS. Recently, the American College of Chest Physicians (ACCP) has recommended that all women with aPL in pregnancy be treated with a combination of low-dose aspirin and subcutaneous, unfractionated heparin, in either thromboprophylactic or anti-coagulation doses. According to the ACCP, women with APS and a previous venous thrombosis should be treated with subcutaneously administered heparin every 12 hours to prolong the activated partial thromboplastin time (aPTT) in the therapeutic range [51]. The ACCP recommends that thromboprophylactic doses be used in women with aPL and recurrent pregnancy loss and should at least be considered in women with aPL and history of pregnancy loss or venous thrombosis. The favored thromboprophylactic regimen includes subcutaneously administered heparin (15 000 to 20 000 units per day of unfractionated sodium heparin) and low-dose aspirin (60–100 mg per day) [31, 34–36]. Low-molecular-weight heparin may also be used in pregnancy, and it will likely replace unfractionated sodium heparin in APS. Doses of low-molecular-weight heparin that produce trough anti-Factor Xa activity levels of 0.1 to 0.15 U/ml would seem reasonable for patients requiring prophylactic doses [59].

It is important to counsel the patient regarding the potential adverse effects of heparin. Heparin-induced osteoporosis with fracture occurs in 1–2% of women treated during pregnancy with unfractionated heparin [60]. For this reason, women treated with heparin should be encouraged to take supplemental calcium and vitamin D (e.g., prenatal vitamins) daily. It is prudent to encourage axial skeleton weight-bearing exercise (e.g., walking) daily.

Heparin is also associated with an uncommon idiosyncratic thrombocytopenia known as heparin-induced thrombocytopenia (HIT). This complication is immune mediated, and usually has its onset 3–15 days after initiation of therapy. The frequency is difficult to determine, but probably occurs in less than 5% of patients treated with heparin, with most cases being relatively mild in nature. A more severe form of HIT, paradoxically involving venous and arterial thromboses, may occur in up to 0.5% of patients treated with unfractionated sodium heparin. It has recently been shown that low-molecular-weight heparin is much less likely to be associated with HIT [61], a major safety feature compared to unfractionated sodium heparin.

The use of high-dose intravenous immune globulin (IVIG) has generated interest because of anecdotal reports of successful pregnancy outcomes [62–66]. The literature contains nearly a dozen APS pregnancies treated with IVIG, but all but one were also treated with prednisone, heparin, or low-dose aspirin. For the most part, the reported cases appear to involve more severe cases of aPL-related pregnancy loss ("refractory" cases), who had failed other therapies. In a retrospective analysis of selected cases, some of whom had failed other therapies, patients treated with monthly IVIG infusions, unfractionated heparin, and low-dose aspirin had few pregnancy-related complications [66] None of 16 pregnancies had fetal growth restriction, all were delivered after 34 weeks' gestation, and pre-eclampsia was diagnosed in only 25%. In a small, uncontrolled trial, investigators noted no cases of pre-eclampsia and few preterm deliveries in women with APS treated with a regimen that included IVIG [67]. However, a prospective, randomized, controlled pilot study of women with APS, all of whom were given heparin and low-dose aspirin, found no difference in obstetric or maternal outcomes between those who received IVIG versus placebo (5% albumin solution) [68]. This study included only 16 patients, and though they met stringent criteria for APS, all had live births with few obstetric complications. The authors attributed this to receiving treatment early in the course of gestation. The likelihood of a successful pregnancy outcome with any treatment appears to depend in part upon the number of pregnancy losses or fetal deaths suffered in the past [69, 70]. For clinicians experienced in the evaluation and treatment of women with recurrent pregnancy loss, these observations come as no surprise. Regardless of etiology, the more consecutive pregnancy losses a woman has had, the worse her prognosis for future pregnancies. The reason for this is unknown, but this observation may influence a patient's decision to pursue additional pregnancies.

Infertility and aPL

It is now common practice in the United States to test infertile women, particularly those undergoing in vitro fertilization and embryo transfer (IVF-ET) for aPL, usually in a "panel" assay of any one of five to seven aPL. The obvious implication is that these antibodies have scientifically validated prognostic significance, impacting treatment in a way proven to be efficacious. In fact, this is hotly debated among experts, and infertile women testing positive for aPL may be exposed to potentially dangerous medications without reasonable scientific support.

Antibodies directed toward gametes or other critical components could inhibit fertilization, impair early embryo development, or hinder implantation or post-implantation/placental development. One group coined the term "reproductive autoimmune failure syndrome" to designate the entire spectrum of the reproductive process that may be susceptible to immunological disruption in clinically asymptomatic women [71]. They also hypothesized that an unknown stimulus causes a general polyclonal B-cell activation resulting in the production of a variety of autoantibodies. Depending on the specific autoantibodies formed, and perhaps the genetic vulnerability of the individual, failure of reproduction at assorted stages might result. One way to explain the development of aPL is that pelvic tissue damage due to such clinical entities as endometriosis, IVF-ET, or pelvic inflammatory disease might incite their formation.

Much of the evidence linking aPL and infertility is confined to retrospective serological studies of patients with other potentially confounding conditions such as endometriosis, unexplained infertility, pelvic disease, and IVF-ET failure. Gleicher and colleagues [71] performed 33 separate assays in infertility patients (including IgM, IgA, and IgG for antibodies against two phospholipid, five histone and four polynucleotide antigens), and 23 of 26 women with unexplained infertility were positive for at least one autoantibody. However, it is unclear whether the proportion of infertile women positive for aPL reached statistical significance, and the control group included males. Another group found that a significant proportion of 41 women with unexplained infertility had either LA or aCL antibodies, but the control group consisted of 80 pregnant women [72]. A third group, who reported the presence of aPL in infertile patients, used no controls at all [58]!

Aoki and co-investigators assayed stored sera from 65 women with unexplained infertility and 64 women with endometriosis (many of whom had recurrent pregnancy loss) for multiple aPL and compared them to 97 women with infertility of unknown cause and without a history of recurrent pregnancy loss [73]. A greater proportion of women with unexplained infertility and endometriosis was positive for (1) two or more of either aCL, antiphosphatidylserine, or antiphosphatidyinositol (5 versus 0% for controls) and (2) β_2-glycoprotein I-dependent aCL antibodies (5.4 versus 0% for controls). However, the study sera were selected from a bank enriched with patients who had previously demonstrated positive autoimmune test results, and the proportion of positive antiphospholipid test results among the infertile patients differed remarkably from a previous report by the same group. In a serologically blinded study in which investigators attempted to control for the potential problem of interassay variation, the prevalence of aPL in women with unexplained infertility was no different than that of fertile controls [74]. There also was no difference in the mean normalized antibody results.

Several groups have studied aPL in women undergoing IVF-ET. In the first report, investigators found that sera from 10 of 26 women undergoing IVF were positive for at least one of 11 autoantibodies, including antibodies to aCL and phosphatidylserine [76]. The subjects with positive and negative results were similar in regard to the number of IVF attempts, number of oocytes retrieved, fertilization rates, pregnancy rates, cleavage rates, number of abnormal oocytes, or clinical infertility diagnosis. The pregnancy rates were no different between autoantibody positive and negative women. The same group has recently confirmed that no combination of 15 autoantibody tests, including aPL, predicts the frequency of chemical or clinical pregnancy losses or successes [77].

Kutteh et al found that 19% of women undergoing IVF-ET tested positive for one or more of five aPL compared to only 5.5% of normal controls ($P < 0.05$) [78]. However, neither pregnancy rates nor implantation rates differed between the groups. Nip and colleagues studied a large number of autoantibodies, including aPL, in sera and follicular fluids from women with unexplained infertility, endometriosis, tubal factor infertility, and normal, non-pregnant, fertile controls and found no relationship between autoantibodies and IVF-ET outcome [79]. Another group of investigators found that 6.9 and 11.2% of 500 women undergoing IVF-ET had positive tests for aCL and antiphosphatidylserine, respectively [80]. However, there was no difference in pregnancy success rates between women with positive and negative results. These findings were confirmed by separate investigators. A third group measured IgG, IgM, and IgA autoantibodies to seven phospholipid antigens in 793 women undergoing assisted reproduction for a variety of reasons [81]. They found no relationship between aPL or antibody threshold and pregnancy rates. Porter and colleagues studied seven aPL in 167 women undergoing IVF-ET comparing them to 188 fertile women and 50 women with confirmed APS [82]. Only patients with bona fide APS had significantly higher levels of all seven of the antibodies. In a comparison of women with successful IVF-ET versus failed IVF-ET, none of the seven antibodies could be consistently correlated to pregnancy failure. Moreover, there were no differences in mean antibody levels between the groups.

The evidence linking IVF-ET failure and aPL is even less convincing. Birkenfeld and co-investigators measured LA and aCL antibodies in women undergoing IVF-ET for tubal infertility [83]. Sixteen of the 56 patients who failed to conceive were positive for one or both autoantibodies compared to none of 14 women who successfully implanted. However, it is uncertain whether or not the two groups were comparable with regard to number of prior cycles, timing of blood sampling, and other factors. In the same paper, the authors reported that less than 11% of 69 women undergoing their first IVF cycle were positive for LA, aCL, or antinuclear antibodies (ANA). This suggested the possibility that prior ovulation induction, ovum retrieval, or embryo transfers might increase the likelihood of antiphospholipid positivity. Results of other studies, however, do not support this hypothesis [84, 85].

Proposed Treatment for Infertile Women with aPL

Though a relationship between aPL and infertility is far from secure, several groups have performed unblinded, non-randomized, studies of treatment of aPL-positive women undergoing IVF-ET. In the first published study, investigators treated 15 women who had failed to conceive during prior IVF cycles and who were positive for LAC, aCL, or ANA with 10 mg of prednisone and low-dose aspirin daily starting two weeks before cycle initiation [83]. Seven of the women became pregnant, but there no control patients. Another group treated 19 women positive for aCL or other phospholipid-binding antibodies with subcutaneously administered heparin and low-dose aspirin [78]. Ten (53%) achieved pregnancies compared to 8 of 17 (47%) untreated women. A third group also treated aPL-positive IVF patients with subcutaneously administered heparin and low-dose aspirin starting the day of oocyte retrieval [86]. Neither found a difference in implantation rates between the treated women and aPL-negative patients (13 versus 8%). Furthermore, neither the clinical nor ultimate ongoing pregnancy rates differed according to apL status or treatment.

Sher et al found conflicting results in aPL-positive IVF patients with documented pelvic pathology who were treated with subcutaneously administered heparin and aspirin starting the day of cycle initiation [87, 88]. Clinical pregnancies were established in 49% of treated patients compared to 16% of untreated aPL-positive women ($P < 0.05$). However, assignment to treatment was neither randomized nor explained and when patients were divided into disease categories (i.e., endometriosis, pelvic inflammatory disease, or pelvic adhesions), there were no significant differences in pregnancy rates between treated and untreated patients. Live birth rates were not reported. It is interesting that the 49% pregnancy rate among the treated aPL-positive patients was comparable to that expected from women undergoing IVF-ET for pelvic pathology in experienced centers. But the 16% pregnancy rate among non-treated women was somewhat lower than expected if aPL status were unknown. Recently, the same group reported similar results in a three part trial of 687 women who tested positive for at least one of several aPL [89]. Again, some patients were treated with heparin and aspirin and appeared to have improved pregnancy rates over those who were untreated (46 versus 17%). Antibodies directed against phosphatidylserine and phosphatidylethanolamine appeared to be associated with treatment failure. Subsequently, these women had their treatment expanded to include IVIG which resulted in improved pregnancy rates (41 versus 17%). However, it is unclear from the paper how patients were assigned to treatment, what threshold of positivity was necessary for inclusion, why patients were retested for other aPL, and how other confounding variables were controlled. In contrast, other studies failed to demonstrate consistent correlations between antiphosphatidylserine and antiphosphatidylethanolamine and IVF-ET failure in untreated patients [82].

The concept of aPL-mediated infertility is popular and hypothetically attractive. Many investigators have found a statistically higher rate of aPL in women with infertility, though not all agree. Any proof that aPL are associated with a specific type of infertility or influence pregnancy outcome with assisted reproductive technology is insubstantial at best. Most extant studies lack scientific rigor – in particular, many studies have used poorly selected controls for comparison. A more fundamental problem is the lack of aPL assay standardization and standard calibration sera.

The idea that heparin treatment of women with aPL undergoing IVF-ET is beneficial is based on a series of hypotheses, none of which have been adequately substantiated by scientific evidence. As noted by Hatasaka and colleagues, studies regarding both the diagnosis and treatment of female immune-mediated infertility fall into the lowest quality category (opinions of respected authorities, based on clinical experience, descriptive studies, or reports of expert committees) when evaluated according to the five levels of evidence quality established by the US Preventive Services Task Force [74].

References

1. Harris EN. Syndrome of the black swan. Br J Rheumatol 1987;26:324–326.
2. Wilson WA, Gharavi AE, Koike T et al. International consensus statement on preliminary classification criteria for definite antiphospholipid syndrome: report of an international workshop. Arthritis Rheum 1999;42:1309–1311.
3. Boklage CE. Survival probability of human conceptions from fertilization to term. Int J Fertil 1990;35:75–93.
4. Wilcox AJ, Weinberg CR, O'Connor JF et al. Incidence of early loss of pregnancy. N Engl J Med 1988; 319:189–194.
5. Goldstein SR. Embryonic death in early pregnancy: a new look at the first trimester. Obstet Gynecol 1994;84:294–297.
6. Miller JF, Williamson E, Glue J, Gordon YB, Grudzinskas JG, Sykes A. Fetal loss after implantation: a prospective study. Lancet 1980;ii:554–556.
7. Edmonds DK, Lindsay KS, Miller JF, Williams E, Wood PJ. Early embryonic mortality in women. Fertil Steril 1982;38:447–453.
8. Whitaker PG, Taylor A, Lind T. Unsuspected pregnancy loss in healthy women. Lancet 1983;i:1126–1127.
9. Regan L. A prospective study of spontaneous abortion. In: Beard RW, Sharp F, editors. Early pregnancy loss. London: Springer-Verlag, 1988;23–37.
10. Warburton D, Fraser FC. Spontaneous abortion risks in man: data from reproductive histories collected in a medical genetics unit. Am J Hum Genet 1964;16:1–25.
11. Fitzsimmons J, Jackson D, Wapner R, Jackson L. Subsequent reproductive outcome in couples with repeated pregnancy loss. Am J Med Genet 1983;16:583–587.
12. Stirrat GM. Recurrent miscarriage I: definition and epidemiology. Lancet 1990;336:673–675.
13. Oyen N, Skjaerven R, Irgens LM. Population-based recurrence risk of sudden infant death syndrome compared with other infant and fetal deaths. Am J Epidemiol 1996;144:300.
14. Samueloff A, Xenakis E, Berkus MD, Huff RW, Langer O. Recurrent stillbirth: significance and characteristics. J Reprod Med 1993;38: 883–886.
15. Stern JJ, Dorfmann AD, Gutierrez-Najar AJ, Cerrillo M, Coulam CB. Frequency of abnormal karyotypes among abortuses from women with and without a history of recurrent spontaneous abortion. Fertil Steril. 1996;65(2):250–253.
16. Fox H. Histological classification of tissue from spontaneous abortions: a valueless exercise? Histopathology 1993;.22:599–600.
17. De Wolf F, Carreras LO, Moerman P, Vermylen J, Van Assche A, Renaer M. Decidual vasculopathy and extensive placental infarction in a patient with repeated thromboembolic accidents, recurrent fetal loss, and a lupus anticoagulant. Am J Obstet Gynecol 1982;142:829–834.

18. Rushton DI. Examination of products of conception from previable human pregnancies. J Clin Pathol 1981;34:819–835.
19. Infante-Rivard C, David M, Gauthier R, Rivard GE. Lupus anticoagulants, anticardiolipin antibodies, and fetal loss. A case control study. N Engl J Med 1991;325:1063–1066.
20. Petri M, Golbus M, Anderson R, Whiting-O'Keefe Q, Corash L, Hellmann D. Antinuclear antibody, lupus anticoagulant, and anticardiolipin antibody in women with idiopathic habitual abortion. A controlled, prospective study of forty-four women. Arthritis Rheum 1987;30:601–606.
21. Out HJ, Bruinse HW, Christiaens GCML et al. Prevalence of aPL in patients with fetal loss. Ann Rheum Dis 1991;50:553–557.
22. Parazzini F, Acaia B, Faden D, Lovotti M, Marelli G, Cortelazzo S. APL and recurrent abortion. Obstet Gynecol 1991;77:854–858.
23. Parke AL, Wilson D, Maier D. The prevalence of aPL in women with recurrent spontaneous abortion, women with successful pregnancies, and women who have never been pregnant. Arthritis Rheum 1991;34:1231–1235.
24. Plouffe L Jr, White EW, Tho SP et al. Etiologic factors of recurrent abortion and subsequent reproductive performance of couples: have we made any progress in the past 10 years? Am J Obstet Gynecol 1992;167:313–320.
25. MacLean MA, Cumming GP, McCall F, Walker ID, Walker JJ. The prevalence of lupus anticoagulant and anticardiolipin antibodies in women with a history of first trimester miscarriages. Br J Obstet Gynaecol 1994;101:103–106.
26. Yetman DL, Kutteh WH. Antiphospholipid antibody panels and recurrent pregnancy loss: prevalence of anticardiolipin antibodies compared with other aPL. Fertil Steril 1996;66:540–546.
27. Branch DW, Silver RM, Pierangelli SS, van Leeuwen I, Harris EN. APL other than lupus anticoagulant and anticardiolipin antibodies in women with recurrent pregnancy loss, fertile controls, and antiphospholipid syndrome. Obstet Gynecol 1997;89:549–555.
28. Oshiro BT, Silver RM, Scott JR, Yu H, Branch DW. APL and fetal death. Obstet Gynecol 1996;87:489–493.
29. Silver RM, Porter TF, van Leeuwen I, Jeng G, Scott JR, Branch DW. Anticardiolipin antibodies: clinical consequences of "low titers." Obstet Gynecol 1996;87:494–500.
30. Aoki K, Hayashi Y, Hirao Y, Yagami Y. Specific aPL as a predictive variable in patients with recurrent pregnancy loss. Am J Reprod Immunol 1993a;29:82–87.
31. Branch DW, Silver RM, Blackwell JL, Reading JC Scott JR. Outcome of treated pregnancies in women with antiphospholipid syndrome: an update of the Utah experience. Obstet Gynecol 1992;80:614–620.
32. Branch DW, Dudley DJ, Scott JR, Silver RM. APL and fetal loss. N Engl J Med 1992;326:952.
33. Lima F, Khamashta MA, Buchanan NM, Kerslake S, Hunt BJ, Hughes GR. A study of sixty pregnancies in patients with the antiphospholipid syndrome. Clin Exp Rheumatol 1996;14:131–136.
34. Cowchock FS, Reece EA, Balaban D, Branch DW, Plouffe L. Repeated fetal losses associated with aPL: a collaborative randomized trial comparing prednisone to low-dose heparin treatment. Am J Obstet Gynecol 1992;166:1318–1327.
35. Rosove MH, Tabsh K, Wasserstrum N, Howard P, Hahn BH, Kalunian KC. Heparin therapy for pregnant women with lupus anticoagulant or anticardiolipin antibodies. Obstet Gynecol 1990;75:630–634.
36. Kutteh WH, Ermel LD. A clinical trial for the treatment of antiphospholipid antibody-associated recurrent pregnancy loss with lower dose heparin and aspirin. Am J Reprod Immunol 1996;35:402–407.
37. Lockshin MD, Druzin ML, Goei S et al. Antibody to cardiolipin as a predictor of fetal distress or death in pregnant patients with systemic lupus erythematosus. N Engl J Med 1985;313:152–156.
38. Branch DW, Scott JR, Kochenour NK, Hershgold E. Obstetric complications associated with the lupus anticoagulant. N Engl J Med 1985;313:1322–1326.
39. Caruso A, De Carolis S, Ferrazzani S, Valesini G, Caforio L, Mancuso S. Pregnancy outcome in relation to uterine artery flow velocity waveforms and clinical characteristics in women with antiphospholipid syndrome. Obstet Gynecol 1993;82:970–977.
40. Kutteh WH. Antiphospholipid antibody associated recurrent pregnancy loss:treatment with heparin and low-dose aspirin is superior to low dose aspirin alone. Am J Obstet Gynecol 1996;174:1584–1589.
41. Scott RAH. Anticardiolipin antibodies and pre-eclampsia. Br J Obstet Gynecol 1987;94:604.
42. Branch DW, Andres R, Digre K,B , Rote NS, Scott JR. The association of aPL with severe pre-eclampsia. Obstet Gynecol 1989;73:54.
43. Milliez J, Lelong F, Bayani N et al. The prevalence of autoantibodies during third-trimester pregnancy complicated by hypertension or idiopathic fetal growth retardation. Am J Obstet Gynecol 1991;165:51–55.
44. Sletnes KE, Wisloff F, Moe N, Dale PO. APL in pre-clamptic women: relation to growth retardation and neonatal outcome. Acta Obstet Gynecol Scand 1992;71:112–117.

45. Moodley J, Bhoola V, Duursma J, Pudifin D, Byrne S, Kenoyer DG. The association of aPL with severe early-onset pre-eclampsia. S Afr Med J 1995;85:105–107.
46. Pattison NS, Chamley LW, McKay EJ, Liggins GC, Butler WS. APL in pregnancy: prevalence and clinical associations. Br J Obstet Gynaecol 1993;100:909–913.
47. Yasuda M, Takakuwa K, Tokunaga A, Tanaka K. Prospective studies of the association between anticardiolipin antibody and outcome of pregnancy. Obstet Gynecol 1995;86:555–559.
48. Lynch A, Marlar R, Murphy J et al. APL in predicting adverse pregnancy outcome. A prospective study. Ann Intern Med 1994;120:470–475.
49. Polzin WJ, Kopelman JN, Robinson RD, Read JA, Brady K. The association of aPL with pregnancies complicated by fetal growth restriction. Obstet Gynecol 1991;78:1108–1111.
50. Branch DW, Silver RM. Criteria for antiphospholipid syndrome: early pregnancy loss, fetal loss, or recurrent pregnancy loss. Lupus 1996;5:409–413.
51. Ginsberg JS, Hirsh J. Use of antithrombotic agents during pregnancy. Chest 1998;114(5 Suppl): 524S–530S.
52. Lubbe WF, Butler WS, Palmer SJ et al. Lupus anticoagulant in pregnancy. Br J Obstet 1984;91:357–363.
53. Nayar R, Lage JM. Placental changes in a first trimester missed abortion in maternal systemic lupus erythematosus with antiphospholipid syndrome: a case report and review of the literature. Hum Pathol 1996;27:201–206.
54. Silver RM, Draper ML, Scott JR et al. Clinical consequences of aPL: an historic cohort study. Obstet Gynecol 1994;83: 372–377.
55. Khong TY, DeWolf F, Robertson WB et al. Inadequate maternal vascular response to placentation in pregnancies complicated by pre-eclampsia and by small for gestational age infants. Br J Obstet Gynecol 1986;93:1049–1059.
56. Salafia CS, Parke AL. Placental pathology in systemic lupus erythematosus and phospholipid antibody syndrome. Rheum Dis Clin North Am 1997;23:85–97.
57. Druzin ML, Lockshin M, Edersheim TG, Hutson JM, Krauss AL, Kogut E. Second-trimester fetal monitoring and preterm delivery in pregnancies with systemic lupus erythematosus and/or circulating anticoagulant. Am J Obstet Gynecol 1987;157:1503–1510.
58. Roussev RG, Kaider BD, Price DE, Coulam CB. Laboratory evaluation of women experiencing reproductive failure. Am J Reprod Immunol 1996;35:415–420.
59. Dulitzki M, Pauzner R, Langevitz P, Pras M, Many A, Schiff E. Low-molecular-weight heparin during pregnancy and delivery: preliminary experience with 41 pregnancies. Obstet Gynecol 1996;87:380–383.
60. Dahlman TC. Osteoporotic fractures and the recurrence of thromboembolism during pregnancy and the puerperium in 184 women undergoing thromboprophylaxis with heparin. Am J Obstet Gynecol 1993;168:1265–1270.
61. Warkentin TE, Levine MN, Hirsh J et al. Heparin-induced thrombocytopenia in patients treated with low-molecular-weight heparin or unfractionated heparin. N Engl J Med 1995;332:1330–1335.
62. Scott JR, Branch DW, Kochenour NK, Ward K. Intravenous immunoglobulin treatment of pregnant patients with recurrent pregnancy loss caused by aPL and Rh immunization. Am J Obstet Gynecol 1988;159:1055–1056.
63. Wapner RJ, Cowchock FS, Shapiro SS. Successful treatment in two women with aPL and refractory pregnancy losses with intravenous immunoglobulin infusions. Am J Obstet Gynecol 1989;161:1271–1272.
64. Katz VL, Thorp JM Jr, Watson WJ, Fowler L, Heine RP. Human immunoglobulin therapy for preeclampsia associated with lupus anticoagulant and anticardiolipin antibody. Obstet Gynecol 1990;76:986–988.
65. Kaaja R, Julkunen H, Ammala P, Palosuo T, Kurki P. Intravenous immunoglobulin treatment of pregnant patients with recurrent pregnancy losses associated with aPL. Acta Obstet Gynecol Scand 1993;72:63–66.
66. Clark AL, Branch DW, Silver RM, Harris EN, Pierangeli S, Spinnato JA. Pregnancy complicated by the antiphospholipid syndrome: outcomes with intravenous immunoglobulin therapy. Obstet Gynecol 1999; 93:437–441.
67. Spinnato JA, Clark AL, Pierangeli SS, Harris EN. Intravenous immunoglobulin therapy for the antiphospholipid syndrome in pregnancy. Am J Obstet Gynecol 1995;172:690–694.
68. Pregnancy Loss Study Group. A multicenter, controlled, pilot study of intravenous immune globulin treatment of antiphospholipid syndrome in pregnancy.
69. Glueck HI, Kant KS, Weiss MA et al. Thrombosis in systemic lupus erythematosus: Relation to the presence of circulating anticoagulant. Arch Intern Med 1985;145:1389–1395.
70. Branch DW, Scott JR. Clinical implication of anti-phospholipid antibodies: the Utah experience. In: Harris EN, Exner T, Hughes GRV, Asherson RA, editors. Phospholipid-binding antibodies. Boca Raton, FL: CRC Press, 1990;335–346.

71. Gleicher N, El-Roeiy A, Confino E, Friberg J. Reproductive failure because of autoantibodies: Unexplained infertility and pregnancy wastage. Am J Obstet Gynecol 1989;160:1376–1385.

72. Taylor PV, Campbell JM, Scott JS. Presence of autoantibodies in women with unexplained infertility. Am J Obstet Gynecol 1989;161: 377–379.

73. Aoki K, Dudkiewicz AB, Matsuura E, Novotny M, Kaberlein G, Gleicher N. Clinical significance of β_2-glycoprotein I-dependent anticardiolipin antibodies in the reproductive autoimmune failure syndrome: correlation with conventional antiphospholipid antibody detection systems. J Obstet Gynecol 1995b;172:926–931.

74. Hatasaka H, Porter TF, Silver RM, Lee RM, Ricks C, Branch DW. Antiphospholipid antibody levels are not elevated among women with tubal factor and unexplained infertility. Annu Proc Am Soc Reprod Med 1997.

75. Hatasaka HH, Branch DW, Kutteh WH, Scott JR. Autoantibody screening for infertility: explaining the unexplained? J Reprod Immunol 1997;34:137–153.

76. El-Roey A, Gleicher N, Friberg J, Confino E, Dudkiewicz AB. Correlation between peripheral blood and follicular fluid autoantibodies and impact on in vitro fertilization. Obstet Gynecol 1987;70: 163–170.

77. Gleicher N, Liu HC, Dudkiewicz A et al. Autoantibody profiles and immunoglobulin levels as predictors of in vitro fertilization success. Am J Obstet Gynecol 1994;170:1145–1149.

78. Kutteh WH, Yetman DL, Chantilis SJ, Crain J. Effect of aPL in women undergoing in vitro fertilization: role of heparin and aspirin. Hum Reprod 1997;12:1171–1175.

79. Nip MMC, Taylor PV, Rutherford AJ, Hancock KW. Autoantibodies and antisperm antibodies in sera and follicular fluids of infertile patients; relation to reproductive outcome after in-vitro fertilization. Hum Reprod 1995;10:2564–2569.

80. Kowalik A, Vichnin M, Liu H-C, Branch DW, Berkeley AS. Mid-follicular anticardiolipin and antiphosphatidylserine antibody titers do not correlate with IVF outcome. Fertil Steril 1997;68:298–304.

81. Denis AL, Guido M, Adler RD, Bergh PA, Brenner C, Scott RT. APL and pregnancy rates and outcome in in vitro fertilization patients. Fertil Steril 1997;67: 1084–1090.

82. Porter TF, Branch DW, Silver RM, Hatasaka HH, Cramer DW, Hill JA. APL are not related to the success of implantation in infertile women undergoing in vitro fertilization–embryo transfer.

83. Birkenfeld A, Mukaida T, Minichiello L, Jackson M, Kase NG, Yemini M. Incidence of autoimmune antibodies in failed embryo transfer cycles. Am J Reprod Immunol 1994;31:65–68.

84. Fisch B, Fried S, Manor Y, Ovadia J, Witz IP, Yron I. Increased antiphospholipid antibody activity in in-vitro fertilization patients is not treatment-dependent but rather an inherent characteristic of the infertile state. Am J Reprod Immunol 1995;34:370–374.

85. Birdsall MA, Lockwood GM, Ledger WL, Johnson PM, Chamley LW. APL in women having in-vitro fertilization. Human Reprod 1996;11:1185–1189.

86. Schenk LM, Butler L, Morris JP, Cox B, Leete J, Abuhamed A et al. Heparin and aspirin treatment yields higher implantation rates in IVF patients with antiphospholipid antibody seropositity compared to untreated seronegative patients (abstract). Proceedings of the Annual Meeting of the American Society of Reproductive Medicine, Boston, 1996.

87. Sher G, Feinman M, Zouves C, Kutter G, Maassarani G, Salem R et al. High fecundity rates following antiphospholipid antibody seropositive women treated with heparin and aspirin. Hum Reprod 1994;9:2278–2283.

88. Sher G, Matzner W, Feinman M et al. The selective use of heparin/aspirin therapy, alone or in combination with intravenous immunoglobulin G, in the management of antiphospholipid antibody-positive women undergoing in vitro fertilization. Am J Reprod Immunol 1998;40:74–82.

89. Sher G, Zouves C, Feinman M et al. A rational basis for the use of combined heparin/aspirin and IVIG immunotherapy in the treatment of recurrent IVF failure associated with aPL. Am J Reprod Immunol 1998;39:391–394.

20 Imaging of Microemboli in Antiphospholipid Syndrome

Ch. Specker, M. Siebler and M. Schneider

Identification and acknowledgement of the antiphospholipid syndrome (APS) led to a revised view of neuropsychiatric manifestations in systemic lupus erythematosus (SLE) [1]. Evidence came up that there are at least two different pathophysiological concepts of central nervous system (CNS) involvement in this condition. Beyond "vasculitic" manifestation as a consequence of immunologically induced inflammation ("cerebritis"), mostly accompanied by systemic activity of underlying lupus with other organs affected and serological signs of increased immune response, there is in addition a "vasculopathic" CNS manifestation caused by obliteration of small- or medium-sized cerebral arteries leading to various neurologic symptoms of cerebrovascular ischemia [2–4]. The latter form could be identified as the underlying mechanism of CNS disease in APS [5], and indeed it could be the main cause of CNS involvement in SLE [6]. Differentiation of these distinct states in a patient with CNS disease is essential for appropriate treatment.

Patients with SLE or APS may present with a wide array of neuropsychiatric clinical symptoms [4, 6, 7]. As there is no single diagnostic "gold standard" for CNS involvement in SLE or APS, the assessment of individual patients is mostly dependent upon clinical evaluation [8]. Thereafter, information about autoantibodies, brain lesions and dysfunction may support the diagnosis. Certain autoantibodies (i.e., aPL) can be regarded as highly specific and rather sensitive for cerebrovascular disease in SLE/APS, unlike the case for vasculitic CNS involvement in SLE without APS. Diagnostic methods evaluating the structure or function of the CNS are more or less sensitive but not specific [7–9].

Magnetic resonance imaging (MRI) is a highly sensitive method to detect cerebral lesions and its capability to identify small parenchymal defects or local disturbance of brain tissue lies far beyond that of computed tomography. Since non-specific "white matter lesions" and minimal parenchymal changes can be also detected using MRI in normal controls [10, 11], the lack of specific findings providing additional clinical information in non-CNS patients with SLE [12] is not confounding. When an alteration of the brain is clinically considered, MRI is the method of choice to look for structural abnormalities; their formation and distribution allow conclusions concerning the underlying mechanisms (Fig. 20.1). Additional procedures (angiography, electroencephalography) provide little additional information and are restricted to special indications (i.e., diagnosis of vascular malformations, epileptic potentials).

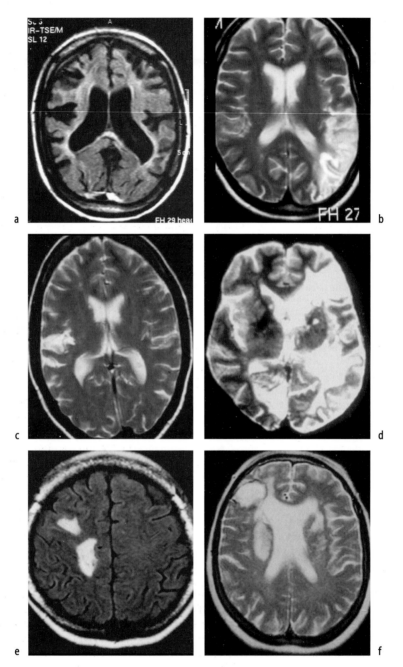

Figure 20.1. Different MRI scans in patients with SLE / APS: **a** diffuse cerebral atrophy in a 42-year-old woman with secondary APS; **b** territorial infarction of the left MCA in a 29-year-old woman with primary APS; **c** cortical infarction in a 28-year-old woman with secondary APS; **d** multiple cerebral infarctions in a 37-year-old woman with secondary APS; **e** biopsy proven vasculitic cerebral lesions in a 43-year-old woman with SLE; **f** cerebral abscesses in a 65 yr. old woman with SLE.

Ultrasound Doppler technique has been applied to investigate first extracranial and subsequently intracranial arteries using pulse waved transcranial insonation [13]. This transcranial Doppler sonography (TCD) is a standard technique allowing non-invasive investigation of the intracerebral arteries. Stenoses, occlusions, and blood-flow abnormalities can be quite easily detected as well as in extracranial sites.

In the late 1960s transient, high, intense ultrasonic signals within the velocity spectrum of insonated arteries have been detected in the aortic arch of divers during hyperbaric decompression and were attributed to air bubbles arising in the blood under this condition [14]. Similar signals were found in the intracranial arteries using TCD monitoring in cardiopulmonary bypass operations [15] and carotid endarterectomy [16]. As inclusions of air in liquids cause high intense acoustic reflection signals, these findings were not surprising; but since those so called "microemboli" were also detectable *before* incision of blood vessels in the preoperative phase rendering air bubbles unlikely, formed particles were postulated as another cause of those signals [17]. That experimental emboli can induce micro-embolic signals (MES) in blood vessels was shown by Russel and co-workers in 1991. They injected emboli of thrombotic components sized about 500 to 1500 μm into the aorta of rabbits and detected characteristic high energetic acoustic signals in the downstream blood velocity spectrum [18].

Beside the extraordinary conditions of hyperbaric decompression and air "contamination" during operations, MES have been described in two different states [19]: patients with artificial heart valves (AHV), which are supposed to generate air bubbles by cavitations [20], and patients with internal carotid stenosis in which the MES were considered as thrombogenic microparticles [21]. Since then a number of studies suggested that detectability of MES may be associated with cerebrovascular ischemia (CVI) occurring in these states [22]. Indeed, MES proved to be of predictive value not only for former [23, 24] but also for subsequent [25, 26] CVI in patients with stenosis of the internal carotid artery, allowing for therapeutic stratification (i.e., endarterectomy) [27].

Outside these established indications microemboli detection was first applied in an interdisciplinary study on patients with Sneddon's syndrome. Interestingly, some patients showed MES and they were found to have a significantly shorter time elapse since the last ischemic symptom than those without [28]. Because as well as atherosclerosis and hypertension antiphospholipid antibodies (aPL) have also been considered to play a role in Sneddon's syndrome [29], it was of special interest that the two patients with the highest event rates of MES turned out to be aPL positive.

Long-term (60 minutes) TCD monitoring is usually performed with a 2-MHz pulsed-wave transducer with the Doppler probe being fixed bilaterally by a head-tape to the temporal region of a resting patient for insonation of the middle cerebral artery (MCA). The sample volume is set at an axial width of 10–15 mm and an insonation focus depth of 45–55 mm. TCD session is recorded digitally on tape (DAT) for further off-line analyses. The analogous Doppler signal is processed by 128-point fast-Fourier transformation (FFT) with a 75% overlapping signal analysis to increase time resolution and ensure that any TCD epoch of interest is within one time frame, thereby avoiding FFT inaccuracy caused by sampling gaps [30]. The calculated power spectrum of the audible shift is visualized color-coded on screen. TCD signals indicating microemboli are defined according to the following criteria: (1) high-intensity unidirectional signal within the blood flow velocity spectrum; (2) short duration of less than 100 ms; (3) signal intensity greater than 1 dB compared with the background blood flow signal; and (4) characteristic "chirping" sound. Although discrimination between so-defined embolism, artefacts, and normal spectra remains a principal problem, all published clinical studies thus far have relied on human observers. In an intercenter study a high level of agreement in the identification of MES was found between (experienced) observers (0.89–0.94) suggesting that the technique is sufficiently reproducible for clinical use [31]. Duration of TCD monitoring required to detect MES depends on their frequency which seems to vary considerably in repeated investigations of individual patients. A typical example of a recorded microembolic event and a corresponding auto-mated analysis by a neural network trained for MES-pattern detection is shown in Fig. 20.2.

Microemboli detection using TCD in a first cohort of 46 patients with SLE and five with primary APS (PAPS) revealed MES in a range of 2–70 events/hour in 14 of 16 patients with a history of CVI (88%) versus only one out of 35 (3%) patients without CVI ($P < 0.001$) [32]. Concerning the combination of MES and aPL, 12/16 patients with a history of CVI had both, two patients had MES and another two aPL only. One of 15 patients with MES (2 events/hour) had no history of CVI and no aPL. All patients with aPL and MES ($n = 12$) and none of those without aPL and without MES ($n = 18$) had a history of CVI ($P < 0.001$). No MES were found in 22 normal controls. Interestingly, the rate of MES correlated with the titer of IgG aCL arguing for a pathophysiological association between aPL and MES. The prevalence of MES in more than 120 SLE patients investigated was 28% in SLE, 13% in SLE without APS and 44% with APS ($P < 0.005$).

Until now, studies on MES in APS have not been designed to address possible treatment effects. Repeated TCD monitoring in some patients under different treat-ment however, revealed cessation of MES in three out of 10 patients after adminis-tration of low-dose aspirin and in seven out of 12 after coumadin. Among the patients with ongoing MES despite treatment one died from "catastrophic" APS.

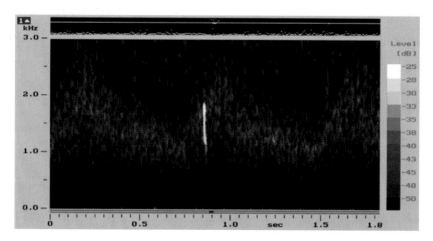

Figure 20.2. A 128-point fast Fourier transformed Doppler velocity spectrum obtained from the middle cerebral artery over two heart cycles. The sharp bright signal corresponds to a characteristic high pitched acoustic signal in the audible Doppler shift. The output of a neural network trained for detection of MES-patterns is depicted in the upper panel (yellow line: decision threshold).

The finding of MES in patients with APS and their correlation to a history of CVI raise many further questions and some theoretical considerations. One question is: where these microemboli derive from. In analogy to the known generation of MES on AHV and the association of APS with heart valve thickening [33], one might expect altered heart valves to be the source of MES in APS. Using transthoracic echocardiography in our patients, the rate of valvular changes in particular of the mitral valve was considerable and in the same range as in a study performing repeated transoesophageal examination in SLE patients [34]. However, only mitral valve prolapse tended to be more frequent in the MES-positive than in the MES-negative group, and many patients with cerebral MES had no signs of cardiac valvular alteration. On the other hand, MES in patients with carotid artery disease (CAD) are generated on atherosclerotic plaques of the internal carotid artery. In this condition, their detectability depends on the site, degree, extent, and surface of stenosis [35]. In an experimental model Kessler and co-workers implanted a rough-surfaced Dacron® graft in the internal carotid artery of baboons and detected MES by TCD in the downstream cerebral vasculature. Histologically proven infarctions were due to thromboses generated on the vessel graft [36]. In the APS patients investigated by TCD, carotid artery disease was excluded by cervical Doppler and duplex sonography. To further address the question of the source, we analysed the "acoustic energy" of MES found in APS, AHV and CAD. In this aspect, the signals of APS patients were nearly identical to those in CAD whereas the signals from patients with AHV showed a much higher energy (Fig. 20.3).

The question of which size or constitution these microemboli have is obvious, but difficult to answer. For physical reasons Doppler signal properties (i.e., the reflected energy) do not allow for direct calculation of embolus size or composition. Derived from experimental models, physical conditions of the method used and the fact that MES do not cause neurological symptoms of actual vascular occlusion, it is speculated that they are in a range of about 50 to 500 μm [37]. This does not imply that particles of other size will not occur in APS patients.

Detectability of MES favors thromboembolic vasculopathy rather than vasculitis as the underlying mechanism of CVI in APS. Most theories about induction and forming of thrombi and emboli in APS suppose an interaction of aPL with endothelial cells

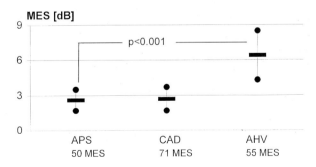

Figure 20.3. Energy (in dB) of microembolic signals (MES) in patients with APS, carotid artery disease (CAD), and artificial heart valves (AHV). Mean, SD and number of MES analysed is given. "Embolic signal power" was the average of four FFT lines including the MES and "background power" was the average of 2 seconds Doppler signal FFT lines without MES.

and/or thrombocytes [38,39], and aPL are discussed as "a link between thrombosis and atherosclerosis" [40]. In analogy to atherosclerosis, it can be hypothesized that the signals detected in SLE/APS patients are aPL-induced microaggregates emerging within the blood flow or on endothelial surfaces, leading to clinically silent microembolism as a possible precursor of the "macroembolism" with the well-known clinical manifestations of APS. This is supported by the following findings: (1) a strong association of MES with CVI and aPL; (2) a significant direct correlation between frequency of MES and the titer of aPL; (3) a very similar acoustic energy of the MES in APS and atherosclerotic patients (in contrast to significantly higher energy of MES evolving from artificial heart valves); (4) a significant inverse association between the time elapsing since the last ischemic event and the detectability of MES; and (5) possible dependence of continuing cerebral symptoms on the frequency of MES recorded by repeated TCD monitoring in individual patients.

From the present data it can not be decided to what extent detection of cerebral MES using TCD offers a potential tool for screening APS patients at risk for developing CVI and for assessing treatment strategies. Even though the retrospective results are promising, these have to be verified by prospective controlled investigations. However, detection of MES in APS using TCD is an inexpensive, non-invasive method offering a new approach in risk stratification and possibly therapy monitoring in patients with aPL [41] and encourages elucidation of some pathophysiological aspects in APS.

References

1. Hughes GRV. The antiphospholipid syndrome: ten years on Lancet 1993;342: 341–344
2. The Antiphospholipid Antibodies in Stroke Study Group (APASS). Clinical and laboratory findings in patients with antiphospholipid antibodies and cerebral ischemia. Stroke 1990;21:1268–1273.
3. Meroni PL, Rivolta R, Ghidoni P. Histopathological findings in cases of systemic lupus erythematosus-associated antiphospholipid syndrome. Clin Rheumatol 1991;10:211–214
4. Levine SR, Brey RL. Neurological aspects of the antiphospholipid antibody syndrome. Lupus 1996;5:347–353.
5. Lie JT. Vasculopathy of the antiphospholipid syndromes revisited: thrombosis is the culprit and vasculitis the consort. Lupus 1996;5:368–371.
6. Hess DC. Cerebral lupus vasculopathy: mechanisms and clinical relevance. Ann N Y Acad Sci 1997;823:154–168.
7. Brey RL, Escalante A. Neurological manifestations of antiphospholipid antibody syndrome. Lupus 1998;7 (Suppl 2): S67–S74.
8. Hanly JG. Evaluation of patients with CNS involvement in SLE. Baillières Clin Rheumatol 1998;12:415–431.
9. Sabbadini MG, Manfredi AA, Bozzolo E et al. Central nervous system involvement in systemic lupus erythematosus patients without overt neuropsychiatric manifestations. Lupus 1999;8:11–19.
10. Gerard G, Weisberg LA. MRI periventricular lesions in adults. Neurology 1986;36:998–1001
11. Fazekas F. Magnetic resonance signal abnormalities in asymptomatic individuals: their incidence and functional correlates. Eur Neurol 1989;29:164–168.
12. Kozora E, West SG, Kotzin BL, Julian L, Porter S, Bigler E. Magnetic resonance imaging abnormalities and cognitive deficits in systemic lupus erythematosus patients without overt central nervous system disease. Arthritis Rheum 1998;41:41–47.
13. Aaslid R, Markwalder TM, Nornes H. Noninvasive transcranial Doppler ultrasound recording of flow velocity in basal cerbral arteries. J Neurosurg 1982;57:769–774.
14. Spencer MP, Campell SD, Sealey JL, Henry FC, Lindbergh J. Experiments on decompression bubbles in the circulation using ultrasonic and electromagnetic flowmeters. J Occupat Med 1969;11:238–244.

15. Padayachee TS, Parsons S, Theobald R, Linley J, Gosling RG, Deverall PB. The detection of micro-emboli in the middle cerebral artery during cardiopulmonary bypass: a transcranial Doppler ultrasound investigation using membrane and bubble oxygenators. Ann Thorac Surg 1987;44:298–302.

16. Padayachee TS, Parsons S, Theobald R, Linley J, Gosling RG, Deverall PB. Monitoring middle cerebral artery blood velocity during carotid endarteryectomy. Br J Surg 1986;73:98–100.

17. Spencer MP, Thomas GI, Nicholls SC, Sauvage LR. Detection of middle cerbral artery emboli during carotid artery endarterectomy using transcranial Doppler ultrasonography. Stroke 1990;21:415–423.

18. Russel D, Madden KP, Clark WM, Sandset PM, Zivin JA. Detection of arterial emboli using Doppler ultrasound in rabbits. Stroke 1991;22:253–258.

19. Grosset DG, Georgiadis D, Kelman AW et al. Quantification of ultrasound emboli signals in patients with cardiac and carotid disease. Stroke 1993;24:1922–1924.

20. Georgiadis D, Mackay TG, Kelman AW, Grosset DG, Wheatley DJ, Lees KR. Differentiation between gaseous and formed embolic materials in vivo: application in prosthetic heart valve patients. Stroke 1994;25:1559–1563.

21. Siebler M, Sitzer M, Steinmetz H. Detection of intracranial emboli in patients with symptomatic extracranial carotid artery disease. Stroke 1992;23:1652–1654.

22. Markus H. Transcranial Doppler detection of circulating cerebral emboli: a review. Stroke 1993;24:1246–1250.

23. Siebler M, Kleinschmidt A, Sitzer M, Steinmetz H, Freund HJ. Cerebral microembolism in symptomatic and asymptomatic high-grade internal carotid stenosis. Neurology 1994;44:615–618.

24. Tong DC, Albers GW. Transcranial Doppler-detected microemboli in patients with acute stroke. Stroke 1995;26:1588–1592.

25. Siebler M, Nachtmann A, Sitzer M, Rose G, Kleinschmidt A, Rademacher J et al. Cerebral microembolism and the risk of ischemia in asymptomatic high-grade internal carotid artery stenosis. Stroke 1995;26:2184–2186.

26. Babikian VL, Wijman CAC, Hyde C, Cantelmo NL, Winter MR, Baker E et al. Cerebral microembolism and early recurrent cerebral or retinal ischemic events. Stroke 1997;28:1314–1318.

27. Siebler M, Sitzer M, Rose G, Steinmetz H. Microembolism in carotid artery disease. Echocardiography 1996;13:529–535.

28. Sitzer M, Söhngen D, Siebler M, Specker C, Rademacher J, Ianda I et al. Cerebral microembolism in patients with Sneddon's syndrome. Arch Neurol 1995;52:271–275.

29. Söhngen D, Wehmeier A, Specker C, Schneider W. Antiphospholid antibodies in systemic lupus erythematosus and Sneddon's syndrome. Semin Thromb Hemostasis 1994;20:55–63.

30. Siebler M, Rose G, Sitzer M, Bender A, Steinmetz H. Real-time identification of cerebral microemboli with US feature detection by a neural network. Radiology 1994;192:739–742.

31. Markus H, Bland M, Rose G, Sitzer M, Siebler M. How good is intercenter agreement in the identification of embolic signals in carotid artery disease. Stroke 1996;27:1249–1252.

32. Specker Ch, Rademacher J, Söhngen D, Sitzer M, Janda I, Siebler M et al. Cerebral microemboli in patients with antiphospholipid syndrome. Lupus 1997;6:638–644.

33. Khamashta MA et al. Association of antibodies against phospholipids with heart valve disease in systemic lupus erythematosus. Lancet 1990;335:1541–1544.

34 Roldan CA, Shively BK, Crawford MH. An echocardiographic study of valvular heart disease associated with systemic lupus erythematosus. N Engl J Med 1996;335:1424–1430.

35. Sitzer M, Müller W, Siebler M, Hort W, Kniemeyer HW, Jäncke L, Steinmetz H. Plaque ulceration and lumen thrombus are the main sources of cerebral microemboli in high-grade internal carotid artery stenosis. Stroke 1995;26:1231–1233.

36. Kessler C, Kelly AB, Suggs WD, Weissmann JD, Epstein CM, Hanson SR et al. Induction of transient neurological dysfunction in baboons by platelet microemboli. Stroke 1992;23:697–702

37. Markus H, Loh A, Brown MM. Detection of circulating cerebral emboli using Doppler ultrasound in a sheep model. J Neurol Sci 1994;122:117–124.

38. Simantov R, LaSala JM, Lo SK, Gharavi AE, Sammaritano LR, Salmon JE et al. Activation of cultured vascular endothelial cells by antiphospholipid antibodies. J Clin Invest 1995;96:2211–2219.

39. Lockshin MD. Pathogenesis of the antiphospholipid antibody syndrome. Lupus 1996;5:404–408.

40. Vaarala O. Antiphospholipid antibodies and atherosclerosis. Lupus 1996;5:442–447.

41. Brey RL, Carolin MK. Detection of cerebral microembolic signals by transcranial Doppler may be a useful part of the equation in determining stroke risk in patients with antiphospholipid antibody syndrome. Lupus 1997;6: 621–624.

Section 2
Laboratory Investigation

21 Anticardiolipin Testing

S. S. Pierangeli, A. E. Gharavi and E. N. Harris

Introduction

Anticardiolipin antibody (aCL) tests are important to aid the physician in diagnosis of antiphospholipid syndrome (APS) [1]. Patients affected with APS are subject to episodes of thrombosis in arteries and/or veins, pregnancy loss (probably secondary to thrombosis of vessels in the placenta), and thrombocytopenia, associated with antiphospholipid (aPL) antibodies [1, 2]. aPL antibodies are autoantibodies directed against anionic phospholipids or protein–phospholipid complexes [3–5], measured by solid-phase immunoassays as anticardiolipin (aCL) [6], or as an activity which prolongs phospholipid-dependent coagulation assays, the so-called lupus anticoagulants (LA) [7].

Diagnosis of APS is based on finding a "moderate to high" positive aCL test and/or a LA test with any one of the characteristic clinical features presented above [1, 2].

aCL enzyme-linked immunosorbent assay (ELISA) test is not only positive in patients with APS but also in a variety of disorders, including connective tissue diseases, infectious disorders such as syphilis [8, 9], Q fever [10] and acquired immune deficiency syndrome (AIDS) [11, 12], and some drug-induced disorders [13]. It is generally believed that aCL antibodies are clinically significant only when present in APS; thus, there have been continuous attempts to modify the assay to make it more specific for APS. In addition, based on an early observation that patients with high positive IgG aCL tests were more likely to have APS [14], efforts have been devoted to quantifying the aCL ELISA test in a standardized manner. Because these antibodies are heterogeneous and are measured by a variety of techniques, great efforts have been made to standardize the assays for aCL and LA tests [15–18]. This chapter will discuss the various techniques used in the diagnosis of APS, a series of aCL workshops that have been used to validate and improve measurement of aCL antibodies, as well as issues concerning aCL specificity. An overview of new and more specific tests for diagnosis of APS will also be included.

Historical Background of the aCL Test

Conley and Hartmann noticed in 1952 that some patients with systemic lupus erythematosus (SLE) had a rather uncommon coagulation abnormality called "lupus anticoagulant" (LA); this was due to the abnormal prolongation of the partial thromboplastin time (PTT) [19]. Investigators also established that instead of abnormal bleeding, these patients were subject to thrombosis [20]. Soon thereafter, the LA phenomenon was known to be caused by an autoantibody believed to bind phospholipids, because they inhibited two phospholipid dependent coagulation reactions in the clotting-cascade – the prothrombin–thrombin conversion and the activation of factor X activation [21]. In addition, about 25–50% of patients with the LA reaction also had a biological false-positive test for syphilis (BFP-STS). Antibodies responsible for the BFP-STS were known to bind CL, a negatively charged phospholipid. The LA test had some drawbacks: it was a functional assay affected by a number of variables, including preparation and storage of samples, type of reagent used, etc. In addition, the test lacked sensitivity and could not be readily standardized [21]. Thus, in 1983 a group of investigators at the Hammersmith Hospital in London, UK reasoned that use of a solid-phase immunoassay with cardiolipin as antigen might be one way of detecting antibodies with LA activity. They thought that such a test would have the advantages of greater sensitivity, more reproducibility, better quantitation, and the possibility of standardization. The group succeeded in establishing a solid phase radioimmunoassay with cardiolipin as antigen, and the antibodies were termed "anticardiolipin antibodies" [6]. Hence, the first aCL test [6] was established in 1983. The test proved more sensitive than the LA assay and enabled diagnosis of a much larger number of patients with the APS. Also, the investigators soon noticed that aCL antibodies cross-reacted with negatively charged phospholipids, such as phosphatidylserine (PS) and phosphatidylglycerol (PG) [22]. Thus, the name aCL antibodies was changed to antiphospholipid antibodies (aPL) [2], and the disorder with which these antibodies were associated was called the "antiphospholipid syndrome (APS)" [2].

Widespread adoption of the solid phase aCL assay led to several potential problems. These antibodies were soon reported in several disorders such as syphilis [8, 9] AIDS [11, 12] connective tissue diseases, as well as in normal individuals who did not have the features of the disorder. However, methods of performing the test also varied and results were questionable in some instances. Fortunately, it was recognized that the majority of the patients with APS tended to have high aCL antibody levels, usually of the IgG isotype (however, some patients were only IgM positive) [23]. To ensure that the aCL test would retain its value in diagnosis APS, it would be necessary to identify antibodies by isotype and to quantify results using some reliable unit of measurement. There was also a need to establish which testing methods were valid as well as standard procedures for performing the solid phase immunoassay [24]. To achieve these goals, an international standardization workshop was first conducted in 1986 [15] and subsequently some other workshops were conducted.

Tests Used in Diagnosis of APS

The aCL Test

Association of a positive aCL test with clinical manifestations of APS occurs principally with persistent medium to high levels of aCL (or aPL) antibodies and IgG is more prevalent than IgM [23]. However, there are reports that IgM and occasionally IgA aCL are also associated with clinical manifestations of APS [23]. Frequently, the results of the test are reported by ranges of positivity in addition to G phospholipid (*GPL*) and M phospholipid (*MPL*) units. In addition, if results are reported by ranges of positivity, the interlaboratory agreement is better [16]. The aCL test is sensitive and is positive in more than 80–90% of patients with the disorder. The problem has been that this test may be positive in a number of diseases other than APS [8–13]. However, because patients with APS usually have higher aCL levels [23], greater specificity in diagnosis has been enabled by the use of higher cut off points. Alternatively, the use of other antigens to coat the ELISA has improved specificity [25–27].

The first aCL assay was a radioimmunoassay [6]. Since the test was first developed, several changes and improvements have been made to reduce the background binding, to quantitate the results in units and with respect to incubation times and temperatures [24]. The introduction of adult bovine or fetal calf serum [24] was found to enhance antibody binding to cardiolipin, and this enhancing effect has been attributed to a serum protein termed β_2-glycoprotein I [27–29]. It is because antibody levels are so important to diagnosis that considerable effort has been spent in standardizing test procedures and defining antibody levels [15–18].

Standardization of the aCL Test

In the first anticardiolipin workshop, the assay methods that enabled valid measurements of aCL antibody levels were determined [15]. In addition, units of measurement were established, and six calibrator standards were introduced to assist laboratories worldwide in establishing the aCL assay. The second workshop demonstrated that semiquantitative measures of aCL levels enabled the best agreement between laboratories [16]. The third and fourth workshops sought to settle controversial issues regarding anticardiolipin specificity, but also sought to examine some of the newly introduced commercial kits [17, 18]. Together these workshops have demonstrated that investigators working collaboratively can contribute to improvement in testing methods, and to greater understanding of scientific issues such as those related to aCL specificity. Despite these efforts in standardization, a considerable degree of interlaboratory variation still exits [30, 31]. National and international organizations have also contributed to the standardization of the aCL test: the College of American Pathologists enrolls laboratories in quality control surveys for aCL testing and requires participation in the program for accreditation purposes; the National Committee for Clinical Laboratory Standards (NCCLS) will soon publish and distribute the first proposed guidelines for the determination of aCL antibodies.

The LA Test

The LA test is less frequently positive in APS and is regarded as a more specific test for detection of aPL [32]. This specificity derives from the fact that the LA reaction is found much less frequently in non-APS disorders. The LA test measure the ability of aPL autoantibodies to prolong phospholipid-dependent clotting reactions. The aPL antibodies detected in aCL and LA tests are specific for phospholipids, phospholipid-binding proteins, or a complex of these molecules. These antibodies are heterogeneous; the two tests (aCL and LA) do not necessarily identify the same antibodies [33]. Recent studies indicate LA and aCL antibodies to be distinct entities [12, 13].

Furthermore, although the majority of the patients with APS have positive aCL and LA tests, approximately 10–16% of them are positive for LA and negative for aCL, and 25% are positive for aCL and negative for LA.

More Specific Tests for APS

One of the major drawbacks of the aCL ELISA test is that it is not only positive in APS patients. Binding of sera to cardiolipin coated plates from patients with a variety of diseases, other than APS is frequent [8–13]. Recently, new assays that utilize phosphatidylserine [25], mixture of negatively charged phospholipids (APhL® ELISA Kit Louisville APL Diagnostics, Inc.) [26] or β_2-glycoprotein I [34–36] have been proposed for a more specific measurement of antibodies present in APS. Some reports now suggest that both the aCL and a more specific test (antiphosphatidylserine, APhL® ELISA, or anti-β_2-GP1), be run in patients suspected of having APS to confirm diagnosis [37].

Ideally, these tests using more specific antigens should also be sensitive. Two antigen preparations are likely candidates. The first and most extensively studied is β_2-GPI [34–36, 38]. The second is the APhL® phospholipid mixture utilized as the antigen in an ELISA Kit (APhL® ELISA Kit, Louisville, KY [26, 39, 40].

Recently, some studies show that binding of APS sera to β_2-GPI by ELISA occurs when "high binding" or oxidized microtiter plates are used [34–36]. Reports from several laboratories indicate that the sensitivity of the anti-β_2-GP1 test for APS vary from 40 to 90% [34–36, 41]. Our experience after testing 54 APS samples suggest that the sensitivity of antiβ_2-GPI is 74% [42] (Table 21.1). However, this needs to be confirmed by studies using a larger number of patients and controls. Some investigators argue that the anti-β_2-GPI test is more specific than the aCL ELISA for diagnosis of APS. The clinical specificity of the anti-β_2-GPI assay also varies among groups of investigators and publications [39, 43], depending on the selection patient sera and the technique utilized. In a series of experiments performed by our group, in 184 samples from non-APS patients who had syphilis or other autoimmune disorders [42]. Eighteen out of 184 samples were positive, yielding a specificity of 82% (Table 21.2).

The second antigen is the APhL® phospholipid mixture prepared as a kit (The APhL® ELISA Kit,). Two of the authors of this review were principals (ENH and SP) in developing both the antigen and the kit, and any evaluation of data presented in this report must be mindful of this fact. A mixture of phospholipids was identified

Table 21.1. Clinical sensitivity of two antiphospholipid assays and one anti-β_2 GPI assay.

Assay	No. APS samples that tested + total no. APS samples tested	Sensitivity (%)
aCL ELISA	54/54	100
APhL® ELISA	53/54	98
aβ_2 GPI ELISA	40/54	74

Note: aCL ELISA, anticardiolipin ELISA, APhL® ELISA Kit (Louisville APL Diagnostics, Inc); aβ_2GPI ELISA, QUANTA LITE β_2GP1 INOVA Diagnostics, Inc kits for anti-β_2GP1 antibodies. Positive sample: above the cut-off point for each assay. Sensitivity for given assay was calculated as follows: (no. of samples that tested positive/no. of samples tested) × 100.

Table 21.2. Clinica1 specificity of two antiphospholipid assays and one anti-β_2 GPI assay.

Assay	No. of non APS samples that tested + total no. APS samples tested	Specificity (%)
aCL ELISA	74/184	60
APhL® ELISA	1/184	99.9
aβ_2 GP1 ELISA	18/84	82

Note: aCL ELISA, anticardiolipin ELISA, APhL® ELISA Kit (Louisville APL Diagnostics, Inc);
aβ_2GPI ELISA, QUANTA LITE β_2GP1 (INOVA Diagnostics, Inc) kit for anti-β_2GP1 antibodies.
Positive sample, above the cut-off point for each assay.
Specificity for a given assay was calculated as follows: 1 − (no. of non-APS samples that
tested positive/no. of samples tested) × 100.

that enabled better distinction of APS and non-APS sera (infectious, autoimmune disorders) distinction, while retaining sensitivity for detection of APS. Studies by our group (same series of experiments, described in the previous paragraph), the APhL®ELISA Kit was shown to be 98% sensitive and 99% specific [42]. Four published studies have examined this kit [18, 26, 39, 40]. The largest is one from 438 patients with various connective tissue diseases, 33 patients with APS, and 200 healthy controls were examined using the aCL bench assay and the APhL® ELISA Kit [40]. The sera were prepared and labeled in one center and tested blind in another laboratory; results were analyzed in the center where the samples were labeled. In that study, all patients with APS were positive for aCL antibodies and 30/33 were positive utilizing the APhL® ELISA kit (90.9% sensitivity). In patients without APS, 45/438 were aCL positive but only nine of 438 sera were positive in the APhL® ELISA kit. (99.5% specific)[40]. These data suggest that the APhL®ELISA Kit may be a sensitive and relatively specific means of identifying patients with APS.

In September 1996, a fourth anticardiolipin workshop was conducted [18]. The objective of this most recent workshop was to compare four techniques for measurement of aCL antibodies to determine which was more specific for identification of APS. Samples tested were eight APS, four aCL positive syphilis, two aCL positive (one obtained from a patient with Q fever and the other from a patient with SLE, neither of whom had features of APS), and six from normal healthy controls. Techniques evaluated were the aCL bench method; two commercial aCL ELISA kits (INOVA Diagnostics, Inc), and Incstar Corp; the APhL® ELISA Kit), an anti-β_2-GPI Kit (INOVA Diagnostics, Inc.) and a flow-cytometric technique in which IgG and IgM aCL and to phosphatidylserine can be determined simultaneously.

The results obtained by this workshop were noteworthy. All techniques tested were 90–100% sensitive, correctly identifying almost all sera from patients with APS [18]. However, results varied with respect to specificity. The APhL® ELISA Kit, utilizing a mixture of phospholipids as antigens was most specific (100%), the anti-β_2-GPI (INOVA Diagnostics, Inc.) was nearly as specific, with only the Q fever sample (but not the syphilis or SLE samples) "falsely" identified as positive. The flow cytometric assay method with PS as antigen showed the third best specificity, "falsely" identifying only two samples [18]. None of the aCL assays, whether bench method or ELISA kit, proved to be 100% specific; the syphilis, Q fever, and SLE samples were all reported as positive.

Finally, there have been an increasing number of reports from some various centers suggesting that patients with APS have antibodies that bind proteins other than β_2-GPI in recently developed ELISA tests. These include prothrombin [44, 45], protein C, protein S [46], and annexins [47]. Reports showing the diagnostic value of these assays remain controversial. Determination of the value of ELISA tests utilizing protein antigens other than β_2-GPI will require validation and standardization of the techniques and testing of large numbers of sera from patients with APS as well as with other disorders to determine their diagnostic and predictive values.

Use of Flow Cytometry for Detection of aPL

Recently Stewart et al, reported a new method of detection of aPL antibodies. These authors described a rapid and sensitive method of detecting aPL using phospholipid-coated polystyrene beads and flow cytometry [48]. The study showed that aPL bind to CL and phosphatidylserine (PS) beads and this binding can be detected by utilization of labeled conjugates and flow cytometry. By utilizing beads of two different sizes, aCL and aPS antibodies can be detected simultaneously in a single tube. Our group adapted this method and constructed the aCL/aPS ®FACS Kit (Louisville APL Diagnostics, Inc). This kit, now cleared by the FDA to be used for "in vitro diagnostic" purposes was evaluated during the Anticardiolipin Wet Workshop at the 7th International Symposium on aPL antibodies [18]. The assay showed to be sensitive and more specific than the aCL ELISA for detection of autoimmune aPL.

What Test(s) Should Be Used for Diagnosis of APS?

Correct identification of patients with APS is important, since prophylactic anticoagulant therapy can prevent thrombosis from recurring, and treatment of affected women during pregnancy can result in live births. Since there are many causes of thrombosis, and of pregnancy loss, the confirmation of diagnosis of APS is dependent on finding a positive aPL antibody or LA test. The LA and aCL tests are generally accepted confirmatory tests for APS. Recently, a forum of antiphospholipid experts gathered at a special session during the 8th International Symposium on aPL antibodies agreed that these two tests should be used primarily in the diagnosis of APS [49]. In summary, a diagnosis of APS can be made with confidence in patients who present with well-documented clinical features (venous or arterial thrombosis and/or pregnancy loss) characteristic of APS, and a moderate to high positive IgG aCL.(above 40 GPL units) or LA test. However, there are a number of situations in which the anti-β_2GPI of the APhL® ELISA Kit might be utilized to confirm diagnosis of the APS.

These are as follows:

1. Patients with venous or arterial thrombosis or with pregnancy loss who are low positive for IgG aCL, or only IgM or IgA aCL positive.
2. Patients presenting with equivocal features of APS. Examples include idiopathic thrombocytopenia, thrombophlebitis, atherosclerosis, first trimester pregnancy losses or instances in which venous or arterial thrombosis or recurrent pregnancy loss may be attributable to factor other than APS.

3. Unusual presentations of APS. Examples include chorea, transverse myelopathy, livedo reticularis, leg ulcers, or cardiac valvular lesions presenting in the absence of pregnancy loss or thrombosis.
4. Patients with clinical features that are very suggestive of APS, but are aCL and LA negative.

Based on the knowledge and experience accumulated up to date we are proposing that in the initial stages, the aCL and LA tests should be performed as a first line of testing for APS. If any of these tests are negative or both, then a more specific test should be performed such as the β_2GPI or the APhL® ELISA Kit.

Summary

The first aCL solid-phase immunoassay test was developed in 1983 and subsequently standardized [15–18]. Although in the last 6–7 years, new and more specific tests have become available, the aCL ELISA and the LA tests are still the first choice to be used in diagnosis of APS [49]. The development of newer tests such as the β_2GPI ELISA and the APhL® ELISA Kit, utilizing the phospholipid mixture, or the new flow-cytometric assay (using PS- and CL- coated beads) may provide a more specific, and reliable diagnosis of APS, while retaining good sensitivity. Other tests such as ELISA for prothrombin antibodies and annexin V antibodies are still under development and will require extensive evaluation.

References

1. Harris EN. Antiphospholipid syndrome. In: Klippel JH, Dieppe PA, editors Rheumatology. London: Mosby-Year Book, 1994;Section 6, 32.1–32.6.
2. Harris EN, Gharavi AE, Hughes GRV. Antiphospholipid antibodies. Clin Rheum Dis 1985;11:591–601.
3. Pierangeli SS, Davis SA, Harris EN and DeLorenzo G. β_2-glycoprotein 1 (β_2GP1) enhances cardiolipin binding activity but it is not the target antigen for antiphospholipid antibodies. Br J Haematol 1992;82:565–570.
4. McNeil HP, Simpson RJ, Chesterman CN, Krilis SA. Anti-phospholipid antibodies are directed against a complex antigen that includes a lipid-binding inhibitor of coagulation: $\beta_2$glycoprotein I. Proc Natl Acad Sci USA 1990;87:4120–4124.
5. Roubey RA. Autoantibodies to phospholipid binding-plasma proteins: a new view of lupus anticoagulants and other "antiphospholipid" autoantibodies. Blood 1994;84:2854–2867.
6. Harris EN, Gharavi AE, Boey ML, Mackworth-Young CG, Loizou S, Hughes GR. Anticardiolipin antibodies: detection by radioimmunoassay and association with thrombosis. Lancet 1983;ii:1211–1214.
7. Triplett DA, Brandt JT. Lupus anticoagulants: misnomer, paradox, riddle, epiphenomenon. Hematol Pathol 1988;2:121–143.
8. Harris EN, Gharavi AE, Wasley GD, Hughes GRV. Use of an enzyme-linked immunosorbent assay and of inhibition studies to distinguish between antibodies to cardiolipin from patients with syphilis or autoimmune disorders. J Infect Dis 1988;157:23–31.
9. Moritsen S, Hoier-Madsen M, Wiik A, Orum O, Strandberg-Pedersen N. The specificity of anticardiolipin antibodies from syphilis patients and from patients with systemic lupus erythematosus. Clin Exp Immunol 1989;76:178–183.
10. Galvez J, Martin I, Medino D, Pujol E. Thrombophlebitis in a patient with abute Q fever and anticardiolipin antibodies. Med Clin (Barc) 1997;15;108:396–397.
11. Intrator L, Oksenhendler E, Desforges L, PB. Anticardiolipin antibodies in HIV infected patients with or without autoimmune thrombocytopenia purpura. Br J Haematol 1988; 67:269–270.
12. Canoso RT, Zon LI, Groopman JE. Anticardiolipin antibodies associated with HTLV-III infection. Br J Haematol 1987;65: 495–498.

13. Canoso RT. Sise HS. Chlorpromazine-induced lupus anticoagulant and associated immunologic abnormalities. Am J Hematol 1982;13:121-129.
14. Harris EN, Chan JKH, Asherson RA, Aber VR, Gharavi AE, Hughes GRV. Thrombosis, recurrent fetal loss and thrombocytopenia Predictive value of the anti-cardiolipin test. Arch Intern Med 1986;146:2153-2156
15. Harris EN, Gharavi AE, Patel S, Hughes GRV. Evaluation of the anti-cardiolipin antibody test: report of an international workshop held April 4 1986. Clin Exp Immunol 1987;68:215-222.
16. Harris EN. The second international anticardiolipin standardization workshop/the Kingston Antiphospholipid Antibody study (KAPS) group. Am J Clin Pathol. 1990;94:476-484.
17. Harris EN, Pierangeli SS, Birch D. Anticardiolipin wet workshop report: Vth International Symposium on Antiphospholipid Antibodies. Am J Clin Pathol 1994;101:616-0624.
18. Pierangeli SS, Stewart M, Silva LK, Harris EN. Report of an anticardiolipin wet workshop during the VIIth International Symposium on antiphospholipid antibodies. J Rheumatol 1998;25:156-162.
19. Conley CL, Hartmann RC. A hemorrhagic disorder caused by circulating anticoagulant in patients with disseminated lupus erythematosus. J Clin Invest 1952; 31:621-622.
20. Boey MD. Colaco CB, Gharavi AE. Thrombosis in SLE: striking association with the presence of circulating " lupus anticoagulant". BMJ 1983;287:1088-1089.
21. Shapiro SS. Thiagarajan P. Lupus anticoagulant. Prog Haemost Thromb 1982;6:263-285.
22. Harris EN, Gharavi AE, Loizou S, Derue G, Chan JKM, Patel BM et al. Crossreactivity of anti-phospholipid antibodies. J Clin Lab Immunol. 1985;16:1-6.
23. Gharavi AE, Harris EN, Asherson RA, Hughes GRV Anticardiolipin antibody isotype distribution and phospholipid specificity. Ann Rheum Dis 1987;46:1-6.
24. Gharavi AE, Harris EN, Asherson R, Hughes GRV. Antiphospholipid antibodies. Ann Rheum Dis 1987;46:1-8.
25. Rote NS, Dostal-Johnson D, Branch DW. Antiphospholipid antibodies and recurrent pregnancy loss: correlation between the activated partial thromboplastin time and antibodies against phosphatidylserine and cardiolipin. Am J Obstet Gynecol 1990;163:575-584.
26. Harris EN. Pierangeli SS. A more specific ELISA assay for the detection of antiphospholipid antibodies. Clin Immunol Newslet 1995;15:26-28.
27. Matsuura E, Igarashi Y, Fujimoto M. Anticardiolipin antibodies directed not to cardiolipin but to a plasma protein cofactor. Lancet 1990;336:1547.
28. Galli M, Comfurius P, Maassen C, Hemker HC, de Baets MH, van Breda-Vriesman PJ et al. Anticardiolipin (ACA) antibodies directed not to cardiolipin but to a plasma protein cofactor. Lancet 1990;336:1544-1547.
29. McNeil HP, Simpson RJ, Chesterman CN, Krilis S. Anti-phospholipid antibodies are directed against a complex antigen that includes a lipid binding inhibitor of coagulation: β_2 glycoprotein I (apolipoprotein H). Proc Natl Acad Sci USA 1990;87:4120-4124.
30. Peaceman AH, Silver RK, MacGregor SN, Scool ML. Interlaboratory variation in antiphospholipid antibody testing. Am J Obstet Gynecol 1992;144:1780-1784.
31. Reber G, Arvieux J, Comby E, Degenne D, de Moerloose P, Sanmarco M et al. Multicenter evaluation of nine commercial kits for the quantitation of anticardiolipin antibodies. Thromb Haemost 1995;73:444-452.
32. Derksen RH, Hasselaar P, Blokzijl L, Gmelig Meyling FH, de Groot PG. Coagulation screen is more specific than the anticardiolipin antibody ELISA in defining a thrombotic subset of lupus patients. Ann Rheum Dis 1988;47:364-371.
33. Walton SP, Pierangeli SS, Campbell A, Klein E, Burchitt B, Harris EN. Demonstration of antiphospholipid antibodies heterogeneity by phospholiphid column chromatography and salt gradient elution. Lupus 1995;4:26.
34. Matsuura E. Igarashi Y, Yasuda Triplett DA, Koike T. Anticardiolipin antibodies recognize β_2 glycoprotein 1 structure altered by interacting with an oxygen modified solid phase surface. J Exp Med 1994;179:457-462.
35. Forastiero RR, Martinuzzo ME, Kordich LC, Carreras LO. Reactivity to β_2 glycoprotein I clearly differentiates anticardiolipin antibodies from antiphospholipid syndrome and syphilis. Thromb Haemost 1996;75:717-720.
36. Roubey RAS, Eisenberg RA, Harper MF, Winfield JB. "Anticardiolipin" antibodies recognize β_2-glycoprotein 1 in the absence of phospholipid. J Immunol 1995;154:954-960.
37. Harris EN, Pierangeli SS, Gharavi AE. Diagnosis of the antiphospholipid syndrome: A proposal for use of laboratory tests. Lupus 1998;7:S144-S148.
38. Balestrieri G, Tincani A, Spatola L, Allegri F, Prati E, Cattaneo R et al. Anti-β_2 glycoprotein I antibodies: a marker of antiphospholipid syndrome? Lupus 1995;4:122-130.

39. Day HM, Thiagarajan P, Ahn C, Reveille JD, Tinker KF, Arnett FC. Autoantibodies to β_2 glycoprotein I in systemic lupus erythematosus and primary antiphospholipid sybndrome: clinical correlations in comparison with other antiphospholipid antibody tests. J Rheumatol 1998;4:667–674.
40. Merkel PA, Chang Y, Pierangeli SS, Harris EN, Polisson RP. Comparison between the standard anticardiolipin antibody test and a new phospholipid test in patiens with a variety of connective tissue diseases. J Rheumatol 1999;26:591–596.
41. Pengo V, Biasiolo A, Fior MG. Autoimmune antiphosphoilipid antibodies are directed against a cryptic epitope expressed when the β_2 glycoprotein I is bound to suitable surface. Thromb Haemost 1995;89:397–402.
42. Abreu I, Pierangeli SS, Harris EN. Comparison of three assays for the detection of antiphospholipid and anti-β_2 glycoprotein I antibodies. Lupus 1998;7:S211.
43. Guerin J, Feighery C, Sim RB, Jackson J. Antibodies to β_2 glycoprotein I, a specific marker for the antiphospholipid syndrome. Clin Exp Immunol 1997;109:304–309.
44. Bevers E, Galli M, Barbui T, Comfurius P, Zwaal RF. Lupus anticoagulant IgG's (LA) are not directed to phospholipids only, but to a complex of lipid-bound human prothrombin. Thromb Haemost 1991;66:629–632.
45. Rao LVM, Hoang AD, Rapaport SI. Differences in interactions of lupus anticoagulant IgG with human prothrombin and bovine prothrombin. Thromb Haemost. 1995;73:668–674.
46. Oosting JD, Derksen RH, Bobbink IW, Bouma BN, deGroot PC. Antiphospholipid antibodies directed against a combination of phospholipids with prothrombin, protein C or protein S: an explanation for their pathogenic mechanism? Blood. 1993;81:2618–2625.
47. Matsuuda J, Saitoh N, Gohchi K, Gotoh M, Tuskamoto M. Anti-annexin V antibody in systemic lupus erythematosus patients with lupus anticoagulant and/or anticardiolipin antibody. Am J Hematol 1994;47:56–58.
48. Stewart MW, Gordon PA, Etches WS, Marusyk H, Poppema S, Bigam et al. Binding of cardiolipin to polystyrene beads: evidence for a lamelar phase orientation. Br J Haematol 1995;90:900–905.
49. Wilson W. International consensus statement on preliminary classification criteria for definite antiphospholipid syndrome: report of an international workshop. Arthritis Rheum 1999;42:1309–1311.

22 Lupus Anticoagulant Measurement

I. J. Mackie, S. Donohoe and S. J. Machin

Introduction

In 1952, Conley and Hartman described patients with haemorrhagic symptoms, whose plasma prolonged the whole blood clotting time and failed to correct on the addition of normal plasma. Further patients were reported and in 1972 the term "lupus anticoagulant" was coined [1], as the apparent inhibitor of coagulation had been observed in patients with systemic lupus erythematosus (SLE). Unfortunately, the term lupus anticoagulant (LA) is a misnomer, as delayed coagulation is only observed in vitro, and hemorrhage in patients with LA is rare. The phenomenon is not confined to SLE and has been observed in patients with a wide range of disease states as well as asymptomatic, apparently healthy subjects. LA appears to be due to certain acquired immunoglobulins of varying class that interact with prothrombin/phospholipid and β_2-glycoprotein I/phospholipid complexes in a manner that influences phospholipid-dependent in vitro coagulation tests. There may also be additional target proteins involved.

The laboratory diagnosis of the antiphospholipid syndrome (APS) relies predominantly on coagulation-based assays for LA and solid-phase assays (enzyme-linked immunosorbent assays; ELISA) employing cardiolipin. Most antibodies to cardiolipin actually interact with β_2-glycoprotein I, and a subset of these also express LA activity. However, not all patients with cardiolipin antibodies have LA, and vice versa. It is therefore essential that both types of test are available for adequate detection of the APS. Transient LA-positive results are sometimes encountered, particularly after severe infections, where they are not usually associated with thrombosis. It is therefore important to demonstrate persistence of the positive tests, by collecting further blood samples after at least 6 weeks.

Lupus Anticoagulant Tests

Guidelines and criteria for the detection of LA have been published by both National [2, 3] and International [4, 5] bodies. The basic criteria for the presence of LA are as follows.

1. Prolongation of a phospholipid-dependent coagulation test.
2. Evidence of an inhibitor demonstrated by mixing studies.
3. Confirmation of the phospholipid-dependent nature of the inhibitor.

Further criteria that have been recommended are the failure to demonstrate any inhibitory activity directed against a specific coagulation factor, and purification of immunoglobulin with LA activity. These remain beyond the scope of most clinical hematology departments. Another important factor is the demonstration of persistence; transient antiphospholipid antibodies (aPL) are known to occur after certain infections and do not appear to be associated with any of the clinical consequences of APS. A large number of diagnostic tests have been described, and many of these are widely available as commercial kits and reagents. The laboratory investigation employs a screening stage and confirmation stage, each of which may utilize more than one type of test.

LA Screening

Phospholipid-dependent coagulation tests must be used in the screening stage. Many laboratories use an activated partial thromboplastin time (aPTT) test, or a modification of this, for their front line investigation of LA. It is also possible to use a modified prothrombin time with diluted thromboplastin reagent, or a dilute Russell's viper venom time (DRVVT) for this purpose. The screening stage must be as sensitive as possible, and sometimes reduced specificity must be accepted in order to maximize detection. A high degree of specificity is therefore essential in confirmation stages. Unfortunately, no LA test has yet been described that has 100% specificity and sensitivity during routine use. It is unlikely that these ideals will be achieved, because of the heterogeneous nature of aPL. The particular characteristics of some samples mean that they will give normal results in certain tests, and it is therefore useful to employ more than one type of screening test when a LA is strongly suspected. The interpretation of the screening test is complimented by measurement of the prothrombin time, as well as the thrombin clotting time and/or fibrinogen assay. These tests provide information about possible coexistent coagulation defects and the presence of anticoagulants (about which the laboratory technologist may be unaware), which influence the interpretation of LA tests. A variety of screening and correction tests are listed in Table 22.1.

Determination of the Presence of an Inhibitor

The performance of mixing studies in screening tests usually provides evidence of an inhibitor. Normal plasma is mixed with patient plasma and the test is performed. The normal plasma will correct coagulation deficiencies, so that the clotting time

Table 22.1.

LA screening tests	Confirmation tests
aPTT	Use of LA insensitive reagents
aPTT with dilute phospholipid	Hexagonal phase lipids
DRVVT with dilute phospholipid	Platelet neutralization procedures
KCT and colloidal silica clotting time	High concentration phospholipid
Dilute thromboplastin time test	Comparison with a similar, insensitive test (e.g, Ecarin time)
Textarin time	
Taipan Time	

will return to normal. However, if an inhibitor is present, such as LA, the clotting time will remain prolonged and may even show a further prolongation (the lupus cofactor effect). One problem with performing and interpreting mixing tests is that the addition of normal plasma or other reagents has the effect of diluting the immmunoglobulins responsible for LA. If these are weak or low titer, their effect may be reduced and in some cases this can lead to the loss of detectable LA activity and a false negative test result.

Confirmation of the Phospholipid Dependence of an Inhibitor

Tests that confirm the phospholipid dependence of an inhibitor, or confirm that it is a LA, must have a high degree of specificity, but need not necessarily be highly sensitive, provided that a suitable (and complimentary) screening test is used. Confirmation of the phospholipid-dependent nature of the inhibitor is usually obtained using correction or confirmation procedures relying on washed, activated platelets or reagents with a high concentration of phospholipid, and demonstrating correction of the coagulation time.

Preanalytical Variables and Normal Ranges

It is essential to establish the normal reference range in each laboratory for each type of method. This should be accomplished by performing tests on at least 20 healthy normal subjects with no known hemostatic defect or illness. Patients should not be used for this purpose, even if they are attending the hospital for relatively minor complaints, since stress, as well as chronic illness, pregnancy and other factors cause changes in the levels of certain coagulation factors. Reference ranges vary according to the type of coagulometer used, as well as the reagent formulation [6], and some laboratories will find it necessary to have separate normal ranges for each analyzer and commercial kit. Blood samples for the establishment of the normal range, for quality control purposes and from patients must be obtained by clean venepuncture, with minimal venous stasis. The blood should be collected into tri-sodium citrate and processed within 1 hour of collection. The blood should be centrifuged at 2000 g for 15 minutes. To minimize platelet contamination, the supernatant plasma should be removed to a clean polypropylene tube and centrifuged again. The final supernatant plasma should be tested immediately, or stored at –70 °C for later analysis. Plasma samples should not be repeatedly thawed and refrozen, as this will lead to the deterioration of labile coagulation factors. The plasma must be handled with plastic pipettes and tubes to avoid contact activation of the sample. Alternative methods of platelet depletion are to place the plasma in a conical microcentrifuge tube and spin for 5 minutes at 10 000 g, or to slowly express the plasma through a 0.2 μm cellulose acetate syringe filter. A platelet count of $<10 \times 10^9$/l in the plasma sample must be achieved in order to have a sensitive test of LA.

Activated Partial Thromboplastin Time (aPTT)

The aPTT has been extensively employed, since it is widely available as part of a general hemostatic screen. There are numerous commercial aPTT reagents available, which show considerable variation in content and performance. The characteristics of the phospholipid component of the reagent are critical in determining its LA sensitivity and reagents vary in both the type of phospholipid present as well as in their relative concentrations [7]. Some reagents have been shown to have very poor LA sensitivity [8–12]. In plasma from patients with an acute phase reaction, or with pregnancy, there may be increased levels of fibrinogen and factor VIII, which may shorten the aPTT, and mask a LA.

Modified aPTT

A number of modifications of the aPTT have been described, to improve its performance for LA detection. In some cases, the results with two aPTT reagents have been compared, one with good and one with poor LA sensitivity [9, 11–12]. In this type of test, it is essential that both reagents have similar sensitivities to clotting factor deficiency, otherwise false comparisons may be obtained. A similar approach has been used with hexagonal-phase lipids added to a LA sensitive aPTT reagent. Hexagonal-phase lipids appear to neutralize LA and correct the clotting time [13]. In the dilute aPTT method [14], the aPTT reagent is diluted so that greater sensitivity to LA is achieved. In some variant methods, two or more dilutions of the aPTT reagent are used and the ratio of the clotting times of test plasma between each dilution are calculated and compared to control plasma ratios. This type of method has also been proposed as a way of studying LA potency [15].

The Platelet Neutralization Procedure

A platelet neutralization procedure (PNP) has been described, which improves the specificity of the aPTT [16]. Washed normal platelets are activated with calcium ionophore or lysed by repeated freezing and thawing to expose their procoagulant phospholipid. These platelets are added to plasma, and their effect is compared to a buffer control. Platelets appear to bypass the LA (although the mechanism of the effect is not completely understood) in the aPTT, and will correct the aPTT value, whereas in factor deficiency, the aPTT remains prolonged. This approach has also been used in the DRVVT and other LA tests.

The Kaolin Clotting Time (KCT)

The KCT or Exner's test [17] may be considered as a modified aPTT, since an activator and calcium ions are added to plasma in the absence of any phospholipid reagent. The generation of thrombin is thought to be supported by the presence of residual cell membranes and plasma lipids. This is probably why the KCT is particularly sensitive to platelet contamination of the plasma sample, which greatly reduces the sensitivity of the test, especially after cell membranes are disrupted by freezing and thawing. In the original description of the test, a number of different proportion mixtures of test and control plasma were tested and the clotting time was plotted against the test plasma concentration. This allowed LA to be identified by the failure of the KCT to correct even when relatively large proportions of normal plasma were added, whereas with factor deficiency, the KCT was corrected by adding small amounts of normal plasma. The performance of the KCT on large numbers of test and control plasma mixtures is now thought to be too time consuming, and most laboratories only test one mixture (80% control: 20% test). A test : control ratio of >1.2 indicates an abnormal result, and a mixture ratio of >1.2 is considered as indicative of LA, while a ratio of 1.1–1.2 is considered equivocal. In manual tests, a clotting time of < 60 seconds usually indicates platelet contamination of the sample and invalidates the result.

The KCT is not suitable for all types of coagulometer, particularly some photo-optical devices, owing to the particulate nature of the kaolin reagent, which tends to scatter light, while the stock reagent needs constant and effective stirring to prevent sedimentation. A variant of the KCT using colloidal silica (CSCT) instead of kaolin has recently been described [18]. This has the dual benefits of good optical clarity, and low sedimentation, since it is a colloid rather than a simple suspension. The sensitivity and specificity of the CSCT for LA appear to be very similar to the KCT.

A further problem with both the KCT and CSCT is that they require the presence of most coagulation factors to obtain a normal clotting time, which means that there are a number of points at which specificity may be reduced by factor deficiency or the presence of inhibitors and anticoagulants.

Modified Prothrombin Time (PT) Methods

The prothrombin time is usually normal in patients with LA, and rarely shows any gross prolongation unless anticoagulants are used, or the prothrombin concentration is low due to the presence of a specific inhibitor (hypoprothrombinemia). Part of the reason for this is the relatively high concentration of phospholipid in the reagent. However, when the thromboplastin reagent is diluted, the concentration of the phospholipid component becomes a rate-limiting factor for thrombin generation, and therefore any inhibition of prothrombinase function by LA will cause a prolongation of the modified PT. This principle has been used in a test known by various names: the tissue thromboplastin inhibition test [19], dilute thromboplastin time test (DTT), thromboplastin dilution curve, etc. In the DTT, a prothrombin time is performed using a several different dilutions of thromboplastin reagent. The clotting time of test plasma is divided by the clotting time of control plasma to give a ratio. A progressive increase in the ratio as the thromboplastin is diluted is suggestive of LA. However, the potency of thromboplastin reagents and the concentration and characteristics of their phospholipid component show considerable variability. This means that the sensitive dilution range for LA varies considerably between PT reagents. Generally this test shows poor sensitivity and specificity and with some thromboplastins, factor deficiency can mimic the LA pattern. There has recently been a resurgence of interest in the DTT, with the observation that a thromboplastin reagent comprising recombinant human tissue factor mixed with synthetic phospholipids (Innovin) is particularly sensitive to LA [20, 21]. The formulation of the phospholipid component probably accounts for the sensitivity of Innovin to LA, and only a small dilution of the reagent leads to a gross prolongation of the clotting time in the presence of LA.

Dilute Russell's Viper Venom Time (DRVVT)

Russell's viper venom (RVV) contains an enzyme that cleaves and activates factor X. The factor Xa generated is able to activate prothrombin in the presence of calcium ions, factor V and phospholipid, leading to the formation of a fibrin clot. In the

DRVVT [22] system the phospholipid reagent is diluted such that its concentration becomes rate limiting. If there is any inhibition of the coagulant active phospholipid, the DRVVT clotting time becomes prolonged.

The DRVVT offers greater specificity than the KCT, since fewer coagulation reactions are involved. However, it is not completely specific for LA, since deficiency of fibrinogen, prothrombin, factors V or X, will also cause a prolongation of the clotting time. To some extent, the possibility of these influencing the test can be eliminated by the performance of coagulation screening tests (PT, aPTT, thrombin time and fibrinogen assay). Most workers combine the DRVVT test with a confirmation step for LA, which utilizes either a high concentration of phospholipid or a platelet neutralization procedure. In this confirmation step, the dilute phospholipid reagent is replaced with the correction or neutralization reagent. If there is a LA, the clotting time is reduced or normalized in this confirmation step. A neutralization test based on platelet-derived microvesicles has also been described [23].

There are many different commercial reagents available for the DRVVT, and these generally overcome the need to titrate each reagent, and avoid problems of instability of the venom. These kits vary in sensitivity and specificity [24], and the degree of variability is influenced by the type of coagulometer used [6]. Some washed platelet preparations are contaminated with platelet factor 4, released from platelet granules after lysis or activation. This can cause false positive LA tests in samples containing therapeutic levels of heparin. However, this is rarely a clinical problem, as LA tests can usually be performed once patients have ceased heparin therapy. It is unclear whether high phospholipid concentration reagents or platelet neutralization reagents are most suitable for confirmation tests. This probably depends on the exact preparation and characteristics of the given reagent as well as the test system or type of coagulometer in use.

Some RVV preparations show poor stability and confirmation reagents can themselves alter the actual clotting time of LA negative plasmas. For this reason, it is generally advisable to work with DRVVT ratios rather than raw clotting times in the interpretation of the test; thus:

DRVVT ratio = clotting time of test plasma/clotting time of normal plasma

Such ratios should be determined separately for the dilute phospholipid reagent and for the confirmation step; the two ratios can then be compared. A correction of the DRVVT ratio is generally accepted as a reduction of >10% in the ratio obtained with dilute phospholipid or to within the normal range, when the confirmation reagent is used. However, there is little objective information to support any exact percentage. Obviously where the ratio corrects back to within the normal range, that is evidence for the presence of LA. Several methods for calculating the degree of DRVVT correction (with the confirmation reagent) have been suggested by "expert" bodies and commercial manufacturers [3, 24]; three of these are as follows.

1. Percentage Correction of Ratio

The DRVVT ratio of test/control plasma for the dilute phospholipid reagent (DPL ratio) and for the correction [confirm] reagent (CORR ratio) are calculated. The percentage correction is equal to [(DPL ratio – CORR ratio) × 100]/DPL ratio. A result above the normal range (e.g., >1.1) with dilute phospholipid, which corrects to within the normal range, or by >10%, with the high phospholipid reagent or platelet neutralization procedure, is considered indicative of LA.

2. Percentage Correction of Clotting Time

The control DRVVT clotting time is subtracted from the test DRVVT, and the product is divided by the control DRVVT, to yield a weighted ratio for the diluted phospholipid (DPL) and for the correction reagent (CORR). The percentage correction is then calculated as [(DPL – CORR) × 100]/DPL. In general, corrections of >65% are indicative of LA.

3. Test : Confirm Ratio

The DRVVT clotting time with dilute phospholipid is divided by the DRVVT with the correction reagent. A test : confirm ratio > 2 SD above the mean normal ratio indicates the presence of LA.

There is little objective information to support any exact percentage correction as indicative of LA, and the above limits are largely arbitrary. Correction back to within the normal range is strong evidence for the presence of LA. The use of the test : confirm ratio does not take into account any variation in the normal clotting time with the reagent, differences in operator performance, and changes in reagent stability, and therefore cannot be recommended for general use. The method is improved by normalising, where the patient clotting times are divided by control times, prior to ratio calculation. The percentage correction of ratio and the percentage correction of clotting time gives the most reliable results, although the latter is slightly more cumbersome [24].

Great care must be taken when mixing tests with normal plasma are performed. The addition of normal plasma results in a dilution of the LA immunoglobulin, and this can result in an apparent correction, particularly with samples having very weak LA. Where patients are known to be factor deficient (e.g., patients receiving oral anticoagulants), the confirm step of the DRVVT should also be performed on a mixture of patient and control plasma, and the two modified ratios compared. Failure to do this may result in an erroneous interpretation of results.

Other Snake Venoms Used for LA Testing

Several venoms containing prothrombin activators have been assessed for LA testing, with the principle that they should offer greater specificity than the DRVVT since less clotting factors are involved. Two venoms have been shown to be useful in this regard: that of *Oxyuranus scutellatus* (Taipan venom) [25, 26], and the venom of *Pseudonaja textilis* (Textarin®) [27]. Taipan venom activates prothrombin in the presence of phospholipid and calcium ions, so that if a suitable phospholipid reagent is used, and its concentration is made rate limiting, the test becomes sensitive to LA. The specificity of the test can be improved by the use of mixing tests and/or a confirmation procedure. The latter usually employs a platelet neutralization procedure, although there is no obvious reason why a high phospholipid concentration should not be used.

The Textarin venom acts in a similar fashion, but also requires the presence of factor V. The specificity is again improved by mixing tests, although the performance of an additional test using a different snake venom, the Textarin/Ecarin ratio, has been recommended [27]. Ecarin is an enzyme purified from the venom of *Echis carinatus*, which activates prothrombin, but with no requirement for phospholipid. Thus, the test is not affected by the presence of LA, and the clotting time will therefore be prolonged with Textarin, but normal with Ecarin, giving a high Textarin/Ecarin ratio.

An unexpected advantage of both Taipan and Textarin venom times is that they appear to be particularly useful in patients receiving oral anticoagulants. Under the conditions suitable for LA testing, they are not very sensitive to prothrombin deficiency, and since no other vitamin K dependent factors are required, the clotting time in oral anticoagulant patients lacking LA, remains normal. However, unless a mixing test or confirmation procedure is used, their specificity is not as high as that generally found with the DRVVT.

The Textarin/Ecarin ratio has been criticized because of the use of two different test systems, rather than modifications of a single reaction. This may be important when the test is applied to certain automates, and the relative performance of one of the venoms may be different to that observed manually.

Quality Control

The inclusion of quality control (QC) systems (Table 22.2) is important in all LA tests, regardless of the instrumentation used and the source of reagents. At the simplest level, aliquots of known LA-positive and -negative plasmas collected from local patients should be used. These should ideally be stored at –70 °C, and a separate aliquot thawed each time and included in every batch of LA tests. Where storage is only available at higher temperatures, the plasmas may only be viable for short periods of time. The collection and preparation of the QC plasmas is just as important as that for patient plasmas. Care should be taken to avoid loss of factor activity, and that suitable platelet depletion has been achieved. This is also true for pooled normal plasmas used for the calculation of LA clotting time ratios. These normal plasmas should be collected with minimal stasis from at least 12 healthy normal subjects and definitely not from any type of patient.

Alternatively, some lyophilized commercial LA-positive plasmas are available. However, these are often very potent and therefore give little information about the sensitivity of the LA test at a given time. A set of LA-positive and -negative reference plasmas have recently been prepared [28] by the LA working party of the British Society for Haematology, and are available to UK laboratories from the National Institute for Biological Standards and Control (NIBSC). These were prepared by pooling several LA-positive plasmas and diluting them in LA-negative plasma to achieve a range of potencies for LA. It was hoped that by pooling the plasmas, a

Table 22.2. Quality control reagents.

Reference plasmas ("in house", commercial, NIBSC)
Plasmas spiked with monoclonal antibodies
Arachnase
Polymixin B
Phospholipase A_2
Cetylpyridinium chloride
Other positively charged amphiphilic compounds.

mixture of LA immunoglobulin types would be obtained and that this might reflect the different specificities of LA found in different patients.

Plasmas spiked with certain murine monoclonal antibodies against β_2-glycoprotein I have also been suggested as suitable QC materials [29]. The advantage of these would be that a consistent supply of material would be available, since the same antibodies would be mixed with every batch of normal plasma.

The National External Quality Assessment Scheme (NEQAS) for blood coagulation provides a means of external quality assessment of LA tests, by the distribution of plasma samples to all participating centers. Recent exercises have highlighted ongoing problems in the accurate identification of LA [30].

A variety of other artificial LA-positive or mimicking reagents have been suggested for QC purposes. Arachnase is a QC material prepared by spiking normal plasma with the venom of the Brown Recluse spider, which has antiphospholipid properties. Polymixin B, an antibiotic has a similar property of interfering in phospholipid-dependent reactions. However, both of these reagents fail to work consistently in all LA test systems and have therefore not enjoyed widespread acceptance [5].

Recommended Approach for the Detection of LA

Laboratory testing for both lupus anticoagulant (LA) and IgG and IgM anticardiolipin antibodies should be used in patients suspected of having APS. A thorough medical history must be taken and the use of anticoagulants noted. A coagulation screen should be performed including a sensitive aPTT, with a mixing test if the aPTT is prolonged (Table 22.3). The DRVVT with a platelet neutralization procedure or a high concentration phospholipid confirm step, appears to be more sensitive than the kaolin clotting time in detecting LA in women with recurrent miscarriage [31, 32]. A second confirmatory test should be performed after at least 6 weeks in those with an initial positive test result to exclude transient positive test results, found in one-third to a half of patients [33]. Maternal aPL may be downregulated during pregnancy [34], and therefore, ideally, diagnostic tests should not be performed during pregnancy and for 6 weeks postpartum. The DRVVT also appears to be more specific than the KCT for detecting LA related to thrombosis [35]. Taipan and Textarin times may be helpful in patients receiving oral anticoagulants.

Table 22.3. Summary of recommended approaches to the detection of LA.

Stage 1
Clotting screen (PT, aPTT, thrombin time and/or fibrinogen assay)
LA sensitive aPTT

Stage 2
Mixing tests (with normal plasma)
Modified aPTT or DTT (with suitable reagent) for interim confirmation

Stage 3
More sensitive screening test (DRVVT, KCT, Taipan time, Textarin time)
Confirmation step (high phospholipid concentration or platelet neutralization)

Stage 4
Further sensitive screening and confirmation steps (alternative tests from Stage 3).

References

1. Feinstein DI, Rapaport SI. Acquired inhibitors of blood coagulation. Prog Hemost Thromb 1972;1:75–95.
2. Lupus Anticoagulant Working Party on behalf of the BCSH Haemostasis and Thrombosis Task Force. Guidelines on testing for the lupus anticoagulant. J Clin Pathol 1991;44:885–889.
3. Lupus Anticoagulant Working Party on behalf of the BCSH Haemostasis and Thrombosis Task Force. Guidelines on the investigation and management of the antiphospholipid syndrome. Br J Haematol 2000;108:in press.
4. Exner T, Triplett DA, Taberner D et al. Guidelines for testing and revised criteria for lupus anticoagulants. SSC Subcommittee for the Standardization of Lupus Anticoagulants. Thromb Haemost 1991;65:320–322.
5. Brandt JT, Triplett DA, Alving B et al. Criteria for the diagnosis of lupus anticoagulants: an update. On behalf of the Subcommittee on Lupus Anticoagulant/Antiphospholipid Antibody of the Scientific and Standardisation Committee of the ISTH. Thromb Haemost 1995;74:1185–1190.
6. Lawrie A., Mackie I, Purdy G et al. The sensitivity and specificity of commercial reagents for the detection of lupus anticoagulant show marked differences in performance between photo-optical and mechanical coagulometers. Thromb Haemost 1999;81:758–762.
7. Kelsey PR, Stevenson KJ, Poller L. The diagnosis of lupus anticoagulants by the activated partial thromboplastin time – the central role of phosphatidylserine. Thromb Haemost 1984;52:172–175.
8. Brandt JT, Triplett DA, Musgrave K et al. The sensitivity of different coagulation reagents to the presence of lupus anticoagulants. Arch Pathol Lab Med 1987;111:120–124.
9. Brandt JT, Triplett DA, Rock WA et al. Effect of lupus anticoagulants on the activated partial thromboplastin time. Results of the College of American Pathologists survey program. Arch Pathol Lab Med 1991;115:109–114.
10. Denis-Magdelaine A, Flahault A, Verdy E. Sensitivity of sixteen aPTT reagents for the presence of lupus anticoagulants. Haemostasis 1995;25:98–105.
11. Brancaccio V, Ames PR, Glynn J et al. A rapid screen for lupus anticoagulant with good discrimination from oral anticoagulants, congenital factor deficiency and heparin, is provided by comparing a sensitive and an insensitive aPTT reagent. Blood Coagul Fibrinolysis 1997;8:155–160.
12. Lawrie AS, Purdy G, Mackie IJ et al. Monitoring of oral anticoagulant therapy in lupus anticoagulant positive patients with the anti-phospholipid syndrome. Br J Haematol 1997;98:887–892.
13. Rauch J., Tannenbaum M, Janoff AS. Distinguishing plasma lupus anticoagulants from anti-factor antibodies using hexagonal (II) phase phospholipids. Thromb Haemost 1989;62:892–896.
14. Alving BM, Barr CF, Johansen LE et al. Comparison between a one-point dilute phospholipid aPTT and the dilute Russell viper venom time for verification of lupus anticoagulants. Thromb Haemost. 1992;67:672–678.
15. Jacobsen EM, Barna-Cler L, Taylor JM et al. Lupus ratio: an international inter-laboratory study using an intergrated test for lupus anticoagulant (LA). Lupus 1998;7 (Suppl 2):S216.
16. Triplett DA, Brandt JT, Kaczor D et al. Laboratory diagnosis of lupus inhibitors: a comparison of the tissue thromboplastin inhibition procedure with a new platelet neutralization procedure. Am J Clin Pathol 1983;79:678–682.
17. Exner T, Rickard A, Kronberg H. A sensitive test demonstrating lupus anticoagulant and its behavioral patterns. Br J Haematol 1979;40:143–151.
18. Chantarangkul V, Tripodi A, Arbini A et al. Silica clotting time (SCT) as a screening and confirmatory test for detection of the lupus anticoagulants. Thromb Res 1992;67:355–365.
19. Schleider MA, Nachman RL, Jaffe EA et al. A clinical study of the lupus anticoagulant. Blood 1976;48:499–509.
20. Arnout J, Vanrusselt M, Huybrechts E et al. Optimization of the dilute prothrombin time for the detection of the lupus anticoagulant by use of a recombinant tissue thromboplastin. Br J Haematol 1994;87:94–99.
21. Forastiero RR, Cerrato GS, Carreras LO. Evaluation of recently described tests for detection of the lupus anticoagulant. Thromb Haemost 1994;72:728–733.
22. Thiagarajan P, Pengo V, Shapiro SS. The use of the dilute Russell viper venom time for the diagnosis of lupus anticoagulants. Blood 1986;68:869–874.
23. Arnout J, Huybrechts E, Vanrusselt M et al. A new lupus anticoagulant neutralization test based on platelet-derived vesicles. Br J Haematol 1992;80:341–346.
24. Medical Devices Agency (MDA) Evaluation of lupus anticoagulant kits. London: Department of Health, MDA, ISDN No. 1 85839 918 1, 1998, No 43.

25. Speijer H, Govers-Riemslag JW, Zwaal RF et al. Prothrombin activation by an activator from the venom of *Oxyuranus scutellatus* (Taipan snake). J Biol Chem 1986;261:13258–13267.
26. Rooney AM, McNally T, Mackie IJ et al. The Taipan snake venom time: a new test for lupus anticoagulant. J. Clin. Pathol 1994;47:497–501.
27. Triplett DA, Stocker KF, Unger GA et al. The Textarin/Ecarin ratio: a confirmatory test for lupus anticoagulants. Thromb Haemost 1993;70:925–931.
28. Gray E, Mackie I, Greaves M. Calibration of the 1st British reference plasma panel for lupus anticoagulants. Br J Haematol 1998;105 (suppl 1):97.
29. Arnout J, Vanrusselt M, Wittevrongel C et al. Monoclonal antibodies against beta-2-glycoprotein I: use as reference material for lupus anticoagulant tests. Thromb Haemost 1998;79:955–958.
30. Jennings I, Kitchen S, Woods TA et al. Potentially clinically important inaccuracies in testing for the lupus anticoagulant: an analysis of results from three surveys of the UK National External Quality Assessment Scheme (NEQAS) for Blood Coagulation. Thromb Haemost 1997;77:934–937.
31. MacLean MA, Cumming GP, McCall F et al. The prevalence of lupus anticoagulant and anticardiolipin antibodies in women with a history of first trimester miscarriages. Br J Obstet Gynaecol 1994;101:103–106.
32. Rai RS, Regan L, Clifford K et al. Antiphospholipid antibodies and β_2-glycoprotein-1 in 500 women with recurrent miscarriage: results of a comprehensive screening approach. Hum Reprod 1995;10:2001–2005.
33. Rai RS, Clifford K, Cohen H et al. High prospective fetal loss in untreated pregnancies of women with recurrent miscarriage and antiphospholipid antibodies. Hum Reprod 1995;10:3301–3304.
34. Kwak JYH, Barini R, Gilman-Sachs A et al. Down-regulation of maternal antiphospholipid antibodies during early pregnancy and pregnancy outcome. Am J Obstet Gynaecol 1994;171:239–246.
35. Galli M, Finazzi G, Norbis F et al. The risk of thrombosis in patients with lupus anticoagulants is predicted by their specific coagulation profile. Thromb Haemost 1999;81:695–700.

23 Lupus Anticoagulants: Mechanistic and Diagnostic Considerations

J. Arnout and J. Vermylen

Introduction

The antiphospholipid syndrome (APS) is defined as the association of antiphospho-lipid antibodies (aPL) with arterial or venous thrombosis, recurrent fetal loss, thrombocytopenia or neurologic disorders [1–3]. The gradual development of the notion of the APS started in the 1950s with the recognition of two laboratory curiosities in a subset of patients with systemic lupus erythematosus (SLE). In these patients, rheumatologists frequently found a chronic biological false positive test for syphilis whereas hematologists described a non-specific coagulation inhibitor manifested by prolongation of the whole blood clotting time and the prothrombin time, without reduction of any specific clotting factor then measurable [1–3]. The coagulation inhibitor which appeared not to be associated with a bleeding tendency was named the "lupus anticoagulant" (LA) by Feinstein and Rapaport [4] and was regarded as a laboratory curiosity until Bowie et al [5] drew the attention to the high prevalence of thrombotic complications in SLE patients with this "anticoagu-lant". The LA was later also found to be associated with obstetric complications and thrombocytopenia [6].

Only in the 1980s did it became clear that antibodies interacting with anionic phospholipids are responsible for the in vitro LA effect and the chronic biological false positive syphilis serology [7]. This led to the development of better-defined LA tests and the so-called anticardiolipin test in which antibodies binding to solid-phase cardiolipin (aCL) are measured [8, 9]. With these improved assays, the majority of SLE patients with a LA also had elevated aCL levels and a statistically significant relation between these two types of aPL was observed. It is now well established that persistently present aCL and LAs in patients with SLE are associ-ated with thrombosis, cerebral infarction, fetal loss and thrombocytopenia [10]. This association is now termed the APS [11]. Some patients with similar clinical symptoms and laboratory findings but not suffering from SLE or a closely related autoimmune disease are diagnosed as having a "primary APS" [12]. The availablity of a sensitive assay for aCL has been crucial for the further characterization of aPL. Affinity purification of aCL led to the discovery that, in contrast to what the term aPL could suggest, these autoimmune antibodies do not bind to negatively charged phospholipids per se but to phospholipid-binding proteins eventually bound to phospholipid surfaces [13–15]. β_2-glycoprotein I (β_2GPI) and prothrombin appear to be the major proteins involved in the binding of aPL to phospholipid surfaces [16] but other phospholipid-binding proteins such as protein C, protein S, high- and low-molecular-weight kininogens, factor XI and annexin V, have been described as target antigens for aPL [17]. β_2GPI is an absolute requirement for the binding of auto-immune aCL to cardiolipin [18]. LAs have been found to depend for their in vitro anticoagulant activity either on prothrombin [19] or on β_2GPI [20–22]. Most patients with LA appear to have both β_2GPI- and prothrombin-dependent antibodies [23]. β_2GPI-dependent aPL have been studied in most detail. Epidemiological retrospective studies described a significant relationship between a history of thrombosis and the presence of high-titer aCL [10]. A similar relationship has been found with antibodies directly binding to β_2GPI in the absence of phospholipids [24]. There are also a few prospective trials that provide evidence that elevated aPL are a real risk factor for thrombosis. A substudy of the Physicians Health Study found a relationship between the aCL titer at entry to the study and the subsequent risk for thrombosis and pulmonary embolism in healthy adult men [25]. Another prospective cohort study of unselected patients with suspected deep venous thrombosis or pulmonary embolism showed a strong association between proven venous thromboembolism and the presence of a LA [26]. Animal experimental work provided more direct evidence for a pathogenic role of aPL. Passive and active immunization of mice with such antibodies results in the induction of an experimental APS [27–29]. In addition, several groups have demonstrated that an APS can be induced in animals upon immunization with β_2GPI alone [30, 31]. Pierangeli et al recently reported on the thrombogenic effects of murine and human aCL which suggests that these antibodies may be pathogenic in patients with APS [32]. However, whereas clinical and animal experimental data clearly suggest a role for β_2GPI-dependent aPL in the development of the APS, the pathogenic mechanism is not known.

Pathogenetic Mechanism of aPL

The interest in aPL was kindled by early reports suggesting that these antibodies could be pathogenic. In 1980, Carreras et al showed that plasma of a patient with a strong LA, arterial thromboses and recurrent intrauterine death impeded the production of prostacyclin by rat aorta rings, human myometrial tissue, and bovine endothelial cells in culture and suggested that the LA would decrease the production of antithrombotic prostacyclin by interfering with the phospholipid substrate from which arachidonic acid is released [33]. However, even in this early work, it became apparent that not all plasmas containing a LA reduce prostacyclin formation [34]. A few years later, the LA was reported to inhibit protein C activation in the presence of thrombin, thrombomodulin and phospholipid [35–37]. In addition, LA have been found to prevent inactivation of factor Va by activated protein C on a phospholipid surface [38]. However, again not all aPL impede the protein C anticoagulant pathway. Other proposed mechanisms to explain the way by which aPL could cause hyper-coagulability include interference with the function of antithrombin [39, 40], impeding the fibrinolytic potential [41] and reducing the anticoagulant potential of annexin V [42]. However, none of these proposed mechanisms received general acceptance.

While reviewing the literature, a number of striking similarities between APS and heparin-induced thrombocytopenia (HIT), another condition in which antibodies lead to thrombosis, became clear [43]. Characteristic of both APS and HIT is a paradoxical association of thrombocytopenia and thrombosis. The site of thrombosis, which may be arterial and venous, appears to depend on patient related factors. In both syndromes, the target antigen is a complex formed on cell membranes.

The pathogenesis of HIT has recently been elucidated. Thrombosis in this syndrome is caused by an immunoglobulin, usually IgG, that becomes detectable 5 or more days following first exposure to heparin. The major target antigen is a macromolecular complex of acidic heparin with the basic protein called platelet factor 4, which is secreted by activated platelets and binds to the platelet membrane and to endothelium [44]. Binding of heparin–platelet factor 4-antibody complexes to the platelet surface leads to tight occupancy of the platelet FcγRII receptors by the IgG's Fc moiety [45]. Strong platelet activation results, with generation of procoagulant platelet-derived microparticles [46]. Binding of IgG or IgM antibodies to platelets [47], or to platelet factor 4-proteoglycan complexes on the endothelial cell [48], may also result in activation of complement and cellular stimulation; C5a has recently been shown to induce tissue factor expression in endothelial cells [49]. Local generation of tissue factor could obviously promote thrombosis.

aPL have also been shown to promote platelet activation and tissue factor expression on endothelial cells. Limited evidence indicated that at least some of the observed effects are dependent upon the binding to the platelet FcγRII receptor. Based on these similarities the following hypothesis was formulated for the pathogenesis of the APS (Fig. 23.1). As a consequence of an initial damage or activation,

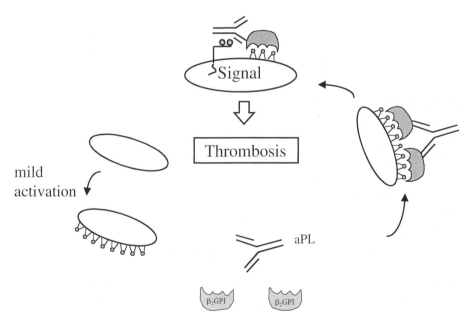

Figure 23.1. Putative pathogenic mechanism in the APS: as a consequence of an initial damage, anionic phospholipids are exposed on cells of the blood, on endothelium or on trophoblasts. These potentially reactive phospholipids are covered up by phospholipid-binding proteins (PL-binding protein), such as β_2GPI or prothrombin. If, however, aPL are present against such surface-bound proteins, these immunoglobulins concentrate on the cell surface, bind to cellular Fcγ receptors (FcR) and induce strong thrombosis-promoting modifications such as release of ADP, serotonin and microvesicles, TxA_2 biosynthesis, tissue factor expression, removal of endothelial heparan sulfate, etc. (Reproduced with permission, see ref 43.)

anionic phospholipids are exposed on cells of the blood, on endothelium or on trophoblasts. These potentially reactive phospholipids are covered up by phospholipid-
binding proteins, such as β_2GPI or prothrombin. If, however, antibodies are present
against such surface-bound proteins, these immunoglobulins concentrate on the cell
surface, bind to cellular FcγRII receptors and induce strong thrombosis-promoting
modifications. In contrast to previous hypotheses, the pathogenesis would seem to
be more related to tight cellular binding of immunoglobulin than to interference by
antibody with the activity of specific antigens. The hypothesis, comparable to the
mechanism currently accepted to account for heparin-induced thrombocytopenia
and thrombosis, is compatible with a "double hit" mechanism leading to thrombosis.

The proposed model, although supported by a number of experimental observations, does not, however, provide a direct explanation for the recent observation that
LA are more strongly associated with thrombosis than aCL [50, 51]. In order to study
this we raised murine monoclonal antibodies (moab) against human β_2GPI [52].
Eight of the 21 anti-β_2GPI moabs, obtained from two fusions, fulfilled the criteria
for LA activity as tested with a variety of sensitive screening assays and several
confirmatory tests. Seven moabs did not influence any clotting test.

Study of the Mechanism of Action of β_2GPI-dependent LA

Two moabs with potent LA activity and one moab without LA activity were selected
to study the interaction between aCL, β_2GPI and phospholipid. Interactions were
investigated by real-time biospecific interaction analysis (BIA) based on plasmon
surface resonance technology on a BIA-core instrument using a sensor chip coated
with a commercial phospholipid mixture used in coagulation assays. When 22 F6,
our moab with the most pronounced LA activity, was allowed to interact with the
phospholipid surface at concentrations between 0 and 400 nmol/l, no appreciable
binding could be detected. Likewise, no binding could be measured when β_2GPI at
concentrations between 0 and 400 nmol/l was passed over the phospholipid-coated
sensor chip. Significant binding was only observed when combinations of β_2GPI
and 22 F6 were allowed to interact simultaneously. Similar results were obtained
with 22 B3, another moab with LA activity. A LA negative moab, 16 B3, did not
cause binding of antibody–β_2GPI complexes. From these experiments we could
conclude that the affinity of β_2GPI for coagulation active phospholipids is enhanced
by LA-positive anti-β_2GPI moabs. Whether this enhanced affinity was due to conformational changes induced by monovalent antibody binding or by the formation
of bivalent complexes was investigated using Fab' fragments derived from the same
moab. Fab fragments derived from moab 22 F6, although reacting with high affinity
with β_2GPI, were unable to induce binding of β_2GPI to phospholipid. On the contrary, 22 F6 Fab' fragments, by preventing the formation of bivalent β_2GPI–22 F6 or
β_2GPI–22 B3 complexes, neutralized the stimulatory effect of the intact anti-β_2GPI
moabs on β_2GPI binding to phospholipid. The availability of large quantities of LA-
positive moabs also allowed us to study the importance of bivalent antibody–β_2GPI
complex formation for the LA activity of moabs in plasma. Fab' fragments of moab
22 F6 had no LA activity by themselves but inhibited the LA activity of both moab
22 F6 and 22 B3 in a concentration-dependent fashion. These results clearly show
that the LA activity of certain anti-β_2GPI moabs depends on the formation of bivalent β_2GPI–antibody complexes that bind with high affinity to phospholipids. The

importance of bivalent binding of aCL has been suggested by others. Roubey et al have indicated that autoimmune aCL are low-affinity antibodies that bind to β_2GPI on oxidized plastic surfaces through a bivalent interaction promoted by the enhanced surface density of the antigen [53]. Using ellipsometry, Willems et al [54] studied the interaction of β_2GPI, affinity purified aCL with LA activity from a single patient with a primary APS, and artificial bilayer membranes with physiological concentrations of phosphatidylserine. They reported high-affinity binding of aCL–β_2GPI complexes to phospholipids and provided strong evidence that this high-affinity interaction was the consequence of bivalent interactions between the antibody and lipid-bound β_2GPI. After finishing our study, another paper appeared showing that only LA positive anti-β_2GPI moabs enhanced the binding of β_2GPI to phospholipids [55]. This appeared to depend on the capability of these antibodies to form bivalent complexes as F(ab')$_2$ fragments also promoted β_2GPI binding to phospholipids whereas Fab fragments did not. Our study was the first one to show that Fab fragments of an anti-β_2GPI moab with LA activity inhibit the high-affinity binding of such β_2GPI–antibody complexes to phospholipids by impeding bivalent complex formation.

Our study also indicated that, in contrast to what is generally accepted, β_2GPI by itself only binds with low affinity to coagulation-active phospholipid mixtures. Physiological coagulation promoting phospholipid surfaces only contain low concentrations of negatively charged phospholipids. However, phospholipid-binding studies with β_2GPI, showing high-affinity interactions with dissociation constants (K_d) in the order of 10 to 20 nM, were initially done using pure cardiolipin immobilized onto microtiter plates or using multilamellar vesicles composed entirely of anionic phospholipids [56]. Such high-affinity interaction would suggest β_2GPI to compete with vitamin K-dependent clotting factors for the same catalytic surface and therefore to behave as a relatively potent anticoagulant. This, however, does not seem the case. Physiological concentrations of β_2GPI only have a weak effect on in vitro coagulation reactions, as indicated by the observation that coagulation reactions in normal plasma and β_2GPI-depleted plasma are hardly different [20, 21]. Data on the affinity of β_2GPI for more physiologic phospholipid surfaces only very recently became available and it appears that the affinity of β_2GPI for phospholipids highly depends on the phospholipid composition. Willems et al [54], using ellipsometry, reported dissociation constants of 3.9 and 14 μM for membranes containing 20 and 10 mol % phosphatidylserine, respectively. Harper et al [57] reported apparent K_d values ranging from approximately 5 to 0.5 μM over a range of 5 to 20 mol % anionic phospholipid. The affinity of clotting factors for similar phospholipid surfaces is one to two orders of magnitude higher [57]. These data help explain why β_2GPI by itself is indeed only a very weak anticoagulant protein that, however, can become a potent anticoagulant protein upon formation of antibody-linked bivalent complexes.

From the above mentioned studies, the binding of β_2GPI-dependent LA to phospholipid surfaces could be summarized as shown in Fig. 23.2. Depending on the affinity of these antibodies for β_2GPI (high affinity in the case of moabs and probably low affinity for human autoantibodies), monovalent antibody–β_2GPI complexes may or may not be formed in solution. Both free β_2GPI and monovalent complexes bind with a weak affinity to negatively charged phospholipid surfaces, such as activated cell membranes. On such a surface, the mobility of β_2GPI is high since its binding is based on ionic interaction. aPL can also form low affinity monovalent complexes with lipid bound β_2GPI. Depending on the epitope recognized, the mobility of the antibody hinge region, the lipid-bound β_2GPI density, and its mobility, stable bivalent

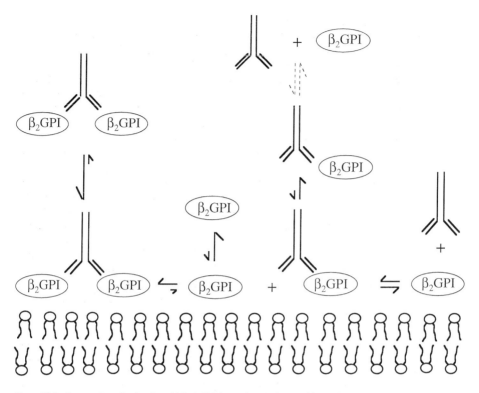

Figure 23.2. Proposed mechanism by which β_2GPI-dependent LA form stable bivalent antibody-β_2GPI complexes on phospholipid surfaces. Depending on the affinity of the antibody for β_2GPI, monovalent antibody-β_2GPI complexes are formed in solution. Both free β_2GPI and monovalent complexes bind to negatively charged phospholipid surfaces, such as activated cell membranes, with a weak affinity. On such a surface, the mobility of β_2GPI is high since its binding is based on ionic interaction. aCL can also form low-affinity monovalent complexes with lipid bound β_2GPI. Depending on the epitope recognized, the mobility of the antibody hinge region, the lipid-bound β_2GPI density, and its mobility, stable bivalent complexes are formed. (Reproduced with permission, see ref 52.)

complexes are formed. These complexes, with high affinity for phospholipids, can then compete with coagulation factors for the available catalytic surface and retard procoagulant and anticoagulant reactions. Such complexes, which may also remain tightly bound on activated cell membranes, also might potentiate cell activation via Fc receptor binding or possibly other mechanisms such as complement activation as is currently under investigation (see Ongoing Research).

Monoclonal Antibodies Against β_2GPI: Use as Reference Material for LA Tests

The availability of LA-positive anti-β_2GPI moabs prompted us to study their potential use for the production of control specimens for LA testing. Despite internationally accepted guidelines [58, 59] and many efforts to better standardize LA assays, several national and international inter-laboratory surveys and workshops have shown that the accuracy of LA testing is still far from optimal [60–62]. To date, it is almost impossible to formulate precise recommendations on which assays or combination of assays to use. Only a few comparative studies are available evaluating the differences in sensitivity or responsiveness among various tests. These studies have several limitations such as the small number of patients included, differences in inclusion criteria, instruments, reagent sources or batches, plasma preparation, etc. Moreover, there is no gold standard patient population available against which assays can be evaluated. Also for internal quality assessment, laboratories and reagent manufacturers still have to rely on LA-positive patient samples. The supply of these is, however, usually very limited and therefore does not allow profound study of the performance of different assay systems and reagent batches. Alternatives such as plasma spiked with polymyxin B, an antibiotic interfering with phospholipid-dependent clotting assays, or Arachnase, a spider venom, failed as so-called surrogate positive control plasmas [62]. Monoclonal antibodies with similar activities as human autoantibodies have never been tested in this regard. As the LA-positive anti-β_2GPI moabs that we generated lengthen phospholipid-dependent clotting reactions similarly as to what has been reported for affinity-purified human LA-positive aCL, they can be considered as representative for β_2GPI-dependent LA; normal plasma pools spiked with certain amounts of these moabs have the potential to serve as reference and control materials for LA testing.

With such plasmas, we studied the relative LA responsiveness of screening assays used in the laboratory diagnosis of LA [63]. A high LA responsiveness was found for the dilute prothrombin time (dPT), the kaolin clotting time (KCT), the dilute Russell's viper venom time (DRVVT) and the activated partial thromboplastin time (aPTT) using PTT–LA (Stago). Most routine aPTT reagents were only weakly influenced by the LA-positive moabs. This ranking of LA responsiveness compares well with several reports in the literature. Of particular interest is the finding that the prothrombin time using Simplastin™ (Organon Teknika) and the aPTT using Actin FS™ (DADE-Behring) are almost completely uninfluenced by the moabs. To further validate the potential role of our moabs to serve as reference materials, we compared the relative responsiveness of different reagents for LA positive anti-β_2GPI moabs with those found on samples from patients with a known LA. Also here, the dPT, the KCT, the DRVVT and the aPTT using PTT–LA showed high responsiveness. These results seem to indicate that LA-positive anti-β_2GPI moabs can be used to study the relative sensitivity of different clotting assays for β_2GPI-dependent LA. To assess interassay precision of LA tests, most hemostasis laboratories have to rely on positive patient samples. In a next part of our study, plasma pools spiked with LA-positive anti-β_2GPI moabs were used as control specimens. Interassay variability with these control specimens proved to be acceptably low.

In a final study, a normal plasma pool, and the same pool spiked with LA-positive anti-β_2GPI antibodies at two potency levels, were used as control materials in an external quality assessment scheme organized by the European Concerted Action on Thrombosis (ECAT) [64]. Fifty-nine laboratories participated in the ECAT pilot trial on LA and were asked to test for the presence of a LA in the three samples submitted. The majority (82%) of the participants found the high-potency LA sample to be positive. Only 37% of the laboratories considered the weak-potency LA sample to be positive. The submission of a normal sample, a weak positive sample and a clearly positive sample enabled us to compare the relative LA responsiveness of the different screening assays used. This analysis of the data indicates that many laboratories still rely on poorly responsive screening assays for their LA tests. Other laboratories rely on sensitive and specific modern integrated test systems based on a highly sensitive screening assay with a low phospholipid content and a confirmatory test employing high phospholipid concentrations.

These two studies indicate that LA-positive anti-β_2GPI moabs have a potential for the production of LA control specimens, that could be made available to routine hemostasis laboratories to assess intra-laboratory precision of LA testing, to manufacturers to produce highly sensitive assay systems and to control batch-to-batch variability of their reagents and to organizations involved in external quality assessment.

Ongoing Research

Thrombogenicity of LA-positive and LA-negative anti-β_2GPI Antibodies

Our preceding study has shown that only LA-positive anti- β_2GPI antibodies can form stable antigen–antibody complexes on phospholipid surfaces. One can therefore assume that these antibodies would have a more pronounced effect on cellular activation and would be more thrombogenic than LA-negative ones. Several of the available moabs recognize cardiolipin-bound hamster β_2GPI, and one of these, 5H2, also behaves as a LA in hamster plasma. The availability of large quantities of these moabs allows us to study their potential differential prothrombotic effects using a thrombosis model in the hamster that has been developed in our laboratory [65]. In this model, a carotid artery is dissected and placed on a transilluminator. Vessel damage is caused by infusion of Rose Bengal and critical exposure of the carotid artery to green light from a xenon light source. Thrombus formation is monitored with a video camera and quantitated. Preliminary experiments indicate that 5H2 promotes thrombus formation in a dose-dependent way (see Fig. 23.3). The role of bivalent antigen–antibody complex formation for cellular Fc receptor activation and thrombus formation will be evaluated using Fab′ and F(ab′)$_2$ fragments of this antibody. Comparative experiments will be carried out with similar doses of LA-negative antibodies.

Study of the Epitopes Involved in the Formation of Bivalent Antigen–Antibody Complexes on Phospholipid Surfaces

β_2GPI is composed of five repeating "sushi" domains of some 60 amino acids with a number of characteristic disulfide bridges. The only so far well-characterized phospholipid binding domain is located on the fifth domain. There is some evidence that this domain also contains binding sites for aPL. Data on the precise binding sites for aPL are, however, very limited. Specific domain-deletion mutants of β_2GPI are being constructed which will be used to determine against which "sushi" domain the different monoclonal antibodies are directed.

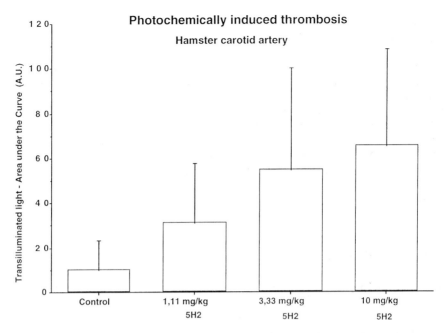

Figure 23.3. Thrombogenicity of 5H2, an anti-β_2GPI monoclonal antibody with LA activity. Cumulative thrombus formation over 40 min following a mild carotid artery photochemical injury and expressed as total light intensity for animals treated with 5H2 at the indicated doses. Data are presented as mean and SEM obtained with 10 animals per dose.

Summary

The APS is defined as the association of aPL with arterial or venous thrombosis, recurrent fetal loss, thrombocytopenia or neurologic disorders. Some aPL can be detected via phospholipid-dependent coagulation assays where they present as a non-specific coagulation inhibitor termed the LA. Other antibodies can be measured via immunologic assays mostly via their capability to bind to immobilized cardiolipin and are therefore called anticardiolipin antibodies (aCL). Affinity purification of aCL led to the discovery that, in contrast to the term suggested by aPL, these autoimmune antibodies do not bind to negatively charged phospholipids per se but to β_2GPI, a phospholipid-binding protein eventually bound to phospholipid surfaces. LAs have been found to be directed towards either prothrombin or β_2GPI bound to anionic phospholipids. Whereas clinical and animal experimental data clearly suggest a role for β_2GPI-dependent aPL in the development of the APS, the pathogenic mechanism is not known. Interference with several phospholipid-dependent anticoagulant pathways have been proposed but none of these has received general acceptance. Based on clinical and experimental similarities with heparin-induced thrombocytopenia, another syndrome of antibody-mediated thrombosis, we proposed a model of prothrombotic cellular activation. This model, although supported by a number of experimental observations, does not provide a direct explanation for the recent observation that LA are more strongly associated with thrombosis than aCL. In order to study this, we raised murine monoclonal antibodies (moab) against human β_2GPI. These antibodies, of which some had LA activity and others not, enabled us to study the interaction between β_2GPI, antibody and phospholipids. In contrast to what was generally accepted, β_2GPI appeared to have only low affinity for coagulation promoting phospholipids. In the presence of LA-positive anti-β_2GPI moabs, the affinity of β_2GPI for phospholipids increased significantly. This appeared to be dependent on the formation of bivalent β_2GPI–antibody complexes on the phospholipid surface. It is conceivable that such bivalent complexes also remain tightly attached to membranes of activated cells enabling further thrombosis promoting activation via Fc receptor interaction or the complement system, a hypothesis that is currently being investigated. Further studies also showed that our LA-positive anti-β_2GPI moabs have a potential for the production of LA control specimens, that could be made available to routine hemostasis laboratories, to manufacturers, and to organizations involved in external quality assessment.

In conclusion, this work has enabled us to understand the molecular mechanism by which certain autoimmune antibodies found in patients with APS prolong coagulation assays in vitro. The antibodies generated are an important tool to improve the laboratory diagnosis of the LA and may help us clarify the pathogenic role of autoimmune anti-β_2GPI antibodies.

References

1. Moore JE, Mohr CF. Biologically false-positive serologic tests for syphilis: type, incidence, and cause. JAMA 1952;150:467–473.
2. Moore JE, Lutz WB. The natural history of systemic lupus erythematosus: an approach to its study through chronic biologic false-positive reactions. J Chronic Dis 1955;1:297–316.
3. Conley CL, Hartmann RC. A hemorrhagic disorder caused by circulating anticoagulant in patients with disseminated lupus erythematosus. J Clin Invest 1952;31:621–622.
4. Feinstein DI, Rapaport SI. Acquired inhibitors of blood coagulation. Prog Hemost Thromb 1972;1:75–95.
5. Bowie EJW, Thompson JH Jr, Pascuzzi CA, Owen CA Jr. Thrombosis in systemic lupus erythematosus despite circulating anticoagulants. J Lab Clin Med 1963;62:416–430.
6. Laurell AB, Nilsson IM. Hypergammaglobulinaemia, circulating anticoagulant, and biologic false positive Wassermann reaction: a study of 2 cases. J. Lab Clin Med 1957;49:694–707.
7. Thiagarajan P, Shapiro SS, De Marco L. Monoclonal immunoglobulin M coagulation inhibitor with phospholipid specificity. Mechanism of lupus anticoagulant. J Clin Invest 1980;66:397–405.
8. Harris EN, Gharavi AE, Boey ML, Patel BM, Mackworth-Young CG, Loizou S et al. Anticardiolipin antibodies: detection by radioimmunoassay and association with thrombosis in systemic lupus erythematosus. Lancet 1983;ii:1211–1214.
9. Triplett DA, Brandt JT, Kaczor D, Schaeffer J. Laboratory diagnosis of lupus inhibitors: a comparison of the tissue thromboplastin inhibition procedure with a new platelet neutralization procedure. Am J Clin Pathol 1983;79:678–682.
10. Love PE, Santoro SA. Antiphospholipid antibodies: anticardiolipin and the lupus anticoagulant in systemic lupus erythematosus (SLE) and in non-SLE disorders. Ann Intern Med 1990;112:682–698.
11. Hughes GRV, Harris EN, Gharavi AE. The anticardiolipin syndrome. J Rheumatol 1986;13:486–489.
12. Alarcon-Segovia D, Sanchez-Guerrero J. Primary antiphospholipid syndrome. J Rheumatol 1989;16:482–488.
13. McNeil HP, Simpson RJ, Chesterman CN, Krilis SA. Anti-phospholipid antibodies are directed against a complex antigen that includes a lipid-binding inhibitor of coagulation: beta-2-glycoprotein I (apolipoprotein H). Proc Natl Acad Sci USA 1990;87:4120–4124.
14. Galli M, Comfurius P, Maassen C, Hemker HC, de Baets MH, van Breda-Vriesman PJC et al. Anticardiolipin antibodies (ACA) directed not to cardiolipin but to a plasma protein cofactor. Lancet 1990;335:1544–1547.

15. Matsuura E., Igarashi Y, Fujimoto M, Ichikawa K, Koike T. Anticardiolipin cofactor(s) and differential diagnosis of autoimmune disease. Lancet 1990;336:177–178.
16. McIntyre JA, Wagenknecht DR, Sugi T. Phospholipid binding plasma proteins required for antiphospholipid antibody detection-an overview. Am J Reprod Immunol 1997;37:101–110.
17. Oosting JD, Derksen RH, Bobbink IW, Hackeng TM, Bouma BN, de Groot PG. Antiphospholipid antibodies directed against a combination of phospholipids with prothrombin, protein C, or protein S: an explanation for their pathogenic mechanism? Blood 1993;81:2618–2625.
18. Hunt JE, McNeil HP, Morgan GJ, Crameri RM, Krilis SA. A phospholipid-beta 2-glycoprotein I complex is an antigen for anticardiolipin antibodies occurring in autoimmune disease but not with infection. Lupus 1992;1:75–81.
19. Bevers EM, Galli M, Barbui T, Comfurius P, Zwaal RF. Lupus anticoagulant IgGs (LA) are not directed to phospholipids only, but to a complex of lipid-bound human prothrombin. Thromb Haemost 1991;66:629–632.
20. Oosting JD, Derksen RH, Entjes HT, Bouma BN, de Groot PhG. Lupus anticoagulant activity is frequently dependent on the presence of beta 2-glycoprotein I. Thromb Haemost 1992;67:499–50.
21. Roubey RA, Pratt CW, Buyon JP, Winfield JB. Lupus anticoagulant activity of autoimmune antiphospholipid antibodies is dependent upon beta 2-glycoprotein I. J Clin Invest 1992;90:1100–1104.
22. Galli M, Comfurius P, Barbui T, Zwaal RF, Bevers EM. Anticoagulant activity of beta 2-glycoprotein I is potentiated by a distinct subgroup of anticardiolipin antibodies. Thromb Haemost 1992;68:297–300
23. Horbach DA, van Oort E, Derksen RHWM, de Groot PhG. The contribution of anti-prothrombin-antibodies to lupus anticoagulant activity. Discrimination between functional and non-functional anti-prothrombin antibodies. Thromb Haemost 1998;79:790–795.
24. Martinuzzo ME, Forastiero RR, Carreras LO. Anti beta 2 glycoprotein I antibodies: detection and association with thrombosis. Br J Haematol 1995;89,397–402.
25. Ginsburg KS, Liang MH, Newcomer L, Goldhaber SZ, Schur PH, Hennekens CH et al. Anticardiolipin antibodies and the risk for ischemic stroke and venous thrombosis. Ann Intern Med 1992;117:997–1002.
26. Ginsberg JS, Wells PS, Brill-Edwards P, Donovan D, Moffatt K, Johnston M et al. Antiphospholipid antibodies and venous thromboembolism. Blood 1995;86:3685–3691.
27. Branch DW, Dudley DJ, Mitchell MD, Creighton KA, Abbott TM, Hammond EH et al. Immunoglobulin G fractions from patients with antiphospholipid antibodies cause fetal death in BALB/c mice: a model for autoimmune fetal loss. Am J Obstet Gynecol 1990;163:210–216.
28. Blank M, Cohen J, Toder V, Shoenfeld Y. Induction of anti-phospholipid syndrome in naive mice with mouse lupus monoclonal and human polyclonal anti-cardiolipin antibodies. Proc Natl Acad Sci USA 1991;88:3069–3073.
29. Bakimer R, Fishman P, Blank M, Sredni B, Djaldetti M, Shoenfeld Y. Induction of primary antiphospholipid syndrome in mice by immunization with a human monoclonal anticardiolipin antibody (H-3). J Clin Invest 1992;89:1558–1563.
30. Gharavi AE, Sammaritano LR, Wen J, Elkon KB. Induction of antiphospholipid autoantibodies by immunization with β_2-glycoprotein I (apolipoprotein H). J Clin Invest 1992;90:1105–1109.
31. Blank M, Faden D, Tincani A, Kopolovic J, Goldberg I, Gilburd B et al. Immunization with anticardiolipin cofactor (beta-2-glycoprotein I) induces experimental antiphospholipid syndrome in naive mice. J Autoimmunity 1994;7:441–455.
32. Pierangeli SS, Liu XW, Anderson G, Barker JH, Harris EN. Thrombogenic properties of murine anticardiolipin antibodies induced by β_2-glycoprotein I and human immunoglobulin G antiphospholipid antibodies. Circulation 1996;94:1746–1751.
33. Carreras LO, Defreyn G, Machin SJ, Vermylen J, Deman R, Spitz B et al. Arterial thrombosis, intrauterine death and "lupus" anticoagulant: detection of immunoglobulin interfering with prostacyclin formation. Lancet 1981;i:244–246.
34. Carreras LO, Vermylen JG. Lupus anticoagulant and thrombosis – possible role of inhibition of prostacyclin formation. Thromb Haemost 1982;48:38–40.
35. Comp PC, De Bault LE, Esmon NL, Esmon CT. Human thrombomodulin is inhibited by IgG from two patients with non specific anticoagulants. Blood 1983;62 (Suppl I):299.
36. Freyssinet JM, Cazenave JP. Lupus-like anticoagulants, modulation of the protein C pathway and thrombosis. Thromb Haemost 1987;58:679–681.
37. Cariou R, Tobelem G, Bellucci S, Soria J, Soria C, Maclouf J et al. Effect of lupus anticoagulant on antithrombogenic properties of endothelial cells – inhibition of thrombomodulin-dependent protein C activation. Thromb Haemost 1988;60:54–58.
38. Marciniak E, Romond EH. Impaired catalytic function of activated protein C: a new in vitro manifestation of lupus anticoagulant. Blood 1989;74:2426–2432.
39. Cosgriff TM, Martin BA. Low functional and high antigenic antithrombin III level in a patient with the lupus anticoagulant and recurrent thrombosis. Arthritis Rheum 1981;24:94–96.

40. Shibata S, Harpel P, Gharavi A, Rand J, Fillit H. Autoantibodies to heparin from patients with antiphospholipid antibody syndrome inhibit formation of antithrombin III–thrombin complexes. Blood 1994;83:2532–2540.
41. Tsakiris DA, Marbet GA, Makris PE, Settas L, Duckert F. Impaired fibrinolysis as an essential contribution to thrombosis in patients with lupus anticoagulant. Thromb Haemost 1989;61:175–177.
42. Sammaritano LR, Gharavi AE, Soberano C, Levy RA, Michael D. Lockshin MD. Phospolipid binding of antiphospholipid antibodies and placental anticoagulant protein. J Clin Immunol 1992;12:27–35.
43. Arnout J. The pathogenesis of the antiphospholipid syndrome: a hypothesis based on parallelisms with heparin-induced thrombocytopenia. Thromb Haemost 1996;75:536–541.
44. Amiral J. Bridey F, Dreyfus M, Vissoc AM, Fressinaud E, Wolf M et al. Platelet factor 4 complexed to heparin is the target for antibodies generated in heparin-induced thrombocytopenia. Thromb Haemost 1992,68:95–96.
45. Chong BH, Castaldi PA, Berndt MC. Heparin-induced thrombocytopenia: effects of rabbit IgG, and its Fab and Fc fragments on antibody-heparin-platelet interaction. Thromb Res 1989,55,291–295.
46. Warkentin TE, Hayward CPM, Boshkov LK, Santos AV, Sheppard JA, Bode AP et al. Sera from patients with heparin-induced thrombocytopenia generate platelet-derived microparticles with procoagulant activity: an explanation for the thrombotic complications of heparin-induced thrombocytopenia. Blood 1994;84:3691–3699.
47. Brandt JT. Platelet aggregation in heparin-induced thrombocytopenia is dependent on complement activation. Blood 1996;88:517a.
48. Visentin GP, Ford SE, Scott JP, Aster RH. Antibodies from patients with heparin-induced thrombocytopenia/thrombosis are specific for platelet factor 4 complexed with heparin or bound to endothelial cells. J Clin Invest 1994;93:81–88.
49. Ikeda K, Nagasawa K, Hiriuchi T, Tsuru T, Nishizaka H, Niho Y. C5a induces tissue factor activity on endothelial cells. Thromb Haemost 1997;77:394–398.
50. Horbach DA, van Oort E, Donders RCJM, Derksen RHWM, de Groot PG. Lupus anticoagulant is the strongest risk factor for both venous and arterial thrombosis in patients with systemic lupus erythematosus. Comparison between different assays for the detection of antiphospholipid antibodies. Thromb Haemost 1996;76:916–924.
51. Swadzba J, Declerck LS, Stevens WJ. Association of anticardiolipin anti-β_2-glycoprotein I, antiprothrombin antibodies, and lupus anticoagulants in patients with systemic lupus erythematosus with a history of thrombosis. J. Rheumatol 1997;24:1710–1715.
52. Arnout J, Wittevrongel C, Vanrusselt M, Hoylaerts M, Vermylen J. Beta-2-glycoprotein I dependent lupus anticoagulants form stable bivalent antibody–beta-2-glycoprotein I complexes on phospholipid surfaces. Thromb Haemost 1998;79:79–86.
53. Roubey RAS, Eisenberg RA, Harper MF, Winfield JB. "Anticardiolipin" autoantibodies recognize β_2-glycoprotein I in the absence of phospholipid. Importance of Ag density and bivalent binding. J Immunol 1995;154:954–960.
54. Willems GM, Janssen MP, Pelsers MMAL, Comfurius P, Galli M, Zwaal RFA et al. Role of divalency in the high-affinity binding of anticardiolipin antibody–β_2-glycoprotein I complexes to lipid membranes. Biochemistry 1996;35:13833–13842.
55. Takeya H, Mori T, Gabazza EC, Kuroda K, Deguchi H, Matsuura E et al. Anti-β_2-glycoprotein I (b$_2$GPI) monoclonal antibodies with lupus anticoagulant-like activity enhance the β_2GPI binding to phospholipids. J Clin Invest 1997;99:2260–2268.
56. Wurm H. Beta 2-glycoprotein I (apolipoprotein H) interactions with phospholipid vesicles. Int J Biochem 1984;16:511–515.
57. Harper MF, Hayes PM, Lentz B, Roubey RAS. Characterization of β_2-glycoprotein I binding to phospholipid membranes. Thromb Haemost 1998;80:610–614.
58. Exner T, Triplett DA, Taberner D, Machin SJ. Guidelines for testing and revised criteria for lupus anticoagulants. Thromb Haemost 1991;65:320–322.
59. Brandt JT, Triplett DA, Alving B, Scharrer I. Criteria for the diagnosis of lupus anticoagulants: an update. Thromb Haemost 1995;74:1185–1190.
60. Roussi J, Roisin JP, Goguel A. Lupus anticoagulant. First French Interlaboratory Etalanorme Survey. Am J Clin Pathol 1996;105:788–793.
61. Jennings I, Kitchen S, Woods TAL, Preston FE, Greaves M. Clinically important inaccuracies in testing for the lupus anticoagulant: an analysis of results from three surveys of the UK national external quality assessment scheme (NEQAS) for blood coagulation. Thromb Haemost 1997;77:934–937.
62. Brandt JT, Barna K, Triplett DA. Laboratory identification of lupus anticoagulants: results of the second international workshop for identification of lupus anticoagulants. Thromb Haemost 1995;74:1597–603.
63. Arnout J, Vanrusselt M, Wittevrongel C, Vermylen J. Monoclonal antibodies against Beta-2-glycoprotein I: Use as reference material for lupus anticoagulant tests. Thromb Haemost 1998;79:955–958.

64. Arnout J, Meijer P, Vermylen J. Lupus anticoagulant testing in Europe: an analysis of results from the first European concerted action on thrombophilia (ECAT) survey using plasmas spiked with monoclonal antibodies against human beta-2-glycoprotein I. Thromb Haemost 1999;81:929–934.
65. Kawasaki T, Kaida T, Arnout J, Vermylen J, Hoylaerts M. A new animal model of thrombophilia confirms that high plasma factor VIII levels are thrombogenic. Thromb Haemost 1999;81:306–311.

24 Measurement of Anti-β_2-glycoprotein I Antibodies

A. Tsutsumi and T. Koike

Introduction

The importance of anticardiolipin antibody (aCL) detection for predicting thrombotic symptoms, and fetal loss has been established by a number of studies. Binding to cardiolipin of the aCL present in patients with the antiphospholipid syndrome (APS) depends on existence of the cofactor, β_2-glycoprotein I (β_2GPI) [1–3]. The aCL in patients with APS ("pathogenic" aCL) binds to a complex of β_2GPI and negatively charged phospholipids, in contrast to the aCL present in patients with infectious diseases ("non-pathogenic" aCL), which recognizes cardiolipin, independent of β_2GPI [4, 5]. It is now considered that the major antigenic target for "pathogenic" aCL resides on β_2GPI itself; hence, it may be more appropriate to rename aCL "anti-β_2GPI antibody (anti-β_2GPI)". Studies have shown that measurement of anti-β_2GPI may be of value in determining the risk of thrombotic episodes in patients with autoimmune diseases, and that the anti-β_2GPI assays may have better specificities than do the aCL assays.

Structure of β_2-glycoprotein I

β_2GPI (apolipoprotein H) was first described by Schulze et al in 1961 [6]. β_2-GPI is a glycoprotein consisting of a single polypeptide chain of 326 amino acids, which contains five potential N-glycosylation sites [7, 8]. β_2GPI forms five homologous domains of approximately 60 amino acids, designated short consensus repeats/complement control protein repeats, or "sushi" domains [8–11]. These domains are designated as domain I to domain V, from the N terminus to the C terminus. Each domain has two disulfide bonds, with the exception of domain V, which has an extra "tail" consisting of 20 amino acids (Fig. 24.1). Domain V has the major phospholipid binding site at C[281]KNKEKK[288] [12].

β_2-glycoprotein I–anti-β_2-glycoprotein I interaction

In a normal setting of anti-β_2GPI enzyme immunoassays (EIA) using plain polystyrene plates, with exceptions described in some reports [13], anti-β_2GPI present

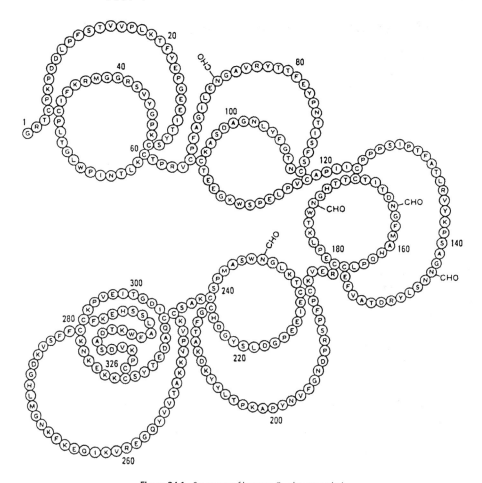

Figure 24.1. Structure of human β_2-glycoprotein I.

in patients with APS does not bind solid-phase β_2GPI. On the other hand, binding to solid phase of anti-β_2GPI created by active immunization of β_2GPI is readily detectable. Anti-β_2GPI in patients with APS will bind solid-phase β_2GPI, but only when (1) β_2GPI is coated on plates which have been pre-coated with cardiolipin, or (2) β_2GPI is coated on irradiated or oxygenated plates. Two theories may explain why anti-β_2GPI can be detected only on "high-binding" or oxygenated plates. (1) Binding of anti-β_2GPI to solid-phase β_2GPI requires a high density of the antigen, and this can be achieved only using oxygenated plates. (2) When β_2GPI is coated on oxygenated plates, C-O and C=O bonds on these plates induce conformational changes of β_2GPI, events which lead to exposure of normally cryptic epitope(s). Evidence supporting the first theory was reported by Roubey et al [14], who observed that bivalent binding was essential for the binding of anti-β_2GPI to solid phase β_2GPI. Their interpretation is that "pathogenic" IgG aCL are intrinsically low affinity antibodies to β_2GPI, and that antibody binding to β_2GPI on a microtiter plate or an anionic phospholipid membrane depends on the marked increase in avidity provided by engagement of both antigen-binding sites of the antibody molecule. Tincani et al [15] reported that anti-β_2GPI from patients with APS have a relatively low affinity, but are capable of binding soluble β_2GPI. On the other hand, Guerin et al [16] reported that fluid phase β_2GPI will not absorb anti-β_2GPI activity in sera from patients with APS. Further support for the first theory was reported by Sheng et al [17]. These authors developed mutant β_2GPI that naturally forms a dimer, and they showed that anti-β_2GPI antibodies have a higher affinity for this dimerized mutant than to wild-type β_2GPI or a control mutant which does not dimerize.

In one of the first documentations on β_2GPI as the aCL cofactor, McNeil et al [1] reported that aCL recognizes β_2GPI bound to cardiolipin, but not to heparin. This observation is consistent with the idea that anti-β_2GPI recognizes either a complex epitope formed by β_2GPI and phospholipids, or that a new epitope is exposed on β_2GPI upon binding to cardiolipin. We [18] extended this idea, and demonstrated that while anti-β_2GPI from mice immunized with human β_2GPI recognized β_2GPI coated on both normal or irradiated plates, anti-β_2GPI from APS patients recognizes β_2GPI coated on irradiated plates, but not on normal plates. It has been shown that a comparable amount of β_2GPI was coated on either of the plates [18, 19], thus suggesting that a new epitope exposed on β_2GPI upon binding to cardiolipin or oxygenated surfaces is important for anti-β_2GPI present in patients with APS. In contrast, anti-β_2GPI created by artificial immunization of β_2GPI can bind native β_2GPI in the absence of anionic phospholipids or oxygenated surfaces. Other laboratories reported results supporting the second theory [20, 21]. Recently, we [22, and manuscript submitted for publication] constructed a three dimensional model of β_2GPI, by computerized calculation from nuclear magnetic resonance (NMR) coordinates of a sushi domain of human factor H, and we searched for putative epitopes of monoclonal anti-β_2GPI established from APS patients or APS model mice, using this model (Fig. 24.2). Epitope candidates for these antibodies, obtained from random peptide libraries, resided on the 4th domain of β_2GPI. Based on this model, these epitopes are usually covered by the 3rd domain, and would require conformational alteration to be recognized by specific antibodies. These results support the notion that conformational changes are of central importance in the expression of epitopes for pathogenic anti-β_2GPI.

The problem of "antigenic density" and "conformational alteration" remains unsolved. However, it should be noted that either theory does not exclude the other.

Epitopes present on β_2GPI are reported to be on the 4th [23] or the 5th [12] domain of β_2GPI, determined by analysis using domain deleted mutants of β_2GPI and monoclonal anti-β_2GPI antibodies established from patients wth APS. In contrast, a recent study using purified polyclonal anti-β_2GPI from APS patients indicated that the major antigenic epitopes reside on the 1st domain of β_2GPI [24]. This discrepancy remains to be addressed.

Clinical Significance of the Measurement of Anti-β_2GPI Antibodies

Reports [16, 25–32] have shown that detection of IgG, and possibly IgM anti-β_2GPI is significantly related to the history of thrombosis. In particular, studies in which

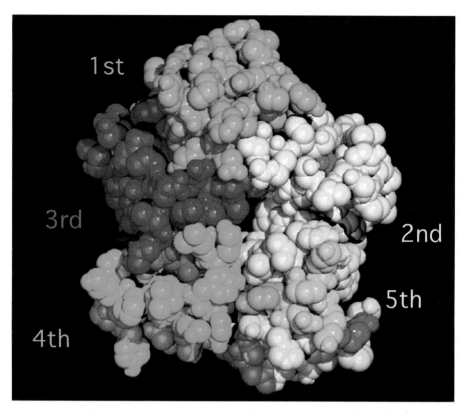

Figure 24.2. Three-dimensional model of human β_2-glycoprotein I, based on NMR coordinates of human factor H. The five domains are shown in different colors. The light blue colored area on the 5th domain indicates the phospholipid-binding region.

investigators utilized both anti-β_2GPI and conventional aCL assays have shown that IgG anti-β_2GPI assays have improved specificities over the conventional aCL assays [16, 27, 31, 33, 34]. This improvement probably relates to the fact that conventional aCL assays will detect "β_2GPI-independent aCL" frequently present in patients with infectious diseases such as syphilis [16, 26, 30], Lyme disease [35], hepatitis C virus infection [36], and acquired immune deficiency syndrome [16, 37]. The superiority of IgM anti-β_2GPI assays over IgM aCL assays has yet to be determined. The incidence of IgG anti-β_2GPI in SLE patients ranges from 10.8% [29], 29.5% [38] to 39.3% [33]. These differences may relate to differences in patient populations, protocols used for detection, and the cut-off levels set by individual investigators.

The significance of IgA class anti-β_2GPI has not been clearly established. We [39] detected IgA anti-β_2GPI in 25% of Japanese systemic lupus erythematosus (SLE) patients and we found that the presence of IgA anti-β_2GPI correlates with the thrombotic history. However, most patients with IgA anti-β_2GPI were also positive for IgG and/or IgM anti-β_2GPI. Fanopoulos et al [40] found that the sensitivity of the anti-β_2GPI test for APS in patients with SLE is significantly increased with measurement of IgA anti-β_2GPI, in addition to IgG and IgM isotypes. These reports findings lend support to the notion that IgA anti-β_2GPI may have a role in the pathogenesis of APS, and that measurement of IgA anti-β_2GPI may be useful in practice. Large scale prospective studies will of course be needed.

The lack of a standardized method and standard material is a serious drawback in the clinical evaluation of anti-β_2GPI measurement. It has been shown that commercially available enzyme immunoassay plates differ greatly regarding detectability of anti-β_2GPI [41]. In addition, individual researchers are using their own standards to quantify anti-β_2GPI antibodies, thus making it almost impossible to compare data obtained in different institutes. Efforts are now being made to construct a chimeric monoclonal anti-β_2GPI antibody consisting of V regions from monoclonal aCL derived from an APS model mouse and Fc portions of human IgG [41,42]. This chimeric antibody, which can be produced in large quantities and distributed to interested laboratories, should aid in standardizing procedures used for anti-β_2GPI assays.

Future Studies

Anti-β_2GPI assays are an important improvement and have several advantages compared to conventional aCL assays. Future prospective studies using standardized methods will more clarify the value of anti-β_2GPI measurement for evaluating the risk of symptoms related to APS. Basic studies dealing on β_2GPI–anti-β_2GPI interactions and specificities of anti-β_2GPI will further our understanding of the pathogenesis of APS and may even pave a way toward development of specific therapies.

The relationship between the presence of anti-β_2GPI and the development of atherosclerosis is also a problem which warrants more attention. A recent in vitro study has shown that β_2GPI binds to oxidized low-density lipoprotein (oxLDL) and inhibits the uptake of oxLDL by macrophages. Anti-β_2GPI was found to enhance the uptake of oxLDL by macrophages in the presence of β_2GPI [43]. Clinical studies will be necessary to determine if the presence of anti-β_2GPI is a risk factor for accelerated atherosclerosis.

References

1. McNeil HP, Simpson RJ, Chesterman CN, Krilis SA. Anti-phospholipid antibodies are directed against a complex antigen that includes a lipid-binding inhibitor of coagulation: β_2-glycoprotein I (apolipoprotein H). Proc Natl Acad Sci USA 1990;87:4120–4124.
2. Galli M, Comfurius P, Maassen C et al. Anticardiolipin antibodies (ACA) directed not to cardiolipin but to a plasma cofactor. Lancet 1990;335:1544–1547.
3. Matsuura E, Igarashi Y, Fujimoto M, Ichikawa K, Koike T. Anticardiolipin cofactor(s) and differential diagnosis of autoimmune disease. Lancet 1990;336:177–178.
4. Koike T, Matsuura E. What is the "true" antigen for anticardiolipin antibodies? Lancet 1991;337:671–672.
5. Matsuura E, Igarashi Y, Fujimoto M et al. Heterogeneity of anticardiolipin antibodies defined by the anticardiolipin cofactor. J Immunol 1992;148:3885–3891.
6. Schultze HE, Heide K, Haupt H. Uber ein bisher ubekanntes niedermolekulars β_2-Globulin des Humanserums. Naturwissenschften 1961;48:719.
7. Lozier J, Takahashi N, Putnam FW. Complete amino acid sequence of human plasma β_2-glycoprotein I. Proc Natl Acad Sci USA 1984;81:3640–3644.

8. Kato H, Enjyoji K. Amino acid sequence and location of the disulfide bonds in bovine β_2 glycoprotein I: the presence of five Sushi domains. Biochemistry 1991;30:11687–11694.
9. Matsuura E, Igarashi M, Igarashi Y et al. Molecular definition of human β_2-glycoprotein I (β_2.GPI) by cDNA cloning and inter-species differences of β_2 GPI in alternation of anticardiolipin binding. Int Immunol 1991;3:1217–1221.
10. Steinkasserer A, Estaller C, Weiss EH, Sim RB, Day AJ. Complete nucleotide and deduced amino acid sequence of human β_2-glycoprotein I. Biochem J 1991;15:387–391.
11. Mehdi H, Nunn M, Steel DM et al. Nucleotide sequence and expression of the human gene encoding apolipoprotein H (β_2-glycoprotein I). Gene 1991;108:293–298.
12. Hunt J, Krilis S. The fifth domain of β_2-glycoprotein I contains a phospholipid binding site (Cys281–Cys288) and a region recognized by anticardiolipin antibodies. J Immunol 1994;152:653–659.
13. Arvieux J, Regnault V, Hachulla E, Darnige L, Roussel B, Bensa JC. Heterogeneity and immunochemical properties of anti-beta2-glycoprotein I autoantibodies. Thromb Haemost 1998;80:393–398.
14. Roubey RA, Eisenberg RA, Harper MF, Winfield JB. "Anticardiolipin" autoantibodies recognize β_2-glycoprotein I in the absence of phospholipid. Importance of Ag density and bivalent binding. J Immunol 1995;154:954–960.
15. Tincani A, Spatola L, Prati E et al. The anti-β_2-glycoprotein I activity in human anti-phospholipid syndrome sera is due to monoreactive low-affinity autoantibodies directed to epitopes located on native β_2-glycoprotein I and preserved during species' evolution. J Immunol 1996;157:5732–5738.
16. Guerin J, Feighery C, Sirı RB, Jackson J. Antibodies to β_2-glycoprotein I – a specific marker for the antiphospholipid syndrome. Clin Exp Immunol 1997;109:304–309.
17. Sheng Y, Kandiah DA, Krilis SA. Anti-beta 2-glycoprotein I autoantibodies from patients with the "antiphospholipid" syndrome bind to beta 2-glycoprotein I with low affinity: dimerization of beta 2-glycoprotein I induces a significant increase in anti-beta 2-glycoprotein I antibody affinity. J Immunol 1998;161:2038–2043
18. Matsuura E, Igarashi Y, Yasuda T, Triplett DA, Koike T. Anticardiolipin antibodies recognize β_2-glycoprotein I structure altered by interacting with an oxygen modified solid phase surface. J Exp Med 1994;179:457–462.
19. Koike T, Tsutsumi A, Ichikawa K, Matsuura E. Antigenic specificity of the "anticardiolipin" antibodies. Blood 1995;85:2277–2278.
20. Wagenknecht DR, McIntyre JA. Changes in β_2-glycoprotein I antigenicity induced by phospholipid binding. Thromb Haemost 1993;9:361–365.
21. Pengo V, Biasiolo A, Fior MG. Autoimmune antiphospholipid antibodies are directed against a cryptic epitope expressed when β_2-glycoprotein I is bound to a suitable surface. Thromb Haemost 1995;73:29–34
22. Koike T, Ichikawa K, Kasahara H, Atsumi T, Tsutsumi A, Matsuura E. Epitopes on β_2-GPI recognized by anticardiolipin antibodies. Lupus 1998;7 Suppl 2:S14–S17
23. George J, Gilburd B, Hojnik M et al. Target recognition of β_2-glycoprotein I (β_2GPI)-dependent anticardiolipin antibodies: evidence for involvement of the fourth domain of β_2GPI in antibody binding. J Immunol 1998;160:3917–23
24. Iverson GM, Victoria EJ, Marquis DM. Anti-β_2 glycoprotein I (β_2GPI) autoantibodies recognize an epitope on the first domain of β_2GPI. Proc Natl Acad Sci USA 1998;95:15542–6
25. Martinuzzo ME, Forastiero RR, Carreras LO. Anti β_2-glycoprotein I antibodies: detection and association with thrombosis. Br J Haematol 1995;89:397–402.
26. McNally T, Purdy G, Mackie IJ, Machin SJ, Isenberg DA. The use of an anti-β_2-glycoprotein-I assay for discrimination between anticardiolipin antibodies associated with infection and increased risk of thrombosis. Br J Haematol 1995;91:471–473.
27. Balestrieri G, Tincani A, Spatola L et al. Anti-beta 2-glycoprotein I antibodies: a marker of antiphospholipid syndrome? Lupus 1995;4:122–130.
28. Cabral AR, Cabiedes J, Alarcon-Segovia D. Antibodies to phospholipid-free β_2-glycoprotein-I in patients with primary antiphospholipid syndrome. J Rheumatol 1995;22:1894–1898.
29. Tsutsumi A, Matsuura E, Ichikawa K et al. Antibodies to β_2-glycoprotein I and clinical manifestations in patients with systemic lupus erythematosus. Arthritis Rheum 1996;39:1466–1474.
30. Forastiero RR, Martinuzzo ME, Kordich LC, Carreras LO. Reactivity to β_2 glycoprotein I clearly differentiates anticardiolipin antibodies from antiphospholipid syndrome and syphilis. Thrombosis Haemost 1996;75:717–720.
31. Roubey RAS, Maldonado MA, Byrd SN. Comparison of an enzyme-linked immunosorbent assay for antibodies to β_2-glycoprotein I and a conventional anticardiolipin immunoassay. Arthritis Rheum 1996;39:1606–1607.
32. Amengual O, Atsumi T, Khamashta MA, Koike T, Hughes GRV. Specificity of ELISA for antibody to β_2-glycoprotein I in patients with antiphospholipid syndrome. Br J Rheumatol 1996;35:1239–1243.

33. Cabiedes J, Cabral AR, Alarcon-Segovia D. Clinical manifestations of the antiphospholipid syndrome in patients with systemic lupus erythematosus associate more strongly with anti-beta 2-glycoprotein-I than with antiphospholipid antibodies. J Rheumatol 1995;22:1899–1906

34. Sanmarco M, Soler C, Christides C et al. Prevalence and clinical significance of IgG isotype anti-beta 2-glycoprotein I antibodies in antiphospholipid syndrome: a comparative study with anticardiolipin antibodies. J Lab Clin Med 1997;129:499–506.

35. Garcia Monco JC, Wheeler CM et al. Reactivity of neuroborreliosis patients (Lyme disease) to cardiolipin and gangliosides. J Neurol Sci 1993;117:206–214.

36. Cacoub P, Musset L, Amoura Z et al. Anticardiolipin, anti-β_2-glycoprotein I, and antinucleosome antibodies in hepatitis C virus infection and mixed cryoglobulinemia. J Rheumatol 1997;24:2139–2144.

37. Viscarello RR, Williams CJ, DeGennaro NJ, Hobbins JC. Prevalence and prognostic significance of anticardiolipin antibodies in pregnancies complicated by human immunodeficiency virus-1 infection. Am J Obst Gynecol 1997;167:1080-1085.

38. McNally T, Mackie IJ, Machin SJ, Isenberg DA. Increased levels of beta 2 glycoprotein-I antigen and beta 2 glycoprotein-I binding antibodies are associated with a history of thromboembolic complications in patients with SLE and primary antiphospholipid syndrome. Br J Rheumatol 1995;34:1031–1036.

39. Tsutsumi A, Matsuura E, Ichikawa K, Fujisaku A, Mukai M, Koike T. IgA class anti-β_2-glycoprotein I in patients with systemic lupus erythematosus. J Rheumatol 1998;25:74–78.

40. Fanopoulos D, Teodorescu MR, Varga J, Teodorescu M. High frequency of abnormal levels of IgA anti-β_2-glycoprotein I antibodies in patients with systemic lupus erythematosus: relationship with antiphospholipid syndrome. J Rheumatol 1998;25:675–680.

41. Tsutsumi A, Ichikawa K, Matsuura E, Koike T. Anti-β_2-glycoprotein I antibodies. Lupus 1998;7 Suppl 2:S98–102.

42. Ichikawa K, Tsutsumi A, Atsumi T et al. A chimeric antibody with the human γ_1 constant region as a putative standard for assays to detect IgG β_2-glycoprotein I-dependent anticardiolipin anti-β_2-glycoprotein I antibodies. Arthritis Rheum 1999;42:2461–2470.

43. Hasunuma Y, Matsuura E, Makita Z, Katahira T, Nishi S, Koike T. Involvement of beta 2-glycoprotein I and anticardiolipin antibodies in oxidatively modified low-density lipoprotein uptake by macrophages. Clin Exp Immunol 1997;107:569–573.

25 Antiprothrombin Antibodies

M. L. Bertolaccini, O. Amengual and T. Atsumi

Introduction

In clinical practice, anticardiolipin antibody (aCL) detected by enzyme-linked immunosorbent assay (ELISA) and lupus anticoagulant (LA) detected by clotting assays have been standardized for the diagnosis of Hughes syndrome (antiphospholipid syndrome). However, the family of antiphospholipid antibodies (aPL) has recently expanded to include a heterogeneous group of autoantibodies whose specificity is directed against proteins involved in coagulation or a complex of the former with phospholipids.

Amongst phospholipid binding proteins, the best studied is β_2-glycoprotein I (β_2GPI), which bears the cryptic epitope(s) for aCL binding. These epitopes are exposed when β_2GPI binds to negatively charged phospholipids such as cardiolipin, or irradiated plastic plates [1], behaving thus as a cofactor for aCL binding. Several studies have highlighted the significance of anti-β_2-glycoprotein I antibodies (anti-β_2GPI) as an alternative ELISA with higher specificity than the conventional aCL ELISA [2–4].

Prothrombin, another phospholipid binding protein, was first proposed as a possible cofactor for LA by Loeliger in 1959 [5]. In subsequent years, the interest regarding this protein has increased and several groups have investigated the significance of antiprothrombin antibodies (aPT).

Prothrombin

Prothrombin is a single chain glycoprotein synthesized in the liver whose plasma concentration is around of 2.5 μmol/l. Its gene spans 21-kilobase-pairs [6] on chromosome 11. Mature prothrombin contains 579 amino acid residues with a molecular mass of 72 kDa, including three carbohydrate chains and ten γ-carboxyglutamic acid residues [7].

Prothrombin is physiologically activated by the tenase complex, that is a complex of factor Xa, with factor V, calcium and phospholipids as cofactors (Fig. 25.1). Once negatively charged phospholipids bind prothrombin, tenase converts prothrombin to thrombin which triggers fibrinogen polymerization into fibrin [8]. In addition, thrombin binds thrombomodulin on the surface of endothelial cells and activates protein C which then exerts its anticoagulant activity by digesting factor V and

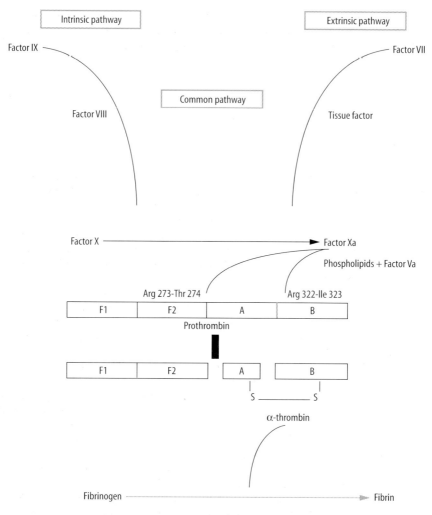

Figure 25.1. Schematic representation of the coagulation cascade and prothrombin degradation.

depriving the tenase complex of its most important cofactor. Because of this negative feedback pathway prothrombin/thrombin behaves as an "indirect" anticoagulant.

During its liver biosynthesis, prothrombin undergoes γ carboxylation (10 glutamic acid residues in proximity of its amino terminus). These γ-carboxyglutamic residues, known as a Gla-domains, are located on fragment 1 of the prothrombin molecule. Gla-domains are essential for the calcium dependency of phospholipid binding to prothrombin, necessary for the conversion of prothrombin to biologically active α-thrombin. Two kringle domains follow this region and are involved in pro(thrombin) binding to fibrin [6]. Tenase selectively hydrolyzes two peptide bonds on the prothrombin molecule. Cleavage at Arg 273–Thr 274 results in the liberation of prothrombin fragment 1+2 (residues 1–273) and prethrombin 2 (residues

274–581); further cleavage at Arg 322–Ile 323 results in the formation of α-thrombin. The latter, one of the most potent enzymes known, not only converts fibrinogen to fibrin (Fig. 25.1) but acts upon factors V, VIII, XIII, protein C, platelets [9] or endothelial cells.

Antiprothrombin Antibodies

History

In 1959, Loeliger [5] was the first to describe the "LA cofactor phenomenon". The addition of normal plasma to that of a patient with LA increased the degree of co-agulation inhibition. A low plasma level of prothrombin was also found, suggesting that the cofactor associated with the expression of the LA activity was most likely prothrombin. One year later, Rapaport et al [10] described the case of a child with LA who underwent recurrent bleeding episodes. Further investigations showed a severe prothrombin deficiency, a prolonged prothrombin time and a prolonged activated partial thromboplastin time (aPTT). In 1983, Bajaj et al [11] were the first to ascertain the presence of prothrombin-binding antibodies in two patients with LA and hypoprothrombinemia. They inferred that hypoprothrombinemia resulted from the binding of aPT to prothrombin in vivo and showed that the decreased concentrations of prothrombin could be caused by enhanced clearance of prothrombin–aPT complexes from plasma.

In 1984, Edson et al [12] demonstrated prothrombin–aPT complexes by crossed-immunoelectrophoresis (CIE) in 67% of 21 patients with the LA. Ten of these patients had quantitatively normal prothrombin. In 1988, Fleck et al [13] found that 72% of the LA population under study had prothrombin–aPT complexes by CIE and showed that aPT had LA activity. Subsequently, circulating prothrombin–aPT complexes were also observed in patients with LA and normal prothrombin levels. In 1991, Bevers et al [14] highlighted the importance of aPT in causing LA activity when they studied 16 patients with both aCL and LA. After incubation with cardiolipin-containing liposomes, the LA activity remained in the supernatant in 11/16 patients. These 11 samples demonstrated LA activity in a phospholipid-bound prothrombin dependent fashion. Subsequently, Oosting et al [15] showed that 4/22 LA inhibited endothelial cell-mediated prothrombinase activity and the IgG fraction containing LA activity bound to phospholipid–prothrombin complex. In 1995, Arvieux et al [16] showed that aPT could be detected by a standard ELISA using prothrombin coated onto irradiated plates.

Immunological Characteristics

A number of uncertainties exist regarding the immunological specificities and properties of aPT. Antiprothrombin antibodies are commonly detected by ELISA methods, using irradiated plates [16] or in complex with phosphatidylserine. The mode of presentation of prothrombin in solid phase seems to influence its recognition by aPT. In fact, aPT cannot bind when prothrombin is immobilized onto non-irradiated plates [16, 17], but does so if prothrombin is immobilized on a suitable anionic surface, adsorbed on gamma irradiated plates or exposed to immobilized anionic phospholipids. An analogy between the behavior of these antibodies and anti-β_2GPI has been hypothesized. aPT may be directed against cryptic or neoepitopes (antigens) exposed when prothrombin binds to anionic phospholipids, and/or may be low affinity antibodies binding bivalently to immobilized prothrombin.

Hexagonal (II) phase phosphatidylethanolamine is used as excess of phospholipids in the clotting assay to confirm LA [18]. Not only phosphatidylserine-bound prothrombin but hexagonal (II) phase phosphatidylethanolamine bound prothrombin may expose the epitope to aPT [19]. There still are some discrepancies regarding whether aPT are directed against neoepitopes or are low affinitty antibodies. Wu et al [20] observed that human prothrombin undergoes a conformational change upon binding to phosphatidylserine-containing surfaces in the presence of calcium. On the other hand, Galli et al [17] demonstrated that aPT could be of low affinity and suggested that prothrombin complexed with phosphatidylserine could allow clustering and better orientation of the antigen, offering optimal conditions for antibody recognition.

A high percentage of aPT has species-specificity for the human protein [14], and a minority of aPT reacts with bovine prothrombin [21]. The epitope(s) recognised by aPT is being investigated. Rao et al [22], by using purified IgG preparations from LA-positive patients demonstrated binding of aPT to prethrombin 1 and fragment 1, as well as to the whole prothrombin molecule. However, none of the antibodies reacted with immobilized thrombin. These data were later confirmed by Malia et al [23] who demonstrated binding of aPT to prothrombin fragment 1+2. These findings suggest that dominant epitopes are likely to be located near the phospholipid-binding site of prothrombin molecule, although they may have heterogeneous distribution. More recently it was reported that most LA depend on the presence of phospholipid-bound prothrombin, as well as of phospholipid-bound β_2GPI, and the anticoagulant properties of aPT have been studied by several groups. Permpikul et al [24] purified IgG fractions from 10 patients with LA, showing that LA activity was due to aPT in at least nine of the samples. Galli et al [17] and Horbach et al [25] reported the existence of two types of circulating aPT which may be distinguished on the basis of their effect in coagulation assays: (1) functional, which cause LA activity; and (2) non-functional which do not contribute to the LA activity, probably caused by a difference in epitope specificities between different aPT [26]. Horbach et al [25] also described that the majority of LA-positive samples were represented by a combination of antibodies with specificity for prothrombin and for β_2GPI, suggesting that the detection of specific aPT might be hampered by the possible presence of anti-β_2GPI antibodies in the same plasma sample.

Clinical Significance

It appears that prothrombin is a common antigenic target of aPL, since aPT are detected in about 28–90% of the patients, depending on the assay performed and the population under study. As they display rather heterogeneous immunological and functional properties, their clinical significance is far from clear.

Petri et al [27] reported that aPT have potential predictive value for thrombosis in a cohort of patients with systemic lupus erythematosus (SLE). At variance Pengo et al [28] found no correlation between the presence of aPT and thrombosis in 22 APS patients with thrombosis. Galli et al [17] found aPT in 58% of APS patients, but they found no correlation between thrombotic events and aPT. Outside the auto-

Table 25.1. Correlation between the presence of aPT and thrombosis – clinical data reported in the literature.

Author	Population	Correlation between aPT and thrombosis
Petri et al [27]	SLE (n = 100)	Potential predictive value for thrombotic events
Pengo et al [28]	aPL (n = 22)	No correlation with thrombosis
Vaarala et al [29]	Myocardial infarction (n = 106)	2.5-fold increase in the risk of myocardial infarction or cardiac death
Puurunen et al [30]	SLE (n = 139)	Positive correlation with DVT
Horbach et al [25]	SLE (n = 175)	Positive correlation with venous thrombosis
Galli et al [17]	aPL (n = 59)	No correlation with thrombosis
Palosuo et al [31]	DVT or PE (n = 265)	Positive correlation with DVT and PE
Forastiero et al [32]	aPL (n = 233)	Positive correlation with venous thrombosis
Swadzba et al [34]	SLE (n = 100) LLD (n = 27)	No correlation with thrombosis
Bertolaccini et al [33]	SLE (n = 207)	Positive correlation with thrombosis
Guerin et al [35]	Infectious disease, SLE, APS, RA, thrombosis (n = 265)	No association with thrombosis
Sorice et al [36]	SLE (n = 38)	Positive correlation with clinical features of APS

SLE, systemic lupus erythematosus; aPL, antiphospholipid antibodies positive patients; APS, antiphospholipid syndrome; DVT, deep vein thrombosis; PE, pulmonary embolism; LLD, lupus-like disease; RA, rheumatoid arthritis.

immune setting, Vaarala et al [29] showed that high levels of aPT confer a 2.5-fold increase in the risk of myocardial infarction or cardiac death in middle-aged men. Puurunen et al [30] also found a positive correlation between the presence of aPT and deep vein thrombosis (DVT) in a SLE population. Horbach et al [25] investigated the clinical significance of aPT in 175 patients with SLE and found that both IgG and IgM aPT were more frequent in patients with a history of venous thrombosis. Palosuo et al [31] studied 265 cases of DVT or pulmonary embolism and found that the risk of thrombotic events was significantly increased in carriers of aPT. Forastiero et al [32] reported an association between the presence of aPT and venous thrombosis in 233 patients with LA and/or aCL. In our study, we found correlation between the presence of aPT and the occurrence of vascular events in 207 patients with SLE [33]. Therefore, most of the available data would support a correlation between aPT and thrombosis as a whole, without a clear cut discrimination between arterial and venous thrombosis (data summarized in Table 25.1).

Pathogenetic Role of aPT

Despite uncertainties regarding the pathogenetic mechanism of aPT, there is increasing evidence that they have a role to play in the hypercoagulable state of APS. First, the antigens are present in plasma or on cell surfaces that are exposed to plasma, therefore accesible to circulating antibodies. Secondly, many of these antigens are molecules involved in coagulation.

Some effects on endothelial cells have been proposed: (1) aPT inhibit thrombin-mediated endothelial cell prostacyclin release and hamper protein C activation [37]; (2) aPT could recognize the prothrombin–anionic phospholipid complex on endothelial cell surface, activating endothelial cells and inducing procoagulant substances via prothrombin [38] (Fig. 25.2) or 3) aPT could increase the affinitty of

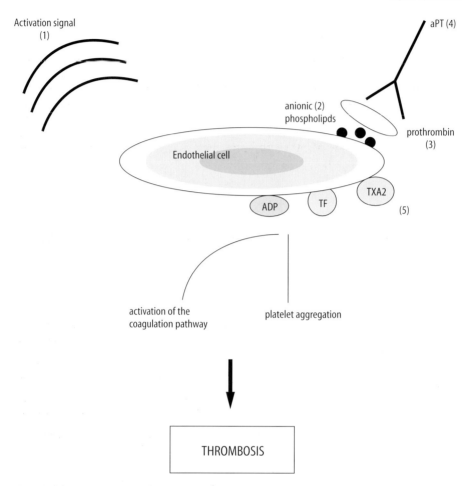

aPT antiprothrombin antibodies; ADP: adenosine diphosphate; TF: tissue factor; TXA2: thromboxane A2. After an activation signal or damage (1), anionic phospholipids are exposed at the endothelial cell level (2). Prothrombin, a phospholipid-binding protein, binds to them on the surface (3). Circulating aPT recognize these complexes binding to them (4). The endothelial cell is thus activated inducing release of procoagulant substances as TXA2, TF and ADP (5), with the consequent activation of the coagulation pathway, platelet aggregation and thrombosis.

Figure 25.2. Hypothetical mechanism at the endothelial cell level.

prothrombin for negatively charged phospholipids [22]. Thus, the prothrombin–aPT complexes would compete with the binding of other coagulation factors for the available surface, resulting in a prolongation of clotting assays that can be neutralised by the addition of extra phospholipids. This in vitro phenomenon could be extrapolated to an in vivo scenario: membrane binding of aPT–prothrombin complexes could decrease the concentration of prothrombin and/or phospholipid sites available for optimal assembly of the prothrombinase complex [39], leading to an hypercoagulable state and consequently to a thrombotic tendency.

Conclusion

It has been demonstrated that the interaction between aPL and anionic phospholipids is mediated by plasma proteins, one of them identified as prothrombin. aPT are frequently found in patients with aPL but the immunological characteristics and mechanisms of action are not completely understood. As thrombotic mechanisms are multifactorial and complex, further investigations are required to define the role of aPT in the pathogenesis of thrombosis. Knowledge of the behavior of specific aPL would aid in defining specific thrombogenic pathways and improved management of patients with Hughes syndrome.

Acknowledgment

The authors wish to thank Dr Paul R.J. Ames, Haematology Department, St. Thomas' Hospital for helpful discussion of this manuscript.

References

1. Matsuura E, Igarashi Y, Yasuda T, Triplett DA, Koike T. Anticardiolipin antibodies recognised β_2-glycoprotein I structure altered by interacting with an oxygen modified solid phase surface. J Exp Med 1994;179:457–462.
2. Roubey RAS, Maldonado MA, Byrd SN. Comparison of an enzyme-linked immunosorbent assay for antibodies to β_2 Glycoprotein I and a conventional anticardiolipin immunoassay. Arthritis Rheum 1996;39:1606–1607.
3. McNally T, Mackie IJ, Machin SJ, Isenberg DA. Increased levels of β_2 glycoprotein antigen and β_2 glycoprotein binding antibodies are associated with a history of thromboembolic complications in patients with SLE and primary antiphospholipid syndrome. Br J Rheumatol 1995;34:1031–1036.
4. Amengual O, Atsumi T, Khamashta MA, Koike T, Hughes GRV. Specificity of an ELISA for antibody to β_2-glycoprotein I in patients with antiphospholipid syndrome. Br J Rheumatol 1996;35:1239–1243.
5. Loeliger A. Prothrombin as a co-factor of the circulating anticoagulant in systemic lupus erythematosus?. Thromb Diath Haemorrh 1959;3:237–256.
6. Degen SJ, Davie EW. Nucleotide sequence of the gene for human prothrombin. Biochemistry 1987;26:6165–6177.
7. Chow BKC, Ting V, Tufaro F, MacGillivray RTA. Characterization of a novel liver-specific enhacer in the human prothrombin gene. J Biol Chem 1991;266:18927–18933.
8. Mann KG, Nesheim ME, Church WR, Haley P, Krishnaswamy S. Surface dependent reactions of the vitamin K-dependent enzyme complexes. Blood 1990;76:1–16.
9. Pelzer H, Schwarz A, Stuber W. Determination of human prothrombin activation fragment 1+2 in plasma with an antibody against a synthetic peptide. Thromb Haemost 1991;65:153–9
10. Rapaport SI, Ames SB, Duvall BJ. A plasma coagulation defect in systemic lupus erythematosus arising from hypoprothrombinemia combined with antiprothrombinase activity. Blood 1960;15:212–27.
11. Bajaj SP, Rapaport SI, Fierer DS, Herbst KD, Schwartz DB. A mechanism for the hypoprothrombinemia of the acquired hypoprothrombinemia-lupus anticoagulant syndrome. Blood 1983;61:684–92.
12. Edson JR, Vogt JM, Hasegawa DK. Abnormal prothrombin crossed-immunoelectrophoresis in patients with lupus inhibitor. Blood 1984;64:807–16.
13. Fleck RA, Rapaport SI, Rao LV. Antiprothrombin antibodies and the lupus anticoagulant. Blood 1988;72:512–9.
14. Bevers EM, Galli M, Barbui T, Comfurius P, Zwaal RFA. Lupus anticoagulant IgGs (LA) are not directed to phospholipid only, but to a complex of lipid-bound human prothrombin. Thromb Haemost 1991;66:629–32.
15. Oosting JD, Derksen RHWM, Bobbink IWG, Hackeng TM, Bouma BN, de Groot PG. Antiphospholipid antibodies directed against a combination of phospholipids with prothrombin, protein C, or protein S: an explanation for their pathogenic mechanism?. Blood 1993;81:2618–25.

16. Arvieux J, Darnige L, Caron C, Reber G, Bensa JC, Colomb MG. Development of an ELISA for autoantibodies to prothrombin showing their prevalence in patients with lupus anticoagulant. Thromb Haemost 1995;74:1120–1125.
17. Galli M, Beretta G, Daldossi M, Bevers EM, Barbui T. Different anticoagulant and immunological properties of anti-prothrombin antibodies in patients with antiphospholipid antibodies. Thromb Haemost 1997;77:486–491.
18. Tripplet DA. Many faces of lupus anticoagulants. Lupus 1998;7:S18-S22.
19. Rauch J, Tannenbaum M, Neville C, Fortin PR. Inhibition of lupus anticoagulant activity by hexagonal phase phosphatidylethanolamine in the presence of prothrombin. Thromb Haemost 1998;80:936–941.
20. Wu JR, Lenz BR. Phospholipid-specific conformational changes in human prothrombin upon binding to procoagulant acid lipid membranes. Thromb Haemost 1994;71:596–604.
21. Rao LVM, Hoang AD, Rapaport SI. Differences in the interactions of lupus anticoagulant IgG with human prothrombin and bovine prothrombin. Thromb Haemost 1995;73:668–674.
22. Rao LVM, Hoang AD, Rapaport SI. Mechanism and effects of the binding of lupus anticoagulant IgG and prothrombin to surface phospholipid. Blood 1996;88:4173–4182
23. Malia RG, Brooksfield C, Bulman I, Greaves M. Prothrombin fragment F1-2: the epitope for antiphospholipid antibody expression. XVIth Congress of the International Society of Thrombosis and Haemostasis, Florence, Italy, June 6–12, 1997 (abstract 689)
24. Permpikul P, Rao LVM, Rapaport SI. Functional and binding studies of the roles of prothrombin and β_2-glycoprotein I in the expression of lupus anticoagulant activity. Blood 1994;83:2878–2892.
25. Horbach DA, Van Oort E, Donders RCJM, Derksen RHWM, De Groot PG. Lupusanticoagulant is the strongest risk factor for both venous and arterial thrombosis in patients with systemic lupus erythematosus – comparison between different assays for the detection of antiphospholipid antibodies. Thromb Haemost 1996;76:916–924.
26. Horbach DA, Van Oort E, Derksen RHWM, de Groot PG. The contribution ofanti-prothrombin-antibodies to lupus anticoagulant activity. Discriminationbetween functional and non-functional anti-prothrombin-antibodies. Thromb Haemost 1998;79:790–795.
27. Petri M, Miller J, Goldman D, Ebert R. Anti-plasma protein antibodies are predictive of thrombotic events [abstract]. Arthritis Rheum 1994;37 Suppl:S281.
28. Pengo V, Biasolo A, Brocco T, Tonetto S, Ruffatti A. Autoantibodies to phospholipid-binding plasma proteins in patients with thrombosis and phospholipid reactive antibodies. Thromb Haemost 1996;75:721–724.
29. Vaarala O, Puurunen M, Manttari M, Manninen V, Aho K, Palosuo T. Antibodies to prothrombin imply a risk of myocardial infarction in middle-aged men. Thromb Haemost 1996;75:456–459.
30. Puurunen M, Vaarala O, Julkunen H, Aho K, Palosuo T. Antibodies to phospholipid-binding plasma proteins and occurrence of thrombosis in patients with systemic lupus erythematosus. Clin Immunol Immunopathol 1996;80:16–22.
31. Palosuo T, Virtamo J, Haukka J, Taylor PR, Aho K, Puurunen M et al. High antibody levels to prothrombin imply a risk of deep venous thrombosis and pulmonary embolism in middle-aged men. A nested case–control study. Thromb Haemost 1997;78:1178–1182.
32. Forastiero RR, Martinuzzo M, Cerrato GS, Kordich LC, Carreras LO. Relationship of anti β_2-glycoprotein I and antiprothrombin antibodies to thrombosis and pregnancy loss in patients with antiphospholipid antibodies. Thromb Haemost 1997;78:1008–1014.
33. Bertolaccini ML, Atsumi T, Amengual O, Khamashta MA, Hughes GRV. Autoantibodies to human prothrombin and clinical manifestations in 207 patients with systemic lupus erythematosus. J Rheumatol 1998;25:1104–1108.
34. Swadzba J, De Clerks LS, Stevens WJ, Bridts CH, van Cotthem KA, Musial J et al. Anticardiolipin, anti-beta(2)-glycoprotein I, antiprothrombin antibodies, and lupus anticoagulant in patients with systemic lupus erythematosus with a history of thrombosis. J Rheum at 1997;24:1710–1715.
35. Guerin J, Smith O, White B, Sweetman G, Feighery C, Jackson J. Antibodies to prothrombin in antiphospholipid syndrome and inflammatory disorders. Br J Haematol 1998;102:896–902.
36. Sorice M, Pittoni V, Circella A, Misasi R, Conti F, Longo A et al. Anti-prothrombin but not "pure" anti-cardiolipin antibodies are associated with the clinical features of the antiphospholipid antibody syndrome. Thromb Haemost 1998;80:713–715.
37. Roubey R. Autoantibodies to phospholipid-binding plasma proteins: a new view of lupus anticoagulant and other "antiphospholipid" antibodies. Blood 1994;84:2854–2867.
38. Arnout J. The pathogenesis of the antiphospholipid syndrome: a hypothesis based on parallelisms with heparin-induced thrombocytopenia. Thromb Haemost 1996;75:536–541.
39. Roubey RAS. Immunology of the antiphospholipid antibody syndrome. Arthritis Rheum 1996;39:1444–1454.

26 Antiphospholipid Antibody-negative Syndrome – Other Phospholipids

R. A. S. Roubey

Introduction

Literally speaking, an antiphospholipid antibody (aPL)-negative antiphospholipid syndrome (APS) is an oxymoron, given that aPL positivity is considered to be a sine qua non of APS. Nonetheless, the term has acquired meaning and refers to patients with clinical manifestations of APS, who are thought to have the syndrome despite negative results in conventional aPL tests (anticardiolipin and lupus anticoagulant assays). There are several possible rationales for including such patients under the rubric of APS. Conceptually, the most important explanation, and the focus of this chapter, is laboratory evidence of autoantibodies thought to be associated with APS, but not detected in conventional aPL assays. These include autoantibodies to certain phospholipid-binding plasma proteins, as well as antibodies detected in immunoassays using phospholipids other than cardiolipin. A second possibility suggested by several reports is that conventional aPL tests may be transiently decreased or negative during an acute episode of thrombosis, presumably due to tissue deposition of circulating antibodies [1, 2]. More trivial explanations include inadequacies in the performance of conventional aPL assays, e.g., use of an insensitive lupus anticoagulant assay, and incomplete use of conventional assays, e.g., failure to test for IgA anticardiolipin antibodies in selected patients.

The existence of aPL-negative APS highlights the unusual relationship of conventional aPL tests to the syndrome. APS is currently defined as the association of certain clinical events, e.g., thrombosis, recurrent fetal loss, with a positive anticardiolipin or lupus anticoagulant assay. Positivity in an aPL test is therefore an essential element of the syndrome, rather than a diagnostic test for the syndrome. There is no independent "gold standard" for APS by which one can assess the diagnostic sensitivity or specificity of aPL tests. Positive aPL assays are probably best thought of as risk factors for the clinical manifestations of APS. An aPL assay should not be considered a "false positive" if the patient does not have a history of thrombosis or another clinical feature of APS. Further, there are no established exclusion criteria for APS. A patient with thrombosis and a positive aPL test would be considered to have APS whether or not other important risk factors for thrombosis were present. In fact, secondary factors may be critical in determining which individuals with aPL will have a thrombotic event or miscarriage.

Autoantibodies Associated with APS

In considering aPL negative APS, it should be keep in mind that conventional anti-cardiolipin enzyme-linked immunosorbent assays (ELISA) and lupus anticoagulant assays were developed based on an inaccurate or incomplete understanding of the specificities of the antibodies detected in these tests. Elucidation of these specificities, and the discovery of additional autoantibodies potentially associated with thrombosis and/or fetal loss, provide the basis for understanding both the limitations of conventional aPL tests and the serological evidence for aPL-negative APS. This process is evolutionary. As more data are collected it is likely that the serological criteria for APS will expand beyond conventional anticardiolipin and lupus anticoagulant assays.

Antibodies Detected in Conventional aPL Assays

Before discussing APS-associated antibodies that may not be detected in conventional aPL assays it is necessary to understand the antibodies that are detected in these tests. The specificities of aPL are reviewed in detail elsewhere in this volume. Briefly, in APS patient sera, the large majority of antibodies detected in anticardiolipin ELISAs recognize epitopes on the phospholipid-binding plasma protein β_2-glycoprotein (β_2GPI), not cardiolipin. β_2GPI in these assays derives from bovine serum, a component of the blocking buffer/sample diluent. Antibodies directed against cardiolipin may also be detected in anticardiolipin assays, but do not appear to be associated with the clinical manifestations of APS. Lupus anticoagulant activity in most APS patient plasmas is due to autoantibodies directed against β_2GPI and/or prothrombin. Although lupus anticoagulant activity is commonly thought of as an intrinsic property of certain antibodies, differences in the various assays used to detect lupus anticoagulants may be critically important in determining whether a given patient sample will exhibit lupus anticoagulant activity in a particular assay. For example, the lupus anticoagulant activity of certain anti-β_2GPI monoclonal antibodies derived from APS patients was found to be dependent on the concentration of β_2GPI in the lupus anticoagulant assay [3]. Certain antibodies may be detected in one type of lupus anticoagulant assay but not another. Galli and colleagues found that the dilute Russell's viper venom time was more sensitive to prolongation by anti-β_2GPI antibodies, whereas, the kaolin clotting time was more sensitive to prolongation by antiprothrombin antibodies [4].

Antibodies Detected in Immunoassays Using Other Anionic Phospholipids

Early in the development of anticardiolipin immunoassays, it was observed that most APS-associated "anticardiolipin" antibodies appeared to be broadly cross-reactive with other anionic phospholipids, e.g., phosphatidylserine, phosphatidylinositol, phosphatidic acid, and phosphatidylglycerol. With the discovery that bovine β_2GPI was the key antigen in anticardiolipin ELISAs, this apparent cross-reactivity is currently best understood in terms of β_2GPI binding similarly to the various anionic phospholipids. Bovine serum is commonly used in the assays with other anionic phospholipids and β_2GPI binds reasonably well to microtiter plates coated with any negatively charged phospholipid [5]. Accordingly, most anti-β_2GPI antibodies can be detected in any of the anionic phospholipids ELISAs. The generally good correlation among ELISAs using different anionic phospholipids has led many investigators to conclude that the anticardiolipin assay, along with lupus anticoagulant testing, are adequate for evaluation of APS. Routine testing of patient samples against panels of other anionic phospholipids is expensive and usually provides little additional clinical information [6, 7].

Although most anticardiolipin-positive APS patient sera react in assays using other anionic phospholipids, anticardiolipin-positive sera from patients with infectious diseases, such as syphilis, do not [8]. These infection-associated antibodies are specific for cardiolipin and do not recognize phosphatidylserine, other anionic phospholipids, or β_2GPI [9]. In light of this observation, it may be argued that ELISAs using phosphatidylserine or one of the other anionic phospholipids would be preferable to the anticardiolipin ELISA in evaluating patient for APS. With nearly 15 years of clinical experience behind it, the justification for the routine use of the anticardiolipin ELISA is in large part historical. Additionally, several international standardization workshops have served to improve the performance and interlaboratory reproducibility of anticardiolipin ELISAs [10–12]. There have not been similar efforts focused on assays using the other anionic phospholipids.

Relevant to aPL-negative APS, there are a number of reports in which sera from patients with clinical features of APS are negative in anticardiolipin ELISAs but positive in one or more assays utilizing other anionic phospholipids. The molecular basis for the this pattern of reactivity and the antigenic specificities of the "non-anticardiolipin" antibodies detected in the other phospholipid ELISAs are both unclear. Like anticardiolipin ELISAs, bovine serum is typically present in these assays. It is not known whether antibodies detected in antiphosphatidylserine, antiphosphatidylinositol, or similar assays are directly binding to phospholipids or to a phospholipid-binding component of bovine or human serum. Detailed studies using highly purified antibodies and antigens, similar to the experiments demonstrating the role of β_2GPI in the anticardiolipin assay, have not been performed. Limited studies using patient sera suggest that at least some antibodies detected in the presence of other phospholipids depend upon the presence of β_2GPI [13–15]. Why such antibodies would not be detectable in standard anticardiolipin assays is not known. The antibodies might be specific for conformational determinants on β_2GPI that are dependent upon the type of phospholipid. Other factors to be considered include differential clustering patterns of β_2GPI on different phospholipids, and differences in phospholipid fatty acid composition and oxidation status which could influence how β_2GPI binds to the phospholipid-coated plate.

In the absence of a positive anticardiolipin or lupus anticoagulant test, an association between positivity in one or more ELISAs utilizing phosphatidylserine, phosphatidylinositol, phosphatidylglycerol, or phosphatidic acid, and the clinical manifestations of APS is not well established [6, 7]. Toschi and colleagues observed that reactivity in non-cardiolipin anionic phospholipid assays was associated with thrombosis and stroke [15, 16]. Interestingly, antibody binding in these assays was β_2GPI dependent. The largest studies evaluating panels of non-cardiolipin anionic phospholipids have been conducted with obstetric patients. Yetman and Kutteh found that 10% of women with recurrent pregnancy loss were negative in the anti-cardiolipin assay but tested positive in another phospholipid assay, including both anionic phospholipids and phosphatidylethanolamine (see below) [17]. Aoki et al. compared a (β_2GPI-dependent) anticardiolipin ELISA with a panel of phospholipid assays in a large group of women with reproductive failure [18]. The anticardiolipin assay was more frequently positive in patients than controls, whereas no difference between patients and controls was observed with any of the other assays alone. Positivity in more than one other assay was more frequent among patients; however, most of these patients were also positive in the anticardiolipin assay.

The performance of ELISAs using anionic phospholipids other than cardiolipin is difficult to assess. As noted above, these assays have not been subjected to rigorous interlaboratory evaluation or national/international standardization efforts. Monospecific reference material for each antiphospholipid assay are not widely available. Accordingly, it is difficult, at best, to make a valid clinical decision based on an isolated positive result in one of these assays.

Antibodies Detected in Immunoassays Using Phosphatidylethanolamine

Antibodies detected in antiphosphatidylethanolamine assays are a different story. Phosphatidylethanolamine is a zwitterionic phospholipid normally present in the outer leaflet of cell membranes. It has recently been shown to play an important role in phospholipid-dependent reactions of the protein C pathway [19] and may be the only autoantibody detectable in a small number of patients with clinical features of the APS [20–22]. Careful studies of the specificity of antiphosphatidylethanolamine antibodies have recently been reported. Most of these antibodies do not bind to phosphatidylethanolamine itself but to a complex of phosphatidylethanolamine and certain proteins present in bovine serum, i.e., high- and low-molecular-weight kininogens (HMWK, LMWK) and/or factor XI and prekallikrein, proteins that bind to HMWK [23–25]; β_2GPI is not involved. Recent data suggest that these antibodies may exert a thrombogenic effect by enhancing thrombin-induced platelet aggregation [25, 26].

Although larger studies to date have not demonstrated the clinical utility of the antiphosphatidylethanolamine ELISA, the case reports and antibody studies cited above support further study and efforts toward standardization. On a research basis it is reasonable to consider antiphosphatidylethanolamine testing in evaluating patients suspected of having APS, who are negative in the standard aPL assays.

Species-specific Autoantibodies to Human β_2GPI

Data accumulated over the past decade indicate that autoantibodies to β_2GPI are among the most important antibodies associated with APS. Conventional anticardiolipin ELISAs and lupus anticoagulant assays detect many anti-β_2GPI antibodies but have some limitations. An important limitation of standard anticardiolipin ELISAs is the species of β_2GPI. As previously mentioned, the predominant species of β_2GPI in anticardiolipin assay is bovine. Whereas, anti-β_2GPI antibodies from most APS patients recognize β_2GPI from many species , some recognize only the human protein. Although a small amount of human β_2GPI is present in anticardiolipin assays (from the diluted serum sample being tested), anticardiolipin assays may miss these antibodies [27, 28]. Species specificity seems to be occur more frequently among IgM anti-β_2GPI antibodies than IgG anti-β_2GPI antibodies. This issue is directly addressed in newly available anti-β_2GPI ELISAs in which the human protein is the antigen. Several groups have reported on the presence of APS clinical manifestations in patients who are positive in the anti-β_2GPI assay but negative in anticardiolipin and/or lupus anticoagulant assays [29–33].

Although the anti-β_2GPI ELISA is not yet accepted as a serological criterion for APS or as a first-line laboratory test, most investigators would consider a patient with anti-β_2GPI antibodies and clinical features of APS to have the syndrome. At present, suspicion of APS in the setting of a negative anticardiolipin assay is a reasonable indication for anti-β_2GPI testing. Inter-laboratory evaluation and standardization efforts for the anti-β_2GPI ELISA are currently in progress.

Autoantibodies to Prothrombin

Autoantibodies directed against prothrombin represent a large proportion of lupus anticoagulant antibodies in patients with APS [34–36]. Immunoassays for the detection of antiprothrombin have recently been developed [36–40]. There are significant methodological differences among the antiprothrombin ELISAs that have been reported and optimal assay conditions have not been established. Despite these differences, the various assays demonstrate that, in certain patients, antiprothrombin antibodies may be present in the absence of a positive lupus anticoagulant assay. This may be due to one or more factors including: (1) use of a lupus anticoagulant assay that is relatively insensitive to the effects of antiprothrombin antibodies; (2) greater analytical sensitivity of immunoassays as compared to coagulation assays (immunoassays may detect lower concentrations of antibody than coagulation reactions); and/or (3) an intrinsic characteristic of certain antiprothrombin antibodies (for example, fine specificity) that may be responsible for lupus anticoagulant activity. The small number of studies to date suggest that lupus anticoagulant positivity is more closely associated with thrombosis and fetal loss than a positive antiprothrombin ELISA [37, 39, 41]. Larger studies and optimization/standardization of antiprothrombin ELISAs are needed to evaluate the association of antiprothrombin antibodies with clinical features of APS and determine whether detection of these antibodies in ELISA constitutes a valid basis for aPL-negative APS.

Autoantibodies to Components of the Protein C Pathway

Inhibition of the anticoagulant protein C pathway has long been considered as a possible mechanism predisposing to thrombosis in patients with APS. Recent data suggest that autoantibodies directed against components of this pathway, protein C, protein S, and thrombomodulin, may be associated with clinical features of APS [42–44]. Such antibodies are probably not detectable in standard anticardiolipin and lupus anticoagulant tests. Additionally, autoantibodies to C4b-binding protein, a complement control protein that regulates free protein S levels and has structural similarity to β_2GPI, have been reported [45]. Studies are being conducted to determine whether ELISAs for antibodies to protein C pathway components are clinically useful in evaluating possible aPL-negative APS.

Other Autoantibodies

Limited data suggest the possible association of a number of other autoantibodies with thrombosis and fetal loss. These include autoantibodies to vascular heparan sulfate proteoglycan [46], annexin V [47], complement factor H [45], and factor XII [48, 49]. Pending further study, such antibodies may be considered as evidence for aPL-negative APS in the future.

Summary

The concept of aPL-negative APS has evolved along with a clearer understanding of the antibodies associated with the clinical features of the syndrome, and a better appreciation of the limitations of standard anticardiolipin and lupus anticoagulant assays. The term originally referred to certain patients who were negative in conventional aPL assays but positive in immunoassays utilizing other phospholipids. At the present time antibodies detected in ELISAs using anionic phospholipids other than cardiolipin are of possible interest; however, evidence for the clinical utility of such assays is weak. Future studies elucidating the specificity of these antibodies and inter-laboratory efforts toward assay standardization are needed. Antibodies detected in antiphosphatidylethanolamine assays have been found to be directed against phosphatidylethanolamine-bound kininogens and kininogen-binding proteins. These antibodies may be associated with clinical features of APS and may directly contribute to a prothrombotic state. Lastly, protein-based immunoassays will likely become the most common basis for use of the term aPL-negative APS, and may eventually lead to revisions in the serological criteria for APS.

References

1. Alarcón-Segovia D, Deleze M, Oria CV et al. Antiphospholipid antibodies and the antiphospholipid syndrome in systemic lupus erythematosus. A prospective analysis of 500 consecutive patients. Medicine (Baltimore) 1989;68:353–365.
2. Drenkard C, Sanchez-Guerrero J, Alarcón-Segovia D. Fall in antiphospholipid antibody at time of thromboocclusive episodes in systemic lupus erythematosus. J Rheumatol 1989;16:614.
3. Takeya H, Mori T, Gabazza EC, et al. Anti-β_2-glycoprotein I (β_2GPI) monoclonal antibodies with lupus anticoagulant-like activity enhance the β_2GPI binding to phospholipids. J Clin Invest 1997;99:2260–2268.
4. Galli M, Finazzi G, Bevers EM, Barbui T. Kaolin clotting time and dilute Russell's viper venom time distinguish between prothrombin-dependent and β_2-glycoprotein I-dependent antiphospholipid antibodies. Blood 1995;86:617–623.
5. Jones JV, James H, Mansour M, Eastwood BJ. β_2-glycoprotein I is a cofactor for antibodies reacting with 5 anionic phospholipids. J Rheumatol 1995;22:2009

6. Bertolaccini ML, Roch B, Amengual O, Atsumi T, Khamashta MA, Hughes GR. Multiple antiphospholipid tests do not increase the diagnostic yield in antiphospholipid syndrome. Br J Rheumatol 1998;37:1229–1232.

7. Branch DW, Silver R, Pierangeli S, Harris EN. Antiphospholipid antibodies other than lupus anticoagulant and anticardiolipin antibodies in women with recurrent pregnancy loss, fertile controls, and antiphospholipid syndrome. Obstet Gynecol 1997;89:549–555.

8. Pierangeli SS, Goldsmith GH, Krnic S, Harris EN. Differences in functional activity of anticardiolipin antibodies from patients with syphilis and those with the antiphospholipid syndrome. Infect Immun 1994;62:4081–4084.

9. McNally T, Purdy G, Mackie IJ, Machin SJ, Isenberg DA. The use of an anti-β_2-glycoprotein-I assay for discrimination between anticardiolipin antibodies associated with infection and increased risk of thrombosis. Br J Haematol 1995;91:471–473.

10. Harris EN, Gharavi AE, Patel SP, Hughes GRV. Evaluation of the anti-cardiolipin test: report of an international workshop held 4 April 1986. Clin Exp Immunol 1987;68:215–222.

11. Harris EN. Special report. The Second International Anti-cardiolipin Standardization Workshop/the Kingston Anti-Phospholipid Antibody Study (KAPS) group. Am J Clin Pathol 1990;94:476–484.

12. Harris EN, Pierangeli S, Birch D. Anticardiolipin wet workshop report. Fifth international symposium on antiphospholipid antibodies. Am J Clin Pathol 1994;101:616–624.

13. Matsuda J, Saitoh N, Gotoh M, Gohchi K, Tsukamoto M. Prevalence of β_2-glycoprotein I antibody in systemic lupus erythematosus patients with β_2-glycoprotein I dependent antiphospholipid antibodies. Ann Rheum Dis 1995;54:73–75.

14. Matsuda J, Saitoh N, Gohchi K, Gotoh M, Tsukamoto M. Detection of beta-2-glycoprotein-I-dependent antiphospholipid antibodies and anti-beta-2-glycoprotein-I antibody in patients with systemic lupus erythematosus and in patients with syphilis. Int Arch Allergy Immunol 1994;103:239–244.

15. Toschi V, Motta A, Castelli C, Paracchini ML, Zerbi D, Gibelli A. High prevalence of antiphosphatidylinositol antibodies in young patients with cerebral ischemia of undetermined cause. Stroke 1998;29:1759–1764.

16. Toschi V, Motta A, Castelli C et al. Prevalence and clinical significance of antiphospholipid antibodies to noncardiolipin antigens in systemic lupus erythematosus. Haemostasis 1993;23:275–283.

17. Yetman DL, Kutteh WH. Antiphospholipid antibody panels and recurrent pregnancy loss: prevalence of anticardiolipin antibodies compared with other antiphospholipid antibodies. Fertil Steril 1996;66:540–546.

18. Aoki K, Dudkiewicz AB, Matsuura E, Novotny M, Kaberlain G, Gleicher N. Clinical significance of β_2-glycoprotein I-dependent anticardiolipin antibodies in the reproductive autoimmune failure syndrome: correlation with conventional antiphospholipid antibody detection systems. Am J Obstet Gynecol 1995;172:926–931.

19. Smirnov MD, Esmon CT. Phosphatidylethanolamine incorporation into vesicles selectively enhances factor Va inactivation by activated protein C. J Biol Chem 1994;269:816–819.

20. Karmochkine M, Cacoub P, Piette JC, Godeau P, Boffa MC. Antiphosphatidylethanolamine antibody as the sole antiphospholipid antibody in systemic lupus erythematosus with thrombosis. Clin Exp Rheumatol 1992;10:603–605.

21. Karmochkine M, Berard M, Piette JC et al. Antiphosphatidylethanolamine antibodies in systemic lupus erythematosus. Lupus 1993;2:157–160.

22. Berard M, Chantome R, Marcelli A, Boffa MC. Antiphosphatidylethanolamine antibodies as the only antiphospholipid antibodies. I. Association with thrombosis and vascular cutaneous diseases. J Rheumatol 1996;23:1369–1374.

23. Sugi T, McIntyre JA. Autoantibodies to phosphatidylethanolamine (PE) recognize a kininogen–PE complex. Blood 1995;86:3083–3089.

24. Boffa MC, Berard M, Sugi T, McIntyre JA. Antiphosphatidylethanolamine antibodies as the only antiphospholipid antibodies detected by ELISA. II. Kininogen reactivity. J Rheumatol 1996;23:1375–1379.

25. Sugi T, McIntyre JA. Phosphatidylethanolamine induces specific conformational changes in the kininogens recognizable by antiphosphatidylethanolamine antibodies. Thromb Haemost 1996;76:354–360.

26. Sugi T, McIntyre JA. Autoantibodies to kininogen-phosphatidylethanolamine complexes augment thrombin-induced platelet aggregation. Thromb Res 1996;84:97–109.

27. Arvieux J, Darnige L, Hachulla E, Roussel B, Bensa JC, Colomb MG. Species specificity of anti-β_2-glycoprotein I autoantibodies and its relevance to anticardiolipin antibody quantitation. Thromb Haemost 1996;75:725–730.

28. Arvieux J, Regnault V, Hachulla E, Darnige L, Roussel B, Bensa JC. Heterogeneity and immunochemical properties of anti-β_2-glycoprotein I autoantibodies. Thromb Haemost 1999;80:393–398.

29. Roubey RAS, Maldonado MA, Byrd SN. Comparison of an enzyme-linked immunosorbent assay for antibodies to β_2-glycoprotein I and a conventional anticardiolipin ELISA. Arthritis Rheum 1996;39:1606–1607.

30. Cabiedes J, Cabral AR, Alarcón-Segovia D. Clinical manifestations of the antiphospholipid syndrome in patients with systemic lupus erythematosus associate more strongly with anti-β_2-glycoprotein-I than with antiphospholipid antibodies. J Rheumatol 1995;22:1899–1906.

31. Cabral AR, Cabiedes J, Alarcón-Segovia D. Antibodies to phospholipid-free β_2-glycoprotein-I in patients with the primary antiphospholipid syndrome. J Rheumatol 1995;22:1894–1898.

32. Balestrieri G, Tincani A, Spatola L et al. Anti-beta$_2$-glycoprotein I antibodies: a marker of antiphospholipid syndrome? Lupus 1995;4:122–130.

33. Martinuzzo ME, Forastiero RR, Carreras LO. Anti-β_2-glycoprotein I antibodies: detection and association with thrombosis. Br J Haematol 1995;89:397–402.

34. Bevers EM, Galli M, Barbui T, Comfurius P, Zwaal RFA. Lupus anticoagulant IgGs (LA) are not directed to phospholipids only, but to a complex of lipid-bound human prothrombin. Thromb Haemost 1991;66:629–632.

35. Permpikul P, Rao LVM, Rapaport SI. Functional and binding studies of the roles of prothrombin and b$_2$-glycoprotein I in the expression of lupus anticoagulant activity. Blood 1994;83:2878–2892.

36. Arvieux J, Darnige L, Caron C, Reber G, Bensa JC, Colomb MG. Development of an ELISA for autoantibodies to prothrombin showing their prevalence in patients with lupus anticoagulants. Thromb Haemost 1995;74:1120–1125.

37. Forastiero RR, Martinuzzo ME, Cerrato GS, Kordich LC, Carreras LO. Relationship of anti β_2-glycoprotein I and anti prothrombin antibodies to thrombosis and pregnancy loss in patients with antiphospholipid antibodies. Thromb Haemost 1997;78:1008–1014.

38. Galli M, Beretta G, Daldossi M, Bevers EM, Barbui T. Different anticoagulant and immunological properties of anti-prothrombin antibodies in patients with antiphospholipid antibodies. Thromb Haemost 1997;77:486–491.

39. Horbach DA, van Oort E, Derksen RH, De Groot PG. The contribution of anti-prothrombin-antibodies to lupus anticoagulant activity – discrimination between functional and non-functional anti-prothrombin-antibodies. Thromb Haemost 1998;79:790–795.

40. Swadzba J, De Clerck LS, Stevens WJ et al. Anticardiolipin, anti-β_2-glycoprotein I, antiprothrombin antibodies, and lupus anticoagulant in patients with systemic lupus erythematosus with a history of thrombosis. J Rheumatol 1997;24:1710–1715.

41. Horbach DA, Oort EV, Donders RCJM, Derksen RHWM, De Groot PG. Lupus anticoagulant in the strongest risk factor for both venous and arterial thrombosis in patients with systemic lupus erythematosus: comparison between different assays for the detection of antiphospholipid antibodies. Thromb Haemost 1996;76:916–924.

42. Oosting JD, Derksen RHWM, Bobbink IWG, Hackeng TM, Bouma BN, De Groot PG. Antiphospholipid antibodies directed against a combination of phospholipids with prothrombin, protein C, or protein S: an explanation for their pathogenic mechanism? Blood 1993;81:2618–2625.

43. Pengo V, Biasiolo A, Brocco T, Tonetto S, Ruffatti A. Autoantibodies to phospholipid-binding plasma proteins in patients with thrombosis and phospholipid-reactive antibodies. Thromb Haemost 1996;75:721–724.

44. Carson CW, Comp PC, Esmon NL, Rezaie AR, Esmon CT. Thrombomodulin antibodies inhibit protein C activation and are found in patients with lupus anticoagulant and unexplained thrombosis. Arthritis Rheum 1994;37:S296 (abstract).

45. Guerin J, Sim RB, Feighery C, Jackson J. Antibody recognition of complement regulatory proteins, factor H, CR1 and C4BP in antiphospholipid syndrome patients. Lupus 1998;7:S180 (abstract).

46. Shibata S, Sasaki T, Harpel P, Fillit H. Autoantibodies to vascular heparan sulfate proteoglycan in systemic lupus erythematosus react with endothelial cells and inhibit the formation of thrombin-antithrombin III complexes. Clin Immunol Immunopathol 1994;70:114–123.

47. Matsuda J, Saitoh N, Gohchi K, Gotoh M, Tsukamoto M. Anti-annexin V antibody in systemic lupus erythematosus patients with lupus anticoagulant and/or anticardiolipin antibody. Am J Hematol 1994;47:56–58.

48. A[o]berg H, Nilsson IM. Recurrent thrombosis in a young woman with a circulating anticoagulant directed against factors XI and XII. Acta Med Scand 1972;192:419–425.

49. Jones DW, Gallimore MJ, Harris SL, Winter M. Antibodies to factor XII associated with lupus anticoagulant. Thromb Haemost 1999;81:387–390.

Section 3

Basic Aspects of Antiphospholipid Syndrome

27 Vascular Pathology of the Antiphospholipid Antibody Syndrome

G. A. McCarty

Introduction

The antiphospholipid antibody syndrome (APS) is characterized by vasculopathy, a term often equated with thrombotic microangiopathy (TMA) but unfortunately used interchangeably with vasculitis, where inflammatory cells are present throughout the vessel wall, or perivasculitis, where the infiltrate is adventitial but the vessel wall is intact [1–6]. The identification of a TMA is dependent on many factors: (a) time course from symptomaticity to biopsy; (b) action of naturally occurring anticoagulants; or (c) time course of institution of antithrombotic treatments. TMA may involve changes on the intraluminal side, through the vessel wall, and into the adventitia. At the light-microscopic level, this spectrum involves endothelial cell swelling, thrombosis that is usually bland, but occasionally associated with a reactive cellular infiltrate as part of neoangiogenesis and recanalization, fibrin and/or platelet deposition in the vessel wall, proliferation of myointimal cells with attendant luminal decrease, medial thickening and hyalinization usually with preservation of the internal elastic lamina, and in certain instances, vasculitis or perivasculitis [3, 4–6, 7–14]. Limited electron microscopic studies have in some vessels identified indistinct electron-dense deposits in subendothelial areas that have not yet been fully characterized as representative of antiphospholipid antibodies (aPL) but have been identified as immunoglobulin [1–6]. The eminent vascular pathologist, the late J. T. Lie has eloquently stated that some of the confusion in the APS literature is attributable to (a) poor differentiation of perivasculitis versus panvasculitis, (b) misinterpretation of positive fluorescent antibody (FA) studies for immunoglobulins and complement components as definitive of an immune complex vasculitis, (c) occurrence of coexisting vasculitis in secondary APS, most often in systemic lupus erythematosus (SLE), and (d) anatomic differences between arteries and veins versus capillaries, with their lack of limiting vascular smooth muscle cells and attendant inflammatory cell extravasation or spillage beyond capillary network without identifiable capillary necrosis; our previous studies would also support his contentions [1–3]. Vascular pathology and clinicoserologic correlations in 17 patients with primary (1°) and secondary (2°) syndromes are presented in this chapter relative to the current spectra of APS involvement in the literature, which has expanded to include different combinations of vascular damage including calciphylaxis, and a prospectus is offered regarding processes of endothelial cell-platelet interactions in inflammation, injury, and repair that might help to explain the wide spectrum of vasculopathy in APS.

Methods

Biopsy, surgical, or autopsy specimens were obtained from patients seen in academic and consultative practice. The diagnoses of 1° or 2° APS were made by modified Harris and American College of Rheumatology (ACR) criteria, longitudinal aPL enzyme immunoassays (EIAs) done on at least two occasions 4–6 weeks apart for IgG/M anticardiolipin (aCL), IgG/M antiphosphatidylserine (aPS) performed in a laboratory certified by the aPL Standardization Laboratory of E. Nigel Harris, simultaneous lupus anticoagulant (LA) profile by activated partial thromboplastin time (aPTT) and dilute Russell's viper venom time (DRVVT) performed according to the Standardization Committee's recommendations, and/or a standardized IgG/M/A EIA for aCL, aPS, and antiphosphatidylethanolamine (aPE) [15–17]. Epidemiologic, clinical criteria for the diagnosis of 1° or 2° APS, serologic or coagulation-based tests, and major categories of vascular pathologic involvement with cross reference to photomicrographs comprise Table 27.1. Eleven of the 17 patients had 1° APS, the remaining six had 2° APS due primarily to SLE. Eleven were white females (age range 5 days–67 years); three were white males (age range 23–45 years) and three were black females (age range 28–50 years). Hematoxylin and eosin (H&E) stains were used except where specified: Vierhoeff van Gieson (VVG) for collagen and elastic tissue; Masson's trichrome for elastic tissue (fibrin red to blue-gray); Mallory's phosphotungstic acid hematoxylin (PTAH) for fibrin (purple); modified Giemsa (MG) for cells and bacteria (blue); and glial fibrillary acidic protein (GFAP) immunoperoxidase (brown); in selected skin or renal biopsies, routine FA techniques for immunoglobulins G, M, A, and complement components C3 or C4 [4–6]. A comprehensive Medline literature review was performed cross-referencing APS, aPL, lupus coagulation inhibitor, and vascular pathology categories; all manuscripts available were reviewed for APS diagnostic criteria, EIA and coagulation-based aPL tests, description and photomicrography for review of major components of APS pathology (TMA, endothelial cell swelling/fibrin deposition, perivasculitis, vasculitis, or necrosis). In some instances FA studies for immunoglobulin and/or complement deposition were available. Tables 27.2–27.6 summarize these major pathologic findings grouped by vessel site, APS classification, major pathologic findings, aPL and LA results, and the references from the literature arranged chronologically. Fifty-four original color slides from 17 patients were analyzed, and digitally scanned to make composite Figs 27.1–27.9.

Characteristic Macrovascular Pathologic Findings in APS

The hallmark lesion suggesting APS in all its forms is livedo reticularis, which can be evanescent, intermittent, or sustained, often overlooked by physicians in recorded physical examinations, yet patients and family members often describe its presence as mottling, blotching, or "giraffe skin", and clearly identify it when presented with photographs. Fig. 27.1 shows in 1° APS patients classic distributions

Table 27.1. Clinical, serologic, and pathologic findings in 17 APS patients.

PT.	1°	2°	aPL	LA	RT	RFL	TMA	EC/Fi	PV	FA	Other	Fig.
1–19 years old WF	+		CL, PE	+	CVA REN	+	+	+	+	IgG, C3	LR	27.1a, 27.7a, c
2–23 years old WM	+		CL		PTE REN DVT PVD	n.a.	+	+	–	–	LR	27.1b, 27.7e, 27.6a, b, c, f, 27.8e, 27.9e
3–67 years old WF	+		CL, PS, PE	+	VOD PTE DVT	+	+	+	–	–	Skin Ulcer	27.1c 27.3d
4–44 years old WF	+		PS, PE	+	VOD DVT SKIN	n.a.	+	+	–	–	Skin Ulcer Pap	27.1d 27.2d
5–45 years old WM	+		C		VOD	n.a.	+	+	–	–	Dig. Inf.	27.1e
6–53 years old WM	+		PE	+	VOD DVT SKIN	n.a.	+	+	+	–	LR, Skin Ulcer	27.1f, 27.2c, 27.3a
7–28 years old BF		+	CL	–	SKIN DVT	+	+	+	+	IgG C3	Skin Nod.	27.2a
8–44 years old WF	+		PE	–	SKIN VOD	–	+	+	+	IgG	Bulla. Calci.	27.2b, e 27.4a–f
9–38 years old WF		+	PS, PE	+	PUL HEM DVT CVA	+	+	+	–	+	Skin ulcer	27.2f, 27.6e
10–53 years old WF	+		PE	+	SKIN DVT	+	+	+	+	–	Skin Nod. Gran.	27.3b, e
11-38 years old WF		+	CL, PS	+	CVA TCP SKIN	+	+	+	–	–	Skin ulcer, Calci.	27.3 c, f
12–50 years old BF		+	CL, PS	–	CVA AIHA REN	+	+	+	–	IgG C3	LR	27.7b, 27.8b, 27.9a, c, d, f
13–33 years old WF		+	CL	+	CVA TCP REN	+	+	–	–	IgG C3	GI Inf.	27.7d 27.8a, d 27.9b
14–29 years old BF		+	CL, PE	+	SKIN REN	+	+	+	–	IgG C3	LR	27.7f
15–29 years old WF	+		PE	–	PUL. HEM AIHA TCP	+	+	+	–	–	Capill	27.6d

Table 27.1. *continued.*

PT.	1°	2°	aPL	LA	RT	RFL	TMA	EC/Fi	PV	FA	Other	Fig.
16–5 days old WF	+		PS, PE	–	CVA VOD AMI	+	+	+	–	–	Mat. 1°, Heart Tx	27.5a–f
17–5 days old WF	+		CL, PE	+	VOD TCP	+	+	+	–	–	Mat. 1°, Dig. Inf.	27.8c, f

W = white, B = black, F = female, M = male.
1° = primary APS, 2° = secondary APS
aPL = antiphospholipid antibody specificity; CL = cardiolipin; PS = phosphatidylserine; PE = phosphatidylethanolamine; LA = lupus anticoagulant (activated partial thromboplastin time, aPTT), and dilute Russell viper venom time (DRVVT); RT = recurrent thromboses; CVA = cerebrovascular accident; PTE = pulmonary thromboembolism; REN = renal thrombotic microangiopathy; DVT = deep venous thromboses; PVD = peripheral venous disease; VOD = vaso-occlusive disease, non-atherosclerotic, large vessels; SKIN = skin infarction/nodule/ulcer/papule; PUL HEM = pulmonary hemorrhage; TCP = thrombocytopenia; AIHA = autoimmune hemolytic anemia; AMI = acute myocardial infarction; LR = livedo reticularis; Heart tx = heart transplant; RFL = recurrent fetal loss; TMA = thrombotic microangiopathy; EC/Fi = endothelial cell hyperplasia/fibrin or fibrin thrombi; PV = perivasculitis, lymphocytic (where specified); FA = fluorescent antibody studies (skin vessels or glomeruli); Dig. Inf. = digital infarction; Bulla. = bullous skin disease; Calci. = calciphylaxis; Gran. = granuloma (three or greater nuclei per giant cell); GI Inf. = gastrointestinal infarction; Capill = capillaritis; Lymph-lymphocytic; MΦ = monocytic/macrophagic; Mat. 1° = Maternal primary APS; n.a. = not applicable.

Table 27.2. Cutaneous vascular pathology.

1° APS	2° APS	TMA	EC/Fi	PV	VASC	NEC	aPL	LA+	Ref.
	+	+						+	14
+		+				+		+	18
+		+				+		+	20
	+ (HIV)					+	+	–	21
+						+			22
	+ (RA)								23
+		+		+ Lymph	+ Lymphs	+	+		12
	+ (RA)				+ Nodule	+			24
+	+	+	+	+ MΦ			+		25
+ ×5	+ ×3	+	+		+ ×1 LCV		+ ×3	+ ×5	27
+		+	+				+β2gp		28
	+	+				+	+		29
	+		+				+		30
+		+					+	+	31
	+	+				Calci.		+	32
+		+					+		33
	+					+	+		34
+		+	+	+			CL, PE	+	Patient 1
+		+	+			+	CL		Patient 2
+		+	+			+	CL, PS	+	Patient 3
+		+	+			+	PS, PE	+	Patient 4
+		+					CL		Patient 5
+		+	+		+ Lymphs	+	PE	+	Patient 6
	+		+			+	CL		Patient 7
+		+	+	+ Pannic.			CL		Patient 8
+		+	+	+	+	Calci.	PE		Patient 9
	+	+	+			Calci.	PS, PE	+	Patient 10
+		+	+	+ Lymphs		Gran.	PE		Patient 11

Table 27.3. Cardiovascular pathology.

1° APS	2° APS	TMA	EC/Fi	PV	VASC	NEC	aPL	LA+	Ref.
+			+				+		11
	+	+	+	+ MΦ			+		12
+		+	+				CL		35
+		+	+				+		36
	+		+				+		37
+		+	+				CL	+	38
+ ×6		+ ×1	+ ×5				CL		39
+ ×8		+	+ ×13	+ MΦ			CL, PS		40
	+	+	+				+		41
+			+				+		42
+		+	+	+	+	Calci	PS		Patient 8
+		+	+			+	PS, PE		Patient 16

Table 27.4. Pulmonary vascular pathology.

1° APS	2° APS	TMA	EC/Fi	PV	VASC	NEC	aPL	LA+	Ref.
	+	Capill.	+				CL	+	43
	+	+					+		44
	+	+	+				+		45
+		+	+			+	CL		Patient 2
+		+	+	+ Pann.			CL		Patient 8
+		+	+	+	+	Calci.	PE		Patient 9
+		Capill.	+				PE		Patient 15

Table 27.5. Renovascular pathology.

1° APS	2° APS	TMA	EC/Fi	PV	VASC	NEC	aPL	LA+	Ref.
	+ ×3	+					+		46
	+	+						+	47
+ ×5	+ ×5	+	+	+			CL ×4	+ ×3	48, 49
+		+	+				CL		50
+ ×1	+ ×5				+		CI ×3		51
+		+	+				CL		35
+ ×5			+				CL ×4	+ ×5	52
	+ ×4	+	+	+	+		+		53
+ ×5		+	+				CL ×4	+ ×1	54
+		+	+				CL		55
	+ ×3	+	+				CL		56
+		+	+		+	+	CL		57
	+ ×14	+	+				CL ×13		58
	+ ×8	+					CL ×3	+ ×5	59
	+	+	+	+			CL, PS		Patient 1
+		+	+			+	CL		Patient 2
	+		+			+	CL		Patient 7
	+	+	+				CL, PS		Patient 12
	+	+					CL		Patient 13
	+	+	+				CL, PE	+	Patient 14

Table 27.6. Cerebrovascular and musculovascular pathology.

1° APS	2° APS	TMA	EC/Fi	PV	VASC	NEC	aPL	LA+	Ref.
+		+	+				+		13
+	+	+	+	+ MΦ			+		25
	+	+	+				+		41
+		+	+				CL		62
	+	+	+						63
	+	+	+		+		+		64
+		+	+	+			CL, PE	+	Patient 1
+		+	+			+	CL		Patient 2
	+	+	+				CL, PS		Patient 12
	+	+	+				CL	+	Patient 13
+		+	+			+	CL, PE	+	Patient 17

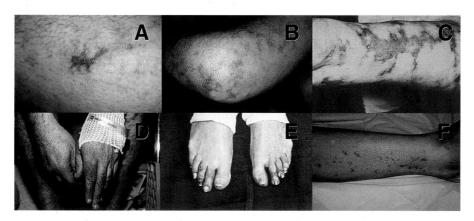

Figure 27.1. Macrovascular cutaneous pathology. **a** Livedo, thigh, Patient 1; **b** livedo, elbow, Patient 2; **c** livedo and necrosis, arm, Patient 3; **d** erythematous papules, livedo, healing ulcerations, hands, and peripheral venous thromboses, legs, Patient 4; **e** livedo and digital infarctions, Patient 5; **f** pyodermatous necrotic papules with infarction and thrombocytopenic bruising, leg, Patient 6. (G. A. McCarty Indiana University APS Database, IUMC Photography Department, and Matrix Digital Photography, Inc., Indianapolis IN.)

over the thigh (a), elbow (b), or accompanied by cutaneous necrosis (b) in Patients 1–3. Livedo and digital infarctions as seen in Patient 5 (e) are a highly specific combination for APS. That pyodermatous necrotic papules, and nodules of varying sizes also occur is increasingly recognized, as exemplified by Patient 6 (f), with bruising due to concomitant severe thrombocytopenia [18, 19].

Cutaneous Vascular Pathology

At the microvascular level, the first major detailed cutaneous pathologic studies were H&E micrographs showing TMA from patients with 2° APS with LA in the setting of SLE, and subsequently in two patients with 1° APS [14, 18, 20]. Next to TMA, which was noted in all these patients in some vessels, endothelial cell changes including variable hypertrophy, positive staining for fibrin in vessel walls, and varying degrees of intraluminal occlusion due to fibrin thrombi were the most commonly noted entities (Patient 3 (Fig. 27.3d), Patients 6, 11 (Fig 27.3a, c); Figs 27.2, 27.3; Patient 8, Fig. 27.4a, d). Because of the short duration of these skin lesions from time of onset to biopsy, necrosis, fibrin staining, perivasculitis, and TMA were noted in many patients, rather than the endothelial cell fibrointimal "cushion" lesions that likely represent a combination of initial vascular injury and response to thrombosis, with reparative attempts at recanalization, and are of myointimal cell origin [1–6]. Since the first case of true vasculitis coexistent in a patient with SLE, APS, and multiple specificity aPLs, other secondary cases have been identified; however, Patient 6 with 1°APS (Figs 27.2c and 27.3a) had a distinctive lymphocytic vascular infiltrate with obliteration in a skin vessel not located underneath a skin ulcer, where this finding could occur due to an infection rather than a true vasculitis [12, 24, 27]. Patients 7 and 8 (Fig. 27.2a, b) had nodular skin infiltrates mimicking a panniculitis. Skin necrosis and ulcerations occur in all forms of APS with usual serologies by Harris criteria [21, 22–24, 27, 29–31, 34]; Patients 3, 4, and 7 (Figs 27.1d, 27.3d, 27.2d, and Fig. 27.2a, respectively) had antibodies to negative phospholipids, while Patients 4 and 6 (Fig. 27.2c and Fig. 27.3a) notably had antibodies to phosphatidylethanolamine (PE). Widespread cutaneous necrosis is now recognized as a reason to prompt an APS workup. Calciphylaxis was noted in a patient with 2° APS and LA with uremia; two patients with 1° APS (Patients 9 (Fig. 27.2f), 11 (Fig. 27.3c) and one with 2° APS (Patient 10, Fig. 27.3b, f) exhibited this finding [32, 34]. The first known report of a giant cell response in a central vessel was a novel finding in Patient 10 (Fig. 27.3e),

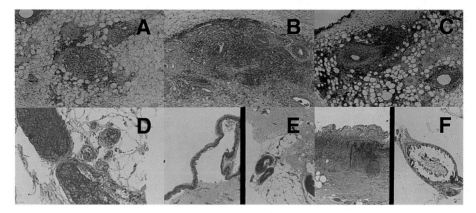

Figure 27.2. Cutaneous vascular pathology. **a** Lymphocytic nodular panniculitis (center), perivasculitis, upper left; lymphocytic perivasculitis with panvasculitis through small vessel wall, upper right, Patient 7; **b** lymphocytic epidermal and subdermal infiltrate (center and right); fibrin thrombi and early perivasculitis, left lower vessel; panvasculitis with red cells in lumen, right central vessel, and two normal vessels, above, right, Patient 8; **c** lymphocytic perivasculitis and panvasculitis with normal lumen, left; mild perivasculitis with early fibrinoid change, right, Patient 6; **d** fibrin thrombi in multiple vessels with varying degrees of luminal occlusion, Patient 4; **e** bullous changes, left, fibrin thrombi and fibrinoid vessel changes, right, Patient 8; **f** pyodermatous skin ulcer above fibrin thrombi in several vessels, left, and bullous changes with early calciphylaxis. Patient 9 (courtesy of Dr. Antoinette Hood). (G. A. McCarty, Indiana University APS Database, IUMC Photography Department, and Matrix Digital Photography, Inc., Indianapolis IN.)

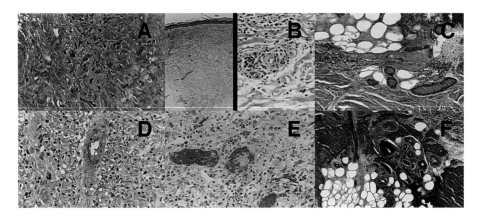

Figure 27.3. Cutaneous vascular pathology. **a** vascular occlusion and obliteration of vascular markings, deep dermis, Patient 6; **b** lymphocytic dermal infiltrate (left), small vessel perivasculitis and panvasculitis, right, Patient 10; **c** multiple fibrin thrombi in deep dermal vessels, Patient 11; **d** fibrin in dermal vessel wall, Patient 3 (courtesy of Dr. Antoinette Hood), Patient; **e** multiple fibrin thrombi and single area of giant cell formation in central vessel (>3 nuclei), Patient 10, (courtesy of Dr. William Caro); **f** multiple fibrin thrombi in deep dermal vessels with hemorrhage, fibrin thrombi, and several vessels with calciphylaxis, Patient 11. (G. A. McCarty, Indiana University APS Database, IUMC Photography Department, and Matrix Digital Photography, Inc., Indianapolis IN.)

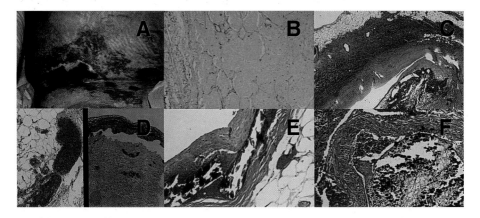

Figure 27.4. Skin, pulmonary, and coronary vascular pathology in catastrophic APS, Patient 8. **a** Skin necrosis, superficial thromboses, and coalescent livedo; **b** pulmonary arteriolar vessels with fibrin and red cells, extensive alveolar hemorrhage (WG); **c** skin arteriole with obliterated vessel markings, adherent old calcified thrombus, and mild subdermal lymphocytic infiltrate; **d** fibrin thrombi in multiple dermal vessels, subcutaneous edema (left), and superficial bulla above thrombosed vessels, right; **e** coronary vein with adherent old thrombi with calciphylaxis; **f** pulmonary arteriolar thrombi with calcified old thrombi and calciphylaxis eroding thru vessel wall (lower left) causing fatal exsanguination (courtesy of Dr. Darrell Davidson). (G. A. McCarty, Indiana University APS Database, IUMC Photography Department, and Matrix Digital Photography, Inc., Indianapolis IN.)

who presented with lower extremity nodules suggestive of a panniculitis but with no obvious drug or infectious etiology. Patient 8 with 1° APS had both classic livedo with coalescence, and skin necrosis, bullous lesions, and obliterated vessel markings (Figs 27.2b, e and 27.4a, c) in the setting of only antibodies to PE, and an overwhelming catastrophic syndrome with severe calciphylaxis. Patient 9 with 2° APS due to SLE presented with necrotic skin ulcers, calciphylaxis, and bullous lesions in the setting of pulmonary hemorrhage, and had antibodies to PE and phosphatidylserine (PS) (Figs 27.2f and 27.6e). Thus, a growing panoply of cutaneous microvascular lesions comprise APS with varying macrovascular presentations.

Cardiovascular Pathology

Major advances in understanding of the vasculopathy of APS were made when the first peripheral vascular photomicrographs of a femoral and an anterior tibial artery were published in two patients with classic positive serologies, although the interpretation at the time was controversial [reviewed in 1–6; 11, 12]. The concept of intimal hyperplastic change in the femoral artery versus simple adherent thrombosis was exemplified by this first report, with a mild focal acute inflammatory infiltrate, whereas a mononuclear vasculitis was demonstrable in the tibial artery [1–3, 11, 12]. In subsequent cases of peripheral vessels, TMA in varying degrees is noted, along with endothelial cell changes and fibrin staining most commonly [11, 12, 35, 37, 38]. Table 27.3 presents comparative data; most cases are valvulopathies occurring in both 1° and 2° APS, with antibodies to classical aPLs, most commonly CL, but also LA and PS [36–42]. In one case, a mononuclear/macrophage cellular infiltrate was noted on the valve, and in another case, calciphylaxis [39, 40]. Platelet-fibrin surface deposition as sources of peripheral emboli, valvulitis with scarring and hypertrophy, and in rare instances calcific changes, are noted. Patient 8 had significant coronary vein thromboses with adherent thrombi and calciphylactic changes at postmortem examination, and calciphylaxis was also noted segmentally in several heart valves (Fig. 27.4e), her death was caused by erosion of a calcified thrombus and calciphylaxis in a pulmonary arteriole causing a fatal exsanguination despite being intubated on an intensive care unit; this patient made antibodies to only PE. Patient 16 was born with significant global livedo reticularis, thrombocytopenia, neonatal small vessel cerebrovascular infarcts in three territories, destruction of several heart valves with APS-related valvulopathy, and underwent open-heart surgery at age 3 days for valvuloplasty complicated by an intraoperative myocardial infarction. Despite the maternal history of prior infertility, thrombocytopenia for the third trimester, and a DVT just prior to labor, maternal APS was not diagnosed prior to birth. Antibodies to PE were defined in both mother and infant when she was 3 days old. At 15 days, a successful heart transplantation was performed, and she remains alive to date; three female family members have APS, and two who have been examined serologically have only antibodies to PE. Figure 27.5(a, b) shows her heart with intramyocardial hemorrhage and infarction, and a minimal polymorphonuclear perivascular infiltrate in the area of the acute myocardial infarction. Figure 27.5(c, d) documents TMA in the infarcted left anterior descending coronary, and necrotic branches with TMA in smaller distal vessels: epicardial vessels with TMA over the area of the acute myocardial infarction are seen in Fig. 27.5f. Figure 27.5e shows the aortic valve with classic fibrin thrombi, valvulitis and early calcification.

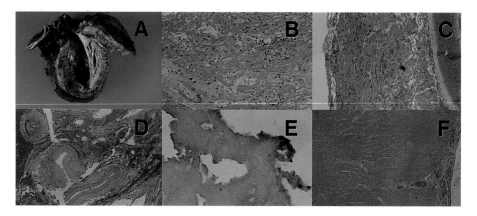

Figure 27.5. Cardiovascular pathology in neonatal APS requiring cardiac transplantation, Patient 16. **a** Left ventricle hypertrophy with visible intramyocardial hemorrhage and infarction; **b** intramyocardial small vessel with minimal polymorphonuclear perivascular infiltrate and dense infiltrate in area of early necrosis and hemorrhage; **c** left anterior descending coronary artery with thrombotic microangiopathy and transmural myocardial infarction; **d** necrotic left anterior descending coronary artery and circumflex branch with thrombotic microangiopathy in small branches; **e** Aortic valve with fibrin thrombi, valvulitis, and early calcification; **f** epicardial surface vessels with thrombotic microangiopathy above transmural myocardial infarction (courtesy of Dr. Mary M. Davis). (G. A. McCarty, Indiana University APS Database, IUMC Photography Department, and Matrix Digital Photography, Inc., Indianapolis IN.)

Pulmonary Vascular Pathology

Arterial and venous TMA occurs in the lungs of patients with APS, as well as capillaritis and pulmonary alveolar hemorrhage, but these latter entities are often go undiagnosed or are attributed to pneumonitis of infectious etiologies, and occur in both adult and pediatric patients (Table 27.4: Figs 27.4b and 27.6a, f) [42–45]. Capillaritis is often not considered on initial pathologic reading of these biopsies, which are often obtained bronchoscopically for the differentiation of bacterial versus pneumocystis pneumonitis so tissue sampling is limited, and prominent hemorrhage can obscure vascular detail such as TMA. That inflammatory cell infiltrate "spillage" in tissue spaces can occur has been cited above due to capillary structural differences. Most of the published cases had classic antibodies to CL and LA. Patient 15 had extensive pulmonary hemorrhage (Fig. 27.4b) with antibodies to PE, thrombocytopenia (TCP)/autoimmune hemolytic anemia (AIHA), infertility, and asymptomatic small vessel ischemic disease of the central nervous system (CNS). Patient 2 had undiagnosed TMA causing recurrent pulmonary emboli misdiagnosed as asthma throughout childhood, and at death in his 20s had pathologic evidence of old and new pulmonary thromboembolism (PTE) and significant microvascular pulmonary hypertension (Fig. 27.6a) [4–6]. Figure 27.6(b, c) show both significant TMA and increased collagenous changes in a pulmonary arteriole, and recanalization processes in other areas of the lungs; resolution of TMA but residual fibrous strands are exemplified in Fig. 27.6f that likely lead to chronic schistocytosis prominent in this patient in his later years. Patient 8 (Fig. 27.4b) had alve-

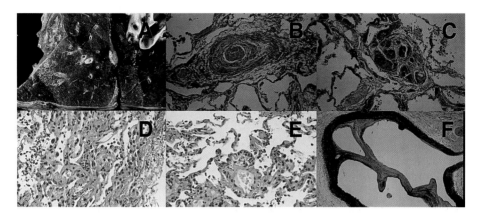

Figure 27.6. Pulmonary vascular pathology. **a** Pulmonary arteriolar hypertrophy, fresh and recanalized thromboses, edema, and hemorrhage, Patient 2; **b** pulmonary arteriole with increased concentric intimal fibrosis and in situ thrombosis (MT), Patient 2; **c** pulmonary arteriole with organizing thrombosis and early recanalization (VVG), Patient 2; **d** pulmonary capillaritis with inflammatory cells "spilling" into alveolar spaces (far left), Patient 15; **e** pulmonary arteriole with fibrinous walls and intraluminal fibrin (center), Patient 9; **f** pulmonary arteriole with fibrous web residual of recanalization of old thrombi (VVG), Patient 2 (courtesy of Dr. Michael Hughson). (G. A. McCarty, Indiana University APS Database, IUMC Photography Department, and Matrix Digital Photography, Inc., Indianapolis IN.)

olar hemorrhage. (Patient 9 had SLE and APS with antibodies to both PE and PS, and a classic pulmonary arteriole with fibrin staining is noted in Fig. 27.6(e), and similar changes with more alveolar capillary infiltrate "spillage" is noted in Patient 15 (Fig. 27.6d).

Renal Vascular Pathology

The first reports of renovascular pathology involved patients with recurrent thrombosis and LA [10, 46, 47]. Renovascular lesions involve afferent arterioles and terminal branches of interlobular arteries, often without eliciting a cellular infiltrate or disruption of internal elastic laminae, but the deposition of hyaline material beneath the endothelium, which is immunoglobulin in nature by previously published electron microscopic studies, has also been noted [1–6, 10, 46, 47]. Table 27.5 collates the vascular pathology, clinical setting of APS independent of type of glomerulonephritis by WHO classification, as clinical renal disease is discussed elsewhere in this book; TMA is characteristic in all cases, as well as endothelial cell hyperplasia and fibrin staining. The earliest reports cite thrombotic thrombocytopenic and/or purpuric presentations which brought patients to early renal biopsy; the first 4 cases were patients with classical serologies, TMA, and SLE [46, 47]. Series of patients have subsequently been identified, with 1° and 2° APS, and a continuing prevalence of antibodies to CL and/or LA 35, 50, 52, 54–56, 58, 59]. Perivasculitis or vasculitis occurred infrequently, primarily in patients with 2° APS, but one case report documents a patient with 1 °APS [51, 52, 57]. Patients. 2, 7, and 12–14 all had

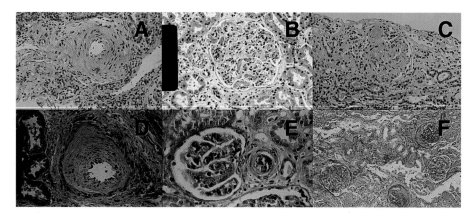

Figure 27.7. Renovascular pathology. **a** Concentric renal arteriolar hypertrophy with mild perivascular but not panvascular inflammatory infiltrate, and normal tubules (top), Patient 1; **b** glomerular capillary loop small thromboses are scattered through the left upper and mid lower quadrants, Patient 12; **c** hyalinized, thickened glomerular capillary loop present superiorly with few inflammatory cells, arteriolar thickening and proliferation; glomerular ischemia, Patient 1; **d** concentric renal arteriolar hypertrophy, Patient 13; **e** glomerular capillary loop hypertrophy with eccentric intimal hyperplasia in extraglomerular vessel, Patient 2; **f** renal arteriolar hypertrophy, crescentic glomerulopathy with varying degrees of capillary loop hypertrophy, hyalinization, and fibrosis, Patient 14 (courtesy of Dr. Moo-Nahm Yum). (G. A. McCarty, Indiana University APS Database, IUMC Photography Department, and Matrix Digital Photography, Inc., Indianapolis IN.)

2° APS and antibodies to CL; additionally, Patients 12 and 14 had antibodies to PS, and PE and LAC, respectively. Patient 1 with 1°APS exhibited concentric renal arteriolar hypertrophy with a mild perivascular infiltrate but no true panvascular infiltrate, and normal tubules (Fig. 27.7a); hyalinized thickened capillary loops with mild proliferative changes occur in Fig. 27.7(c) and she had antibodies to CL and PE. Patient 2 showed glomerular capillary loop hypertrophy with eccentric intimal hyperplasia in an extraglomerular vessel (Fig. 27.7e). Patient 12 had small glomerular capillary loop thromboses and antibodies to CL and PS (Fig. 27.7b). Patient 13 showed concentric arteriolar hypertrophy (Fig. 27.7d), and Patient 14 had crescentic glomerulopathy with varying degrees of hyalinization and fibrosis, and antibodies to CL and PE (Fig. 27.7f). Expected frequencies of IgG and/or C3 by FA studies were noted relative to lupus nephritis classification in some cases (data not shown). Fibrin, erythrocytes, and erythrocyte fragments are often components of a thickened media and effacement with hyaline material is common. The renovascular pathology of APS likely represents the culmination of endothelial cell effector functions in regulation of response to immune injury of various types in recent reviews [4, 60].

Cerebrovascular and Muscular Vascular Pathology

Early studies associated small vessel cerebrovascular ischemic lesions, usually of a multiple territory nature causing multi-infarct dementia, classic antibodies to CL, and coexistent cardiac sources of microemboli due to APS valvulopathy [61–64]. A true TMA with vasculitis was noted in two cases, one with a monocytic/macrophagic perivascultis in a patient with 1° APS, and coexistent intimal hyperplasia, and a transmural lymphocytic infiltrate consistent with true vasculitis in another patient with 1°APS also with antibodies to CL. Three of the four patients here had 1°APS (Patients 1 (Fig. 27.9a), Patients 2 (Fig. 27.8e and 27.9e) and 17 (Fig. 27.8c, f) with antibodies to CL, or CL and PE (Patients 1 and 17). Patient 1 (Fig. 27.9a) additionally had significant endothelial cell swelling and the novel finding of a mitotic figure, with almost complete obliteration of vascular lumen, and a mild periadventitial cellular infiltrate. Patient 12 (Figs 27.8b and 27.9c, d, f) showed a wide variety of TMA with varying webs of recanalization in several sites in both gray and white matter vessels. Special stains showed cortical ribbon infarction proceeding downwards from cortical meningeal arterioles. Patients 12, 13 and 2 also showed similar lesions in areas not underlying a cortical meningeal infarct (Fig. 27.9a, b and e, respectively). TMA characterized all the reports and significant endothelial cell changes were apparent [13, 25, 41, 61–64]. Intraluminal platelet deposition in cerebral vasculopathy is important, and only recently have CNS lesions been identified with characteristic TMA changes in murine models of APS [65, 66]. Two patients have recently been seen at IUMC with multiple isotype aPLs to PE whose review of nerve biopsies previously read as normal were shown to have classic TMA in arterioles (data not shown); their diagnoses were chronic demyelinating immunologic peripheral neuropathy ("CDIP") but they both have multiple criteria for 1° APS [31]. Patient 17 (Fig. 27.8c, f) is a neonate with unilateral cutaneous gangrene and four digital infarctions requiring amputation due to maternal APS that was not recognized despite maternal–fetal TCP and LR; muscular infarction due to TMA and subsequent necrosis is depicted from hand muscle biopsy, but the digital arteries were not examined distally. Both her mother and this baby girl had antibodies to CL, PE, and LAC.

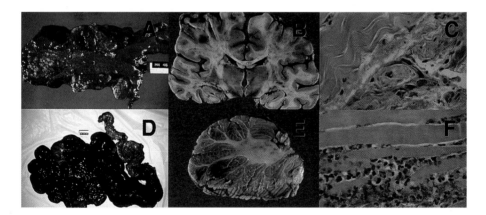

Figure 27.8. Mesenteric, cerebrovascular, and muscular vascular pathology. **a** Mesenteric arterial thrombosis is present and distinct from proximal atherosclerosis, Patient 13 (courtesy of Dr. Michael Hughson); **b** multiple territory cerebral meningeal, gray and white matter small vessel ischemic disease of varying ages, Patient 12; **c** muscle arteriolar thrombosis and muscle fiber necrosis in left forearm, Patient 17; **d** intestinal ischemia due to mesenteric thrombosis in **a**, Patient 13; **e** multiple areas of cerebellar small vessel ischemic disease, Patient 2; **f** muscle necrosis with acute inflammatory infiltrate from small vessel thrombosis in c, Patient 17 (courtesy of Dr. Mary M. Davis). (G. A. McCarty, Indiana University APS Database, IUMC Photography Department, and Matrix Digital Photography, Inc., Indianapolis IN.)

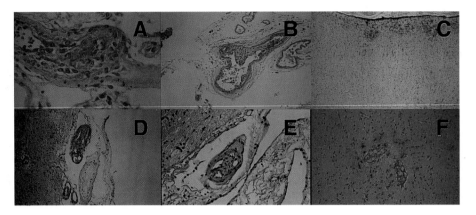

Figure 27.9. Cerebrovascular pathology. **a** Cerebral arteriolar endothelial cell edema and mitotic figure with intimal hyperplasia, fibrin, and major luminal occlusion, Patient 12; **b** intimal fibrous proliferation extending intraluminally in cortical arteriole, Patient 13; **c** cortical infarct confined to cortical ribbon (GFAP), Patient 12; **d** meningeal arteriolar intimal hyperplasia with thrombotic microangiopathy and recanalization, Patient 12; **e** meningeal arteriolar intimal hyperplasia in vessel not overlying a cortical infarct, Patient 2; **f** deep cerebral cortical vessels with fibrous webs and thrombotic microangiopathy with recanalization, Patient 12 (courtesy of Dr. Michael Hughson). (G. A. McCarty, Indiana University APS Database, IUMC Photography Department, and Matrix Digital Photography, Inc., Indianapolis IN.)

Vascular Pathology in Other Organs

Isolated reports of TMA and endothelial cell changes with and without fibrin staining have been reported in other organs; an arterial occlusion in APS causing large bowel infarction similar to the gross aortic/mesenteric arterial occlusive disease is shown in Patient 13 (Fig. 27.8a, d) who had SLE and APS, and died of bowel gangrene; a patient with 1° APS and giant ulcerations with a lymphocytic infiltrate in involved areas near an ulceration, but also around vessels not underlying an ulcer [67–69]; adrenal insufficiency due to vessel thrombosis, hemorrhage, and eventual atrophy with antibodies to CL primarily [70, 71]; bladder infarction in a patient with criteria for 1°APS and antibodies to CL [72], and lastly, pituitary vascular infarction resulting in a maternal death due to TMA and antibodies to CL [73].

Prospectus

The spectra of vascular pathology in APS likely reflects the time course of initial versus chronic vascular injury, host response to immunologic perturbation, and the continual adjustment from a prothrombotic to non-thrombotic milieu of endothelial cells and platelets [1–6, 74–76]. TMA has been considered to be the hallmark pathologic finding for APS. That vasculitis and perivasculitis can occur with APS, even in primary forms, or where autoantibodies are directed to phospholipids other than cardiolipin, is apparent in these cases and from the literature, and might likely reflect the finding that antibodies to phospholipids are enriched in circulating immune complexes found in APS patients [77]. Platelet activation and/or CD40 ligand expression has been shown to cause an inflammatory reaction in endothelial cells and increased platelet–leukocyte aggregation, which would favor thrombosis [78–80]. Endothelin-1, adhesion molecule and monocyte-tissue factor expression upregulation also likely contribute to the ultimate expressions of immune mediated vascular injury, thrombosis, inflammation, and repair [81–84]. That both the clinical features and pathologic findings of APS occur in patients who test consistently negative for aPLs by EIA or LA methodologies is important to recognize, as exemplified by both the new and published cases reviewed here, and may represent circulating aPL in immune complexes unavailable for detection by routine testing, or aPLs being deposited in tissues [77, 85]. Future histopathology in APS will likely include new phenotypic and molecular markers for further characterization and understanding of microvascular events as knowledge progresses.

References

1. Lie JT. Vasculopathy in the antiphospholipid antibody syndrome – thrombosis or vasculitis or both? J Rheumatol 1989;16:713–715.
2. Lie JT. Vasculitis in the antiphospholipid antibody syndrome – culprit or consort? J Rheumatol 1994;21:397–399.
3. Lie JT. Vasculopathy of the antiphospholipid syndromes revisited: thrombosis is the culprit and vasculitis the consort. Lupus 1996;5:368:71.
4. Hughson MD, Nadasdy T, McCarty GA, Sholer C, Min KW, Silva F. Renal thrombotic microangiopathy in patients with systemic lupus erythematosus and the antiphospholipid syndrome. Am J Kid Dis 1992;20(2):150–158.
5. Hughson MD, McCarty GA, Sholer CM, Brumback RA. Thrombotic cerebral arteriopathy in patients with the antiphospholipid syndrome. Mod Pathol 1993;6(6):644–653.
6. Hughson MD, McCarty GA, Brumback RA. Spectrum of vascular pathology affecting patients with the antiphospholipid syndrome. Hum Pathol 1995;26(7):716–724.
7. Cervera R, Asherson RA, Lie JT. Clinicopathological correlations of antiphospholipid antibody syndrome. Semin Arthritis Rheum 1995;24:262–272.
8. Bathena DB, Fobel, BJ, Migdahl SO. Noninflammatory renal microangiopathy of systemic lupus erythematosus, "lupus vasculitis". Am J Nephrol 1985;44:81–84.
9. Bachrach JR, Lie JT. The prevalence of vascular occlusive disease associated with antiphospholipid antibody syndrome. Int Angiol 1992;11:51–56.
10. Asherson RA, Noble, GA, Hughes GRV. Hypertension, renal artery stenosis, and primary antiphospholipid antibody syndrome. J Rheumatol 1991;18: 1413–1415.
11. Alarcon-Segovia D, Cardiel MH, Reyes E. Antiphospholipid arterial vasculopathy. J Rheumatol 1989;16:762–767.
12. Goldberger E, Elder RC, Schwartz RA, Phillips PE. Vasculitis in the antiphospholipid syndrome. A cause of ischemia responding to corticosteroids. Arthritis Rheum 1992;35:569–572.
13. Westerman EM, Miles JM, Backonja M, Sundstrom WR. Neuropathologic findings in multi-infarct dementia associated with anticardiolipin antibody. Evidence for endothelial injury as the primary event. Arthritis Rheum 1992;35:1038–1041.
14. Winklemann RK, Alegre VA. Histopathologic and immunofluorescence study of skin lesions associated with circulating lupus anticoagulant. J Am Acad Dermatol 1988;19:117–124.
15. Ingram SB, Goodknight SH, Bennett RM. An unusual syndrome of devastating noninflammatory vasculopathy associated with anticardiolipin antibody – report of 2 cases. Arthritis Rheum 1987;30:1167–1172.
16. Triplett DA. Many faces of lupus anticoagulants. Lupus 1998;7 (Suppl 2): S18–22.
17. McIntyre JA, Wagenknecht DR, Sugi T. Phospholipid binding plasma proteins required for antiphospholipid antibody detection: an overview. Am J Reprod Immunol 1997;37: 101–107.
18. Frances C, Tribout B, Boisnic S. Cutaneous necrosis associated with the lupus anticoagulant. Dermatologica 1989;178:194–201.

19. Asherson RA, Cervera R. Antiphospholipid syndrome. J Invest Dermatol 1993;100:21S–27S.
20. Dodd HJ, Sarkany I, O'Shaughnessy D. Widespread cutaneous necrosis associated with the lupus anticoagulant. Clin Exp Dermatol 1985;10:581–586.
21. Smith KJ, Skelton HG, James WD et al. Cutaneous histopathologic findings in "antiphospholipid syndrome": correlation with disease, including human immunodeficiency virus disease. Arch Dermatol 1990;126:1176–1183.
22. O'Neill A, Gatenby PA, McGaw B, Painter DM, McKenzie PR. Widespread cutaneous necrosis associated with cardiolipin antibodies. J Am Acad Dermatol 1990;22:356–359.
23. Wolf P, Soyes,HP, Aver Grunbach P. Widespread cutaneous necrosis in a patient with rheumatoid arthritis associated with anticardiolipin. Arch Dermatol 1991;127: 1739–1740.
24. Elkayam O, Yaron M, Brasoush E, Carpi D. Rheumatoid nodules in a patient with primary antiphospholipid antibody syndrome (Hughes' syndrome) Lupus 1998;7:488–491.
25. Macucci M, Dotti MT, Battistini S, De Stefano, N, Vecchione V, Orefice G et al. Primary antiphospholipid syndrome: two case reports, one with histological examination of skin, peripheral nerve and muscle. Acta Neurol 1994;16:87–96.
26. Lalova A, Popov I, Dourmishev A, Baleva M, Nikolov K. Dramatic vasculopathy in a patient with antiphospholipid syndrome [letter]. Acta Derm Venerol 1996;76:406.
27. Abernethy ML, McGuinn JL, Callen JP. Widespread cutaneous necrosis as the initial manifestation of the antiphospholipid antibody syndrome. J Rheumatol 1995;22:1380–1383.
28. Katayama I, Nishioka K, Otoyama K. Clinical analysis of anti-cardiolipin.beta 2 glycoprotein 1 antibody positive patients in anti-phospholipid syndrome. J Dermatol Sci 1995;9:215–220.
29. Frances C, Piette JC. Cutaneous manifestation of Hughes syndrome occurring in the context of lupus erythematosus. Lupus 1997;6:139–144.
30. van Genderen PJ, Michiels JJ. Erythromyalgia: a pathognomonic microvascular thrombotic complication in essential thrombocythemia and polycythemia vera. Semin Thromb Hemost 1997;23:357–361.
32. McCarty GA. Indiana Antiphospholipid Antibody Center Database. 1999, unpublished.
32. Coates T, Kirkland GS, Dymock RB, Murphy BF, Brealey JK Mathew TH et al. Cutaneous necrosis from calcific uremic arteriolopathy. Am J Kidney Dis 1998;32:384–391.
33. Grone HJ. Systemic lupus erythematosus and antiphospholipid syndrome. Pathologe 1996;17:405–416.
34. Hill VA, Whittaker SJ, Hunt BJ, Liddell K, Spittle, MF, Smith NP. Cutaneous necrosis associated with the antiphospholipid syndrome and mycosis fungoides. Br J Dermatol 1994;130:92–96.
35. Kniaz D, Eisenberg GM, Elrad H, Johnson CA, Valaitis J, Bregman H. Postpartum hemolytic uremic syndrome associated with antiphospholipid antibodies. Am J Nephrol 1992;12:126.
36. Alvarez-Blanco A, Egurbide-Arberas MV, Aguirre-Errasti C. Severe valvular heart disease in a patient with primary antiphospholipid syndrome. Lupus 1994;3:433–434.
37. Trent K, Neustater BR, Lottenberg R. Chronic relapsing thrombotic thrombocytopenic purpura and antiphospholipid antibodies: a report of two cases Am J Hematol 1997;54:155–159.
38. Hohlfeld J, Schneider M, Hein R, Barthels M, von der Lieth H, Rosenthal HLW et al. Thrombosis of terminal aorta, deep vein thrombosis, recurrent fetal loss, and antiphospholipid antibodies. Case report. Vasa 1996;25:194–199.
39. Garcia-Torres R, Amigo MC, de la Rosa A, Moron A, Reyes PA. Valvular heart disease in primary antiphospholipid syndrome (PAPS): clinical and morphological findings. Lupus 1996;5:56–61.
40. Ziporen L, Goldberg L, Arad M, Hojnik M, Ordi-Ros J, Afek A et al. Libman-Sacks endocarditis in the antiphospholipid syndrome immunopathologic findings in deformed heart valves. Lupus 1996;5:196–205.
41. Borowska-Lehman J, Bakowska A, Michowska M, Rzepko R, Izycka E, Chrostowski L. Antiphospholipid syndrome in systemic lupus erythematosus – immunomorphological study of the central nervous system; case report. Fol Neuropathol 1995;33:231–233.
42. Hojnik M, George J, Ziporen L, Shoenfeld Y. Heart valve involvement Libman–Sacks endocarditis) in the antiphospholipid syndrome. Circulation 1996;93:1579–1587.
43. Asherson RA, Cervera R. Antiphospholipid antibodies and the lung (editorial). J Rheumatol 1995;22:62–66.
44. Falcini F, Taccetti G, Ermini M, Trapani S, Matucci Cerinic M. Catastrophic antiphospholipid antibody syndrome in pediatric systemic lupus erythematosus. J Rheumatol 1997;24:389–392.
45. Yokoi T, Tomita Y, Fukaya M, Ichihara S, Kakudo K, Takahashi Y. Pulmonary hypertension associated with SLE: predominantly thrombotic arteriopathy accompanied by plexiform lesions. Arch Pathol Lab Med 1998;122:467–470.
46. D'Agati V, Kunis C, William G et al. Anticardiolipin antibody and renal disease – a report of three cases. J Am Soc Nephrol 1980;1:777–784.
47. Kleinknecht D, Bobrie G, Meyer O, Noël LH, Callard P, Ramdane M. Recurrent thrombosis and renal vascular disease in patients with a lupus anticoagulant. Nephrol Dial Transplant 1989;4:854–858.

48. Asherson RA, Hughes GRV, Derksen RHWM. Renal infarction associated with antiphospholipid antibodies in systemic lupus erythematosus and "lupus-like" disease. J Urol 1988;140:1028.
49. Asherson RA, Cervera R, Piette JC, Font J, Lie JT, Burcoglu A et al. Catastrophic antiphospholipid antibody syndrome: clinical and laboratory features of 50 patients. Medicine 1998;77:195–207.
50. Legerton CW, Leaker B, McGregor A, Griffiths M, Snaith M, Neild GH et al. Insidious loss of renal function in patients with anticardiolipin antibodies and the absence of overt nephritis. Br J Rheumatol 1991;30:422–425.
51. Cacoub P, Wechsler B, Piette JC , Beaufils H, Herreman G, Bletry O et al. Malignant hypertension in antiphospholipid syndrome without overt lupus nephritis. Clin Exp Rheumatol 1993;11:479–485.
52. Mandreoli M, Zucchelli P. Renal vascular disease in patients with primary antiphospholipid antibodies. Nephrol Dialysis Transplant 1993;8:1277–1280.
53. Appel GB, Pirani CL, D'Agati V. Renal vascular complications of systemic lupus erythematosus [editorial]. J Am Soc Nephrol 1994;4:1499–1515.
54. Amigo MC, Garcia-Torres R, Robles M, Bochicchio T, Reyes PA. Renal involvement in primary antiphospholipid syndrome. J Rheumatol 1994;19:1181–1185.
55. Petras T, Rudolph B, Filler G, Zimmering M, Ditscherlein G, Loening SA et al. An adolescent with acute renal failure, thrombocytopenia, and femoral vein thrombosis. Nephrol Dialysis Transplant 1998;13: 480–483.
56. Strief W, Monagle P, South M, Leaker M, Andrew M. Arterial thrombosis in children. J Pediatr 1999;134: 110–112.
57. Almeshari K, Alfurayh, Akhtar M. Primary antiphospholipid syndrome and self-limited renal vasculitis during pregnancy: case report and review of the literature. Am J Kidney Dis 1994;24:505–508.
58. Bhandari S, Harnden P, Brownjohn AM, Turney JH. Association of anticardiolipin antibodies with intraglomerular thrombi and renal dysfunction in lupus nephritis. Quart J Med 1998;91: 401–409.
59. Lelievre G, Vanhille P. Renal thrombotic microangiopathy in SLE: clinical correlations and long term renal survival. Nephrol Dialysis Transplant 1998;13:298–304.
60. Nangaku M, Shankland SJ, Couser WG, Johnson RJ. A new model of renal microvascular injury. Curr Opin Nephrol Hypertens 1998;7:457–462.
61. Coull BM, Bourdette DN, Goodnight SH, Briley DP, Hart R. Multiple cerebral infarctions and dementia associated with anticardiolipin antibodies. Stroke 1987;18:1107–1112.
62. Fulham MJ, Gatenby P, Ruck RR. Focal cerebral ischemia and antiphospholipid antibodies: a case for cardiac embolism. Acta Neurol Scand 1994;90:417–423.
63. Futrell N, Asherson RA, Lie JT. Probable antiphospholipid syndrome with recanalization of occluded blood vessels mimicking proliferative vasculopathy. Clin Exp Rheumatol 1994;12:230–231.
64. Belmont HM, Abramson SB, Lie JT. Pathology and pathogenesis of vascular injury in systemic lupus erythematosus. Interaction of inflammatory cells and activated endothelium. Arthritis Rheum 1996;39:9–22.
65. Ellison D, Gatter K, Heryet A, Esiri M. Intramural platelet deposition in cerebral vasculopathy of systemic lupus erythematosus. J Clin Pathol 1993;46:37–40.
66. Nowacki P, Ronin-Walknowska E, Ossowicka-Stepinska J. Central nervous system involvement in pregnant rabbits with experimental model of antiphospholipid syndrome. Fol Neuropathol 1998;36:38–44.
67. Asherson R, Morgan S, Harris E et al. Arterial occlusion causing large bowel infarction: a reflection of clotting diathesis in SLE. Clin Rheumatol 1986;5:102–106.
68. Kallman DR, Khan A, Romain PL, Nompleggi DJ. Giant gastric ulceration associated with antiphospholipid antibody syndrome. Am J Gastroenterol 1996;91(6):1244–1247.
69. Dessailloud R, Papo T, Vaneecloo S, Gamblin C, Vanhille P, Piette JC. Acalculous ischemic gallbladder necrosis in the catastrophic antiphospholipid syndrome. Arthritis Rheum 1998;41:1318–1320.
70. Arnason JA, Graziano FM. Adrenal insufficiency in the antiphospholipid antibody syndrome. Semin Arthritis Rheum 1995;25:109–116.
71. Alperin N, Babu, S, Weinstein A. Acute adrenal insufficiency and the antiphospholipid antibody syndrome. Ann Int Med 1989;110:950.
72. Brooks MD, Fletcher MS, Melcher DH. Venous thrombosis of the bladder associated with antiphospholipid syndrome. J Roy Soc Med 1994;87:633–634.
73. Bendon RW, Wilson J, Getahun B, van der Bel-Kahn J. A maternal death due to thrombotic disease associated with anticardiolipin antibody. Arch Pathol Lab Med 1987;111:370–373.
74. Cockwell P, Tse WY, Savage CO. Activation of endothelial cells in thrombosis and vasculitis. Scand J Rheumatol 1997;26:145–150.
75. Kandiah DA, Sali A, Yonghua S, Victoria EJ, Marquis DM, Coutts SM et al. Current insights into the "antiphospholipid" syndrome: clinical, immunological, and molecular aspects. Adv Immunol 1998;70:507–563.

76. Bordron A, Dueyemes M, Levy Y, Jamin C, Ziporen L, Piette JC et al. Antiendothelial cell antibody binding makes negatively charged phospholipids accessible to antiphospholipid antibodies. Arthritis Rheum 1998;41:1738–1741.

77. Arfors L, Lefvert VK. Enrichment of antibodies against phospholipids in circulating immune complexes (CIC) in the anti-phospholipid syndrome (APLS). Clin Exp Immunol 1996;108:47–51.

78. Henn V, Slupsky JR, Grafe M, Anagnostopoulos I, Forster R, Muller-Berghaus G et al. CD40 ligand on activated platelets triggers an inflammatory reaction of endothelial cells. Nature 1998;391:591–594.

79. Josephs JE, Donohoe S, Harrison P, Mackie IJ, Machin SJ. Platelet activation and turnover in the primary antiphospholipid antibody syndrome. Lupus 1998;7:333–340.

80. Ford I, Urbaniak S, Greaves M. IgG from patients with antiphospholipid antibody syndrome binds to platelets without induction of platelet activation. Br J Haematol 1998;102:841–849.

81. Voelkel NF, Tuder RM. Cellular and molecular mechanisms in the pathogenesis of severe pulmonary hypertension Eur J Respir J 1995;8: 2129–2138.

82. Brey RL, Amato AA, Kagan-Hallett K, Rhine CB, Stallworth CL. Anti-intercellular adhesion molecule-1 (ICAM-1) antibody treatment prevents central and peripheral nervous system disease in autoimmune-prone mice. Lupus 1997;6:645–651.

83. Cuadrado MJ, Lopez-Pedrera C, Khamashta MA, Camps MT, Tinahones F, Torres A et al. Thrombosis in primary antiphospholipid antibody syndrome: a pivotal role for monocyte tissue factor expression. Arthritis Rheum 1997;40:834–841.

84. Kaminski WE, Jendraschak E, Silverstein RL, von Schacky C. Thrombosis and inflammation as multicellular processes: significance of cell–cell interactions. Thromb Haem 1995;74:240–245.

85. Miret C, Cervera R, Reverter JC, Garcia-Carrasco M, Ramos M, Molla M et al. Antiphospholipid syndrome without antiphospholipid antibodies at the time of the thrombotic event: transient "seronegative" antiphospholipid syndrome? Clin Exp Rheumatol 1997;15:541–544.

28   Placental Pathology in Antiphospholipid Antibody Syndrome

A. L. Parke

Introduction

Recurrent fetal wastage is a major clinical feature of antiphospholipid antibody syndrome (APS)[1–3]. Ware Branch has suggested that fetal wastage should be divided into pre-embryonal, embryonal and fetal (more than 10 weeks' gestation), and has concluded that more than 70% of fetal wastage (more than 10 weeks gestation) occurs in women with APS [4]. Fetal wastage in normal women who happen to have antibodies to negatively charged phospholipids is about 10% [5], but women with APS can expect a fetal loss rate of 80% [6]. Many of these women will experience recurrent fetal wastage with some of them never successfully completing pregnancy [7]. Other obstetric problems that occur in patients with APS include; prematurity and preterm delivery (less than 36 weeks gestation) as well as intrauterine growth restriction (IUGR) and hypertension including toxemia of pregnancy [7–9].

   This chapter will describe the pathological changes that occur in the placenta of patients with APS, and will discuss the potential mechanisms that contribute to this pathology in antiphospholipid antibody (aPL) patients.

Antiphospholipid Antibody Syndrome

The basic pathological process found in APS is that of a bland thrombosis in both the arterial and venous systems [10]. Even though this syndrome is almost certainly an antibody mediated process, thrombosis is the primary pathology. Recent studies have determined that certain proteins are required as cofactors for the binding of antibody to negatively charged phospholipid and that some of these protein cofactors are natural anticoagulants [11, 12], or components of the coagulation cascade [13]. Approximately 50% of patients with APS who have experienced a clinical thrombosis will rethrombose [14, 15], and several retrospective studies have suggested that the only way to prevent rethrombosis in APS patients is to treat these patients with high dose, life long anticoagulation [15, 16]. Our recent findings do not completely agree with these previous studies [17] and as it is now known that thrombosis in these patients can be triggered by other pathological and physiological events, i.e., "second

Table 28.1. Triggers for thrombosis in antiphospholipid antibody syndrome patients.

Pregnancy and postpartum state

Oral contraceptives

Lupus flares in patients who also have SLE

Infection

Elective surgical procedures

Invasive vascular studies, i.e., cardiac catherization

hit phenomenon" [18, 19], we feel that it is extremely important to identify specific known triggers for specific patients (Table 28.1) . One of these known triggers is pregnancy and the postpartum period, a complication which makes pregnancy a rather dangerous time for patients with APS. Some patients only thrombose when they are pregnant, or during the postpartum period [20]. Others will rethrombose recurrently and in some patients anatomical defects may contribute to the recurrent problem.

The factors that determine whether women with aPL will have a problem successfully completing pregnancy are not clear. Previous studies have determined that previous fetal losses and aPL predict poor fetal outcome in lupus patients [21]. Our study which addressed the prevalence of aPL in women with recurrent fetal wastage, normal mothers and women who had never been pregnant, showed that women with more than one positive test for aPL are more likely to experience fetal wastage especially if they have high titers of IgG aCL [22]. Others have shown that antibodies to high levels of IgG aCL and a lupus anticoagulant (LA) are also predictors of problems with pregnancy [3, 9, 23].

Uterine Physiological Changes of Pregnancy

Many physiological changes must occur in the uterine wall in order to allow the fetal semi-allograph to persist and grow. These include dilation and enormous growth of the spiral arteries, destruction of the spiral artery endothelium with exposure of the vascular basement membrane and decidual invasion by interstitial trophoblast [24, 25]. Placental growth and development will only continue if an adequate blood supply is provided by the maternal vessels. In diseases like systemic lupus erythematosus (SLE) and APS where there are a variety of pathologies that compromise blood supply, it is not surprising that the placenta exhibits significant pathological changes and that these patients experience considerable difficulties in successfully completing pregnancy.

Placental Pathology

Fetal wastage is increased in patients who have SLE [26, 27] and it has been determined that disease activity at the time of conception or throughout pregnancy is one of the most important factors contributing to the observed increase in fetal losses [26, 27). This is so much of a problem that we advise our patients to plan for months ahead prior to conception and prefer that they have an inactive disease for approximately 6 months before attempting to become pregnant. SLE can also flare during pregnancy (28, 29) and it is our policy in SLE patients who become pregnant on antimalarial drugs to maintain these medications, as it has been determined that stopping antimalarial drugs can provoke a flare of disease [30, 31] and therefore put the pregnancy at risk.

The pathological changes found in the placenta of SLE patients reflect the inflammation of the underlying disease, with deposition of antibodies and immunoglobulin in various parts of the placenta, including the trophoblast and the trophoblast basement membranes [32]. Lupus placentas are small, and demonstrate placental infarction, decidual vessel thrombosis, atherosis of uterine vessels (Fig. 28.1) chronic villitis and intervillisitis (Fig. 28.2] and lack of physiological change [33, 34]. A prospective study by Hanly et al determined that lupus placentas were smaller than normal and that low placental weight correlated with; active SLE, a LA, thrombocytopenia and hypocomplementemia. Fetal loss was not always associated with reduced placental weight, but did correlate with the presence of a circulating anticoagulant [33].

An earlier study by Abramowsky et al had demonstrated a vasculopathy in decidual vessels that included fibrinoid necrosis, subintimal edema, necrotic breakdown of the vessel wall and an infiltrate of cells with foamy cytoplasm, so called atherosis [34]. Similar changes have been found in the placentas from patients with eclampsia, diabetes and maternal hypertension [36]. In Abramowsky's study this decidual vasculopathy correlated with late fetal death. [35].

Out et al studied placentas from patients who had experienced intrauterine death, some of whom had APS. These authors determined that in addition to areas of gross infarction that there was microscopic evidence of extensive villous ischemia in areas

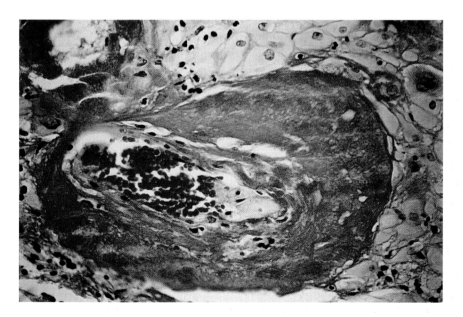

Figure 28.1. Decidual vessel showing fibrinoid necrosis.

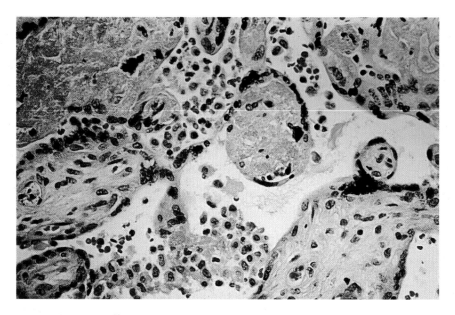

Figure 28.2. Placenta, showing villitis and intervillusitis.

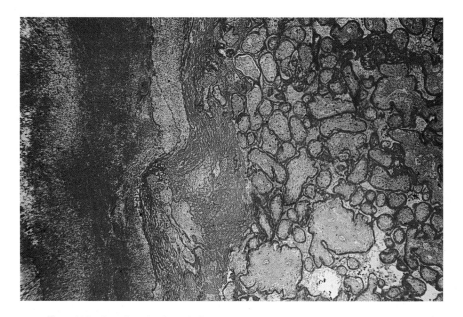

Figure 28.3. Thrombosed, infarcted villi in a patient with phospholipid antibody syndrome.

of villous parenchyma that did not appear to be grossly infarcted. They also determined that so called APS placental pathology could be found in patients that did not have APS [37].

A recent study of 39 pregnancies occurring in 28 aPL positive women determined that excessive perivillous coagulation, avascular terminal villi and chronic villitis and utero placental vasculitis were more common in patients with APS that were being treated, compared to patients who just had aPL antibodies but did not have APS. Multifocal uteroplacental thromboses were a significant feature in both treated (46%) and untreated (60%) patients with APS [38].

In those SLE patients who also have APS, thrombosis and placental infarction may be very extensive. This combination of inflammatory and thrombotic pathologies contribute to the spectrum of obstetric problems seen in these patients including: preterm birth, intrauterine growth restriction, fetal wastage and pre-eclampsia [7–9].

University of Connecticut Experience

At the University of Connecticut Health Center we have a large number of APS patients, and many of these patients have had problems completing pregnancy. It has been our policy to examine all placentas obtained from patients with SLE and patients with APS, and in multiparous patients to obtain the placentas from previous pregnancies. This practice has given us vital information that has been used to determine treatment regimes in subsequent pregnancies.

In order to examine these placentas we have divided placental pathology into three main categories.

1. Coagulation abnormalities; this category included evidence of uteroplacental vascular thrombosis, excessive perivillous deposition of fibrin, and intraplacental thrombosis in chorionic or fetal stem vessels.
2. Uteroplacental vascular pathology and secondary villous damage. This category included lack of physiological change in the spiral vessels, fibrinoid necrosis, and atherosis of the decidual vessels as well as uteroplacental vasculitis. Lesions considered to be a consequence of uteroplacental vascular pathology include; abruption, and infarction, fibrosis, and hypovascularity of villi. Also included are syncytiotrophoblast knotting and cytotrophoblast proliferation.
3. Intraplacental vascular lesions including either thrombotic, vasculitic, atrophic or hyperplastic lesions in the chorionic vessels, fetal stem vessels and the capillaries of the terminal villi.

Using these pathological categories we concluded that:

1. Thrombosis and infarction occur frequently in patients with APS (Fig. 28.3).
2. Treatment with anticoagulants, anti-inflammatory agents and other therapeutic agents was not able to prevent pathological changes in patients with APS.
3. The pathological changes identified in one pregnancy generally would be repeated in subsequent pregnancies in these patients with APS.
4. Some aPL patients who do not meet criteria for SLE also have placental vasculitis as well as the more usual thrombotic pathology associated with APS [39].

These findings suggest that even in treated APS patients who successfully complete pregnancy, the pregnancies are still abnormal as indicated by the persistence of pathological changes found in these placentas. It is our impression that even though these treated pregnancies may result in a live infant, the pathological processes are slowed down so that gestation can progress to the point where a viable baby may be obtained. These placental studies also demonstrate the need for examination of previous placentas in these aPL patients as the original pathological changes will be repeated in subsequent pregnancies.

Pathogenesis

The precise pathogenesis of the thrombotic diathesis associated with aPL remains unknown. The recognition that some aPL require a protein cofactor to augment binding to phospholipid antibodies has helped explain some features [11–13]. However, as it is apparent that these antibodies are a family of antibodies [40] and that the required proteins can also vary [11–13] it would seem that one explanation probably will not suffice.

Animal studies reproducing human disease using passive immunization with aPL-positive immunoglobulin [41, 42,] and active immunization with β_2-glycoprotein I [43, 44] suggest that these antibodies are directly involved in the thrombotic process.

β_2-glycoprotein I (apolipoprotein H) is the most studied of the protein cofactors. This protein is a natural anticoagulant that inhibits platelet aggregation and inhibits protein S binding to its binding protein C4Bp [45]. Several authors have suggested that abnormalities of the protein C and protein S anticoagulant system may contribute to the thrombotic diathesis known to be associated with aPL [46, 47]. In our report we determined that some aPL patients have low levels of free protein S, that was not a consequence of antibodies to protein S or its binding protein [46]. These low levels fell even further when patients became pregnant, a possible explanation for the association of thrombosis with pregnancy that is well described in aPL patients.

β_2-glycoprotein I binds to endothelial cells and therefore may modulate endothelial cell function [48]. Previous studies have demonstrated that sera from APS patients can modulate prostacyclin production from endothelial cells [49, 50] and others have suggested a cross-reactivity between aPL and antiendothelial cell antibodies [51, 52]. Anti-β_2-glycoprotein I antibodies have been demonstrated to react with trophoblast cell membranes and endothelial cell membranes in the placental villi of placentas from aPL patients [53, 54].

The annexins are a recently identified family of proteins with the ability to bind calcium and phospholipids and they appear to have important effects on coagulation [55, 56]. Twenty annexins have been identified and Rand et al have suggested that annexin V (also known placental anticoagulant protein-1) plays a vital role in preventing coagulation reactions within the placenta [57]. These authors have demonstrated that annexin V is normally present on the apical membranes of syncytiotrophoblasts and have also shown that incubating BeWo cells [a placental trophoblast cell line), primary cultured trophoblasts and human umbilical vein endothelial cells with IgG fractions obtained from patients with APS results in reduced levels of annexin V on the cell surfaces of trophoblast and endothelial cells [58]. This reduction in annexin V also correlated with accelerated coagulation times of plasma overlaid on these cells [58].

Annexin V has a very high affinity for phospholipids [59] and Rand suggests that annexin V prevents coagulation by carpeting anionic phospholipids and thus preventing interaction with coagulation proteins [58]. aPL disrupt the ability of annexin V to cluster on the phospholipid surface, providing a possible explanation for the placental insufficiency found in APS patients.

Summary

Until the precise mechanism for the thrombotic diathesis associated with APS is completely understood, the optimum therapy to prevent placental pathology and the associated fetal wastage will remain guesswork. Analyzing previous placentas has been helpful as patients appear to repeat to same pathological process in subsequent pregnancies. Only those patients that demonstrate significant inflammation should be exposed to corticosteroids, particularly as our studies demonstrated the most significant change in placental pathology occurred in patients who had had active SLE in one pregnancy and inactive SLE in a subsequent pregnancy [39]. Heparin, however, does appear to help these patients successfully complete pregnancy [60–62] and should be used in any aPL patient that has sustained a late fetal loss, i.e., more than 10 weeks' gestation, and who wishes to attempt another pregnancy.

References

1. Alarcon-Segovia D, Perez-Vasquez ME, Villa AR et al. Preliminary classification criteria for the antiphospholipid syndrome within systemic lupus erythematosus. Semin Arthritis Rheum 1992;21:275–285.
2. Asherson RA, Cervera R, Piette JC, Shoenfeld Y. The antiphospholipid syndrome: history, definition, classification, and differential diagnosis. The Antiphospholipid Syndrome, Chapter 1. 1996:3–12.
3. Nilsson IM, Astedt B, Hedner U,et al. Intrauterine death and circulating anticoagulant "antithromboplastin". Act Med Scand 1975;197:153–159.
4. Branch WD. Thoughts on the mechanism of pregnancy loss associated with antiphospholipid syndrome. Lupus 1994;3:275–280.
5. Harris EN, Spinnato JA. Should anticardiolipin tests be performed in otherwise healthy pregnant women? Am J Obstet Gynecol 1991;165:1272–1277.
6. Perez MC, Wilson WA, Brown HL et al. Anticardiolipin antibodies in unselected pregnant women in relationship to fetal outcome. J Perinatol 1991;11:33–36.
7. Branch DW et al. Outcomes of treated pregnancies in women with antiphospholipid syndrome: an update of the Utah experience. Obstet Gynecol 1992;80:614–620.
8. Lubbe WF, Butler WS, Palmer SJ et al. Fetal survival after prednisone suppression of maternal lupus anticoagulant. Lancet 1983;i:1361–1363.
9. Out HJ, Bruinse HW, Christiaens GCML et al. A prospective controlled multicenter study on the obstetric risks of pregnant women with antiphospholipid antibodies. Am J Obstet Gynecol 1992;167:26–32.
10. Lie JT. Vasculitis in the antiphospholipid syndrome: culprit or consort? J Rheumatol 1994;21:397–399.
11. McNeil HD, Simpson RJ, Chesterman CN et al. Antiphospholipid antibodies are directed against a complex antigen that included a lipid-binding inhibitor of coagulation: beta-2- glucoprotein I (apolipoprotein H). Proc Natl Acad Sci USA 1990;87:4120–4124.
12. Galli M, Confurius P, Massau C et al. Anticardiolipin antibodies (ACA) directed not to cardiolipin but to a plasma protein cofactor. Lancet 1990;335:1544–1547.

13. Galli M, Barbui T. Prothrombin as cofactor for antiphospholipids. Lupus 1998;7 (suppl 2):S37–S40.
14. McNeil HP, Hunt JE, Krilis SA. Antiphospholipid antibodies – new insights into their specificity and clinical importance. Scand J Immunol 1992;36:647–652.
15. Khamashta M et al. The management of thrombosis in the antiphospholipid antibody syndrome. N Engl J Med 1995;332:993–997.
16. Rosove MH, Brewer P. Antiphospholipid thrombosis: clinical course after the first thrombotic event in 70 patients. Ann Intern Med 1992;117:303–308.
17. Amante EJB, Nasr S, Walsh SJ, Parke AL. Long term follow-up of different therapeutic interventions in patients with the phospholipid antibody syndrome. 1999;submitted.
18. Lockshin MD. New perspectives in the study and treatment of antiphospholipid syndrome. The Antiphospholipid Syndrome Boca Raton, FL: CRC Press, 1996;323–329.
19. Amante E, Sanders MM, Parke AL. "Second hit" phenomenon triggering thrombosis in a patient with SLE and aPL syndrome – a case report. J Rheumatol 1999;in press.
20. Parke AL. Antiphospholipid antibody syndromes. Rheum Dis Clin North Am 1989;15:275.
21. Ramsey-Goldman R, Kutzer JE, Kuller LH et al. Previous pregnancy outcome is an important determinant of subsequent pregnancy outcome in women with systemic lupus erythematosus. Am J Reprod Immunol 1992;28:195–198.
22. Parke AL, Wilson D, Maier D. The prevalence of antiphospholipid antibodies in habitual aborters compared to normal women and women who have never been pregnant. Arthritis Rheum 1991;34:1231–1235.
23. Maclean MA et al. The prevalence of lupus anticoagulant and anticardiolipin antibodies in women with a history of first trimester miscarriages. Br J Obstet Gynecol 1994;101:103–106.
24. Bernirschke K. A review of the pathologic anatomy of the human placenta. Am J Obstet Gynecol 1962;84:1595–1622.
25. Fox H (editor), Bennington JL (consultant). Major problems in pathology. Philadelphia: WB Saunders, 1978;95–148.
26. Zurier RB et al. Systemic lupus erythematosus: management during pregnancy. Obstet Gynecol 1978;51:178–180.
27. Mintz G et al. Prospective study of pregnancy in systemic lupus erythematosus: results of a multi-disciplinary approach. J Rheumatol 1986;13:732–739.
28. Petri M, Howard D, Repke J. Frequency of lupus flare in pregnancy. Arthritis Rheum 1991;34:1538–1545.
29. Hayslett JP. Effect of pregnancy in patients with SLE. Am J Kidney Dis 1982;2:223–228.
30. Rudnicki RD, Gresham GE, Rothfield NF. The efficacy of anti-malarials in systemic lupus erythematosus. J Rheumatol 1975;2:323–330.
31. The Canadian Hydroxychloroquine Study Group. A randomized study of the effect of withdrawing hydroxychloroquine sulfate in systemic lupus erythematosus. N Engl J Med 1991;342:150–154.
32. Grennan DM et al. Immunological studies of the placenta in systemic lupus erythematosis. Ann Rheum Dis 1978;37:129–134.
33. Hanly JG, Gladman DD, Rose TH et al. Lupus pregnancy, a prospective study of placental changes. Arthritis Rheum 1998;31:358–366.
34. Abramowsky CR, Vegas ME, Swinehart G et al. Decidual vasculopathy of the placenta in systemic lupus erythematosus. N Engl J Med 1980;303:668–670.
35. Lowell DM, Kaplan C, Salafia CM, College of American Pathologists Conference XIX on the Examination of the Placenta. Report on the working group on the definition of structural changes associated with abnormal function in the maternal/fetal/placental unit in the second and third trimester. Arch Path Lab Med 1991;115:647.
36. Khong TY, Pearce JM, Robertson WB. Acute atherosis in preeclampsia: Maternal determinants and fetal outcome in the presence of the lesions. Am J Obstet Gynecol 1987;157:360.
37. Out HJ, Kooijman CD, Bruinse HW et al. Histopathological findings in placentas from patients with intra-uterine fetal death and antiphospholipid antibodies. Eur J Obset Gynecol Reprod Biol 1991;41:179.
38. Salafia CM, Cowchock FS. Placental pathology and antiphospholipid: a descriptive study. Am J Perinatol 1997;14:435–441.
39. Salafia CM, Parke AL. Placental pathology in systemic lupus erythematosus and phospholipid antibody syndrome. Clin Rheum Dis 1997;23:85–97.
40. Parke A, Maier D, Hakim C et al. Subclinical autoimmune disease and recurrent spontaneous abortion. J Rheumatol 1986;13:1178–1180.
41. Branch DW, Dudley DJ, Mitchell MD et al. Immunoglobulin G factions from patients with antiphospholipid antibodies cause fetal death in BALB/c mice: a model for autoimmune fetal loss. Am J Obstet Gynecol 1990;163:210–216.

42. Blank M, Cohen J, Toder V et al. Induction of antiphospholipid syndrome by passive transfer of anticardiolipin antibodies. Proc Natl Acad Sci USA 1991;88:3069–3073.
43. Gharavi AE, Sammaritano LR, Wen J et al. Induction of antiphospholipid autoantibodies by immunization with β_2 glycoprotein I (apolipoprotein H). J Clin Invest 1992;90:1105–1109.
44. Blank M, Faden D, Tincani A et al. Immunization with anticardiolipin cofactor (beta 2-glycoprotein I) induces experimental antiphospholipid syndrome in naïve mice. J Autoimmunity 1994;7:441–445.
45. Schousboe I. β_2 glycoprotein-1: a plasma inhibitor of the contact activation of the intrinsic blood coagulation pathway. Blood 1985;66:1086–1091.
46. Parke AL, Weinstein RE, Bona RD et al. The thrombotic diathesis associated with the presence of phospholipid antibodies may be due to low levels of free protein S. Am J Med 1992;93:49–56.
47. Atsumi T, Khamasta MA, Ames PRJ et al. Effect of β_2 glycoprotein-1 and human monoclonal anticardiolipin antibody on the protein-S/C4b-binding protein system. Lupus 1997;6:358–364.
48. Meroni PL, Del Papa N, Beltrami B et al. Modulation of endothelial cell function by antiphospholipid antibodies. Lupus 1996;5:448–450.
49. Carreras LO, Defreyn G, Machin SJ et al. Arterial thrombosis, intrauterine death and "lupus" anticoagulant: detection of immunoglobulin interfering with prostacyclin formation. Lancet 1981;i:244–246.
50. Carreras LO, Vermylen J. Lupus anticoagulant and thrombosis. Possible role of inhibition of prostacyclin formation. Thromb Haemost 1982;48:38–40.
51. Del Papa N et al. Endothelial cells as a target for antiphospholipid antibodies; role of anti β_2 glycoprotein-1 antibodies. Am J Reprod Immunol 1997;38:212–217.
52. Del Papa N et al. Relationship between antiphospholipid and antiendothelial antibodies III: β_2 glycoprotein-1 mediates the antibody binding to endothelial membranes and induces the expression of adhesion molecules. Clin ExpRheumatol 1995;13:179–186.
53. McIntyre JA. Immune recognition at the maternal-fetal interface: overview. Am J Reprod Immunol 1992;28:127–131.
54. La Rosa et al. β_2 Glycoprotein-1 and placental anticoagulant protein-1 in placentae from patients with antiphospholipid syndrome. J Rheumatol 1994;21:1684–1698.
55. Rand JH. "Annexinopathies" – A new class of diseases. N Engl J Med 1999;340:1035–1036.
56. Cesarman GM, Guevara CA, Hajjar KA. An endothelial cell receptor for plasminogen/tissue plasminogen activator (t-PA). II.Annexin II mediated enhancement of t-PA-dependent plasminogen activation. J Biol Chem 1994;269:21 198–203.
57. Rand JH et al. Reduction of annexin-V (placental anticoagulant protein-I) on placental villi of women with antiphospholipid antibodies and recurrent spontaneous abortion. Am J Obstet Gynecol 1994;171:1566–1572.
58. Rand JH, Wu XX, Guller S et al. Antiphospholipid immunoglobulin G antibodies reduce annexin-V levels on syncytiotrophoblast apical membranes and in culture media of placental villi. Am J Obstet Gynecol 1997;177:918–920.
59. Rand JH et al. Pregnancy loss in the antiphospholipid antibody syndrome – a possible thrombogenic mechanism. N Engl J Med 1997;336:154–160.
60. Rosove MH, Tabsh K, Wasserstrum N et al. Heparin therapy for pregnant women with lupus anticoagulant or anticardiolipin antibodies. Obstet Gynecol 1990;75:660–634.
61. Rai R, Cohen H, Dave M et al. Randomized controlled trial of aspirin and aspirin plus heparin in pregnant women with recurrent miscarriage associated with phospholipid antibodies (or antiphospholipid antibodies) Br Med J 1997;314:253–257.
62. Kutteh MD. Antiphospholipid antibody-associated recurrent pregnancy loss: Treatment with heparin and low-dose aspirin is superior to low-dose aspirin alone. Am J Obstet Gynecol 1996;174:1584–1589.

29 Mechanism of Thrombosis in the Antiphospholipid Syndrome: Binding to Platelets

J. C. Reverter and D. Tàssies

Antiphospholipid antibodies (aPL) are related to thrombosis in the antiphospholipid syndrome [1, 2] and numerous pathophysiological mechanisms have been suggested involving cellular effects, plasma coagulation regulatory proteins and fibrinolysis [3]. Among the mechanisms supposed to be involved, platelets have been considered as a promising potential target to circulating aPL in causing antibody-mediated thrombosis.

Platelets play a central role in primary hemostasis involving adhesion to the injured blood vessel wall, followed by platelet activation, granule release, shape change, and rearrangement of the outer membrane phospholipids and proteins transforming them into a highly efficient procoagulant surface [4].

Several facts support platelets as the target of aPL. Studies performed in the aggregometer or in flowing conditions and the evaluation of platelet activation markers in vivo in patients with the antiphospholipid syndrome are used as demonstration.

Activation and spontaneous aggregation of platelets was reported in aggregometric studies to be caused directly by aPL in early reports [5, 6]. Other authors did not found this ability of aPL to initiating platelet activation [7, 8] or reported inhibition of aggregation caused by aPL [9]. However, the most realistic interpretation is that in the aggregometric studies aPL may cooperate in platelet activation by rendering platelets more reactive to the action of weak or low dose agonists [7, 10–12].

Other studies performed using flowing systems that simulate physiological conditions [13, 14] demonstrated, in both systemic lupus erythematosus patients and in "primary" antiphospholipid syndrome patients, increases in the formation of platelet thrombi when small amounts of patients' plasmas or purified immunoglobulins with anticardiolipin activity were added to normal blood, but this increase only occurred when plasma from patients with a thrombotic history was employed. Similar results were obtained in the same system when the experiments were performed using human monoclonal anticardiolipin antibodies [15].

Several studies have been performed to identify platelet activation markers in patients with the antiphospholipid syndrome. The first investigated the eicosanoid regulation in these patients showing inhibition of prostacyclin synthesis [16–18] and/or increased platelet thromboxane production [10, 18–20]. These results were found in in vitro experiments and in vivo in patients with the antiphospholipid syndrome. However, these results have not been confirmed by others [21]. Looking for more direct markers of platelet activation, other authors have found an increase of the CD62p (P-selectin), an integral protein found in the alpha-granules, on platelet surface [22] and/or the soluble CD62 [23], lose from the activated platelet membranes to the plasma pool, in patients with the antiphospholipid syndrome, but not all the authors found the same results [24, 25]. Finally, others have found an increased number of platelet microparticles [26] supporting an increased platelet activation in vivo in these patients.

There are several theoretical mechanisms to explain the action of aPL on hemostasis [3, 27]. aPL may directly inhibit antigen enzymatic or cofactor function of hemostasis, acting as blocking agents. They may bind fluid-phase antigens of hemostasis-involved proteins and then decrease plasma antigen levels by clearance of immune complexes; aPL and their antigens may form immune complexes that may be deposited in blood vessels causing inflammation and tissue injury; aPL may cause dysregulation of antigen–phospholipid binding due to cross-linking of membrane bound antigens; and aPL may trigger cell-mediated events by cross linking of antigen bound to cell surfaces or cell surface receptors [3, 27]. Several characteristics of the aPL – as the concentration, class/subclass, valency, affinity or charge –, and several characteristics of the antigens – concentration, size, valency, location or charge –, may influence which of the theoretical autoantibody actions will occur in vivo [3]. In the present chapter we will focus on platelet membrane interactions of aPL.

The interaction of aPL with platelets can occur in at least three different ways. First, immunoglobulins may bind through the Fab terminus with specific platelet antigens (or with other antigens deposed on platelets) in a classic antigen–antibody reaction; second, immune complexes may bind to platelets via FcγRII receptor; and third, aPL, like other immunoglobulins, may bind to platelets in a non-specific manner by mechanisms not well characterized but probably related to platelet membrane injury [28]. The last mechanism, non-specific binding, does not seem to have a pathophysiological role in antiphospholipid syndrome-related thrombosis.

Normal platelet membranes have a clear phospholipid asymmetry. The outer leaflet of the phospholipid bilayer is rich in choline-phospholipids, whereas aminophospholipids are located in the inner leaflet [29]. Then, in resting platelets phosphatidylserine is predominantly located in the cytoplasmic leaflet of the platelet membranes, but platelets undergoing activation lose their physiological phospholipid asymmetry and increase the exposure of anionic phospholipids, mainly phosphatidylserine, on the external cell membrane [30]. During platelet activation a fast transbilayer movement of phospholipids (flip-flop) is produced [29]. In addition, during platelet activation exposure of anionic phospholipids is accompanied by shedding of procoagulant microvesicles [31]. The extent of the platelet membrane phospholipid expression depends of the type of platelet activator, calcium-ionophore being the most potent, followed in order of potency by the complement complex C5b-9, collagen plus thrombin, collagen and thrombin [29]. ADP and epinephrine are very weak activators considering the induction of the phospholipid flip-flop.

Some studies have demonstrated that aPL may bind to platelet surface, and this binding is higher on activated or damaged platelets than in resting ones [13, 32, 33]. In addition, several agonists, like collagen, may be more able to activate platelets in a way that makes them reactive to aPL than others, like ADP [13]. These results agree with the differential expression of phospholipids during platelet activation.

aPL with lupus anticoagulant activity also bind to platelets and to platelet-derived microvesicles at least in part by membrane-bound prothrombin [34]. However, it has been reported that lupus anticoagulant antibodies can bind to activated platelets in absence of any plasma component, but they can not exclude that the required cofactor may be released from the platelet granules [34].

Membranes from activated platelets are an important source of negatively-charged phospholipids to provide a catalytic surface for interacting coagulation factors [34]. The ability of platelets to support tenase and prothrombinase activity (and also protein C activity) correlates with the extent to the platelet membrane phospholipid asymmetry [29]. By binding to phospholipid surface, aPL may interfere in the prothrombinase activity by hampering the assembly of the prothrombin activating complex (factors Xa and Va, phospholipid and calcium) on the platelet procoagulant surface o by reducing the binding of prothrombin to a otherwise normal prothrombinase complex [35]. The binding of aPL (or at least some of them with lupus anticoagulant activity) to phospholipids causes a decrease in the peak amount of prothrombinase activity that has been attributed to both deficient formation of the complex and to poor prothrombin binding [35]. This effect may be inhibited by the presence of phospholipids depending more on their amount than on their nature and no specific platelet product could be identified responsible for this effect [35]. These effects inhibiting the coagulation pathway may explain the results observed in vitro with lupus anticoagulant, but in vivo aPL cause thrombosis and not bleeding. We can suppose that aPL may interfere with the protein C pathway inhibiting their phospholipid-dependent reactions that occurs on platelet surfaces in the same way in which they act in the prothrombinase reaction [3, 36]. Then, these actions in the regulatory protein C system may lead to a decrease of its physiological anticoagulant activity. It has been suggested that these antibodies that alter protein C pathway may be associated with venous thrombosis [18].

As is known, aPL are in fact directed against phospholipid-binding proteins eventually bound to phospholipids exposed on surfaces [3]. The main protein associated to the anticardiolipin antibody activity is β_2-glycoprotein I bound to phospholipids [37–39]. Anticardiolipin antibodies bind directly to these proteins immobilized on irradiated surfaces [40] constituting the actual epitope of anticardiolipin antibodies. β_2-glycoprotein I, and other phospholipid-binding proteins, could be considered a mechanism to protect the organism from excessive coagulation leading by negatively charged phospholipids exposed on platelet (or other cells) membranes during cell activation or apoptosis [3].

β_2-glycoprotein I is a highly glycosylated single-chain-protein present in plasma that avidly binds to negatively charged phospholipids such as cardiolipin, phosphatidylserine or phosphatidylinositol [41] through their highly positively charged amino acid sequence Cys281–Cys288 [42] located in the fifth domain [43] and the epitope for anticardiolipin antibodies binding located in the fourth domain [44]. The affinity of β_2-glycoprotein I for phospholipid surfaces highly depends on their phospholipid composition. In physiological conditions, β_2-glycoprotein I may inhibit phospholipid-dependent hemostasis reactions, but due to its low affinity for phospholipids [42, 45] β_2-glycoprotein I is by itself only a weak anticoagulant. However, aPL (or at least aPL with lupus anticoagulant activity) may enhance the affinity of β_2-glycoprotein I to phospholipids and, then, β_2-glycoprotein I may become a real competitor to phospholipid-dependent hemostasis reactions. Using artificial bilayer membranes with physiological phosphatidylserine concentration and purified human aPL with lupus anticoagulant activity, a high-affinity interaction was identified in the binding of aPL–β_2-glycoprotein I complexes to phospholipids, due to the bivalent interactions between antibodies and lipid-bound β_2-glycoprotein I [45].

Shi et al [33] observed that human anticardiolipin antibodies only can bind to activated platelets but not to resting platelets and this binding was in a β_2-glycoprotein I–dependent way. In addition, using murine monoclonal antibodies against β_2-glycoprotein I with lupus anticoagulant activity, Arvieux et al [7] demonstrated that these IgG antibodies potentiated the effect of sub-threshold concentrations of aggregation agonists (ADP or adrenaline) but requiring the presence of β_2-glycoprotein I. These data were confirmed by others [10, 11] and it was demonstrated that both Fab and Fc fragments of the antibodies were essentials for this activity and this effect was dependent to the action of the FcγRII receptor, as it could be blocked by inhibitory monoclonal antibodies [7]. In new experiments, the same murine anti-β_2-glycoprotein I antibodies caused activation, degranulation and adherence of neutrophils [46] and these effects were also mediated by the FcγRII receptor.

There are three families of FcγR molecules (RI, RII and RIII) [47], each containing several allelic variants. The only FcγR molecules present on platelets are the FcγRII [48]. The FcγRII (CD32) is present on platelets, neutrophils and monocytes and has weak affinity for the Fc portion of monomeric IgG, but high affinity for the Fc portion of IgG contained in immune complexes or to IgG bound to an antigen on the platelet surface [49]. Activation of the FcγRII receptor causes platelet activation and granule release. This receptor reacts best with murine IgG subclasses 1 and 2b and to human IgG subclasses 1 and 3 [50]. Human subclass IgG2 reacts weakly with the receptor. However, a polymorphism with a single base substitution in the codon for amino acid 131 causing an arginine (Arg) to histidine (His) amino acid change has been described [48, 51]. This polymorphism causes a FcγRII receptor containing the amino acid His at position 131 that reacts much more efficiently to subclass 2 of human IgG than the individuals who have the amino acid Arg at position 131 for this polymorphism [51].

The most interesting proposal to relate anti-β_2-glycoprotein I activity, aPL platelet binding and platelet activation leading to thrombosis suppose a pathogenic scenario very similar to these proposed for heparin-induced thrombocytopenia [50, 52]. In this hypothesis, a small initial platelet activation is produced by physiological or pathological conditions resulting in the expression of phospholipids on the platelet surface. The binding of β_2-glycoprotein I (or in a lesser extent other phospholipid-binding proteins) to these phospholipids may occur. Antiphospholipid antibodies subsequently may bind to the formed β_2-glycoprotein I–phospholipid complexes, and, then, interact with their Fc portion with the platelet surface FcγRII receptors. Through these interaction platelets may be activated and a vicious circle of cellular activation may be created finally ending in a thrombotic event. In the antiphospholipid syndrome, as probably in a similar way in much other situations, thrombosis seems to be a "two hit" phenomenon. Autoantibodies, the first "hit", are continually present in the circulation, but need a local trigger, the second "hit", to produce hemostasis dysregulation leading to a thrombotic event in a particular localization [27]. Thrombosis would require this second "hit", so explaining why patients with persistent plasma antibodies have thrombosis only occasionally and in absence of vascular immunoglobulin deposits [50].

The reason why aPL with anti-β_2-glycoprotein I activity bind to β_2-glycoprotein I bound to platelets but not to free β_2-glycoprotein in plasma needs to be answered. At physiological concentrations of β_2-glycoprotein I, aPL binding to β_2-glyco-protein I in the fluid phase is weak [53]. This fact is due to a low intrinsic affinity of the antibodies to β_2-glycoprotein I. Clustering or a high density of immobilized antigen, as may occur in the surface of activated platelets, allows bivalent or multi-valent antibody binding and then aPL may act locally [3, 53]. In addition, conforma-tional changes induced in β_2-glycoprotein I by its binding to negatively charged surfaces causing the expression of neo-epitopes (or the expression of cryptic epi-topes) have been suggested [40, 54] and aPL could be directed against this neo-epitopes (or cryptic epitopes) but not to free β_2-glycoprotein I. For these reasons aPL need the presence of platelet surfaces to exert their actions through their anti-β_2-glycoprotein I activity.

In this scenario [55] β_2-glycoprotein I may form a small amount of monovalent complexes in the fluid phase, and both free β_2-glycoprotein I and monovalent complexes bind to negatively charged phospholipids on cellular surfaces, such as activated platelet membranes, with low affinity [42, 55]. aPL can then bind to β_2-glycoprotein I bound to membrane phospholipids forming new monovalent aPL–phospholipid complexes [55]. In the platelet membrane, monovalent complexes have high mobility since binding to phospholipids is based on ionic interactions, and due to this mobility and depending on aPL–β_2-glycoprotein I density, bivalent stable complexes may form [55]. Such bivalent complexes have high affinity for phospholipids and may interfere with both anticoagulant and procoagulant reac-tions [42]. Also, aPL could potentiate the inhibitory activity of β_2-glycoprotein I in coagulation by cross-linking membrane-bound β_2-glycoprotein I and enhancing the avidity of the β_2-glycoprotein I–phospholipid interaction [3]. In addition, aPL, in experimental studies using human polyclonal purified antibodies, may enhance β_2-glycoprotein I binding to negatively charged phospholipid surfaces [45].

Activation of the FcγRII receptor by the aPL bound to β_2-glycoprotein I causes platelet activation and thromboxane A$_2$ generation [50]. Activation of FcγRII recep-tor produces intracellular ionic calcium flux, an increase of phosphatidylinositol metabolism and also a rapid phosphorylation of tyrosine residues on a number of molecules [28]. Then, the action of the FcγRII receptors activated by β_2-glycoprotein I–bound aPL may constitute the second "hit" to thrombosis in these patients.

Some other indirect evidence supports this mechanism. The activation of FcγRII by antibodies after their binding to β_2-glycoprotein I, have been highlighted [50]. The need of a initial "triggering" activation to start the process is consistent with the high degree of recurrence of thrombotic events in the same arterial or venous terri-tory [56]. This fact is compatible with a local trigger causing slight activation that can be followed by a secondary amplification due to aPL [50].

However, there are several reasons that do not permit this model to explain all the effects of antiphospholipids in thrombosis. First, anti-β_2-glycoprotein I anti-bodies in autoimmune patients are mainly restricted to the IgG2 subclass [57], and IgG2 subclass antibodies can not efficiently react with the FcγRII receptor if the mutation His–His in the position 131 of the FcγRII receptor is not present. It may be suggested that patients with the form His 131 of the polymorphism may be at greater risk of developing thrombosis by this platelet activation mechanism via the FcγRII receptor [50]. However, this hypothesis has not been sustained by epidemio-logical studies and no increased frequency of the His 131 form of this polymorphism has been found in patients with the antiphospholipid syndrome [58]. Another possible explanation to explain the hypothesis of platelet activation by the FcγRII receptor is that activated platelets express increased number of FcγRII receptors (up to 50%) [59] and by this way the first "triggering" event may improve IgG2 subclass aPL interactions with platelets in the wild type His–His FcγRII polymorphism.

Second, the proposed schema of FcγRII activation may not explain the prothrombotic action of IgM aPL. For this reason, an alternative hypothesis considering the activation of complement by aPL after their attachment to protein-phospholipid complexes on platelet surfaces has been suggested [50], as it will be discussed latter.

In addition, using an in vivo thrombosis model in mice, Gharavi et al [60] suggested that the thrombogenic effect of aPL passively administered is not dependent on their anti-β_2-glycoprotein I activity alone.

Finally, it has been reported very recently an additive effect of lupus anticoagulant and anticardiolipin antibodies that may directly activate platelets [61] and this effect could not be attributed to the FcγRII receptors because separately anticardiolipin antibodies and lupus anticoagulant fractions did not activate platelets.

As mentioned previously, the aPL bound to platelet membranes may also exert their action through the activation of complement. Decreased levels of serum complement in patients with aPL have been described by some authors [62] although others did not support this data [63]. In addition, increased levels of inactivated terminal membrane attack complex of complement (C5b-9) was found in patients with aPL and cerebral ischemia [64]. These data support the possible role of complement activation in the pathophysiology of the antiphospholipid syndrome. It is known that C5b-9 causes platelet activation [65–67], and, in addition, complement activation has been demonstrated by aPL bound to cardiolipin liposomes when these aPL were obtained from antiphospholipid syndrome patients but not when they were obtained from syphilis patients [68]. Then, the complement generated in presence of aPL bound to negatively charged phospholipids may cause platelet activation and, eventually, platelet destruction [69]. Considering this scenario, the "double hit" hypothesis suggested by Arnout in the FcγRII-mediated activation [52] can also be applied to the complement-mediated platelet activation in the antiphospholipid syndrome. First, an initial activation of platelets is needed (provided by local events such as small vascular lesions). Then, negatively charged phospholipid are exposed in a small extent on the platelet surface and aPL may bind to these exposed phospholipids or to proteins bound to these phospholipids. Antiphospholipid antibodies fixed in the platelet surface may induce complement activation in an Fc-independent manner causing more platelet activation [69]. In addition, it has been demonstrated that C5b-9 action may increase the transbilayer migration of phosphatidylserine in the platelet membrane [70] causing increased binding of aPL and, then, C5b-9 activation, and, in a vicious circle, platelet activation.

Finally, the ability of aPL to bind to platelets through different epitopes, like CD36 [71] or glycoprotein IIIa [72], has been reported, and these special bindings have been related to thrombotic phenomena and/or to platelet activation. However, the mechanisms of platelet activation in these peculiar aPL binding sites are not known.

In conclusion, the most reliable explanation for the prothrombotic action of aPL includes a previous platelet activation and the binding of them to platelet membrane phospholipid-bound proteins, mainly β_2-glycoprotein I. Then, in a second step aPL may act activating platelets, via FcγRII receptor or complement C5-9 formation, causing a platelet activation vicious circle, or may act inhibiting the phospholipid-related protein C pathway leading to thrombosis in both cases.

References

1. Hughes GRV, Harris EN, Gharavi AE. The anticardiolipin syndrome. J Rheumatol 1986; 13: 486–489.
2. Love PE, Santoro SA. Antiphospholipid antibodies: anticardiolipin and the lupus anticoagulant in systemic lupus erythematosus (SLE) and in non-SLE disorders. Ann Intern Med 1990;112:682–698.
3. Roubey RAS.Immunology of the antiphospholipid antibody syndrome. Arthritis Rheum 1996;39:1444–1454.
4. Machin SJ. Platelets and antiphospholipid antibodies. Lupus 1996;5:386–387.
5. Wiener HM, Vardinon N, Yust I. Platelet antibody binding and spontaneous aggregation in 21 lupus anticoagulant patients. Vox Sang 1991;61:111–121.
6. Lin YL, Wang CT. Activation of human platelets by the rabbit anticardiolipin antibodies. Blood 1992; 80: 3135–3143.
7. Arvieux J, Roussel B, Pouzol P, Colomb MG. Platelet activating properties of murine monoclonal antibodies to β_2-glycoprotein I. Thromb Haemost 1993;70:336–341.
8. Ford I, Urbaniak S, Greaves M. IgG from patients with antiphospholipid syndrome binds to platelets without induction of platelet activation. Br J Haematol 1998;102:841–849.
9. Ostfeld I, Dadosh-Goffer N, Borokowski S, Talmon J, Mani A, Zor U et al. Lupus anticoagulant antibodies inhibit collagen-induced adhesion and aggregation of human platelets in vitro. J Clin Immunol 1992;12:415–423.
10. Martinuzzo ME, Maclouf J, Carreras LO, Lèvy-Toledano S. Antiphospholipid antibodies enhance thrombin-induced platelet activation and thromboxane formation. Thromb Haemost 1993;70:667–671.
11. Campbell AL, Pierangeli SS, Wellhausen S, Harris EN. Comparison of the effects of anticardiolipin antibodies from patients with the antiphospholipid syndrome and with syphilis on platelet activation. Thromb Haemost 1995;73:529–534.
12. Ichikawa Y, Kobayashi N, Kawada T, Shimizu H, Moriuchi J, Ono H et al. Reactivities of antiphospholipid antibodies to blood cells and their effect on platelet aggregations in vitro. Clin Exp Rheumatol 1990;8:461–465.
13. Reverter JC, Tàssies D, Escolar G, Font J, Lopez-Soto A, Ingelmo M et al. Effect of plasma from patients with primary antiphospholipid syndrome on platelet function in a collagen rich perfusion system. Thromb Haemost 1995;73:132–137.
14. Escolar G, Font J, Reverter JC, Lopez-Soto A, Garrido M, Cervera R et al. Plasma from systemic lupus erythematosus patients with antiphospholipid antibodies promotes platelet aggregation: studies in a perfusion system. Arterioscler Thromb 1992;12:196–200.
15. Reverter JC, Tàssies D, Font J, Khamashta MA, Ichikawa K, Cervera R et al. Effect of human monoclonal anticardiolipin antibodies on platelet function and on tissue factor expression on monocytes. Arthritis Rheum 1998;41:1420–1427.
16. Carreras LO, Defreyn G, Machin SJ, Vermylen J, Deman R, Spitz B et al. Recurrent arterial thrombosis, repeated intrauterine death and "lupus" anticoagulant: detection of immunoglobulin interfering with prostacyclin formation. Lancet 1981;1:244–246.
17. Carreras LO, Vermylen JG, Deman R, Spitz B, Van Asshe A. "Lupus" anticoagulant and thrombosis – possible role of inhibition of prostacyclin formation. Thromb Haemost 1982;48:28–40.
18. Lellouche F, Martinuzzo M, Said P, Maclouf J, Carreras LO. Imbalance of thromboxane/prostacyclin biosynthesis in patients with lupus anticoagulant. Blood 1991;78:2894–2899.
19. Maclouf J, Lellouche F, Martinuzzo M, Said P, Carreras LO. Increased production of platelet derived thromboxane in patients with lupus anticoagulants. Agents Actions Suppl 1992;37:27–33.
20. Forastiero R, Martinuzzo M, Carreras LO, Maclouf J. Anti-β-2-glycoprotein I antibodies and platelet activation in patients with antiphospholipid antibodies: association with increased excretion of platelet-derived thromboxane urinary metabolites. Thromb Haemost 1998;79:42–45.
21. Rustin MHA, Bull HA, Machin SJ. Effects of the lupus anticoagulant in patients with systemic lupus erythematosus on endothelial cell prostacyclin release and procoagulant activity. J Invest Dermatol 1988;90:744–748.
22. Fanelli A, Bergamini C, Rapi S, Caldini A, Spinelli A, Buggiani A et al. Flow cytometric detection of circulating activated platelets in primary antiphospholipid syndrome. Correlation with thrombocytopenia and anticardiolipin antibodies. Lupus 1997;6:261–267.

23. Joseph JE, Donohoe S, Harrison P, Mackie IJ, Machin SJ. Platelet activation and turnover in the primary antiphospholipid syndrome. Lupus 1998;7:333–340.
24. Shechter Y, Tal Y, Greenberg A, Brenner B. Platelet activation in patients with antiphospholipid syndrome. Blood Coag Fibrinol 1998;9:653–657.
25. Out HJ, de Groot P, van Vliet M, de Gast G, Nieuwenhuis K, Derksen RHWM. Antibodies to platelets in patients with antiphospholipid antibodies. Blood 1991;77:2655–2659.
26. Galli M, Grassi A, Barbui T. Platelet-derived microvesicles in the antiphospholipid syndrome. Thromb Haemost 1993;69:541.
27. Roubey RAS. Mechanisms of autoantibody-mediated thrombosis. Lupus 1998;7 (suppl. 2):114–119.
28. Chong BH, Brighton TC, Chesterman CN. Antiphospholipid antibodies and platelets. Semin Thromb Hemost 1995;21:76–84.
29. Bevers EM, Comfurius P, Dekkers DWC, Harmsma M, Zwaal RFA. Regulatory mechanisms of transmembrane phospholipid distributions and pathophysiological implications of transbilayer lipid scrambling. Lupus 1998;7 (suppl. 2):126–131.
30. Schroit AJ, Zwaal RFA. Transbilayer movement of phospholipid in red cell and platelet membranes. Biochim Biophys Acta 1991;1071:313–329.
31. Sims PJ, Wiedmer T, Esmon CT, Weiss HJ, Shattil SJ. Assembly of the platelet prothrombinase complex is linked to vesiculation of the platelet plasma membrane. Studies in Scott's syndrome: an isolated defect in procoagulant activity. J Biol Chem 1989;264:17049–17057.
32. Khamashta MA, Harris EN, Gharavi AE, Derue G, Gil A, Vazquez JJ et al. Immune mediated mechanism for thrombosis: antiphospholipid antibody binding to platelet membranes. Ann Rheum Dis 1988;47:849–854.
33. Shi W, Chong BH, Chesterman CN. β-2-glycoprotein I is a requirement for anticardiolipin antibodies binding to activated platelets: differences with lupus anticoagulants. Blood 1993;81:1255–1262.
34. Galli M, Bevers EM, Comfurius P, Barbui T, Zwaal RFA. Effect of antiphospholipid antibodies on procoagulant activity of activated platelets and platelet-derived microvesicles. Br J Haematol 1993;83:466–472.
35. Galli M, Béguin S, Lindhout T, Hemker CH. Inhibition of phospholipid and platelet-dependent prothrombinase activity in the plasma of patients with lupus anticoagulant. Br J Haematol 1989;72:549–555.
36. Galli M, Ruggeri L, Barbui T. Differential effects of anti-β-2-glycoprotein I and anti-prothrombin antibodies on the anticoagulant activity of activated protein C. Blood 1998;91:1999–2004.
37. McNeil HP, Simpson RJ, Chesterman CN, Krilis SA. Anti-phospholipid antibodies are directed against a complex antigen that includes a lipid-binding inhibitor of coagulation: β_2-glycoprotein I (apolipoprotein H). Proc Natl Acad Sci USA 1990;87:4120–4124.
38. Galli M, Comfurius P, Maassen C, Hemker HC, de Baets MH, van Breda-Vriesman PJ et al. Anticardiolipin antibodies (ACA) directed not to cardiolipin but to a plasma protein cofactor. Lancet 1990;335:1544–1547.
39. Matsuura E, Igarashi Y, Fujimoto M, Ichikawa K, Koike T. Anticardiolipin cofactors and diferential diagnoses of autoimmune diseases. Lancet 1990;336:177–178.
40. Matsuura E, Igarashi V, Yasuda T, Triplett DA, Koike T. Anticardiolipin antibodies recognize β_2-glycoprotein I structure altered by interacting with an oxygen modified solid phase surface. J Exp Med 1994;179:457–462.
41. Wurm H. Beta 2-glycoprotein I (apolipoprotein H) interactions with phospholipid vesicles. Int J Biochem 1984;16:511–515.
42. Arnout J, Vermylen J. Mechanism of action of β-2-glycoprotein I-dependent lupus anticoagulants. Lupus 1998;7 (suppl. 2):23–28.
43. Hunt JE, Krilis S. The fifth domain of β-2-glycoprotein I contains a phospholipid binding site (Cys281–Cys288) and a region recognized by anticardiolipin antibodies. J Immunol 1994;152:653–659.
44. Igarashi M, Matsuura E, Igarashi Y, Nagae H, Ichikawa K, Triplett DA et al. Human β-2-glycoprotein I as an anticardiolipin cofactor determined using deleted mutants expressed by a Baculovirus system. Blood 1996;87:3262–3270.
45. Willems GM, Janssen MP, Pelsers MMAL, Confurius P, Galli M, Zwaal RFA et al. Role of divalency in the high-affinity binding of anticardiolipin antibody-β2-glycoprotein I complexes to lipid membranes. Biochemistry 1996;35:13833–13842.
46. Arvieux J, Jacob MC, Roussel B, Bensa JC, Colomb MG. Neutrophil activation by anti-β_2-glycoprotein I monoclonal antibodies via Fcγ receptor II. J Leukocyte Biol 1995;57:387–394.
47. van de Winkel JGJ, Capel PJA. Human IgG Fc receptor heterogeneity. Immunol Today 1993;14:215–221.
48. Anderson CL, Chacko GW, Osborne JM, Brandt JT. The Fc receptor for immunoglobulin G (FcγRII) on human platelets. Semin Thromb Hemost 1995;21:1–9.

49. De Reys S, Blom C, Lepoudre B, Declerck PJ, De Ley M, Vermylen J et al. Human platelet aggregation by murine monoclonal antibodies is subtype-dependent. Blood 1993;81:1792–1800.

50. Vermylen J, Hoylaerts MF, Arnout J. Antibody-mediated thrombosis. Thromb Haemost 1997;78:420–426.

51. Warmerdam PAM, van de Winkel JGJ, Vlug A, Westerdaal NAC, Capel PJA. A single amino acid in the second Ig-like domain of the FcγRII is critical for human IgG2 binding. J Immunol 1991;147:1338–1343.

52. Arnout J. The pathogenesis of the antiphospholipid syndrome: a hypothesis based on parallelisms with heparin-induced thrombocytopenia. Thromb Haemost 1996;75:536–541.

53. Roubey RAS, Eisenberg RA, Harper MF, Winfield JB. "Anti-cardiolipin" autoantibodies recognize β_2-glycoprotein I in the absence of phospholipid: importance of antigen density and bivalent binding. J Immunol 1995;154:954–960.

54. Wagenknecht DR, McIntyre JA. Changes in β_2-glycoprotein I antigenicity induced by phospholipid binding. Thromb Haemost 1993;69:361–365.

55. Arnout J, Wittelvrongel C, Vanrusselt M, Hoylaerts M, Vermylen J. β_2-glycoprotein I dependent lupus anticoagulants form stable divalent antibody-β_2-glycoprotein I complexes on phospholipid surfaces. Thromb Haemost 1998;79:79–86.

56. Khamashta MA, Cuadrado MJ, Mujic F, Taub NA, Hunt BJ, Hughes GR. The management of thrombosis in the antiphospholipid-antibody syndrome. N Engl J Med 1995;332:993–997.

57. Arvieux J, Roussel B, Ponard D, Golomb MG. IgG subclass restriction of anti β_2-glycoprotein I antibodies in autoimmune patients. Clin Exp Immunol 1994;95:310–315.

58. Atsumi T, Caliz R, Amengual O, Khamashta MA, Hughes GRV. FcγReceptor IIA H/R131 polymorphism in patients with the antiphospholipid syndrome. Thromb Haemost 1998;79:924–927.

59. McCrae KR, Shattil SJ, Cines DB. Platelet activation induces increased Fcγ receptor expression. J Immunol 1990;144:3920–3927.

60. Gharavi AE, Pierangeli SS, Gharavi EE, Hua T, Liu XW, Barker JH et al. Thrombogenic properties of antiphospholipid antibodies do not depend on their binding to β-2-glycoprotein I (β_2GPI) alone. Lupus 1998;7:341–346.

61. Nojima J, Suehisa E, Kuratsune H, Machii T, Koike T, Kitani T et al. Platelet activation induced by combined effects of anticardiolipin and lupus anticoagulant IgG antibodies in patients with systemic lupus erythematosus. Thromb Haemost 1999;81:436–441.

62. Shibata S, Sasaki T, Hirabayashi Y, Seino J, Okamura K, Yoshinaga K et al. Risk factors in the pregnancy of patients with systemic lupus erythematosus: association of hypocomplementaemia with poor prognosis. Ann Rheum Dis 1992;51:619–623.

63. Hess DC, Sheppard JC, Adams RJ. Increased immunoglobulin binding to cerebral endothelium in patients with antiphospholipid antibodies. Stroke 1993;24:994–999.

64. Davis WD, Brey RL. Antiphospholipid antibodies and complement activation in patients with cerebral ischemia. Clin Exp Rheumatol 1992;10:455–460.

65. Rinder CS, Rinder HM, Smith BR, Ficht JC, Smith MJ, Tracey JB et al. Blockade of C5a and C5b-9 generation inhibits leukocyte and platelet activation during extracorporeal circulation. J Clin Invest 1995;96:1564–1572.

66. Solum NO, Rubach-Dahlberg E, Pedersen TM, Reisberg T, Hogasen K, Funderud S. Complement-mediated permeabilization of platelets by monoclonal antibodies to CD9: inhibition by leupeptin, and effects on the GPI-acting-binding protein system. Thromb Res 1994;75:437–452.

67. Wiedmer T, Hall SE, Ortel TL, Kane WH, Rosse WF, Sims PJ. Complement-induced vesiculation and exposure of membrane prothrombinase sites in platelets of paroxysmal nocturnal hemoglobinuria. Blood 1993;82:1192–1196.

68. Santiago MB, Gaburo N, de Oliveira RM, Cossermelli W. Complement activation by anticardiolipin antibodies. Ann Rheum Dis 1991;50:249–250.

69. Stewart MW, Etches WS, Gordon PA. Antiphospholipid antibody-dependent C5b-9 formation. Br J Haematol 1997;96:451–457.

70. Chang CP, Zhao J, Wiedmer T, Sims PJ. Contribution of platelet microparticle formation and granule secretion to the transmembrane migration of phosphatidylserine. J Biol Chem 1993;268:7171–7178.

71. Rock G, Chauhan K, Jamieson GA, Tandon NN. Anti-CD36 antibodies in patients with lupus anticoagulant and thrombotic complications. Br J Haematol 1994;88:878–880.

72. Tokita S, Arai M, Yamamoto M, Katagiri Y, Tanoue K, Igarashi K et al. Specific cross-reaction of IgG antiphospholipid antibody with platelet glycoprotein IIIA. Thromb Haemost 1996;75:168–174.

30 Interaction of Antiphospholipid Antibodies with Endothelial Cells

N. Del Papa, E. Raschi, A. Tincani and P. L. Meroni

Role of Endothelial Cells in the Prothrombotic Diathesis of the Antiphospholipid Syndrome

The presence of circulating anti-phospholipid antibodies (aPL) is associated with a thrombophilic diathesis [1]. Among the proposed mechanisms by which aPL might cause thrombi formation, investigators have considered the relationship between aPL and the surface membranes of cells involved in the coagulation cascade, namely platelets and endothelial cells (EC) [2].

Endothelium is now emerging as a major site of regulation of hemostasis. Normal, unperturbed EC do not support the clotting process and help to maintain blood fluidity by elaborating thrombomodulin, heparan sulfate proteoglycans, protein S and plasminogen activators. However, when perturbed, EC serve as a surface that can support many steps in the coagulation cascade by producing tissue factor and plasminogen-activator inhibitors and synthesizing specific binding sites for several coagulation factors. Altogether these procoagulant events on the endothelium may shift the hemostatic balance towards clot formation [3].

The conversion of the normal antithrombotic endothelial phenotype to a pro-thrombotic surface might be one of the pathological events that causes the hyper-coagulable state of tha antiphospholipid syndrome (APS). Carreras et al. in studies with lupus anticoagulant (LA)-positive plasmas, first suggested that aPL can suppress prostacyclin (prostaglandin I_2; PGI_2) release by vascular endothelium and concluded that this mechanism could be involved in the in vivo thrombotic diathesis [4]. Subsequent studies have found that LA positive plasmas have variable effect on PGI_2 production and a suppressing effect was observed only in a minority of instances. Different sources of EC and aPL (whole sera or plasmas, different immunoglobulin fractions, etc.) and differences in techniques have been regarded as the most likely reasons to explain the discrepancies [5, 6].

Do aPL Bind to Endothelium?

The interaction between aPL and EC assumes that the autoantibodies can recognize phospholipid determinants on endothelial surfaces in order to display the procoagulant effect. Although different groups independently reported a high prevalence of antiendothelial binding activity in sera from both primary and secondary APS, a direct reactivity of purified aPL with EC membranes was not clearly demonstrated [7–13]. For example, absorption studies with phospholipid micelles did inhibit completely aPL reactivity but affected endothelial binding in a minority of sera and only partially [7, 8, 12, 14]. Altogether these findings were quite in line with the fact that EC surface membranes in the resting state do not expose negatively charged phospholipids on the outer leaflet but only on the inner one, as in the majority of cell types. In addition, our own group demonstrated that, differently from platelets [15], endothelial activation following several stimuli (such as cytokines, phorbol esters or lipopolysaccharide; LPS) did not affect at all antiendothelial binding of aPL positive sera, frustating once again the hypothesis that epitopes specific for aPL could be at least available on the surface of activated human EC [9]. In agreement with these data we have been also unable to demonstrate any binding of a human monoclonal antibody (mAb) reactive with anionic phospholipids in a β_2-glycoprotein I (β_2GPI)-independent manner to both resting or cytokine-activated human umbilical vein endothelial cells (HUVEC) (Meroni PL, personal communication).

On the other hand, using an immunoprecipitation assay with radiolabeled HUVEC surface proteins, two groups independently demonstrated that APS sera reacted with endothelial membrane structures [12, 16]. The sera immunoprecipitated proteins with a molecular weight ranging from 200 to 24 kDa, confirming the existence of autoantibodies directed against a heterogeneous family of endothelial constitutive membrane proteins unrelated to the known phospholipid epitopes [12, 16]. Altogether these findings suggest that in APS both aPL and antiendothelial cell antibodies (AECA) could occur as a separate antibody population.

β_2-Glycoprotein I as a Cofactor for aPL Reactivity to Endothelial Cells

Le Tonquèze et al. suggested another possible mechanism to explain the association between anti-endothelial activity and aPL. The authors reported that affinity purified anticardiolipin antibodies (aCL) obtained from sera positive for both AECA and aCL do react with a human endothelioma cell line (EAhy926) only when the IgG fractions were coeluted with β_2GPI, the major plasma cofactor for aPL. Furthermore, the role of β_2GPI in the reaction of aCL with EC was further stressed by the demonstration that the addition of exogenous β_2GPI allowed the endothelial binding of affinity-purified aCL IgG [17]. These data were consistent with the previously reported ability of β_2GPI to bind human EC in vitro (13) and with the in vivo immunohistological demonstration of its binding to EC membranes in trophoblast vessel walls [18, 19].

In 1995 our own group for the first time demonstrated that β_2GPI is able to mediate the binding of aPL to EC surfaces [20]. Actually, whole sera positive for AECA, aCL and anti-β_2GPI antibodies were analyzed for their binding activity to EC; we found that the incubation of EC in serum-free medium significantly reduced the antiendothelial activity, which was restored by the addition of exogenous purified human β_2GPI in a dose-dependent manner. These findings strongly support the hypothesis that fetal calf serum in the cell culturing media could represent a source of β_2GPI taking into account the close homology between bovine and human β_2GPI [21]. In agreement, affinity-purified anti-β_2GPI IgG fractions reacted with EC cultured in the presence of the cofactor but did not with cells in serum-free medium. The addition of purified β_2GPI to the cultures restored the binding once again. Human IgM mAbs – previously characterized as antibodies recognising β_2GPI – showed comparable EC binding [22]. Studies performed with different concentrations of added β_2GPI also demonstrated that the final amount of the cofactor on the cell membranes was a limiting factor for mAb binding [22]. Altogether, these findings suggest that endothelial β_2GPI adherence offers suitable epitopes for anti-β_2GPI antibodies either by making available high density immunogenic epitopes or by displaying new cryptic epitopes comparable to those detectable on γ-irradiated type C plates utilized for anti-β_2GPI detection. Our own group demonstrated that β_2GPI binds to EC membranes in a way similar to that previously found in CL-coated plates. It has been demonstrated that a highly positively charged amino acid sequence, located in the fifth domain of β_2GPI, is the phospholipid-binding site involved in the binding to CL-coated plates [23–25]. A single amino acid substitution from Lys 286 to Glu (mutant 1k) decreased the binding of β_2GPI to CL in a significant manner; further substitutions (mutants 2k, 2ka, 3k) completely abolished the ability of β_2GPI to bind to CL-coated plates [25]. We found that, while the synthetic wild-type molecule was able to bind to EC, mutant 1k binding declined; in contrast, no binding at all was detected with 2k, 2ka and 3k mutants. Altogether, these data suggest that β_2GPI binds to human endothelium by the major phospholipid-binding amino acid sequence in the fifth domain. This observation was further supported by the reactivity of anti-β_2GPI mAbs with EC incubated in the presence of the synthetic P1 peptide, spanning the aminoacid sequence of the phospholipid-binding activity. On the contrary, another peptide (P8), identical to P1 but not displaying any phospholipid-binding activity (because of the substitution of Cys 281 and Cys 288 with serine residues) did not bind to EC. Furthermore, polyclonal anti-β_2GPI IgG fractions from patients with APS were also shown to recognize P1 adhered to endothelial monolayers [26].

Although the above mentioned findings do support the adhesion of β_2GPI to EC membranes, it is still not clear to which structures β_2GPI binds. Since heparan sulfate (HS) – the major proteoglycan of the vascular endothelium – constitutes the majority of the endothelial anionic sites, we investigated whether HS could be involved in the binding of cationic β_2GPI to HUVEC. HUVEC monolayers pretreated with heparitinase I, an enzyme able to cleave specifically the α-N-acetyl-D-glycosaminidic linkage in HS, significantly downregulates their ability to bind β_2GPI (Del Papa et al. unpublished data). It should be pointed out that the effect of heparitinase I on β_2GPI binding was dose dependent and that the highest enzyme concentrations gave an inhibition up to 65%. Taken together, these findings suggest that if it is true that HS is involved in β_2GPI binding, endothelial structures other than HS might be also responsible for the cofactor adhesion.

The most common aPL-associated thrombo-occlusive event occurs in the central nervous system (CNS) [27] suggesting a selective susceptibility of CNS vascular endothelium to aPL. There is increasing evidence that EC are heterogeneous [28] and differ from organ to organ in their antigenic characteristics, secretion of prostaglandins, expression of adhesion molecules, and their thrombogenicity [29]. Hess et al showed that sera from patients with stroke and aPL had increased IgG binding to cultured human microvascular brain endothelial cells (BEC) compared with healthy controls and a group of stroke patients without aPL [30]. However, the same authors could not find any difference in the binding activity to HUVEC or to BEC when sera from aPL-positive patients with cerebral vascular accidents (CVA) were compared with sera from aPL-positive patients without CVA [30]. Our own group recently observed the ability of human polyclonal and monoclonal anti-β_2GPI antibodies to recognize the cofactor adhered to BEC and to induce a proadhesive and a proinflammatory cell phenotype (Del Papa, personal communication). Altogether these data demonstrate that: (i) β_2GPI adhesion to cell membranes is a phenomenon common to both macro- and microvascular EC; and (ii) the binding of antibodies to the adhered cofactor is also able to activate EC from the microvasculature.

Interestingly, anti-β_2GPI mAbs showed a significantly increased binding activity to BEC in comparison to HUVEC suggesting a higher β_2GPI adherence. In addition, at variance with HUVEC, the antibody cell reactivity decreased but did not decline to background levels when BEC were cultured in serum-free medium (Del Papa et al, personal communication).

Functional Modifications Induced by aPL on EC

Proadhesive and Proinflammatory Phenotype

Recently, EC binding of aPL IgG or of both polyclonal and monoclonal anti-β_2GPI antibodies has been shown to induce a phenotypic change in in vitro EC studies. Cells were shown to display a proadhesive surface revealed by the upregulation of E-selectin, intreacellular adhesion molecule-1 (ICAM-1) and vascular cell adhesion molecule-1 (VCAM-1) and to increase the secretion of proinflammatory cytokines such as interleukin (IL)-1β and IL-6 [20, 22, 31, 32]. It should be pointed out that vascular cell activation has been reported to be associated with the appearance of a procoagulant state [33]. In addition, mononuclear leukocytes, adhering to activated endothelium, can be activated by endothelial inflammatory cytokines and induced to display a procoagulant phenotype, further contributing to the thrombophilic state in APS [33]. It is reasonable to speculate that such a series of events might occur not only in vitro but in vivo too. In line with this hypothesis is the demonstration of increased plasma levels of soluble VCAM-1 in patients with primary APS [34]. Actually, adhesion molecules, once upregulated on cell membranes, are shed into the circulation as soluble forms [35]. The hypothesis that aPL can exert their thrombogenicity, at least in part, via EC activation is further supported by the in vivo model of pinch-induced thrombosis described by Pierangeli et al [36]. In this in vivo model the passive transfer of aPL was shown to increase the size of the thrombus and to slow its resolution after a mechanical trauma on the venous vessel wall. Interestingly, these authors also described a locally increased leukocyte adhesion and enhanced adhesion molecule expression [36].

Effect on Endothelial Prostacyclin Metabolism

After the initial report on the inhibitory effect of aPL on endothelial PGI$_2$ production [4] several studies have been focused on the platelet-endothelial cell axis and eicosanoid generation in APS patients. Contrasting data have been reported; a review on the methodological variables that could explain or influence these contradictory results was recently reviewed [4, 5]. In order to reduce the technical variables linked to the use of whole plasmas or sera or polyclonal IgG fractions we evaluated the effect of human anti-β_2GPI mAbs on the production of 6-keto-PGF$_{1\alpha}$ – the main product of arachidonic acid metabolism – by HUVEC monolayers. We found that the mAbs induced a dose-dependent increase of 6-keto-PGF$_{1\alpha}$ that correlated with other parameters of EC activation, such as adhesion molecule upregulation and cytokine secretion [22].

An increase of the inducible cyclo-oxygenase (COX-2) has been reported in HUVEC incubated in the presence of IgG from four APS patients that also displayed an elevated excretion of urinary 11-dehydro-thromboxane B$_2$, an indirect parameter for an in vivo platelet activation [37]. These data might rise the possibility that an antibody-mediated increase in enzyme availability could explain the enhanced metabolic degradation of PGI$_2$. However, the same authors did not find any effect on 6-keto-PGF$_{1\alpha}$ production unless APS IgG were incubated in the presence of thrombin [37].

In addition, an ex-vivo study showed an increase in urinary excretion of thromboxane A (TXA)-platelet-derived metabolites and a smaller increase in 6-keto-PGF$_{1\alpha}$ in APS patients [38]. Such data further underline the difficulty to extrapolate from in vitro studies data that can be applied to in vivo situations in which several variables are present. Moreover, altogether these results support the hypothesis that the TXA$_2$/PGI$_2$ imbalance is apparently more linked to an enhanced TXA$_2$ secretion than to the involvement of vascular PGI$_2$ as a predisposing state for thrombosis.

Effect on Vessel Tone Regulation

Another attractive hypothesis further supporting the dysregulation of EC function has been recently advanced by Atsumi et al [39]. The authors showed that plasma levels of endothelin-1 (ET-1) peptide, the most potent endothelium-derived contracting factor, correlated significantly with the history of arterial thrombosis in APS patients. In addition they demonstrated the in vitro induction of prepro ET-1 mRNA in EC monolayers treated with anti-β_2GPI mAbs. These findings suggest that the aPL-induced endothelial dysfunction might also be related to alterations of the vessel tone (especially in the arterial tree).

Endothelial Apoptosis

aPL bind to apoptotic cells, including EC [40]. The binding might be related to the exposure of plasma membrane phosphatidylserine (PS) in cells undergoing apoptosis [41]. On the other hand, β_2GPI binding to apoptotic cells has recently been reported by several groups [42–45]. Endothelial membrane-bound β_2GPI, either by exposing cryptic epitopes after the formation of a complex with PS or by displaying high antigen density, would satisfy the requisites for the binding of β_2GPI-dependent aPL or of antibodies specifically reacting with β_2GPI.

Conversely, aPL themselves have been reported to be able to induce EC apoptosis [46]. Recently, Bordron et al. showed that some but not all AECA can induce PS exposure and DNA fragmentation in EC suggesting a possible role for AECA to induce endothelial apoptosis [47]. Authors suggested that the AECA-induced EC apoptosis could explain, at least in part, the association between AECA and aPL, since the latter could be produced after the exposure of PS (or PS/phospholipid-binding protein complexes) on EC that are induced to undergo apoptosis by AECA themselves.

Annexin V and aPL Interactions

Annexin V is a phospholipid-binding protein with anticoagulant activity found in different tissues and also in blood. Recently it has been shown that aPL IgG affect the in vitro binding of annexin V both on cultured trophoblasts and HUVEC so increasing the procoagulant activity of these cells [48]. These authors suggested that in physiological conditions a "shield" of annexin V can usually cover the negatively charged structures on the EC membranes (and trophoblast cells) so acting as a natural anticoagulant. Deposition of aPL or aPL/phospholipid-binding protein complexes on the cell membranes would displace such a shield allowing negatively charged molecules to activate the coagulation cascade. Since β_2GPI has been suggested to play a pivotal role in these events, the data further stress the importance of the binding of this " phospholipid-cofactor" to cell membranes.

Conclusion

There is now sound evidence to accept that endothelial cells do play a role in the induction of the prothrombotic diathesis of the APS. The reactivity of aPL with EC membranes appears to be the necessary prerequisite; such an event seems to be strictly related to the involvement of plasma cofactors, especially β_2GPI.

It is not surprising that several pathogenetic mechanisms have been described taking into account the widely accepted heterogeneity of the antibodies belonging to the family of aPL [49] and the several functions that EC are now known to be able to display [3].

References

1. Hughes GRV. Hughes' syndrome: The anti-phospholipid syndrome. A historical view. Lupus 1998;7(Suppl):S1–4.
2. Roubey RAS. Mechanisms of autoantibody-mediated thrombosis. Lupus 1998;7(Suppl):S114–119.
3. Cines D, Pollak E, Buck C et al. Endothelial cells in physiology and in the pathophysiology of vascular disorders. Blood 1998;91:3527–3561.
4. Carreras LO, Vermylen JG. Lupus anticoagulant and thrombosis: possible role of inhibition of prostacyclin formation. Thromb Haemost 1982;48:38–40.
5. Carreras LO, Martinuzzo MO. The lupus anticoagulant and eicosanoids. Prostagland Leukotr Ess Fatty Acids 1993;49:483–488.
6. Carreras LO, Martinuzzo MO, Maclouf J. Antiphospholipid antibodies, eicosanoids and expression of endothelial cyclooxygenase-2. Lupus 1996;5 (Suppl):494–497.
7. Vismara A, Meroni PL, Tincani A, Harris EN, Barcellini W, Brucato A et al. Antiphospholipid antibodies and endothelial cells. Clin Exp Immunol 1988;74:247–253.
8. Hasselaar P, Derksen RHW, Blokzjil L, De Groot PG. Cross-reactivity of antibodies directed against cardiolipin, DNA, endothelial cells and blood platelets. Thromb Haemost 1990;63:169–173.

9. Del Papa N, Meroni PL, Tincani A, Harris EN, Pierangeli SS, Barcellini W et al. Relationship between antiphospholipid and antiendothelial antibodies: further characterization of the reactivity on resting and cytokine-activated endothelial cells. Clin Exp Rheumatol 1992;10:37–42.

10. Le Roux G, Wautier MP, Guillevin L, Wautier JL. IgG binding to endothelial cells in systemic lupus erythematosus. Thromb Haemost 1986;56:144–146.

11. Rosenbaum J, Pottinger BE, Woo P, Black CM, Louzou S, Byron MA et al. Measurement and characterization of circulating anti-endothelial cell IgG in connective tissue diseases. Clin Exp Immunol 1988;72:450–456.

12. McCrae KR, De Michele A, Samuels P, Roth D, Kuo A, Meg QH et al. Detection of endothelial cell reactive immunoglobulin in patients with anti-phospholipid antibodies. Br J Haematol 1991;79:595–605.

13. Del Papa N, Conforti G, Gambini D, Barcellini W, Borghi MO, Fain C et al. Characterization of anti-endothelial cell antibodies in anti-phospholipd syndrome. In: Polli EE, editor. Molecular bases of human diseases. Amsterdam: Excerpta Medica, 1993;67–74.

14. Cervera R, Khamashta MA, Font J, Ramirez J, D'Cruz D, Montalban J et al. Anti-endothelial cell antibodies in patients with the antiphospholipid syndrome. Autoimmunity 1991;11:1–6.

15. Khamashta MA, Harris EN, Gharavi AE, Derue G, Gil A, Vasquez JJ et al. Immune mediated mechanisms for thrombosis: anti-phospholipid antibody binding to platelet membranes. Ann Rheum Dis 1988;47:849–852.

16. Del Papa N, Conforti G, Gambini D, La Rosa L, Tincani A, D'Cruz D et al. Characterization of the endothelial surface proteins recognized by anti-endothelial antibodies in primary and secondary autoimmune vasculitis. Clin Immunol Immunopathol 1994;70:211–216.

17. Le Tonquèze M, Salozhin K, Dueymes M, Piette JC, Lovalev V, Shoenfeld Y et al. Role of b2-glycoprotein I in the anti-phospholipid antibody binding to endothelial cells. Lupus 1995;4:179–186.

18. McIntyre J.A. Immune recognition at the maternal-fetal interface: overview. Am J Reprod Immunol 1992;28:127–131.

19. La Rosa L, Meroni PL, Tincani A, Balestrieri G, Faden A, Lojacono A et al. β_2-glycoprotein I and placental anti-coagulant protein I in placentae from patients with anti-phospholipid syndrome. J Rheumatol 1994;21:1684–1698.

20. Del Papa N, Guidali L, Spatola L, Bonara P, Borghi MO, Tincani A et al. Relationship between antiphospholipid and anti-endothelial antibodies III: β_2-glycoprotein I mediates the antibody binding to endothelial membranes and induces the expression of adhesion molecules. Clin Exp Rheumatol 1995;13:179–186.

21. Kandhia DA, Krilis SA. Beta2-glycoprotein. Lupus 1994;3 (Suppl):207–212.

22. Del Papa N, Guidali L, Sala A, Buccellati C, Khamashta MA, Ichikawa K et al. Endothelial cell as target for antiphospholipid antibodies. Arthritis Rheum 1997;40:551–561.

23. Hunt JE, Simpson RJ, Krilis SA. Identification of a region of β_2-glycoprotein I critical for lipid binding and anti-cardiolipin antibody cofactor activity. Proc Natl Acad Sci USA 1993;90:2141–2149.

24. Hunt JE, Krilis SA. The fifth domain of β_2-glycoprotein I contains a phospholipid binding site (Cys ^{281}–Cys ^{288}) and a region recognized by anti-cardiolipin antibodies. J Immunol 1994;152:653–661.

25. Sheng Y, Sali A, Herzog H, Lahnstein J, Krilis S. Site-directed mutagenesis of recombinant human $\beta_2$glycoprotein I identifies a cluster of lysine residues that are critical for phospholipid binding and anti-cardiolipin antibody activity. J Immunol 1996;157:3744–3751.

26. Del Papa N, Sheng YH, Raschi E, Kandiah DA, Tincani A, Khamashta MA et al. Human β_2-glycoprotein I binds to endothelial cells through a cluster of lysine residues that are critical for anionic phospholipid binding and offers epitopes for anti-β_2-glycoprotein I antibodies. J Immunol 1998;160:5572–5578.

27. Coull BM, Levine SR, Brey RL. The role of anti-phospholipid antibodies and stroke. Neurol Clin 1992;10:125–143.

28. Fajardo LF. The complexity of endothelial cells. Am J Pathol 1989;92:241–250.

29. Page C, Rose M, Yacoub M, Pigott R. Antigenic heterogeneity of vascular endothelium. Am J Pathol 1992;14:673–683.

30. Hess DC, Shepard JC, Adams RJ. Increased immunoglobulin binding to cerebral endothelium in patients with aPL. Stroke 1993;24:994–999.

31. Simantov R, LaSala JM, Lo SK, Gharavi AE, Sammaritano LR, Salmon JE et al. Activation of cultured vascular endothelial cells by antiphospholipid antibodies. J Clin Invest 1995;96:2211–2219.

32. George J, Blank M, Levy Y, Meroni PL, Damianovich M, Tincani A et al. Differential effects of anti-beta 2 glycoprotein I antibodies on endothelial cells and on the manifestations of experimental antiphospholipid syndrome. Circulation 1998;97:900–906.

33. Nawrot P, Stern D. Endothelial cell procoagulant properties and the host response. Semin Thromb Hemost 1987;13:391–398.

34. Kaplanski G. Increased serum soluble VCAM-1 in the anti-phospholipid syndrome. Lupus 1996;5 (Suppl):S548 (abstract).
35. Carlos TM, Harlam JM. Leukocyte-endothelial adhesion molecule. Blood 1994;84:2068–2101.
36. Pierangeli S, Colden Stanfield M, Liu X, Harris EN. Antiphospholipid antibodies activate endothelial cells in vitro and in vivo. Lupus 1998;7 (Suppl):S179 (abstract).
37. Habib A, Martinuzzo M, Carreras LO, Levy-Toledano S, Maclouf J. Increased expression of inducible cyclooxygenase-2 in human endothelial cells by antiphospholipid antibodies. Thromb Haemost 1995;74:770–777.
38. Lellouche F, Martinuzzo ME, Said P, Maclouf J, Carreras LO. Imbalance of thromboxane/prostacyclin biosynthesis in patients with lupus anticoagulant. Blood 1991;78:2894–2899.
39. Atsumi T, Khamashta MA, Haworth RS, Brooks G, Amengual O, Ichikawa K et al. Arterial disease and thrombosis in the anti-phospholipid syndrome: a pathogenic role for endothelin 1. Arthritis Rheum 1998;41:800–807.
40. Goldman D, Philips G, Back K, Petri M. Binding of SLE antibodies on apoptotic cells. Arthritis Rheum 1995;38 (Suppl):S214 (abstract).
41. Fadok VA, Voelker DR, Campbell PA, Cohen JJ, Bratton DL, Henson PM. Exposure of phosphatidylserine on the surface of apoptotic lymphocytes triggers specific recognition and removal by macrophages. J Immunol 1992;148:2207–2215.
42. Casciola-Rosen L, Rosen A, Petri M, Schlissel M. Surface blebs on apoptotic cells are sites of enhanced pro-coagulant activity implications for coagulation events and antigenic spread in SLE. Proc Natl Acad Sci USA 1996;93:1624–1629.
43. Manfredi AA, Rovere P, Galati G, Heltai S, Bozzolo E, Soldini L et al. Apoptotic cell clearance in systemic lupus erythematosus. I. Opsonization by antiphospholipid antibodies. Arthritis Rheum 1998;40:205–214.
44. Manfredi AA, Rovere P, Heltai S, Galati G, Nebbia G, Tincani A et al. Apoptotic cell clearance in systemic lupus erythematosus. II. Role of β_2-glycoprotein I. Arthritis Rheum 1998;40(2):215–222.
45. Rouch J, Subang R, Koh JS, Levine JS. Induction of anti-phospholipid antibodies by β2-glycoprotein I bound to apoptotic thymocytes. Lupus 1998;7(Suppl.):66.
46. Nakamura N, Shidara Y, Kawaguchi N, Azuma C, Mitsuda N, Onishi S et al. Lupus anticoagulant autoantibody induces apoptosis in HUVEC: involvement of annexin V. Biochem Byophis Res Commun 1994;205:1488–1493.
47. Bordron A, Dueymes M, Levy Y, Jamin C, Ziporen L, Piette JC et al. Anti-endothelial cell antibody binding makes negatively charged phospholipids accessible to antiphospholipid antibodies. Arthritis Rheum 1998;41:1738–1747.
48. Rand JH, Wu XX, Andree HAM, Lockwood CJ, Guller S., Scher J et al. Pregnancy loss in the antiphospholipid-antibody syndrome – a possible thrombogenic mechanism. N Engl J Med 1997;337:154–160.
49. Roubey RAS. Immunology of the antiphospholipid antibody syndrome. Arthritis Rheum 1996;39:1444–1454.

31 The Influence of Antiphospholipid Antibodies on the Protein C Pathway

P. G. de Groot and R. H. W. M. Derksen

Introduction

Blood coagulation is the mechanism that maintains the integrity of the high pressure closed circulatory system of blood. To prevent extravasation of the blood after injury, the hemostatic mechanism, which include platelets, plasma coagulation and fibrinolytic proteins and endothelial cells, is activated. A platelet plug will be formed that prevents further blood loss. Subsequently, the coagulation cascade replaces the unstable platelet plug by the stable fibrin clot. An essential feature of the hemostatic reaction is that platelet deposition and fibrin formation is localized and limited to the immediate area of the injury. Therefore, it is essential that different natural anticoagulant mechanisms are operative to regulate coagulation. When the natural anticoagulant mechanisms do not function optimally, this will lead to thrombotic complications. One of the most important natural anticoagulant systems is the protein C pathway [1]. Many patients that have been described with heterozygote protein C deficiency and familial thrombophilia highlight the importance of anticoagulant properties of protein C. Complete protein C deficiency represents a potentially lethal condition. Thrombotic complications can be controlled with protein C replacement [2, 3].

Antiphospholipid antibodies (aPL) are a heterogeneous group of autoantibodies defined by two very distinct assay methods. One group, called lupus anticoagulant (LA), is defined as antibodies that inhibit in vitro phospholipid-dependent coagulation assays. The second group, anticardiolipin antibodies (aCL), is defined by their ability to bind to negatively charged phospholipids in an enzyme-linked immunosorbent assay (ELISA) [4]. Paradoxically, the presence of aPL in plasma is a major risk factor for developing arterial and venous thrombosis and is not correlated with a bleeding diathesis, as should be expected when clotting tests are prolonged [5]. The relation between the aPL in plasma of patients and the risk for thromboembolic complications is still unexplained but an attractive hypothesis is that the aPL interfere with (one of) the natural anticoagulant pathways in the body. In this chapter we will discuss one of these possibilities: a link between aPL and the protein C system.

Protein C Axis

In the early 1980s, a phospholipid dependent antithrombotic pathway was described that shortly turned out to be one of the bodies major defense to uncontrolled coagulation. Vascular endothelium expresses a membrane bound receptor on its surface, thrombomodulin, which binds thrombin and thereby alters its substrate specificity. Thrombin bound to thrombomodulin is no longer able to activate platelets or to convert fibrinogen into fibrin, but it converts a vitamin K-dependent protein, protein C, into activated protein C (APC) [6]. APC is a physiological anticoagulant via its potential to inactivate clotting factors Va and VIIIa, which results in inhibition of further thrombin formation (Fig. 31.1). Thrombomodulin also influences fibrinolysis. Thrombin bound to thrombomodulin activates TAFI (thrombin inducible fibrinolysis inhibitor, carboxypeptidase B). TAFI removes carboxy terminal lysine residues from fibrin, thereby preventing the binding of tissue plasminogen activator (tPA) and plasmin(ogen) to fibrin. TAFI thus reduces fibrinolysis. Activation of TAFI is thought essential for the stability of a fibrin clot [7].

Protein C is a vitamin K dependent glycoprotein with a molecular weight of 62 kDa. In blood it circulates as an inactive zymogen of a serine protease APC, mostly in the form of a two-chain molecule [8]. The thrombin–thrombomodulin complex activates protein C by splitting off a 12-amino acid activation peptide after cleavage at position Arg 169. The plasma concentration of protein C is 4 μg/ml ($\pm$ 65 μM) and the circulating level of APC in healthy subjects is about 2.2 ng/ml [9]. The biological half life of protein C is about 8 hours. In plasma, APC is neutralized by forming complexes with the APC inhibitor (PCI or PAI-3), α_1-antiproteinase (α_1-antitrypsin) and α_2-macroglobulin. The inactivation of APC by PCI is accelerated by heparin [10].

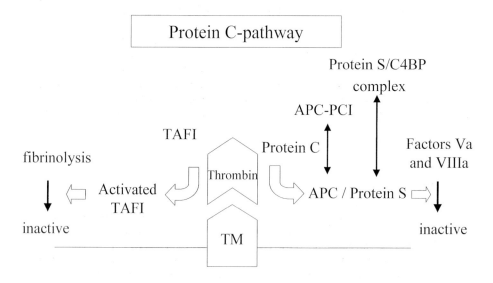

Figure 31.1. The protein C pathway.

Protein S, another vitamin K-dependent protein, amplifies the activity of APC. Protein S is a single chain plasma glycoprotein with a molecular weight of 70 kDa [11]. The total plasma concentration of protein S is about 25 μg/ml (350 μM). The biological half-life of protein S is 42.5 hours. Protein S forms a 1 : 1 complex with APC on phospholipid surfaces. Two independent processes regulate the APC cofactor activity of protein S. First, protein S is cleaved by thrombin, resulting is a molecule that has lost its APC cofactor function [12]. The second inhibition of APC cofactor activity of protein S is the result of its ability to form a 1:1 complex with C4b-binding protein (C4BP). Approximately 60% of plasma protein S circulates in complex with C4BP. Only the free form of protein S has APC cofactor activity [13]. The complex between protein S and C4BP arises by a non-covalent association between protein S and the β-chain of C4BP. About 80% of C4BP in the circulation are composed of seven α-chains and one β-chain, joined together by inter-chain disulfide bridges in the C-terminal region. The remaining C4BP contains only α-chains. During acute-phase reactions the plasma levels of C4BP increases dramatically, however, due to the preferential synthesis of the α-chain, only β-chain free C4BP is synthesized and the levels of free protein S remain stable during inflammation.

The discovery of the concept of activated protein C resistance followed by the explanation of the resistance by a mutation in clotting factor V further emphasizes the importance of the protein C-axis as an antithrombotic pathway [14, 15]. During blood coagulation factor V is converted into factor Va. Factor Va serves as a non-enzymatic cofactor in the prothrombinase complex. The presence of factor Va tremendously accelerates further thrombin formation [16]. Factor Va is inactivated by proteolytic degradation of its heavy chain by APC. The inactivation is a sequential event; the first cleavage takes place at Arg 506, followed by cleavages at Arg 306 and Arg 679. The first cleavage results in a partly inactivated form of factor Va with 30% residual activity, cleavage at Arg 306 results in a completely inactive molecule [17].

In 1993 Dahlbäck and coworkers described patients with thrombophilia whose plasma was resistant to APC [14]. With this APC-resistance test large populations of thrombophilic patients could be characterized. In 1994, a point mutation in factor V gene was identified as the genetic risk factor that described the patients with APC resistance [15]. The point mutation is a G → A transition of nucleotide 1691, which predicts the synthesis of a variant factor V molecule with an Arg 506Gln mutation. Replacement of Arg 506 by Gln will prevent cleavage of factor Va by APC, which results in a delay in the inactivation of factor Va and thus a sustained thrombin formation.

Specificity of APL

Research over the last 10 years has shown that the subset of aPL that are related to the risk for thromboembolic complications do not in fact recognize phospholipids alone. In conventional aCL and LA assays the antibodies are primarily directed towards different phospholipid-binding proteins, most notably β_2-glycoprotein I and prothrombin [18, 19]. Both β_2-glycoprotein I and prothrombin bind to negatively charged phospholipids. When bivalent complexes between two target molecules and one antibody molecule are formed, the affinity for a phospholipid surface of β_2-glycoprotein I and prothrombin increases about 1000 times, which subsequently favors the binding of the complexes to phospholipids over the binding of other phospholipid binding proteins present in plasma [20].

The recognition that, in the classic assays to detect aPL, plasma proteins involved in hemostasis are the real target for aPL logically led to the deduction that the pathogenesis of thrombosis is the result of interference of the antibodies with the biological function of the target proteins. Moreover, the essential role of two plasma proteins in the detection of aPL indicates that, besides β_2-glycoprotein I and prothrombin, other proteins present in plasma and proteins expressed by blood cells and the endothelium may be involved in the pathogenesis of the syndrome. Indeed, a large number of antibodies directed to other phospholipid binding proteins have been identified. The most interesting antibodies found are antibodies directed against protein C, protein S and thrombomodulin, because the presence of these antibodies could immediately link the antibodies to thromboembolic complications [21, 22].

aPL and the Protein C Axis

The assembly of coagulation complexes on negatively charged phospholipid surfaces is a prerequisite for their activity: no exposure of anionic phospholipid binding, no activity. Prolongation of the coagulation assays by aPL is the result of competition between the antibodies and clotting factors for the available catalytic surface. Also, assembly of the APC-protein S complexes on anionic phospholipid surfaces is essential for the catalytic activity. Thus it is logical to assume that when aPL inhibit the binding of the clotting factors, they also inhibit the binding of protein C and protein S and thereby their activity. Extensive investigations, however, have shown that there are more interactions between aPL, their "cofactors", and the protein C axis. Long before the discovery of the role of "cofactors" in the aPL syndrome, Canfield and Kisiel isolated an APC inhibitor with a N-terminal amino acid sequence identical to β_2-glycoprotein I [23]. This original and forgotten observation has been repeated and extended to characterize aPL/β_2-glycoprotein I as an inhibitor to the protein C system.

The antibodies can interfere with the protein C system in different ways [24].

1. The antibodies inhibit the formation of thrombin, the activator of protein C (the *thrombin paradox*)
2. The antibodies inhibit the activation of protein C via interference with thrombomodulin (*antithrombomodulin antibodies*).
3. The antibodies inhibit APC activity (*acquired APC resistance*). This can be achieved:
   a) via inhibition of the assembly of the proteins on the anionic surface;
   b) via direct inhibition of APC activity;
   c) via antibodies against the cofactors Va and VIIIa.
4. The antibodies interfere with the level of protein C and/or S (*acquired protein C/S deficiency*).

The Thrombin Paradox

At first glance it is not easy to understand that inhibition of thrombin formation could cause thrombosis. In 1993, the group of Hanson et al. made an interesting

observation [25]. They infused 2 U/kg/min thrombin in baboons that were connected with an ex vivo thrombosis model. The low doses of thrombin reduced
platelet deposition and fibrin incorporation in the ex vivo thrombus. Circulating
APC levels increased significantly. This suggests that low doses of thrombin preferentially activate protein C.

These and other observations have led to the development of the so-called
"thrombin paradox" [25]: thrombin exerts both anti- and prothrombotic properties
(Table 31.1) and, as a consequence, thrombin is the key factor in the regulation of
hemostasis. When thrombin has so many different activities, its substrate specificity
should be well regulated. One of the fundamental ideas on thrombin activity is that,
due to the affinity of thrombin for its substrates and receptors, the concentration of
the formed thrombin is one of the main factors that determines its substrate
specificity (Fig. 31.2). When only low concentrations of thrombin are formed
protein C is preferentially activated. Thrombin is now an antithrombotic agent.
When more thrombin is formed, fibrinogen is converted into fibrin and factors V
and VIII are activated. Thrombin now expresses prothrombotic properties. When
large amounts of thrombin are formed, TAFI and factor XIII are activated resulting
in an antifibrinolytic response.

An attractive hypothesis to explain the prothrombotic action of aPL relies on its
well-known direct effect on thrombin formation. Low concentrations of APC circulate in normal individuals. This suggests a continuous activation of protein C and
thus a continuous low-level formation of thrombin. It can be hypothesized that the
presence of aPL inhibits this low-level thrombin formation and so decreases circulating APC levels. After damage of a vessel, there now will be insufficient circulating
APC to prevent uncontrolled thrombin formation and a thrombus is formed. In this
way aPL might shift the hemostatic balance to a more prothrombotic state.

Table 31.1. Activities of thrombin related to the hemostatic balance.

Substrate	Product	Activity
Fibrinogen	Fibrin	Prothrombotic
Factor V	Factor Va	Prothrombotic
Factor VIII	Factor VIIIa	Prothrombotic
Factor XI	Factor XIa	Prothrombotic
Platelets	Aggregation	Prothrombotic
Protein S	Inactivation	Prothrombotic
Protein C	APC	Antithrombotic
Endothelial cells	NO & PGI$_2$ production	Antithrombotic
Carboxypeptidase B (TAFI)	Activation	Antifibrinolytic
Urokinase	Inactivation	Antifibrinolytic
Factor XIII	Factor XIIIa	Antifibrinolytic

Antithrombomodulin Antibodies

In 1983, Comp et al described in an abstract that two out of seven IgGs isolated from
LA-positive plasmas inhibited protein C activation by thrombin [27]. They claimed
that the antibodies were directed towards thrombomodulin. Two French groups
using purified thrombomodulin or endothelial cells as source of thrombomodulin
extended these observations [28, 29]. However, other groups did not support these

The thrombin paradox

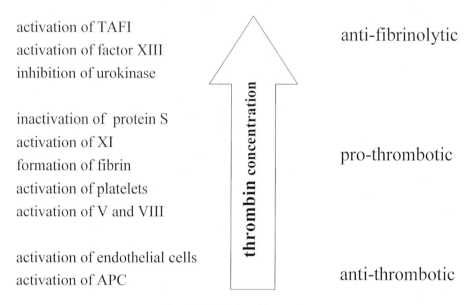

activation of TAFI

activation of factor XIII

inhibition of urokinase

anti-fibrinolytic

inactivation of protein S

activation of XI

formation of fibrin

activation of platelets

activation of V and VIII

pro-thrombotic

activation of endothelial cells

activation of APC

anti-thrombotic

thrombin concentration

Figure 31.2. The thrombin paradox.

observations [30–32]. Pötzsch et al. tested IgGs of 46 different patients with LA and found only two cases with reduced rate of APC formation [33]. The contradictory results are not easy to explain. There is no doubt that in some patients antibodies towards thrombomodulin can be detected. Whether these antibodies always inhibit the functional activity of thrombomodulin is not known. Thrombomodulin activity is regulated by the phospholipid composition in which it is incorporated. Differences in assay conditions might be one explanation for the observed contradictory results. The frequency of antithrombomodulin antibodies in the populations tested, however, is so low that it cannot be the mechanism that will explain the majority of the aPL-related thrombotic events.

A few publications showed raised levels of thrombomodulin in the circulation of patients with the aPL syndrome [34]. Raised levels of thrombomodulin point to an altered endothelial cell metabolism of thrombomodulin, e.g., an increased synthesis or a preferential secretion of newly synthesized molecules. It is not necessarily associated with a decreased expression of thrombomodulin on the endothelial cell surface. Moreover, circulating thrombomodulin might add to APC formation, protecting against thrombosis.

Acquired APC resistance

In a group of 175 patients with systemic lupus erythematosus (SLE) Fijnheer et al. showed that hereditary APC-resistance is not related to aPL [35]. However, a number of publications have shown that aPL inhibit the binding of protein C and protein S, thereby inhibiting their activity [e.g., 36–39]. The antibodies induce an "acquired APC resistance". Smirnov et al showed that aPL required the phospholipid PE to observe anti-APC activity [40]. When the assays were performed in the presence of PE, APL inhibit APC activity more potently than prothrombinase activity. There are enough clinical data that show that a partial reduction of prothrombin activation is not sufficient to induce a bleeding diathesis in patients. However, a partial reduction of APC anticoagulant activity is a major thrombotic risk [41]. These observations indicate that the presence of phosphatidylethanolamine (PE)-dependent antibodies should be a better predictor than other aPL for a thrombotic risk. Studies with PE and APC as antigen for aPL should clarify this point.

In an elegant study, Mori et al. showed that purified β_2-glycoprotein I inhibits the binding of protein C to phospholipids much better than the binding of prothrombin, resulting in a prothrombotic effect [42]. APL recognize protein C only in the presence of β_2-glycoprotein I [43]. These results suggest that aPL-induced protein C dysfunction is mediated by β_2-glycoprotein I. Galli et al suggested that the "APC-resistance" of aPL was strictly β_2-glycoprotein I-dependent and that antibodies directed against prothrombin lack this activity [44]. However, studies with affinity purified anti-β_2-glycoprotein I antibodies and antiprothrombin antibodies showed that there is no difference between both types of antibody [45].

An interesting but insufficiently studied option is that patients may have auto-antibodies directed against factor Va. These autoantibodies against factor Va should not influence its procoagulant function but they should protect factor Va from inactivation by APC.

Acquired Deficiencies of Protein C and/or Protein S

There are a number of publications describing acquired protein C or S deficiencies in isolated patients with aPL syndrome [see e.g., 46, 47]. Studies in larger populations of aPL positive patients failed to show a correlation between decreased protein C plasma levels and the presence of aPL. In one study, a small but significant decrease of plasma protein S levels was found, although protein S levels in the aPL antibody group still were within the normal range [48]. An interesting observation was made by Atsumi et al [49]. They found that β_2-glycoprotein I downregulates the binding between protein S and C4Bp significantly and that aPL abolish the β_2-glycoprotein I inhibitory effect. Thus, aPL increase the affinity of protein S for C4Bp which may result in an acquired free protein S deficiency. These observations warrant further investigations.

In general, no decrease in protein C or protein S were found in patients with aPL, but in some individual cases a combination of low levels of protein C or protein S in combination with the presence of aPL may be found. These cases are probably very susceptible for thrombotic complications.

Concluding Remarks

aPL are a heterogeneous population of antibodies directed against different phospholipid-binding proteins. It is unlikely that a single mechanism is responsible for the thrombogenic activity of all aPL. There are, however, a number of attractive hypotheses indicating that the antibodies selectively inhibit the natural anticoagulant pathways, in particular the protein C pathway. The most attractive hypotheses focussed on the induction of an acquired APC resistance and on a disturbed balance in the thrombin paradox. These concepts can be explained with aPL with different specificity. Deficiencies in the protein C pathway are correlated with venous thrombosis. Although exogenous APC could prevent arterial thrombosis in a number of animal models, it is questionable whether in aPL-related thrombosis, the same antibodies are responsible for both arterial and venous events. A safe conclusion is that interference of the protein C pathway can explain a large part of the venous complications in patients with the antiphospholipid syndrome.

Acknowledgment

Our own studies described in this review were supported by grants from Het Nationaal Reumafonds (grant no 97-1-401) and the Netherlands Heart Foundation (grant no 98.060).

References

1. Esmon CT. The protein C anticoagulant pathway. Arterioscler Thromb 1992;12:135–145.
2. Gresele P, Momi S, Berrettini M, Nenci GG, Schwarz HP, Semeraro N et al. Activated human protein C prevents thrombin induced thromboembolism in mice. J Clin Invest 1998;101:667–676.
3. Taylor FB, Chang A, Esmon CT, D'Angelo A, Vigano-D'Angelo S, Blick KE. Protein C prevents the coagulopathic and lethal effects of *Escherichia coli* infusion in the baboon. J Clin.Invest. 1987;9:918–925.
4. Hughes GRV. Hughes' syndrome: the antiphospholipid syndrome. A historical view. Lupus 1998;7:S1–S7.
5. De Groot PG, Oosting JD, Derksen RHWM. Antiphospholipid antibodies: specificity and pathophysiology. Baillière's Clin Haematol 1993;6:691–709.
6. Esmon CT. Owen WG. Identification of an endothelial cell cofactor for thrombin catalyzed activation of protein C. Proc Natl Acad Sci USA 1981;78:2249–2252.
7. Bajzar L, Morser J, Nesheim ME. TAFI, or plasma procarboxypeptidase B, couples the coagulation and fibrinolytic cascades through the thrombin-thrombomodulin complex. J Biol Chem 1996;271:16603–16608.
8. Lane DA, Mannucci PM, Bauer KA et al. Inherited thrombophilia, part 1. Thromb Haemost 1996;76:651–662.
9. Gruber A, Griffin JH. Direct detection of activated protein C in blood from human subjects. Blood 1992;79:2340–2348.
10. Suzuki K, Nishioka J, Hashimoto S. Protein C Inhibitor. Purification from human plasma and characterization. J Biol Chem 1983;258:163–168.
11. Di Scipio RG, Davie EW. Characterization of protein S, a γ-carboxyglutamic acid containing protein from bovine and human plasma. Biochemistry 1979;18:899–904.
12. Walker FJ. Regulation of vitamin K dependent protein S. Inactivation by thrombin. J Biol Chem 1984;259:10335–10339.
13. Dahlbäck B. Protein S and C4b-binding protein: components involved in the regulation of the protein C anticoagulant pathway. Thromb Haemost 1991;66:49–61.
14. Dahlbäck B, Carlsson M, Svennson PJ. Familiar thrombophilia due to a previous unrecognized mechanism characterized by poor anticoagulant response to activated protein C: prediction of a cofactor to activated protein C. Proc Natl Acad Sci USA 1993;90:1004–1008.
15. Bertina RM, Koeleman BPC, Koster T, Rosendaal FR, Dirven RJ, de Ronde H et al. Mutation in blood coagulation factor V associated with resistance to activated protein C. Nature 1994;369:64–67.

16. Ware AG, Murphy RC, Seegers WH. The function of Ac-globulin in blood clotting. Science 1947;106:618–619.
17. Rosing J, Tans G. Coagulation factor V: an old star shines again. Thromb Haemost 1997;78:427–433.
18. McNeil HP, Simpson RJ, Chesterman CN, Krilis SA. Antiphospholipid antibodies are directed against a complex antigen that includes a lipid binding inhibitor of coagulation: β_2-glycoprotein I (apolipoprotein H). Proc Natl Acad Sci USA 1990;87:4120–4124.
19. Bevers EM Galli M, Barbui T, Comfurius P, Zwaal RFA. Lupus anticoagulant IgG's (LA) are not directed to phospholipids only, but to a complex of lipid bound human prothrombin. Thromb Haemost 1991;66:629–632.
20. Willems GM, Janssen MP, Pelsers MAL, Comfurius P, Galli M, Zwaal RFA et al. Role of divalency in the high affinity binding of cardiolipin antibody-β_2-glycoprotein I complexes to lipid membranes. Biochemistry 1996;35:13833–13842.
21. Oosting JD, Derksen RHWM, Bobbink IWG, Hackeng T, Bouma BN, de Groot PG. Antiphospholipid antibodies are directed to a combination of phospholipids with prothrombin, protein C or protein S. An explanation for their pathogenic mechanism? Blood 1993;81:2618–2625.
22. Oosting JD, Preissner KT, Derksen RHWM, de Groot PG. Autoantibodies directed against the epidermal growth factor-like domains of thrombomodulin inhibit protein C activation in vitro. Br J Haematol 1993;85:761–768.
23. Canfield WM. Kisiel W. Evidence of normal functional levels of activated protein C inhibitor in combined factor V/VIII deficiency disease. J Clin Invest 1982;70:1260–1272.
24. De Groot PG, Horbach DA, Derksen RHWM. Protein C and other cofactors involved in the binding of antiphospholipid antibodies: relation to the pathogenesis of thrombosis. Lupus 1996;5:488–493.
25. Hanson SR, Harker LA, Kelly AB, Esmon CT, Gruber A. Antithrombotic effects of thrombin-induced activation of endogenous protein C in primates. J Clin Invest 1993;92:2003–2012.
26. Griffin JH. Blood coagulation: the thrombin paradox. Nature 1995;23:378 (comment).
27. Comp PC, deBault LE, Esmon NL, Esmon CT. Human thrombomodulin is inhibited by IgG from two patients with non specific anticoagulants. Blood 1983;62:299 (abstract).
28. Freyssinet JM, Weisel JM, Gauchy J, Boneu B, Casanave JP. An IgM lupus anticoagulant that neutralizes the enhancing effect of phospholipids on purified endothelial thrombomodulin activity. A mechanism for thrombosis. Thromb Haemost 1986;55:309–313.
29. Cariou R, Tobelem G, Bellucci S, Soria J, Soria C, Maclouf J et al. Effect of lupus anticoagulant on antithrombotic properties of endothelial cells. Inhibition of thrombomodulin-dependent protein C activation. Thromb Haemost 1988;60:54–58.
30. Oosting JD Derksen RHWM, Hackeng TM, van Vliet M, Preissner KT, Bouma BN et al. In vitro studies of antiphospholipid antibodies and its cofactor, β_2-glycoprotein I, show no effect on endothelial cell mediated protein C activation. Thromb Haemost 1991;66:666–671.
31. Watson KV, Schorer AE. Lupus anticoagulant inhibition of in vitro prostacyclin release is associated with a thrombosis-prone subset of patients. Am J Med 1991;90:47–53.
32. Keeling DM, Wilson AJG, Mackie IJ, Isenberg DA, Machin SJ. Role of β_2-glycoprotein I and antiphospholipid antibodies in activation of protein C in vitro. J Clin Pathol 1993;46:908–911.
33. Pötzsch B, Kawamura H, Preissner KT, Schmidt M, Seelig C, Müller-Berghaus G. Acquired protein C dysfunction but not decreased activity of thrombomodulin is a possible marker of thrombophilia in patients with lupus anticoagulant. J Lab Clin Med 1995;125:56–65.
34. Kawakami M, Kitani A, Hara M, Harigai M, Suzuki K, Kawaguchi Y et al. Plasma thrombomodulin and α2-plasmin inhibitor-plasmin complexes are elevated is systemic lupus erythematosus. J Rheumatol 1992;19:1704–1709.
35. Fijnheer R, Horbach DA, Donders RCJM, Vilé H, van Oort E, Nieuwenhuis HK et al. Factor V Leiden, antiphospholipid antibodies and thrombosis in systemic lupus erythematosus. Thromb Haemost 1996;76:514–517.
36. Kitchen, Malia RG, Preston FE. Inhibition of protein S cofactor activity by antiphospholipid antibodies. Br J Haematol 1989;71:3.
37. Marciniak E, Romond EH. Impaired catalytic function of activated protein C: a new in vitro manifestation of lupus anticoagulant. Blood 1989;74:2426–2432.
38. Malia RG, Kitchen S, Greaves M, Preston FE. Inhibition of activated protein C and its cofactor protein S by antiphospholipid antibodies. Br J Haematol 1989;76:101–107.
39. Borrell M, Sala N, de Castellarnau C, Lopez S, Gari M, Fontcuberta J. Immunoglobulin fractions isolated from patients with antiphospholipid antibodies prevent the inactivation of factor Va by activated protein C on human endothelial cells. Thromb Haemost 1992;68:268–273.
40. Amer L, Kisiel W, Searles RP, Williams RC Jr. Impairment of the protein C anticoagulant pathway in a patient with systemic lupus erythematosus, anticardiolipin antibodies and thrombosis. Thromb Res 1990;57:247–258.

41. Esman NL, Smirnov MD, Esman CT. Thrombogenic mechanisms of antiphospholipid antibodies. Thromb. Haemostas 1997;78:79–82.

42. Mori T, Takeya H, Nishioka, Gabazza EC, Suzuki K. β_2 glycoprotein I modulates the anticoagulant activity of protein C on the phospholipid surface. Thromb Haemost 1996;75:49–55.

43. Atsuma T, Khamashta MA, Amengual O, Donohoe S, Mackie I, Ichikawa K et al. Binding of anti-cardiolipin antibodies to protein C via β_2-glycoprotein I : A possible mechanism in the inhibitory effect of antiphospholipid antibodies on the protein C system. Clin Exp Immunol 1998;112:325–333.

44. Galli M, Ruggeri L, Barbui T. Differential effects of anti-β_2-glycoprotein I and antiprothrombin antibodies on the anticoagulant activity of activated protein C. Blood 1998;91:1999–2004.

45. Horbach DA, van Oort E, Derksen RHWM, de Groot PG. Anti-prothrombin antibodies with LAC activity inhibits tenase, prothrombinase and protein C activity by increasing the affinity of prothrombin for phospholipids. Lupus 1998;7:S209.

46. Harrison RL, Alperin JB. Concurrent protein C deficiency and lupus anticoagulant. Am J Hematol 1992;40:33–37.

47. Parke AL. The thrombotic diathesis associated with the presence of phospholipid antibodies may be due to low levels of free protein S. Am J Med 1992;93:49–56.

48. Hasselaar P, Derksen RHWM, Blokzijl L, Hessing M, Nieuwenhuis HK, Bouma BN et al. Risk factors for thrombosis in lupus patients. Ann Rheum Dis 1989;48:933–940.

49. Atsumi T, Khamashta MA, Ames PRJ, Ichikawa K, Koike T, Hughes GRV. Effect of β_2-glycoprotein I and human monoclonal anticardiolipin antibody on the protein S/C4b-binding protein system. Lupus 1997;6:358–364.

32 Tissue Factor Pathway in Antiphospholipid Syndrome

P. M. Dobado-Berrios, C. López-Pedrera, F. Velasco and M. J. Cuadrado

Introduction

Thrombosis is the key lesion of the antiphospholipid syndrome (APS) [1,2]. Several non-exclusive mechanisms have been proposed to explain the involvement of antiphospholipid antibodies (aPL) in the pathogenesis of thrombosis in APS. These include inhibition of endothelial cell prostacyclin production [3–8], procoagulant effects on platelets [9, 10], impairment of fibrinolysis [11] and interference with the thrombomodulin–protein C–protein S pathway [12–14]. In addition, several studies have suggested that aPL can induce procoagulant activity (PCA) on vascular endothelial cells [9, 15, 16] and monocytes [10, 17–19].

Tissue factor

PCA is mainly a tissue factor (TF)-like activity in that it accelerates clotting through the extrinsic coagulation pathway, it is abolished by phospholipase C and it is inhibited by anti-TF antibodies [9, 15, 17, 20, 21].

TF (previously known as thromboplastin) is a specific transmembrane single-chain glycoprotein composed of 263 amino acids (47 kDa), that requires interaction with specific membrane phospholipids (PL) to become functionally active [22–24]. Unlike other coagulation factors, TF activity does not depend on proteolysis [25], therefore induction of PCA merely requires TF exposure on cell surfaces [26]. TF serves as both high-affinity receptor and enzyme activator for plasma FVII or $FVII_a$ in initiating a localized PCA on the anionic PL cell surface. The bimolecular complex of TF and FVII or $FVII_a$ activates rapidly FX. FX_a is the active enzyme in the prothrombinase complex (X_a-V_a) that converts prothrombin into thrombin (FII_a). Thrombin is the major serine protease that activates platelets and cleaves fibrinogen to form fibrin, leading to clot formation. Besides initiating the extrinsic coagulation pathway, the TF–$FVII_a$ complex activates coagulation through the intrinsic pathway by cleaving FIX to FIX_a, which, when complexed with $FVIII_a$ rapidly activates FX [13, 25, 27–30].

TF is widely accepted to be the major initiator of in vivo coagulation [25]. It is also believed that TF has a key role in fibrin deposition in immunologic disorders, as well as in disseminated intravascular coagulation (DIC) and clot formation in Gram-negative bacterial sepsis, cancer, and inflammatory bowel disease [23, 24, 31].

TF is expressed on the surface of many cell types but, in the resting state, is normally absent from cells in contact with blood [32]. However, TF (or PCA) can be induced, in vitro, to appear on endothelial cells and monocytes in a transcriptionally-regulated manner [33–35] by several physiologic or non-physiologic stimuli including shear stress [36], endotoxin [20], immune complexes [37], and the cytokines interleukin 1 (IL-1) [38] and tumor necrosis factor (TNF) [23, 39, 40].

Soluble TF has been also measured in plasma. Elevated levels have been reported in patients with DIC [41, 42], thrombotic thrombocytopenic purpura (TTP), vasculitis associated with collagen diseases, diabetic microangiopathy, and chronic renal failure receiving haemodialysis [41]. Measurement of soluble TF in plasma may be useful for evaluating the endothelial damage and cell destruction of TF-bearing cells [41].

The catalytic activity of the TF–FVII$_a$ complex to activate FX is inhibited by the TF pathway inhibitor (TFPI, extrinsic pathway inhibitor), a multivalent Kunitz-type plasma proteinase which forms inert and stable quaternary complexes with FX$_a$, FVII$_a$ and TF [25]. Approximately 20% of total TFPI circulates in human plasma as free form, which exhibits anticoagulant effect [43], whereas the remaining of total TFPI circulates as complexes with lipoproteins [44]. Depletion of TFPI sensitizes rabbits to DIC experimentally induced by TF [45] or endotoxin [46]. Infusion of TFPI abrogates DIC induced by these triggers [47, 48] and prevent experimental venous thromboses in rabbits [49]. There are several reports regarding TFPI plasma levels in a range of disorders, particularly low levels in TTP [50] and moderately low TFPI activity in atherothrombotic and lacunar infarction [51]. Elevated plasma levels of TFPI have been found in patients with DIC [50, 52], suggesting that there may be enhanced synthesis and/or release of TFPI in stimulated endothelial cells.

This chapter focuses on the contribution of the TF pathway to the pathogenesis of thrombosis in patients with APS.

TF Pathway in APS

In Vivo Behavior of TF Pathway

Several studies have shown in vivo upregulation of TF pathway in patients with APS. These patients have higher plasma levels of soluble TF than healthy controls [19, 53–55]. There was no difference between those with primary APS (PAPS) and those with APS secondary to systemic lupus erythematosus (SLE) [19]. Among PAPS patients, the highest values of soluble TF have been found in hypertensive men. No significant correlation has been observed between soluble TF and circulating levels of autoantibodies including IgG and IgM anticardiolipin antibodies (aCL) [55].

Soluble TF in APS plasma probably represents molecules coming from TF-producing cells [53]. In 1985, Cole et al [56] demonstrated, in patients with SLE and glomerulonephritis, a marked increase in a partially characterized PCA that spontaneously originated in the monocyte fraction of the mononuclear blood cells (MBC). More recently, we have shown that TF-related PCA and TF mRNA levels in MBC, as well as the cell-surface expression of TF on monocytes, are increased in PAPS patients with thrombosis when compared with those without and with healthy controls [54, 57]. TF expression in these patients has been found to be further increased in those positive for IgG aCL (> 20 IgG PL units), but not in those positive for IgM aCL (> 20 IgM PL units) or Lupus anticoagulant. In addition, TF expression in PAPS does not appear to be related to plasma levels of TNF-α and IL-1β, two inflammatory mediators that influence TF production, suggesting that inflammatory changes do not determine TF production in the steady state[54].

Patients with APS, either primary or secondary to SLE, also have high plasma levels of free and total TFPI [19, 43]. This finding could reflect endothelial activation or damage since, among SLE patients, free TFPI correlates positively with the activity of the disease, and both free and total TFPI correlate with the degree of organic damage [43]. In addition, increased free TFPI might be considered as further evidence of activation of TF pathway in vivo. Since TFPI appears to function as an antithrombotic agent against extrinsic coagulation pathway, increased plasma levels in patients with the APS and a history of thrombosis are a protective effect against the procoagulant tendency seen in this syndrome [19].

In Vitro Studies

TF upregulation in APS is reproducible in vitro. Plasma (or serum) from patients with APS can induce increased PCA on human umbilical vein endothelial cells (HUVEC) [9, 15, 16] and normal donor MBC [18, 19], as well as increased TF expression on normal monocytes [18, 19]. These effects seem to be restricted mostly to the plasma from patients with aPL and a history of thrombosis [9, 18], whereas plasma from individuals with or without aPL but no previous thromboses could have no apparent effect [18]. In addition, a positive correlation can be observed between plasma-induced TF antigen expression on cell surface and plasma levels of soluble TF [19], as well as between MBC PCA and monocyte TF expression induced by patients' plasma [18, 19]. The ability of APS plasma to promote TF-dependent MBC PCA and monocyte TF expression also correlates positively with levels of plasma thrombin-antithrombin III and prothrombin fragment 1+2, suggesting increased turnover of coagulation [18].

Potentiation of HUVEC PCA by aPL-containing sera from SLE patients is strongly decreased after depleting IgG from sera [9]. Fractions of human APS sera containing monomeric IgG, IgM, or IgA, as well as high molecular weight-IgG, or heat-aggregated IgG, each cause HUVEC to increase PCA characteristic of TF [9, 15, 16]. These results indicate that the factor(s) responsible for the induction of TF activity resides, at least in part, in the Ig fraction of the serum. In line with their results obtained with plasmas, Reverter et al [18] have shown that purified IgG aCL from three APS patients with previous thrombotic episodes induce a significant increase in both MBC PCA and monocyte TF expression, as compared with purified IgG aCL from two SLE individuals without thrombosis. The same authors have also reported an increase on TF expression on normal monocytes using affinity-purified IgM aCL (with anti-β_2-glycoprotein I (β_2GPI) activity) from two patients with the APS and a history of thrombosis [10]. IgG monoclonal aCL (Mo-aCL) have been established from mice that had experimental APS [58, 59]. These antibodies, otherwise able to induce APS in mice [58, 59], stimulate normal MBC to increase PCA [17]. Similar results have been reported by Reverter et al [10] and Amengual et al [19] following incubation of normal MBC with human IgM Mo-aCL (with anti-β_2GPI activity) from patients with the APS and a history of thrombosis or fetal loss. In the latter study, human IgM Mo-aCL also induced TF mRNA on HUVEC and normal MBC [19]. All these findings support that, at least, some of aCL are able to induce TF expression in vitro on HUVEC and monocytes. This may be considered as a direct activation at least in the case of monocytes, given that Mo-aCL are not dependent on T lymphocytes for the induction of TF-like activity in normal MBC [17].

Mechanisms for the Induction of TF Expression by aPL

The mechanism(s) by which aPL induce TF expression is unknown. Arnout and coworkers have proposed a hypothesis for antibody-mediated thrombosis in APS based on similarities with the mechanisms involved in the syndrome of heparin-induced thrombocytopenia and thrombosis [60, 61]. An initial damage causing local cell activation is an obvious requirement to trigger the proposed mechanism.

Early studies showed that non-specific antibodies, both polyclonal and mono-clonal, also induce a strong TF-like activity in normal monocytes, in vitro [62], which may suggest that a broad spectrum of IgG (not only IgG aCL) can induce TF-like activity in monocytes through interaction of their Fc region with the surface FcγRII [17]. However, the effects of IgG Mo-aCL are noted with as little as 0.01 to 1 μg/ml [17], whereas the concentration of non-specific antibodies required to induce a similar effect is 100- to 1000-fold higher [62]. This finding may reflect the fact that FcγRII has a much higher affinity for antigen-bound IgG than for monomeric IgG [63], an indirect evidence that also fits Arnout's hypothesis [61].

In at least two studies, the aCL responsible for the in vitro stimulation of TF exhibited anti-β_2GPI activity, and β_2GPI was indeed present in the aCL-containing incubation media [10, 19]. There is evidence for increased β_2GPI deposition in pla-centas obtained from patients with APS [64, 65]. However, β_2GPI binding to mem-branes containing physiologic concentrations of anionic PL appears to be relatively weak [66]. Roubey [67] has suggested that anti-β_2GPI antibodies could stabilize the β_2GPI–anionic PL interaction by cross-linking membrane-bound β_2GPI.

In secondary APS, anti-β_2GPI antibodies are mainly restricted to the IgG2 sub-class [68]. The FcγRII reacts best with murine IgG1 and IgG2b, and human IgG1 and IgG3. However, the binding of human IgG2 is weak except for a FcγRII pheno-type with a single Arg $\rightarrow$ His change at amino acid 131 which allows an efficient interaction [68, 69]. Besides antibody specificity, both IgG subclass and FcγRII phenotype could play therefore a role in IgG aPL-mediated TF expression [61]. However, Atsumi et al [68] have recently shown that FcγRII polymorphism does not correlate with the manifestations of APS (including venous/arterial thrombosis, recurrent pregnancy loss and thrombocytopenia), and that FcγRII genotype is not a genetic marker of APS.

Further questions arise from the study by Kornberg et al [17], in which incuba-tion of normal MBC with F(ab')$_2$ fragments of a Mo-aCL also induced a potent PCA. This finding raises the possibility that binding of aPL to PL-bound proteins on the cell surface, apart from mediating cell activation via the FcγRII, may be in itself a synergistic (or alternative) way by which aPL induce TF expression.

Rand and coworkers have proposed a thrombogenic mechanism [28, 30], in which the high affinity of the aPL for anionic PL-bound proteins on the cell surface may in itself explain the prothrombotic effects including TF expression. They suggest that annexin V has a physiologic role in inhibiting coagulation, by forming clusters that bind with high affinity to anionic PL on cell surfaces exposed to flowing blood, and thus *fully* shielding these surfaces from the assembly of the TF–FVII$_a$ and other coagulation complexes. In the APS, the affinity of the aPL for anionic PL-bound proteins (such as β_2GPI) would be strong enough to disrupt or prevent the assembly of the annexin V protective "carpet" on the PL cell surface. The membrane surface would then exhibit *partial* occupancy by aPL, because of the topographical differences between annexin V- and aPL-binding to PL. This would result in an increased net amount of exposed anionic PL available for the assembly of the TF–FVII$_a$ and other coagulation complexes.

Implications for Therapy

There is no consensus about the secondary prevention of thromboses in the APS [70]. Different therapeutic regimens using immunosuppressive, antiplatelet, and anti-coagulant agents have been performed [1, 2, 71]. Low rates of recurrence have been reported among patients receiving long-term anticoagulation therapy in which an international normalized ratio of ≥ 3 is maintained [72]. Oral anticoagulants act by impairing membrane binding by the vitamin K-dependent coagulation factors [14] including FVII, i.e., the ligand for TF to activate coagulation. Thus, even when high TF activity is present, oral anticoagulants reduce availability of functional FVII, thus minimizing the thrombotic risk.

Conclusions

Increased TF expression may contribute to explain the thrombotic episodes in patients with APS. Mechanism(s) of TF overexpression may involve binding of some aPL to endothelial cells and monocytes. In addition, elevated plasma levels of TFPI in APS patients could reflect either endothelial changes and/or a protective response to reduce their procoagulant tendency. Oral anticoagulants may minimize the thrombotic risk by leaving TF with reduced FVII substrate to activate coagulation.

References

1. Khamashta MA, Asherson RA. Hughes syndrome: antiphospholipid antibodies move closer to thrombosis in 1994. Br J Rheumatol 1995;34:493–494.
2. Lockshin MD. Answers to the antiphospholipid-antibody syndrome? N Engl J Med 1993;332:1025–1027.
3. Carreras LO, Defreyn G, Machin SJ, Vermylen J, Deman R, Spitz B et al. Arterial thrombosis, intrauterine death and lupus anticoagulant: detection of immunoglobulin interfering with prosta-cyclin formation. Lancet 1981;i:244–246.
4. Carreras LO, Vermylen JG. "Lupus" anticoagulant and thrombosis: possible role of inhibition of prostacyclin formation. Thromb Haemost 1982;48:28–40.
5. De Castellarnau C, Vila L, Sancho MJ, Borrell M, Fontcuberta J, Rurlant ML. Lupus anticoagulant, recurrent abortion, and prostacyclin production by cultured smooth muscle cells. Lancet 1983;ii:1137–1138.
6. Cariou R, Tobelem G, Bellucci S, Soria J, Soria C, Maclouf J et al. Effect of lupus anticoagulant on antithrombogenic properties of endothelial cells: inhibition of thrombomodulin-dependent protein C activation. Thromb Haemost 1988;60:54–58.
7. Schorer AE, Wickham NW, Watson KV. Lupus anticoagulant induces a selective defect in thrombin-mediated endothelial prostacyclin release and platelet aggregation. Br J Haematol 1989;71:399–407.

8. Schorer AE, Duane PG, Woods VL, Niewoehner DE. Some antiphospholipid antibodies inhibit phospholipase A_2 activity. J Lab Clin Med 1992;120:67–77.
9. Oosting JD, Derksen RHWM, Blokzijl L, Sixma JJ, de Groot PG. Antiphospholipid antibody positive sera enhance endothelial cell procoagulant activity: studies in a thrombosis model. Thromb Haemost 1992;68:278–284.
10. Reverter J-C, Tàssies D, Font J, Khamashta MA, Ichikawa K, Cervera R et al. Effects of human monoclonal anticardiolipin antibodies on platelet function and on tissue factor expression on monocytes. Arthritis Rheum 1998;41:1420–1427.
11. Ames PRJ, Tommasino C, Iannaccone L, Brillante M, Cimino R, Brancaccio V. Coagulation activation and fibrinolytic imbalance in subjects with idiopathic antiphospholipid antibodies: a crucial role for acquired free protein S deficiency. Thromb Haemost 1996;76:190–194.
12. Freyssinet J-M, Wiesel M-L, Gauchy J, Boneu B, Cazenave J-P. An IgM lupus anticoagulant that neutralizes the enhancing effect of phospholipid on purified endothelial thrombomodulin activity: a mechanism for thrombosis. Thromb Haemost 1986;55:309–313.
13. Oosting JD, Derksen RHWM, Bobbink IWG, Hackeng TM, Bouma BN, de Groot PG. Antiphospholipid antibodies directed against a combination of phospholipids with prothrombin, protein C, or protein S: an explanation for their pathogenic mechanism? Blood 1993;81:2618–2625.
14. Smirnov MD, Triplett DT, Comp PC, Esmon NL, Esmon CT. On the role of phosphatidylethanolamine in the inhibition of activated protein C activity by antiphospholipid antibodies. J Clin Invest 1995;95:309–316.
15. Tannenbaum SH, Finko R, Cines DB. Antibody and immune complexes induce tissue factor production by human endothelial cells. J Immunol 1986;137:1532–1537.
16. Branch DW, Rodgers GM. Induction of endothelial cell tissue factor activity by sera from patients with antiphospholipid syndrome: a possible mechanism of thrombosis. Am J Obstet Gynecol 1993;168:206–210.
17. Kornberg A, Blank M, Kaufman S, Shoenfeld Y. Induction of tissue factor-like activity in monocytes by anti-cardiolipin antibodies. J Immunol 1994;153:1328–1332.
18. Reverter J-C, Tàssies D, Font J, Monteagudo J, Escolar G, Ingelmo M et al. Hypercoagulable state in patients with antiphospholipid syndrome is related to high induced tissue factor expression on monocytes and to low free protein S. Arterioscler Thromb Vasc Biol 1996;16:1319–1326.
19. Amengual O, Atsumi T, Khamashta MA, Hughes GRV. The role of the tissue factor pathway in the hypercoagulable state in patients with the antiphospholipid syndrome. Thromb Haemost 1998;79:276–281.
20. Colucci M, Balconi G, Lorenzet R, Pietra A, Locati D, Donati MB et al. Cultured human endothelial cells generate tissue factor in response to endotoxin. J Clin Invest 1983;71:1893–1896.
21. Williams FMK, Jurd K, Hughes GRV, Hunt BJ. Antiphospholipid syndrome patients' monocytes are "primed" to express tissue factor. Thromb Haemost 1998;80:864–865.
22. Nemerson Y, Gentry R. An ordered addition, essential activation model of the tissue factor pathway of coagulation: evidence for a conformational cage. Biochemistry 1986;25:4020–4033.
23. Nemerson Y. Tissue factor and hemostasis. Blood 1988;71:1–12.
24. Rodgers GM. Hemostatic properties of normal and perturbed vascular cells. FASEB J 1988;2:116–123.
25. Nemerson Y. The tissue factor pathway of blood coagulation. Semin Hematol 1992;29:170–176.
26. Petersen LC, Valentin S, Hedner U. Regulation of the extrinsic pathway system in health and disease: the role of factor VIIa and tissue factor pathway inhibitor. Thromb Res 1995;79:1–47.
27. Galli M, Bevers EM. Inhibition of phospholipid-dependent coagulation reactions by "antiphospholipid" antibodies: possible modes of action. Lupus 1994;3:223–228.
28 Rand JH, Wu X-X, Andree HAM, Ross JBA, Rusinova E, Gascon-Lema MG et al. Antiphospholipid antibodies accelerate plasma coagulation by inhibiting annexin-V binding to phospholipids: a "lupus procoagulant" phenomenon. Blood 1998;92:1652–1660.
29. Mackman N, Morrissey JH, Fowler B, Edgington TS. Complete sequence of the human tissue factor gene, a highly regulated cellular receptor that initiates the coagulation protease cascade. Biochemistry 1989;28:1755–1762.
30. Rand JH, Wu X-X, Andree HAM, Lockwood CJ, Guller S, Scher J et al. Pregnancy loss in the antiphospholipid syndrome: a possible thrombogenic mechanism. N Engl J Med 1997;337:154–160.
31. Weis JR, Pitas RE, Wilson BD, Rodgers GM. Oxidized low-density lipoprotein increases cultured human endothelial cell tissue factor activity and reduces protein C activation. FASEB J 1991;5:2459–2465.
32. Osterud B, Flaegstad T. Increased tissue thromboplastin activity in monocytes of patients with meningococcal infection: related to an unfavourable prognosis. Thromb Haemost 1983;49:5–7.

33. Gregory SA, Morrissey JH, Edgington TS. Regulation of tissue factor gene expression in the monocyte procoagulant response to endotoxin. Mol Cell Biol 1989;9:2752-2755.
34. Mackman N. Regulation of the tissue factor gene. FASEB J 1995;9:883-889.
35. Courtney MA, Haidaris PJ, Marder VJ, Sporn LA. Tissue factor mRNA expression in the endothelium of an intact umbilical vein. Blood 1996;87:174-179.
36. Lin MC, Almus-Jacobs F, Chen HH, Parry GCN, Mackman N, Shyy JYJ et al. Shear stress induction of the tissue factor gene. J Clin Invest 1997;99:737-744.
37. Schwartz BS, Edgington TS. Immune complex-induced human monocyte procoagulant activity: a rapid unidirectional lymphocyte-instructed pathway. J Exp Med 1981;154:892-906.
38. Nawroth PP, Handley DA, Esmon CT, Stern DM. Interleukin 1 induces endothelial cell procoagulant while suppressing cell-surface anticoagulant activity. Proc Natl Acad Sci USA 1986;83:3460-3464.
39. Bevilacqua MP, Pober JS, Majeau GR, Fiers W, Cotran RS, Gimbrone MA Jr. Recombinant tumor necrosis factor induces procoagulant activity in cultured human vascular endothelium: characterization and comparison with the actions of interleukin 1. Proc Natl Acad Sci USA 1986;83:4533-4537.
40. Conway EM, Bach R, Rosenberg RD, Konigsberg WH. Tumor necrosis factor enhances expression of tissue factor mRNA in endothelial cells. Thromb Res 1989;53:231-241.
41. Koyama T, Nishida K, Ohdama S, Sawada M, Murakami N, Hirosawa S et al. Determination of plasma tissue factor antigen and its clinical significance. Br J Haematol 1994;87:343-347.
42. Wada H, Nakase T, Nakaya R, Minamikawa K, Wakita Y, Kaneko T et al. Elevated plasma tissue factor antigen level in patients with disseminated intravascular coagulation. Am J Hematol 1994;45:232-236.
43. Marco P, Roldán V, Fernández C, Verdú J, De Paz F, García C. Niveles del inhibidor del factor tisular (TFPI) en pacientes con lupus eritematoso sistémico (LES): relación con la actividad y daño orgánico. Haematologica 1998;83 (Supl 2):8 (abstract).
44. Hubbard AR, Jennings CA. Inhibition of the tissue factor-factor VII complex: involvement of factor Xa and lipoproteins. Thromb Res 1987;46:527-537.
45. Sandset PM, Warn-Cramer BJ, Rao LVM, Maki SL, Rapaport SI. Depletion of extrinsic pathway inhibitor (EPI) sensitizes rabbits to disseminated intravascular coagulation induced with tissue factor: evidence supporting a physiologic role for EPI as a natural anticoagulant. Proc Natl Acad Sci USA 1991;88:708-712.
46. Sandset PM, Warn-Cramer BJ, Maki SL, Rapaport SI. Immunodepletion of extrinsic pathway inhibitor sensitizes rabbits to endotoxin-induced intravascular coagulation and the generalized Shwartzman reaction. Blood 1991;78:1496-1502.
47. Day KC, Hoffman LC, Palmier MO, Kretzmer KK, Huang MD, Pyla EY et al. Recombinant lipoprotein-associated coagulation inhibitor inhibits tissue thromboplastin-induced intravascular coagulation in the rabbit. Blood 1990;76:1538-1545.
48. Bregengard C, Nordfang O, Wildgoose P, Svendsen O, Hedner U, Diness V. The effect of two-domain tissue factor pathway inhibitor on endotoxin-induced disseminated intravascular coagulation in rabbits. Blood Coag Fibrinol 1993;4:699-706.
49. Holst J, Lindblad B, Bergqvist D, Nordfang O, Ostergaard PB, Peterson JG et al. Antithrombotic effect of recombinant truncated tissue factor pathway inhibitor (TFPI-161) in experimental venous thrombosis: a comparison with low molecular weight heparin. Thromb Haemost 1994;71:214-219.
50. Kobayashi M, Wada H, Wakita Y, Shimura M, Nakase T, Hiyoyama K et al. Decreased plasma tissue factor pathway inhibitor levels in patients with thrombotic thrombocytopenic purpura. Thromb Haemost 1995;73:10-14.
51. Abumiya T, Yamaguchi T, Terasaki T, Kokawa T, Kario K, Kato H. Decreased plasma tissue factor pathway inhibitor activity in ischemic stroke patients. Thromb Haemost 1995;74:1050-1054.
52. Takahashi H, Sato N, Shibata A. Plasma tissue factor pathway inhibitor in disseminated intravascular coagulation: comparison of its behavior with plasma tissue factor. Thromb Res 1995;80:339-348.
53. Atsumi T, Khamashta MA, Amengual O, Hughes GRV. Up-regulated tissue factor expression in antiphospholipid syndrome. Thromb Haemost 1997;77:222-223.
54. Cuadrado MJ, López-Pedrera C, Khamashta MA, Camps MT, Tinahones F, Torres A et al. Thrombosis in primary antiphospholipid syndrome: a pivotal role for monocyte tissue factor expression. Arthritis Rheum 1997;40:834-841.
55. Cuadrado MJ, Dobado-Berrios PM, López-Pedrera C, Gómez-Zumaquero JM, Tinahones F, Jurado A et al. Variability of soluble tissue factor in primary antiphospholipid syndrome. Thromb Haemost 1998;80:712-713.
56. Cole EH, Schulman J, Urowitz M, Keystone E, Williams C, Levy GA. Monocyte procoagulant activity in glomerulonephritis associated with systemic lupus erythematosus. J Clin Invest 1985;75:861-868.

57. Dobado-Berrios PM, Lopez-Pedrera C, Velasco F, Aguirre MA, Torres A, Cuadrado MJ. Increased levels of tissue factor mRNA in mononuclear blood cells of patients with primary antiphospholipid syndrome. Thromb Haemost 1999;82:1578–1582.

58. Blank M, Cohen J, Toder V, Shoenfeld Y. Induction of anti-phospholipid syndrome in naive mice with mouse lupus monoclonal and human polyclonal anti-cardiolipin antibodies. Proc Natl Acad Sci USA 1991;88:3069–3073.

59. Bakimer R, Fishman P, Blank M, Sredni B, Djaldetti M, Shoenfeld Y. Induction of primary antiphospholipid syndrome in mice by immunization with a human monoclonal anticardiolipin antibody (H-3). J Clin Invest 1992;89:1558–1563.

60. Arnout J. The pathogenesis of the antiphospholipid syndrome: a hypothesis based on parallelisms with heparin-induced thrombocytopenia. Thromb Haemost 1996;75:536–541.

61. Vermylen J, Hoylaerts MF, Arnout J. Antibody-mediated thrombosis. Thromb Haemost 1997;78:420–426.

62. Rothberger H, Zimmerman TS, Spiegelberg HL, Vaughan JH. Leukocyte procoagulant activity: enhancement of production in vitro by IgG and antigen antibody complexes. J Clin Invest 1977;59:549–554.

63. De Reys S, Blom C, Lepoudre B, Declerck PJ, De Ley M, Vermylen J et al. Human platelet aggregation by murine monoclonal antiplatelet antibodies is subtype-dependent. Blood 1993;81:1792–1800.

64. Chamley LW, Pattison NS, McKay EJ. Elution of anticardiolipin antibodies and their cofactor β_2-glycoprotein I from placentae of patients with a poor obstetric history. J Reprod Immunol 1993;25:209–220.

65. La Rosa L, Meroni PL, Tincani A, Balestrieri G, Faden D, Lojacono A et al. β_2-glycoprotein I and placental anticoagulant protein I in placentae from patients with antiphospholipid syndrome. J Rheumatol 1994;21:1684–1693.

66. Roubey RAS, Harper MF, Lentz BR. The interaction of β_2-glycoprotein I with phospholipid membranes. Arthritis Rheum 1995;38 (Suppl 9):S211 (abstract).

67. Roubey RAS. Immunology of the antiphospholipid antibody syndrome. Arthritis Rheum 1996;39:1444–1454.

68. Atsumi T, Caliz R, Amengual O, Khamashta MA, Hughes GRV. Fcγ receptor IIA H/R131 polymorphism in patients with antiphospholipid antibodies. Thromb Haemost 1998;79:924–927.

69. Brandt JT, Isenhart CE, Osborne JM, Ahmed A, Anderson CL. On the role of platelet FcγRIIa phenotype in heparin-induced thrombocytopenia. Thromb Haemost 1995;74:1564–1572.

70. Lockshin MD. Which patients with antiphospholipid antibody should be treated and how? Rheum Dis Clin N Am 1993;19:235–247.

71. Asherson RA, Chan JKH, Harris EN, Gharavi AE, Hughes GRV. Anticardiolipin antibody, recurrent thrombosis, and warfarin withdrawal. Ann Rheum Dis 1985;44:823–825.

72. Khamashta MA, Cuadrado MJ, Mujic F, Taub NA, Hunt BJ, Hughes GRV. The management of thrombosis in the antiphospholipid-antibody syndrome. N Engl J Med 1995;332:993–997.

33 Plasminogen Activation and Fibrinolysis in the Antiphospholipid Syndrome

E. Anglés-Cano

Fibrinolysis and Pericellular Proteolysis in the Vascular Wall

The vascular endothelium is a non-thrombogenic surface. This antithrombotic state is maintained by the expression of antiplatelet, anticoagulant and fibrinolytic activities [1]. The contribution of the endothelium to these mechanisms varies with the degree of activation induced by several stimulators including thrombin and cytokines (tumor necrosis factor-α (TNF-α), interleukin-1 (IL-1)) released from inflammatory cells and platelets. The activated phenotype is characterized by the expression of von Willebrand factor, prostacyclin, thrombomodulin, tissue-type plasminogen activator (t-PA, M_r 71 000) and plasminogen activator inhibitor type-1 (PAI–1, M_r 50 000), among other factors [2, 3, 4]. Endothelial cells may also express a receptor for t-PA [5]. PAI-1 released from endothelial cells is very labile and its activity must be stabilized by vitronectin (M_r 75 000) both in plasma and in the extracellular matrix [4]. Active PAI-1 regulates the activity of t-PA through the formation of inactive t-PA–PAI-1 complexes. Alternatively, t-PA released from endothelial cells binds to either its endothelial receptor or to newly formed fibrin and becomes thereby the main plasminogen activator of the intravascular space. The basic mechanism underlying fibrinolysis, the transformation of plasminogen into plasmin, is therefore a fibrin-induced mechanism [6] to which the endothelial cell surface may contribute [1] (Fig. 33.1). Plasmin once formed remains bound to the cell membrane or to the surface of fibrin, a condition that prevents inhibition by α_2-antiplasmin (M_r 71 000). However, plasmin released into the circulation during fibrinolysis is rapidly inhibited by α_2-antiplasmin with a second order rate constant of $2-4 \times 10^7$/M/s. Solid-phase activation and liquid-phase inhibition ensure thereby the specificity of fibrinolysis and control the extent of fibrin degradation.

Other cells in the vascular wall or included in the clot, such as monocytes and leukocytes, may also contribute to fibrinolysis although they are mainly involved in other proteolytic activities of plasmin collectively known as pericellular proteolysis [7] (Fig. 33.1). These cells synthesize prourokinase (single-chain urokinase-type plasminogen activator, scu-PA, M_r 54 000) and its specific receptor u-PAR (urokinase-type plasminogen activator receptor, CD-87, M_r 55 000) [8]. The u-PAR may also be expressed by endothelial cells [9]. It has been well demonstrated that prourokinase is the most important activator for pericellular proteolysis in the extravascular space. Recent studies suggest that prourokinase, which has no affinity for fibrin, may induce

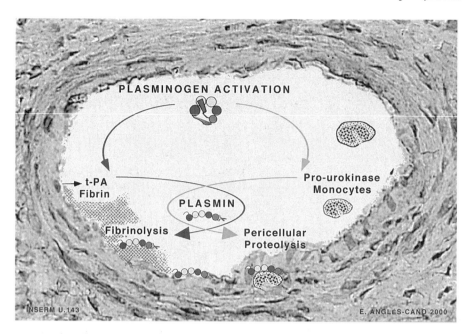

Figure 33.1. Fibrinolysis and pericellular proteolysis in the vascular wall. Cross-section of an arteriole. The endothelial cell lining is marked with a peroxidase-labeled antibody directed against the tissue-type plasminogen activator (t-PA) [2]. Circulating plasminogen bound to fibrin and membrane proteins is transformed into plasmin either at the surface of fibrin by fibrin-bound t-PA released from endothelial cells or by prourokinase bound to its cellular receptor.

fibrin specific lysis by activating plasminogen bound to new binding sites unveiled by plasmin on degrading fibrin [10].

Colocalization of activators and plasminogen on fibrin and cell membranes results in efficient plasmin formation that plays a major role in fibrinolysis as well as in endothelial cell thromboresistance and in a variety of other cellular functions. The latter include tissue remodeling, migration of monocytes to the subendothelium, patency of tissue tubular structures, proteolytic activation of metalloproteinases (collagenase) and growth factors, among others [7, 11]. These mechanisms are regulated at the plasminogen activator level by PAI-1 present in plasma or released from platelets [12]. PAI-1 reacts with single-chain and two-chain t-PA and with two-chain urokinase, but not with single-chain urokinase (prourokinase). The second order rate constant for inhibition of these enzymes is in the order of $10^7/M/s$. A second type of plasminogen activator inhibitor, PAI-2, has been identified and may also play a role in fibrinolysis and pericellular proteolysis [13].

The activation of plasminogen may be abnormally inhibited by other factors. For instance, the atherogenic lipoprotein Lp(a) may interfere with fibrinolysis and pericellular proteolysis by its ability to compete with plasminogen for binding to fibrin and cell membranes [14, 15]. The different population of autoantibodies observed in APS may disturb fibrinolysis and contribute thereby to vascular complications. Thrombosis may therefore result from an impaired or insufficient fibrinolytic cellular response to vascular injury provoked by factors such as Lp(a) and autoanti-bodies. The relationship between autoantibodies and fibrinolysis in APS is analyzed in this chapter.

Protein Interactions with Biological Surfaces: Beyond Fibrinolysis, Autoimmunity

Plasmin is a large spectrum proteolytic enzyme that cleaves lysyl and arginyl peptide-bonds in a number of proteins. Under physiological conditions its activity is, however, specifically restricted to the lysis of fibrin, to extracellular matrix remodeling and to the activation of growth factors and metalloproteinases. To develop these specialized and specific functions, plasmin must be generated at the surface of fibrin or cell membranes. The surface dependence of this reaction is closely related to: (1) the organization of fibrinolytic proteins as an array of struc-tural domains with functional autonomy [16]; (2) the structure of fibrin [17]; and (3) the assembly of phospholipid–protein complexes on the membrane of platelets, monocytes, leukocytes and endothelial cells [18].

Proteins intervening in fibrinolysis are composed of a serine-proteinase region and several distinct domains (Fig. 33.2). Prourokinase is composed of an epidermal growth factor (EGF) and a kringle domain. The EGF domain contains a sequence that is recognized by the urokinase receptor. t-PA contains a domain called "finger", an EGF domain and two kringle domains. The finger domain allows binding of t-PA to fibrin. Plasminogen (M_r 93 000) consists of five homologous triple-loop structures or "kringle" domains and an amino-terminal peptide of 77 residues [19]. A variable

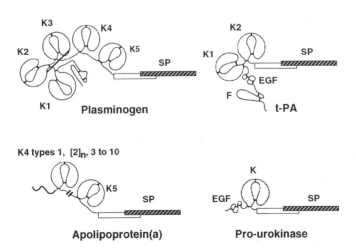

Figure 33.2. Domain structure of apo(a), plasminogen and its activators. The serine-proteinase (SP) region is located at the COO-terminal end. The domains "kringle" (K), finger (F) and epidermal growth factor-like (EGF) are localized in the amino-terminal extension [16]. Apo(a) contains a variable number of a domain homologous to plasminogen kringle 4, and single copies of kringle 5 and the serine-proteinase region.

number (10–40) of copies of kringle 4, and single copies of kringle 5 and the serine-proteinase domain of plasminogen are present in an apolipoprotein [apo(a)] that is disulfide linked to the apo B100 of a low-density lipoprotein (LDL) to form Lp(a) the lipoprotein particle [20]. Kringle 4 in plasminogen and the corresponding kringle 4 copies in apo(a) share functional properties with regard to binding to fibrin and cell surfaces. In contrast, the serine-proteinase domain of apo(a) cannot be cleaved by activators and remains in an inactive state. Apo(a) may therefore inhibit plasminogen binding and thereby fibrinolysis [14, 15].

The formation of fibrin unveils binding sites for t-PA and plasminogen that are buried in fibrinogen. Fibrinogen is a complex molecule composed of three pairs of polypeptide chains, $(A\alpha, B\beta$ and $\gamma)_2$, linked by disulfide bonds and organized in a trinodular structure [21]. The amino-terminal regions form the central domain E that is linked to two globular D domains by a coiled-coil connector region. The binding site for t-PA is most probably located in region D or in D-dimers in a sequence that interacts with the finger domain of t-PA. Binding of plasminogen to fibrin is mediated by interactions between the lysine-binding sites of kringles 1 and 4 and lysine residues of fibrin. Binding of t-PA and plasminogen to fibrin results in a trimolecular complex with catalytic advantages. Plasmin thus formed cleaves lysyl bonds in fibrin and unveils new carboxy-terminal lysine residues [22] to which plasminogen may bind [23] (Fig. 33.3). Since plasminogen bound to carboxy-terminal lysines of progressively degraded fibrin is readily transformed into plasmin by fibrin-bound t-PA, this mechanism represents the most important pathway for the acceleration and amplification of fibrinolysis [24].

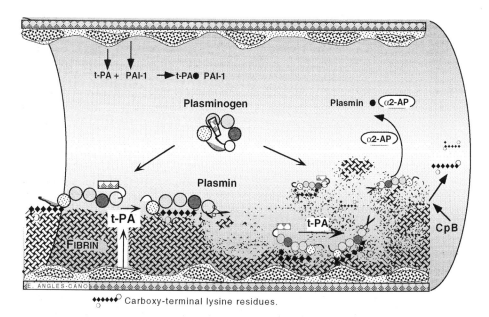

Carboxy-terminal lysine residues.

Figure 33.3. Acceleration of fibrinolysis by carboxy-terminal lysine and regulation by PAI-1 and α2-antiplasmin. Plasmin unveils new carboxy-terminal lysine residues to which plasminogen bind [23]. Plasma carboxypeptidase B (CpB) may regulate fibrinolysis by cleaving these residues [72].

The phospholipid bilayer provides both a hydrophobic milieu and anionic charges for proteins engaged in interactions at the cell surface such as coagulation factors and β_2-glycoprotein I (β_2GPI) [25]. The receptor for prourokinase is attached to the phospholipid bilayer through a glycosylphosphatidylinositol anchor. Plasminogen and t-PA binds to "integral" membrane proteins: a receptor for t-PA (annexin II) [v], and a number of membrane proteins with exposed carboxy-terminal lysine residues to which plasminogen binds [26]. As for the fibrin surface, degradation of membrane proteins by plasmin unveils new carboxy-terminal lysine residues for plasminogen binding [27].

The assembly of activators and plasminogen onto distinct binding sites of these surfaces results in conformational changes that are of physiological significance but also lead to exposure of domains with different antigenic properties. These neo-epitopes may evoke an autoimmune response in patients with immunological dis-orders. Autoantibodies directed against an epitope exposed on fibrin-bound t-PA in the sera of patients with scleroderma [28], systemic lupus erythematosus (SLE) [29] and primary pulmonary hypertension [30] have been described. These observations suggest that conformational changes of molecules upon binding to their ligands results in the expression of conformation-induced neoepitopes. This phenomenon is probably similar to the reactivity of antiphospholipid antibodies against β_2GPI (or other proteins) bound to anionic phospholipid surfaces.

Endothelial Cell Dysfunction and Fibrinolysis in APS

Following the original description 20 years ago, of impaired fibrinolysis associated with thrombosis and antiphospholipid antibodies in SLE [31], a number of reports confirmed these findings [32, 33, 34]. Although these abnormalities were not found in some reports [35], in recent studies it has been further shown that the hypo-fibrinolysis detected in these patients is most probably a manifestation of endo-thelial cell dysfunction, as indicated by increased plasma levels of PAI-1 and t-PA antigens [36, 37, 38, 39]. t-PA thus detected circulates complexed to PAI-1 and is therefore inactive, a condition which explains why hypofibrinolysis is observed in the presence of high t-PA antigenic levels (Fig. 33.4). High levels of PAI-1 have been associated with an increased risk of thromboembolic disease and myocardial infarc-tion [40]. These manifestations of endothelial cell dysfunction have been found in association with antibodies directed against endothelial cells, or with the presence of immune complexes, thus suggesting that endothelial cells are important sites of action for antibodies that have role in the pathogenesis of thrombosis [41]. Of note, patients with primary pulmonary hypertension present signs of endothelial cell dys-function (elevated PAI-1 and t-PA plasma antigens) [42] and may have antiphos-pholipid antibodies [43].

Similar manifestations of endothelial dysfunction have also been found in primary APS [44, 45], though at present there are no solid arguments to propose a direct asso-ciation between aPL and impaired fibrinolysis in the thrombotic manifestation of APS [46, 47, 48]. It has been shown, however, that antiendothelial cell antibodies in sera of patients with SLE and in patients with primary and secondary APS may alter the fibrinolytic activity of endothelial cells [49]. Of note, antiphospholipid and anti-endothelial cell antibodies may coexist in both primary and secondary APS [50, 51].

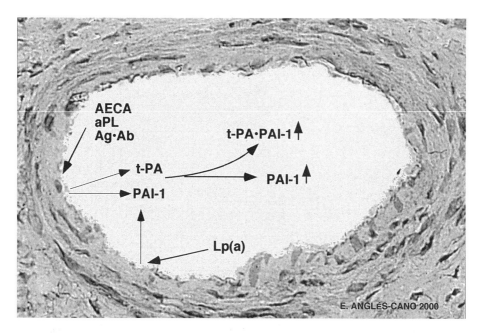

Figure 33.4. Anti-endothelial cell antibodies (AECA), antiphospholipid antibodies (aPL) and immun complexes (Ag–Ab) may stimulate/activate endothelial cells [41, 51–3]. This immuno-stimulation/activation may induce the release of both t-PA and PAI-1. Lp(a) may also stimulate the release of PAI-1 [14]. The t-PA thus released forms inactive complexes with PAI-1, which circulates in excess over t-PA. Thus, increased levels of t-PA and PAI-1 after endothelial cell activation result in low fibrinolytic activity.

Furthermore, cross-reaction between these antibodies has been demonstrated [52]. Whether autoantibodies to phospholipid-binding proteins, i.e., β_2GPI, are able to stimulate cells or platelets bearing the phospholipid–protein complex on their membrane has not as yet been clarified. However, it has been recently reported that antiphospholipid antibodies may directly activate vascular endothelial cells and induce E-selectin expression. The activation requires the presence of β_2GPI [53]. It is possible that such antibodies may induce the secretion of others markers of endothelial cell injury/activation such as t-PA and PAI-1. The increased levels of PAI-1 and t-PA– PAI-1 complexes may explain the low fibrinolytic activity in a similar fashion as in patients with SLE [31].

Current Research: aPL, Lp(a) and the β_2GPI, apo(a) and Plasmin Connections

Recent clinical and experimental evidence suggest that Lp(a), the atherothrombogenic particle, may be implicated in the thrombotic complications of APS (Fig. 33.5). The mechanism by which high Lp(a) levels may favor atherothrombosis is still a matter of debate but the fact that Lp(a) has both LDL and plasminogen-like moieties suggest that Lp(a) may constitute a link between the processes of atherosclerosis and

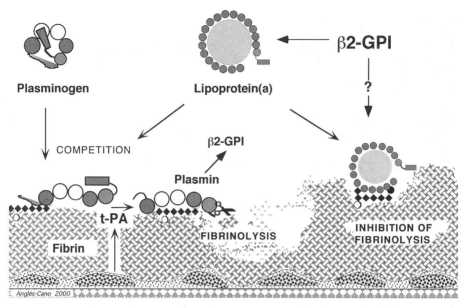

Figure 33.5. Lp(a) effects on fibrinolysis and β_2GPI, apo(a) and plasmin interactions. Apo(a) the characteristic glycoprotein of Lp(a) shares structural homology with plasminogen and impairs its binding to cells and fibrin thus inhibiting fibrinolysis and pericellular proteolysis [55]. β_2GPI may be localized on these surfaces through interactions with apo(a) [67] and may be proteolysed by plasmin [68, 69].

thrombosis. A number of experimental in vitro studies resulted in convincing evidence that Lp(a) binds to the fibrin surface and cell membranes and thereby competes with plasminogen so as to inhibit its activation [54, 55]. Such unique behavior was attributed to the fibrin-binding properties conferred by the kringle 4 repeats of apo(a) [56]. The levels of Lp(a) are under genetic control by the apo(a) gene and are not modified by current pharmacological means employed to decrease LDL. A few pathological conditions (acute-phase reactions, nephrotic syndrome) may produce a transitory increase in Lp(a) levels. Increased levels of Lp(a) has also been reported in autoimmune diseases [57, 58, 59] including primary and secondary APS [60, 61, 62, 63, 64, 65, 66]. Since Lp(a) levels are genetically determined and no correlation between Lp(a) levels and aPL was found, the question remains as whether these patients had already a high Lp(a) before developing the autoimmune disease. The high Lp(a) levels observed in these patients may impair plasminogen binding and/or induce the secretion of PAI-1 by endothelial cells, two mechanisms that may contribute to the thrombotic complications in APS as suggested by Atsumi et al [65]. However, the effect of high Lp(a) levels on plasminogen binding to fibrin or cells in these patients remains to be determined.

Besides being an additional factor for thrombosis, high Lp(a) levels in APS may be of importance within the context of recent data indicating that β_2GPI may interact with distinct kringle 4 domains of apo(a) in a specific manner [67]. The interaction of apo(a) with β_2GPI requires a sequence (181 amino acids) contained in the short consensus repeats (SCR or "sushi" domain) 2 to 4. The interaction was demonstrated with apo(a) in both its free form and as a part of the Lp(a) particle. The role of this interaction remains unknown. It may, however, be of pathophysiological relevance if in the presence of high Lp(a) levels, the β_2GPI-Lp(a) complex could be the trigger of decreased fibrinolytic activity. Binding of the β_2GPI-Lp(a) complex to fibrin and cells may also favor localization of β_2GPI to these surfaces where it may be cleaved by plasmin. Indeed, it has been recently shown that β_2GPI is very sensitive to cleavage by plasmin between Lys 317 and Thr 318 [68]. The resulting forms bind to negatively charge phospholipids with much lower affinity [69]. This phenomenon has been demonstrated in vivo in patients with an activated fibrinolytic system, i.e., disseminated intravascular coagulation and thrombolytic therapy. Plasmin formed on cells membranes may also cleave phospholipid-bound β_2GPI. The implication of this proteolytic processing of β_2GPI by plasmin on the interaction of aPL with β_2GPI–phospholipid complexes remains to be determined. It is possible that the nicked form of β_2GPI may not react with aPL, thus implying that plasminogen activation may function as a mechanism of defense against antibody-mediated thrombosis that, when impaired, may favor the cortege of clinical symptoms of APS.

New Directions and Perspectives in Fibrinolysis and APS

The description of newer autoantibodies and the recognition of other pathways that regulate fibrinolysis may open new directions of research in the pathophysiology of fibrinolysis and antibody-induced thrombosis (Table 33.1). Some of the most recent areas that deserve investigation follows.

It has been proposed that neoepitopes exposed by conformational changes due to surface assembly of components of the fibrinolytic system, may evoke an autoimmune response in patients with immunological disorders [70]. Autoantibodies to fibrin-bound t-PA have been observed in SLE and scleroderma patients with vascular disorders and may be important in the vascular events of APS if they coexist with anti-β_2GPI/phospholipid antibodies. In this light, the reported cross-reaction of aPL with oxidized LDL [71], a major atherosclerotic component, needs to be studied on Lp(a) as this composite LDL- and plasminogen-like particle has been found increased in primary and secondary APS. The fact that Lp(a) interferes with fibrinolysis, and decreases the fibrinolytic potential of endothelial cells, underscores the relevance of these studies.

It has recently been suggested that activated carboxipeptidase B, an exopeptidase present in plasma in a proenzyme form, may play a role in the downregulation of fibrinolysis by cleaving carboxy-terminal lysine residues, the plasminogen binding

Table 33.1. Fribrinolysis in APS: current research and new directions.

1. Relevance of high Lp(a) levels [65].
2. Apo(a)/Lp(a) and β_2GPI interactions [67].
3. Proteolysis of β_2GPI by plasmin [68, 69].
4. Relevance of new autoantibodies [70].
5. The carboxypeptidase B pathway [72]
6. Annexin II and plasminogen activation [5, 73]

sites unveiled by plasmin on fibrin [72] (Fig. 33.3). This mechanism may protect fibrin clots from fibrinolysis. The activation of procarboxypeptidase B requires thrombomodulin–bound thrombin generated through the phospholipid-dependent factor XI activation pathway. The thrombin-thrombomodulin complexes also activate protein C, and aPL have been show to interfere with this mechanism. Impaired protein C activation by aPL may shift the activation effect of the thrombin–thrombomodulin complex to procarboxypeptidase B, and favor the inhibition of fibrinolysis by active carboxypeptidase B. The study of downregulated fibrinolysis by the carboxypeptidase B pathway in patients with APS has not as yet been investigated.

Endothelial cell surface plasmin generation is promoted through the binding of both plasminogen and t-PA to the calcium-dependent phospholipid-binding protein, annexin II [73]. Annexin II tetramer bound to phospholipid vesicles also stimulates the activation of plasminogen [74]. Annexins constitute a family of proteins with homologous amino acid and cDNA sequences. Because both aPL and annexin II have affinity for anionic phospholipids, it is possible that, as recently proposed for annexin V in coagulation [75], aPL may interfere with the t-PA and plasminogen-binding function of annexin II. This mechanism may result in impaired fibrinolysis, a hypothesis that deserves investigation.

References

1. Cines DB, Pollak ES, Buck CA, Loscalzo J, Zimmerman GA, McEver RP et al. Endothelial cells in physiology and in the pathophysiology of vascular disorders. Blood 1998;91:3527–3561
2. Anglés-Cano E, Balaton A, Le Bonniec B, Genot E, Elion J, Sultan Y. Production of monoclonal antibodies to the high fibrin-affinity, tissue-type plasminogen activator of human plasma. Demonstration of its endothelial origin by immunolocalization. Blood 1985;66:913–920.
3. Meidell RS. Endothelial dysfunction and vascular disease. Am J Med Sci 1994;30:7378–389.
4. Stefansson S, Haudenschild CC, Lawrence DA. Beyond fibrinolysis: the role of plasminogen activator inhibitor-1 and vitronectin in vascular wound healing. Trends Cardiovasc Med 1998;8:175–180.
5. Hajjar KA. The endothelial cell tissue plasminogen activator receptor. Specific interaction with plasminogen. J Biol Chem 1991;266:21962–21970.
6. Collen D, Lijnen HR. Fibrin-specific fibrinolysis. Ann NY Acad Sci 1992; 667:259–271.
7. Vassalli JD, Sappino A-P, Belin D. The plasminogen activator/plasmin system. J Clin Invest 1991;88:1067–1072.
8. Behrendt N, Stephens RW. The urokinase receptor. Fibrinol Proteol 1998;12:161–204.
9. Barnathan ES, Kuo A, Kariko K et al. Characterization of human endothelial cell urokinase-type plasminogen activator receptor protein and messenger RNA. Blood 1990;76:1795–1786.
10. Fleury V, Lijnen HR, Anglés-Cano E. Mechanism of the enhanced intrinsec activity of single-chain urokinase-type plasminogen activator during ongoing fibrinolysis. J Biol Chem 1993;2688:18554–18559.
11. Ellis V, Dano K. Plasminogen activation by receptor-bound urokinase. Semin Thromb Haemost 1991;17:194–200.
12. Loskutoff DJ. Regulation of PAI-1 gene expression. Fibrinolysis 1991;5:197–206.
13. Ritchie H, Robbie LA, Kinghorn S, Exley R, Booth NA. Monocyte plasminogen activator inhibitor 2 (PAI-2) inhibits u-PA-mediated fibrin clot lysis and is cross-linked to fibrin. Thromb Haemost 1999;81:96–103.
14. Anglés-Cano E. Structural basis for the pathophysiology of lipoprotein(a) in the athero-thrombotic process. Braz J Med Biol Res 1997;30:1271–1280.
15. Scanu AM. Atherothrombogenicity of lipoprotein(a): the debate. Am J Cardiol 1998;88:26Q–33Q.
16. Patthy L. Evolution of blood coagulation and fibrinolysis. Blood Coag Fibrinol 1990;1:153–166.
17. Doolittle RF, Spraggon G, Everse SJ. Three-dimensional structural studies on fragments of fibrinogen and fibrin. Curr Opin Struct Biol 1998;8:792–798.
18. Zwaal RFA, Schroit AJ. Pathophysiologic implications of membrane phospholipid asymmetry in blood cells. Blood 1997;89:1121–1132.

19. Petersen TE, Martzen MR, Ichinose A, Davie EW. Characterization of the gene for human plasminogen, a key proenzyme in the fibrinolytic system. J Biol Chem 1990;265:6104–6111.
20. McLean J, Tomlinson J, Kuang W, Eaton D, Chen E, Fless G et al. cDNA sequence of apolipoprotein(a) is homologous to plasminogen. Nature 1987;330:132–137.
21. Blombäck B. Fibrinogen and fibrin-proteins with complex roles in hemostasis and thrombosis. Thromb Res 1996;83:1–75.
22. Harpel PC, Chang T-S, Verdeber E. Tissue plasminogen activator and urokinase mediates the binding of Glu-plasminogen to plasma fibrin I. Evidence for new binding sites in plasmin-degraded fibrin. J Biol Chem 1985;260:4432–4440.
23. Fleury V, Anglés-Cano E. Characterization of the binding of plasminogen to fibrin surfaces: the role of carboxy-terminal lysines. Biochemistry 1991;30:7630–7638.
24. Suenson E, Lützen O, Thorsen S. Initial plasmin-degradation of fibrin as the basis of a positive feedback mechanism in fibrinolysis. Eur J Biochem 1984;140:513–522.
25. Zwaal RFA, Comfurius P, Bevers EM. Lipid-protein interactions in blood coagulation. Biochim Biophys Acta 1998;1376:433–453.
26. Felez J. Plasminogen binding to cell surfaces. Fibrinol Proteol 1998;12:183–190.
27. Gonzalez-Gronow M, Stack S, Pizzo S. Plasmin binding to the plasminogen receptor enhances catalytic efficiency and activates the receptor for subsequent ligand binding. Arch Biochem Biophys 1991;286:625–628.
28. Fritzler MJ, Hart DA, Wilson D, Garcia de la Torre I, Salazar-Paramo M, Vazquez del Mercado M et al. J Rheumatol 1995;22:1688–1693.
29. Salazar-Paramo M, Garcia de la Torre I, Fritzler MJ, Loyau S, Anglés-Cano E. Lupus 1996;5:275–2788.
30. Morse JH, Barst RJ, Fontino M, Zhang Y, Flaster E, Gharavi AE et al. Primary pulmonary hypertension, tissue plasminogen activator antibodies, and HLA-DQ7. Am J Resp Crit Care Med 1997;155:274–278.
31. Anglés-Cano E, Sultan Y, Clauvel JP. Predisposing factors to thrombosis in systemic lupus erythematosus. Possible relation to endothelial cell damage. J Lab Clin Med 1979;94:312–323.
32. Glas-Greenwalt P, Kant PS, Allen C, Pollak VE. Fibrinolysis in health and disease: severe abnormalities in systemic lupus erythematosus. J Lab Clin Med 1984;104:962–976.
33. Anglés-Cano E. Endothelial damage and hypofibrinolysis in systemic lupus erythematosus. Thromb Haemost 1989;61:322.
34. Awada H, Barlowatz-Meimon G, Dougados M, Maisonneuve P, Sultan Y, Amor B. Fibrinolysis abnormalities in systemic lupus erythematosus and their relation to vasculitis. J Lab Clin Med 1988;111:229–236.
35. Francis RB, Neely S. Effect of the lupus anticoagulant on endothelial fibrinolytic activity in vitro. Thromb Haemost 1989;61:314–317.
36. Tsakiris DA, Marbet GA, Makris PE, Settas L, Duckert F. Impaired fibrinolysis as an essential contribution to thrombosis in patients with lupus anticoagulant, Thromb Haemost 1989;61:175–177.
37. Violi F, Ferro D, Valesini G, Quintarelli C, Saliola M, Grandilli MA et al. Tissue plasminogen activator inhibitor in patients with systemic lupus erythematosus and thrombosis. Br Med J 1990;300:1099–1102.
38. Jurado M, Paramo JA, Gutierrez-Pimentel M, Rocha E. Fibrinolytic potential and antiphospholipid antibodies in systemic lupus erythematosus and other connective tissue disorders. Thromb Haemost 1992;688:516–520.
39. Ferro D, Pittoni V, Quintarelli C, Basili S, Saliola M, Caroselli C et al. Coexistence of anti-phospholipid antibodies and endothelial perturbation in systemi lupus erythematosus patients with ongoing prothrombotic state. Circulation 1997;95:1425–1432.
40. Rocha E, Paramo JA. The relationship between impaired fibrinolysis and coronary heart disease. A role for PAI-1. Fibrinolysis 1994;8:294–303.
41. Cockwell P, Tse WY, Savage COS. Activation of endothelial cells in thrombosis and vasculitis. Scand J Rheumatol 1997;26:145–150.
42. Boyer-Neumann C, Brenot F, Wolf M, Peynaud-Debayle E, Duroux P, Anglés-Cano E et al. Continuous infusion of prostacyclin decreases plasma levels of t-PA and PAI-1 in primary pulmonary hypertension. Thromb Haemostas 1995;73:735–736.
43. Asherson RA, Cervera Ricard. Review: antiphospholipid antibodies and the lung. J Rheumatol 1995;22:62–66.
44. Ames PRJ, Tommasino C, Iannaccone L, Brillante M, Cimino R, Brancaccio V. Coagulation activation and fibrinolytic imbalance in subjects with idiopathic antiphospholipid antibodies – a crucial role for acquired free protein S deficiency. Thromb Haemostas 1996;75:190–194.
45. Gris J-C, Ripart-Neveu S, Maugard C, Tailland M-L, Brun S, Courtieu C et al. Prospective evaluation of the prevalence of haemostasis abnormalities in unexplained primary early recurrent miscarriages. Thromb Haemost 1997;77:1096–1103.

46. Keeling DM, Campbell SJ, Mackie IJ, Machin SJ, Isenberg DA. The fibrinolytic response to venous occlusion and the natural anticoagulants in patients with antiphospholipid antibodies both with and without systemic lupus erythematosus. Br J Haematol 1991;77:154–159.

47. Patrassi GM, Sartori MT, Ruffatti A, Viero M, Di Lenardo L, Cazzanello D et al. Fibrinolytic pattern in recurrent spontaneous abortions: no relationship between hypofibrinolysis and anti-phospholipid antibodies. Am J Hematol 1994;47:266–272.

48. Mackworth-Young CG, Andreotti F, Harmer I, Loizou S, Pottinger BE et al. Endothelium-derived haemostatic factors in the antiphospholipid syndrome. Br J Rheumatol 1995;34:201–206.

49. McCrae KR, DeMichele A, Samuels P, Roth D, Kuo A, Meng Q-H et al. Detection of endothelial cell-reactive immunoglobulin in patients with anti-phospholipid antibodies. Br J Haematol 1991;79:595–605.

50. Meroni PL, del Papa N, Gambini D, Tincani A, Balestrieri G. Antiphospholipid antibodies and endothelial cells: an unending story. Lupus 1995;4:169–171.

51. Hill MB, Philipps JL, Malia RG, Greaves M, Hughes. Characterization and specificity of anti-endothelial cell membrane antibodies and their relationship to thrombosis in primary antiphospholipid syndrome (APS). Clin Exp Immunol 1995;102:365–372.

52. Lanir N, Zilberman M, Yron I, Tennenbaum G, Shechter Y, Brenner B. Reactivity patterns of antiphospholipid antibodies and endothelial cells: effect of antiendothelial antibodies on cell migration. J Lab Clin Med 1998;131:548–556.

53. Simantov R, LaSala JM, Lo SK, Gharavi AE, Sammaritano LR, Salmon JE et al. Activation of cultured vascular endothelial cells by antiphospholipid antibodies. J Clin Invest 1995;96:2211–2219.

54. Harpel PC, Borth W. Fibrin, lipoprotein(a), plasmin interactions: a model linking thrombosis and atherogenesis. Ann NY Acad Sci 1992;667:233–238.

55. Anglés-Cano E, Hervio L, Rouy D, Fournier C, Chapman JM, Laplaud M et al. Effects of lipoprotein(a) on the binding of plasminogen to fibrin and its activation by fibrin-bound tissue-type plasminogen activator. Chem Phys Lipids 1993;67/68:369–380.

56. Rouy D, Koschinsky ML, Fleury V, Chapman MJ and Anglés-Cano E. Apolipoprotein(a) and plasminogen interactions with fibrin: a study with recombinant apolipoprotein(a) and isolated plasminogen fragments. Biochemistry 1992;3:6333–6339.

57. Rantapää-Dahlqvist S, Wällberg-Jonsson S, Dahlén G. Lipoprotein(a), lipids, and lipoproteins in patients with rheumatoid arthritis. Ann Rheum Dis 1991;50:366–368.

58. Lotz H, Salabè GB. Lipoprotein(a) increase associated with thyroid autoimmunity. Eur J Endocrinol 1997;136:87–91.

59. Seriolo B, Accardo D, Mercuri M, Raurama R. Lipoprotein(a) and anticardiolipin antibodies as risk factors for vascular disease in rheumatoid arthritis. Thromb Haemost 1995;74:799–800.

60. Matsuda J, Gotoh M, Gohchi K, Saitoh N, Tsukamot M. Serum lipoprotein(a) level is increased in patients with systemic lupus erythematosus irrespective of positivity of antiphospholipid antibodies. Thromb Res 1994;73:83–84.

61. Kawai S, Mizushima Y, Kaburaki J. Increased serum lipoprotein(a) levels in systemic lupus erythematosus with myocardial and cerebral infractions. J Rheumatol 1995;22:1210–1211.

62. Yamazaki M, Asakura H, Jokaji H, Saito M, Uotani C, Kumabashiri I et al. Plasma levels of lipoprotein(a) are elevated in patients with the antiphospholipid syndrome. Thromb Haemost 1994;71:424–427.

63. Borba EF, Santos RD, Bonfa E, Vinagre CG, Pileggi FJC, Cossermelli W et al. Lipoprotein(a) levels in systemic lupus erythematosus. J Rheumatol 1994;21:220–223.

64. Levy PJ, Cooper CF, Gonzalez MF. Massive lower extremity arterial thrombosis and acute hepatic insufficiency in a young adult with premature atherosclerosis associated with hyperlipoprotein(a)emia and antiphospholipid syndrome. J Vasc Dis 1995;4:853–858.

65. Atsumi T, Khamashta MA, Andujar C, Leandro MJ, Amengual O, Ames PRJ et al. Elevated plasma lipoprotein(a) level and it s association with impaired fibrinolysis in patients with antiphospholipid syndrome. J Rheumatol 1998;25:69–73.

66. Okawa-Takatsuji M, Aotsuka S, Sumiya M, Ohta H, Kawakami M, Sakurabayashi I. Clinical significance of the serum lipoprotein(a) level in patients with systemic lupus erythematosus: its elevation during disease flare. Clin Exp Rheumatol 1996;14:531–536.

67. Köhl S, Fresser F, Lobentaz E, Baier G, Utermann. Novel interaction of apolipoprotein(a) with β_2-glycoprotein I mediated by the kringle IV domain. Blood 1997;90:1482–1489.

68. Ohkura N, Hagihara Y, Yoshimura T, Goto Y, Kato H. Plasmin can reduce the function of human β_2 glycoprotein I by cleaving domain V into a nicked form. Blood 1998;91:4173–4179.

69. Horbach DA, vanOort E, Lisman T, Meijers JCM, Derksen RHWM, de Groot PF. $\beta(2)$-glycoprotein I is proteolytically cleaved in vivo upon activation of fibrinolysis. Thromb Haemostas 81:87–95.

70. Von Mühlen CA, Chan EKL, Anglés-Cano E, Mamula MJ, Garcia de la Torre I, Fritzler MJ. Advances in autoantibodies in SLE. Lupus 1998;7:507–514.

71. Witztum JL, Horkko S. The role of oxidized LDL in atherogenesis: immunological response and anti-phospholipid antibodies. Ann NY Acad Sci 1997;8811:88–96.
72. Bouma BN, von dem Borne PAK, Meijers JCM. Factor XI and protection of the fibrin clot against lysis – a role for the intrinsic pathway of coagulation in fibrinolysis. Thromb Haemost 1998;80:24–27.
73. Cesarman GM, Guevara CA, Hajjar KA. An endothelial cell receptor for plasminogen/tissue plasminogen activator (t-PA). II. Annexin II-mediated enhancement of t-PA-dependent plasminogen activation. J Biol Chem 1994;269:21198–21203.
74. Kassam G, Choi K-S, Ghuman J, Kang H-M, Fitzpatrick SL, Zackson T et al. The role of annexin II tetramer in the activation of plasminogen. J Biol Chem 1998;273:4790–4799.
75. Rand JH. Antiphospholipid antibody syndrome: new insights on thrombogenic mechanisms. Am J Med Sci 1998;316:142–151.

34 Interaction Between Antiphospholipid Antibodies and Eicosanoids

L. Carreras, R. Forastiero and M. Martinuzzo

Biosynthesis of Eicosanoids and Isoeicosanoids

The arachidonic acid (AA) present in cell membranes is the precursor of a heterogeneous family of compounds with very important in vivo modulating functions (Table 34.1). The oxidative modifications of the AA backbone lead to the formation of enzymatic (eicosanoids) and non-enzymatic (isoeicosanoids) derivatives (Fig. 34.1) [reviewed in 1].

The biosynthesis of eicosanoids depends primarily on the liberation of unesterified AA from membrane phospholipids (PL) as a consequence of the activation of phospholipase A_2 (PLA$_2$) by different cell stimulation agents. Unesterified AA is rapidly transformed into unstable intermediates such as prostaglandin (PG) H_2 (PGH$_2$) by PGH-synthase, leukotriene (LT) A_4 (LTA$_4$) by a 5-lipoxygenase or various (5-, 12-, 15-) hydroperoxides (HPETEs) by corresponding lipoxygenases. PGH-synthase, also referred to as cyclo-oxygenase (COX) has two isoenzymes. COX-1 is a "constitutive" enzyme present in most cells (e.g., platelets, monocytes, vascular cells) and located equally on the luminal side of the endoplasmic reticulum

Table 34.1. Main in vivo effects of eicosanoids and isoeicosanoids.

Metabolite	Physiological role
TXA$_2$	Vasoconstriction Platelet aggregation
PGI$_2$	Vasodilation Inhibition of platelet aggregation
PGE$_2$, PGD$_2$, PGF$_{2\alpha}$	Vasodilation Vascular permeability
LTB$_4$	Chemoattractant
LTC$_4$, LTD$_4$	Vasoconstrictor Permeant
IP-F$_{2\alpha}$	Vasoconstriction Platelet aggregation

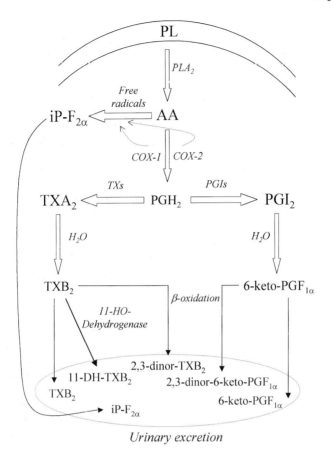

Figure 34.1. Metabolism of eicosanoids and isoeicosanoids. After activation of phospholipases, arachidonic acid undergoes oxidative modifications to enzymatic (eicosanoids) and non-enzymatic (isoeicosanoids) derivatives. The main unstable intermediates generated in platelets (thromboxane A_2) or in endothelial cells (prostacyclin) are transformed by different pathways (hydrolysis, dehydrogenation or β-oxidation) into inactive metabolites. They are excreted in urine along with the free radical-derived compounds of arachidonic acid. See text for abbreviations.

and on the nuclear envelope. On the other hand, most nucleated cells have the gene for the "inducible" COX-2 which is slightly more abundant in the nuclear envelope and can be expressed in response to cell activation [2]. Although practically all cells are capable of synthesizing PGH_2 intermediates, their further metabolism depends on the specific enzymes that are present in each tissue. Platelets contain thromboxane (TX)-synthase (TXs) generating TXA_2 whereas endothelial cells (EC) have prostacyclin-synthase (PGIs) transforming PGH_2 into prostacyclin (PGI_2). These bioactive products (TXA_2 and PGI_2) are chemically unstable and undergo non-enzymatic hydrolysis to TXB_2 and 6-keto-PGF_{1a}, respectively. Both TXB_2 and 6-keto-PGF_{1a} are subsequently transformed by β-oxidation into the inactive metabolites 2,3-dinor-TXB_2 and 2,3-dinor-6-keto-PGF_{1a}. The catabolism of TXB_2

also includes a specific pathway of dehydrogenation by the 11-HO-dehydrogenase resulting in the formation of the product named 11-dehydro-TXB_2 (11-DH-TXB_2). This metabolite is excreted in urine at a higher rate than 2,3-dinor-TXB_2.

Other pathways of AA metabolism are related to the action of lipoxygenases. There are several lipoxygenases which differ in their specificity for placing the hydroperoxy group in different positions of the substrate. Platelets only synthesize 12-HPETE whereas leukocytes produce 5-HPETE and 15-HPETE. All HPETEs are converted into HETEs by a peroxidase. Neutrophils contain the 5-lipoxygenase leading to the formation of LTA_4 from 5-HPETE. LTA_4 is rapidly metabolized into LTB_4 which in turn may be transformed into LTC_4. LTD_4 and LTE_4 derived from the latter. LTE_4 and their metabolites generated by β-oxidation are excreted in urine.

It is nowadays accepted that transcellular metabolism of eicosanoids represents a specialized mode of cell communication. While neutrophils are the main source of LTB_4, LTA_4 represents the most abundant 5-lipoxygenase-derived metabolite released outside the cell. Human red cells, which contain high amounts of LTA_4 hydrolase, convert LTA_4 into LTB_4 although they are devoid of lipoxygenases. In the presence of platelets, EC or smooth muscle cells, LTA_4 can be metabolized efficiently into LTC_4 by such cells, despite neither cell alone can generate LTC_4. It is also well-known that aspirin-treated platelets can metabolize PGH_2 from vascular cells into TXA_2.

Iso-eicosanoids are non-enzymatic, free radical (FR)-derived compounds isomeric with enzymatically formed eicosanoids such as PG, leukotrienes, and TX. In contrast to classic PGs, which are formed through the action of synthases from free AA, isoeicosanoids are generated in situ from the fatty acid backbone esterified in membrane PL or circulating LDLs. Later, they are released in response to cellular activation, circulate in plasma and are excreted by urine. The formation of isoeicosanoids can occur in all cells (e.g., monocytes, EC, neutrophils, platelets) (Fig. 34.2). Isoprostaglandins or isoprostanes (iP) are the best characterized compounds of the isoeicosanoid family. The most extensively investigated are the isomers of PGF_{2a} (iP-F_{2a}). For the time being, four isomers of iP-F_{2a} have been identified and measured in urine [3]. There is recent evidence that iP-F_{2a} can also be produced as a minor product of the platelet COX-1 in response to platelet stimulation with various agonists. Induction of COX-2 in monocytes was also associated with cyclo-oxygenase-dependent formation of iP-F_{2a}.

Measurement of metabolites from eicosanoids and isoeicosanoids in urine provides a reliable indication of their biosynthesis in vivo. Furthermore, this noninvasive approach may be useful to evaluate the pathophysiologic role of these compounds in several multifactorial human diseases and the pharmacological effect of new drugs.

aPL and Eicosanoids

Historical Background

In 1981 it was reported that the IgG with lupus anticoagulant (LA) activity isolated from a patient with thrombosis and repeated intrauterine death was able to interfere with PGI_2 formation by rat aortic rings, bovine EC and pregnant human

340   Hughes Syndrome

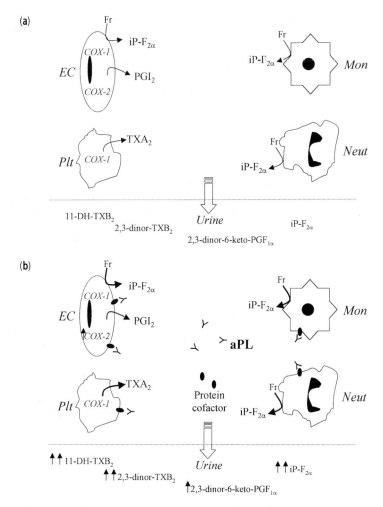

Figure 34.2. Scheme of the effect of antiphospholipid antibodies (aPL) on the eicosanoid and isoeicosanoid metabolism. **a** Endothelial cells (EC) and platelets (Plt), in the absence of aPL, synthesize prostacyclin and thromboxane, respectively, as the main eicosanoids. Given the ubiquitous distribution of arachidonic acid, biosynthesis of isoeicosanoids can occur in virtually all cellular elements, including monocytes (Mon) and neutrophils (Neut). These compounds undergo different transformations and are excreted in the urine. **b** In the presence of protein cofactor-dependent aPL, eicosanoid and isoecosanoid production is enhanced and reflected by a higher rate of their metabolites in urine. Thus, an imbalance of platelet/endothelial cell-derived metabolites and an increase of markers of lipid peroxidation seem to characterise patients with aPL. See text for other abbreviations and details.

myometrium [4]. Moreover, it was suggested that LA could interfere with AA release from PL membranes because the effect was abolished in the presence of AA. Many studies have confirmed this inhibitory mechanism by using EC in culture [5–9]. In addition, the inhibition of PGI$_2$ synthesized by EC has been associated to arterial, but not to venous thrombosis [8]. In a study reported in 1992 Schorer et al [10] have demonstrated that some purified antiphospholipid antibodies (aPL) inhibit the enzymatic activity of PLA_2. Thus, some aPL were able to interfere with thrombin-induced generation of two PLA_2-dependent processes, PGI_2 and platelet-activating factor, in EC. In contrast, some authors obtained discrepant results reporting no inhibition or even an increase of the production of PGI_2 by human umbilical vein EC (HUVEC) [11,12]. Several methodological variables could explain these discrepancies and have been reviewed elsewhere [13].

Regarding the in vitro effect of aPL on platelet-derived eicosanoids, several studies have shown an increase in TXB_2 production by platelets [11, 14, 15]. Initially, it was reported that sera from some patients with systemic lupus erythematosus (SLE) and aPL increase TXB_2 generation by platelet-rich plasma stimulated by collagen or AA [11]. In 1993 we demonstrated that $F(ab')_2$ prepared from IgGs of patients with LA and anticardiolipin antibodies (aCL) induce a direct stimulatory effect on washed human platelets activated by a threshold concentration of thrombin, including an increase in TXB_2 production [14]. It was also shown that affinity-purified aCL raised in rabbits immunised with cardiolipin activate gel-filtered human platelets inducing TXB_2 formation [15]. The enhancement of TX generation without affecting PGI_2 formation in vitro by IgGs from patients with antiphospholipid syndrome (APS) was also observed in normal placental tissue [16].

As mentioned above, the biosynthesis of eicosanoids in vivo can be measured by evaluating the urinary excretion of platelet and vascular cell metabolites. In a series of 25 patients with aCL and LA we found a significantly enhanced excretion of 11-DH-TXB_2, whereas 2,3-dinor-6-keto-PGF_{1a} was much less increased (Fig. 34.2) [17]. Thus, in patients with aPL there is an imbalance of the normal TXA_2/PGI_2 equilibrium. It was reestablished after seven days treatment with low-dose aspirin (20 mg/day), confirming the platelet origin of TX metabolites [17]. A similar increase of urinary TXA_2 products has been shown in patients with aCL of IgG isotype [18], but no correlation was observed between the levels of aCL and 11-DH-TXB_2 as reported in our study [17].

Effects on Thromboxane Production and Platelets

The LA and aCL belong to the heterogeneous group of aPL, which in association with the occurrence of thrombotic episodes, fetal loss and/or thrombocytopenia define the APS [19]. The antiphospholipid–protein cofactor syndrome [20, 21] is a concept introduced after the demonstration that aCL recognize a complex formed by cardiolipin and β_2-glycoprotein I (β_2GPI) [22, 23] and that some LA are antibodies directed against the complex of PL with human prothrombin [24]. Further studies demonstrated the binding of autoimmune aPL to β_2GPI (anti-β_2GPI) or prothrombin (anti-II) in solid-phase immunoassays in the absence of PL by using irradiated plates [25–28]. Moreover, a strong association between the presence of anti-β_2GPI and/or anti-II and the history of thrombosis in patients with APS was found [29–33].

It was suggested that aCL do not bind to intact platelets [34], but other authors have shown that LA antibodies bind to platelets activated by thrombin and aCL bind to thrombin-activated platelets only in the presence of β_2GPI [35]. Moreover, Rote et al [36] by using monoclonal antibodies reacting to phosphatidylserine (PS) or cardiolipin demonstrated that anti-PS antibodies, but not aCL, bind to thrombin-activated platelets and that there are two sequentially immunoreactive forms of PS expressed on platelets during activation. Arvieux et al [37] showed that six murine monoclonal anti-β_2GPI had direct platelet activating properties (demonstrated by platelet aggregation, secretion and calcium mobilisation) synergizing with weak agonists. Aspirin inhibited this effect but did not block it, indicating that thromboxane formation was also enhanced. The presence of β_2GPI and whole IgG was needed to produce the activating effect suggesting a role of Fc fragment binding to Fcg receptor as postulated by Arnout [38]. Recently, Robbins et al [39] showed that control platelets from healthy individuals were activated and produced higher amounts of TXB$_2$ when incubated with thrombin and aCL/β_2GPI complexes obtained from one patient with APS. A lesser effect of aCL alone was seen. They observed that F(ab$'$)$_2$ fragments of IgG aCL in the absence of β_2GPI also enhanced TX formation suggesting the recognition of a PL epitope on the membrane of activated platelets, but some residual β_2GPI has not been ruled out from their experiments. Very recently, Ford et al [40] found higher levels of platelet-associated IgG after incubation of normal platelets with five out of 11 sera from patients with APS compared to normal sera. However, it did not imply higher expression of P-selectin or increased platelet microparticle formation reflecting no direct in vivo activating effect for these autoantibodies, even when platelets were preactivated with subthreshold ADP or thrombin-receptor-activating peptide concentrations.

Concerning ex vivo studies, we previously demonstrated that patients with aPL undergo a state of in vivo platelet activation by measuring urinary excretion of 11-DH-TXB$_2$ but we failed to find any association with aCL titers or coagulation test results [17]. In a more recent work we observed a close correlation between levels of urinary 11-DH-TXB$_2$ and the titer of anti-β_2GPI of IgG isotype from 34 patients with aPL [41]. We showed significantly higher levels of 11-DH-TXB$_2$ in the urine of patients with moderate or high levels of anti-β_2GPI than in those with low titer or negative results. We also found higher levels of this urinary TX metabolite in patients with history of thrombosis. Other group has recently showed increased levels of urinary 11-DH-TXB$_2$ in a small group of patients with APS [39].

Joseph et al [42] found that platelets from patients with primary APS expressed higher levels of CD63 than that from normal controls. They also demonstrated that these patients had increased plasma levels of soluble P-selectin detected by enzyme-linked immunosorbent assay (ELISA) reflecting in vivo platelet activation, but they did not find any difference between patients with or without anti-β_2GPI. In a series of 30 patients with aPL, we also demonstrated that patients with aPL had higher levels of soluble P-selectin compared to 20 normal controls, and this increase was significantly higher in patients with anti-β_2GPI positive results. In a subgroup of 15 patients, a good correlation between levels of soluble P-selectin and the urinary excretion of 11-DH-TXB$_2$ was found (unpublished work).

The formation of TX by other tissues seems also to be important as demonstrated by Peaceman et al [43] who showed that IgGs from patients with LA increase TX production by normal placental tissue. They also demonstrated that aspirin reduced TX production without affecting PGI$_2$ generation in their experiments while indomethacin decreases TX and PGI$_2$ production simultaneously [16, 43]. Moreover, this was confirmed by Shoenfeld and Blank [44] who demonstrated that the treatment with an antagonist of TX receptor (BMS 180,291) suppressed different manifestations of APS (fetal resorption, low embryo weights, thrombocytopenia and activated partial thromboplastin time prolongation) in an experimental model in mice.

Effects on Prostacyclin Formation by Endothelial Cells

PGI_2 is the most important natural inhibitor of platelet aggregation and it is also a vasodilator, being considered as one of the antithrombotic mechanisms of vascular endothelium. Its effect is contrary to that of TXA_2 [45]. We have already indicated that because of these contrasting effects the equilibrium between PGI_2 and TXA_2 could be important to prevent thrombotic events. As mentioned above, many reports since our first one have showed an inhibitory effect of IgG isolated from patients with APS on PGI_2 synthesis by EC, although some contrasting studies have also been published.

In more recent studies we demonstrated that COX-2 expression could be inducible by IgGs from patients with aPL in resting EC (Fig. 34.2) [46]. However, the control HUVEC in culture are in a "low activation state" because of an unavoidable low amount of cytokines and growth factors present in normal human sera used in culture medium. This state is evident by a small amount of COX-2 present in these cells after culture [2]. However, despite inducing COX-2, very little synthesis of 6-keto-PGF_{1a} could be detected in the cell supernatant after incubation with patients' IgGs [46]. It is in contrast to what has been reported for cytokines [2] and growth factors [47]. This could be due to the reported inhibition of PLA_2 by aPL [10]. These results are in accordance to those obtained in our ex vivo studies in which no significant variation in the amount of 2,3 dinor-6-keto-PGF_{1a} excreted by urine of patients with aPL was found [17]. However, we observed a small reproducible increase in the formation of 6-keto-PGF_{1a} by cells incubated with patients' IgGs and thrombin compared to IgGs alone [46]. The absence of correlation between COX-2 expression and PG synthesis has also been shown in other cell types after their stimulation with different substances [48]. Both COX are compartmentalized inside the cell and it has been suggested that this may imply that COX-2 could play a role in nuclear signaling and has other functions different than generating products to be released [1]. However, we did not investigate in our study the localization of these isoenzymes. Furthermore, it is not known whether these findings depend on the cell type studied. Many reports in the literature showed that in different situations (mainly in inflammatory states, in parturition, during labor, etc.) the upregulation of COX-2 is accompanied by the release of high amounts of metabolites suggesting a direct correlation between enzyme mass and products generated outside.

Concerning the target recognized by these antibodies on EC surface, in our experiments the recognition of PL epitopes on EC membrane seemed to be important, as demonstrated by the partial neutralization of the effect of antibodies after preincubation with cardiolipin liposomes [46]. In some experiments performed with bovine serum albumin instead of serum in the culture medium we observed that the EC responses were similar, suggesting that final concentration of β_2GPI did not affect the reactivity of the patients' IgGs [49]. However, residual β_2GPI could still be present on the surface of EC at a concentration allowing a substantial effect on the intensity of response. Recently, Del Papa et al [50, 51] have demonstrated that polyclonal IgG and monoclonal IgM anti-β_2GPI are able to bind EC in a β_2GPI dose-dependent manner. This binding leads to the activation of EC as reflected by the upregulation of adhesion molecules (E-selectin, vascular cell adhesion molecule-1 (VCAM-1) and intracellular adhesion molecule-1 (ICAM-1)), adhesion of leukocytes to EC membrane and increase in interleukins (IL-1b, IL-6) and 6-keto-PGF_{1a} secretion. George et al [52] demonstrated that three different IgM monoclonal antibodies cloned from a patient with APS had different in vitro reactivity against β_2GPI in solid and fluid phase, and different activating effects on EC (measured by the increased adherence of U937 cells to them). In addition, the differential effect of the monoclonal anti-β_2GPI on EC correlates with the induction of clinical features of APS by passive administration to pregnant mice.

Isoeicosanoids: an Emerging Area

Isoeicosanoids are emerging as a new class of biologically active compounds of potential relevance to human vascular disease. Formation of these products seems to reflect a non-enzymatic mechanism of lipid peroxidation in vivo. It has been postulated that lipid oxidation is a key event involved in the development of athero-sclerotic lesions and their superimposed thrombotic complications. One of the main mediators responsible for this process might be the iP-F_{2a}, which was found to be a potent vasoconstrictor and a modulator of platelet activity. Recently, iP-F_{2a} has been observed to increase platelet adhesiveness and the expression of the fibrinogen receptor [53]. The antiplatelet activity of nitric oxide is also reduced by iso-eicosanoids. The ability of iP-F_{2a} to induce platelet secretion and aggregation requires the presence of platelet agonists. These effects can be obtained in vivo in settings where platelet activation and enhanced free-radical formation coincide. Therefore, iP-F_{2a} may alter the equilibrium between prothrombotic and antithrom-botic factors which modulate platelet–endothelium interactions. The contribution of COX-dependent processes to the formation of iP-F_{2a} in vivo and its regulation by therapeutic strategies is a fascinating area, not yet completely understood. Given that aPL have been recently found directed against oxidized PL [54], some investi-gators have evaluated the excretion of iP-F_{2a} as marker of lipid peroxidation. Elevated urinary levels of this isoeicosanoid were clearly found in patients with APS with or without SLE (Fig. 34.2) [55, 56]. Thus, the existence of a close association between aPL and increased in vivo lipid peroxidation, supports the hypothesis that pro-oxidative conditions and inflammation underlie the APS.

Concluding Remarks

Eicosanoids and isoeicosanoids are arachidonic acid derivatives that play an impor-tant role on modulation of cell functions in vivo. On the basis of research performed in this field in patients with aPL it is likely that an imbalance of TXA$_2$/PGI$_2$ ratio observed in vivo contributes to the pathogenesis of the APS. The recently reported correlation between urinary excretion of 11-DH-TXB$_2$ and the titer of anti-β_2GPI suggests that these antibodies may be responsible for platelet activation in vivo. On the other hand, the enhanced expression of the inducible COX-2 by endothelial cells in the presence of aPL may be reflecting endothelial cell perturbation induced by these antibodies. Moreover, recent data showed that the biosynthesis of iso-eicosanoids, indices of lipid peroxidation in vivo, is closely associated to aPL. This finding supports the hypothesis that aPL may result from pro-oxidative conditions. In summary, recent studies remain in agreement with the concept initially proposed in 1981 in the sense that aPL disturb the production of eicosanoids by platelets and endothelial cells. The abnormal eicosanoid biosynthesis in these patients may reflect and potentiate cell activation induced by aPL, leading to a prothrombotic condition.

References

1. Maclouf J, Folco G, Patrono C. Eicosanoids and iso-eicosanoids: constitutive, inducible and transcellular biosynthesis in vascular disease. Thromb Haemost 1998;79:691–705.
2. Habib A, Créminon C, Frobert Y, Grassi J, Pradelles P, Maclouf J. Demonstration of an inducible cyclooxygenase in human endothelial cells using antibodies raised against the C-terminal region of the cyclooxigenase-2. J Biol Chem 1993;268:23448–23454.
3. Lawson JA, Li H, Rokach J et al. Identification of two major F2 isoprostanes, 8,12-iso- and 5-epi-8, 12-iso-isoprostane F2alpha-VI, in human urine. J Biol Chem 1998;273:29295–29301.
4. Carreras LO, Defreyn G, Machin SJ et al. Arterial thrombosis, intrauterine death and lupus anticoagulant: detection of immunoglobulin interfering with prostacyclin formation. Lancet 1981;i:244–246.
5. Carreras LO, Vermylen JG. "Lupus" anticoagulant and thrombosis. Possible role of inhibition of prostacyclin formation. Thromb Haemost 1982;48:38–40.
6. Carreras LO, Vermylen J, Spitz B, van Assche A. Lupus anticoagulant and inhibition of prostacyclin formation in patients with repeated abortion, intrauterine growth retardation and intrauterine death. Br J Obstet Gynaecol 1981;88:890–894.
7. Schörer AE, Wickham NWR, Watson KV. Lupus anticoagulant induces a selective defect in thrombin-mediated endothelial prostacyclin release and platelet aggregation. Br J Haematol 1989;71:399–407.
8. Watson KV, Schorer AE. Lupus anticoagulant inhibition of in vitro prostacyclin release is associated with a thrombosis-prone subset of patients. Am J Med 1991;90:47–53.
9. Elias M, Eldor A. Thromboembolism in patients with the "lupus" type circulating anticoagulant. Arch Intern Med 1984;144:510–515.
10. Schorer AE, Duane PG, Woods VL, Niewoehner DE. Some antiphospholipid antibodies inhibit phospholipase A_2 activity. J Lab Clin Med 1992;120:67–77.
11. Hasselaar P, Derksen RHWM, Blokzijl L, de Groot PG. Thrombosis associated with antiphospholipid antibodies cannot be explained by effects on endothelial and platelet prostanoid synthesiz. Thromb Haemost 1988;59:80–85.
12. Cariou R, Tobelem G, Bellucci S et al. Effect of lupus anticoagulant on antithrombogenic properties of endothelial cells. Inhibition of thrombomodulin-dependent protein C activation. Thromb Haemost 1988;60:54–58.
13. Carreras LO, Maclouf J. The lupus anticoagulant and eicosanoids. Prostagland Leukotr Ess Fatty Acids 1993;49:483–488.
14. Martinuzzo ME, Maclouf J, Carreras LO, Lévy Toledano S. Antiphospholipid antibodies enhance thrombin-induced platelet activation and thromboxane formation. Thromb Haemost 1993;70:667–671.
15. Lin YL, Wang CT. Activation of human platelets by the rabbit anticardiolipin antibodies. Blood 1992;80:3135–3143.
16. Peaceman AM, Rehnberg KA. The effect of immunoglobulin G fractions from patients with lupus anticoagulant on placental prostacyclin and thromboxane production. Am J Obstet Gynecol 1993;169:1403–1406.
17. Lellouche F, Martinuzzo M, Said P, Maclouf J, Carreras LO. Imbalance of thromboxane/prostacyclin biosynthesis in patients with lupus anticoagulant. Blood 1991;78:2894–2899.
18. Arfors L, Vesterqvist O, Johnsson H, Gréen K. Increased thromboxane formation in patients with antiphospholipid syndrome. Eur J Clin Invest 1990;20:607–612.
19. Harris EN. The antiphospholipid syndrome: an introduction. In: Harris EN, Exner T, Hughes GRV, Asherson R, editors. Phospholipid binding antibodies. Boca Raton, FL: CRC Press, 1991;373–376.
20. Vermylen J, Arnout J. Is the antiphospholipid syndrome caused by antibodies directed against physiologically relevant phospholipid–protein complexes? J Lab Clin Med 1992;120:10–12.
21. Roubey RAS. Immunology of the antiphospholipid antibody syndrome. Arthritis Rheum 1996;39:1444–1454.
22. McNeil HP, Simpson RJ, Chesterman CN, Krilis SA. Antiphospholipid antibodies are directed against a complex antigen that includes a lipid-binding inhibitor of coagulation: β_2-glycoprotein I (apolipoprotein H). Proc Natl Acad Sci USA 1990;87:4120–4124.
23. Galli M, Comfurius P, Maassen C et al. Anticardiolipin antibodies (ACA) directed not to cardiolipin but to a plasma protein cofactor. Lancet 1990;335:1544–1547.

24. Bevers EM, Galli M, Barbui T, Comfurius P, Zwaal RFA. Lupus anticoagulant IgGs (LA) are not directed to phospholipids only, but to a complex of lipid-bound human prothrombin. Thromb Haemost 1991;66:629–632.
25. Matsuura E, Igarashi Y, Yasuda T, Triplett DA, Koike T. Anticardiolipin antibodies recognize β_2-glycoprotein I structure altered by interacting with an oxygen modified solid phase surface. J Exp Med 1994;179:457–462.
26. Roubey RAS, Eisenberg RA, Harper MF, Winfield JB. Anticardiolipin autoantibodies recognize β_2-glycoprotein I in the absence of phospholipid. Importance of antigen density and bivalent binding. J Immunol 1995;154:954–960.
27. Arvieux J, Darnige L, Caron C, Reber G, Bensa JC, Colomb MG. Development of an ELISA for autoantibodies to prothrombin showing their prevalence in patients with lupus anticoagulants. Thromb Haemost 1995;74:1120–1125.
28. Forastiero RR, Martinuzzo ME, Kordich LC, Carreras LO. Reactivity to β_2-glycoprotein I clearly differentiates anticardiolipin antibodies from antiphospholipid syndrome and syphilis. Thromb Haemost 1996;75:717–720.
29. Martinuzzo M, Forastiero R, Carreras LO. Anti β_2 glycoprotein I antibodies: detection and association with thrombosis. Br J Haematol 1995;89:397–402.
30. Forastiero RR, Martinuzzo ME, Cerrato GS, Kordich LC, Carreras LO. Relationship of anti β_2 glycoprotein I and anti prothrombin antibodies to thrombosis and pregnancy loss in patients with antiphospholipid antibodies. Thromb Haemost 1997;78:1008–1014.
31. Roubey RAS. Autoantibodies to phospholipid-binding plasma proteins: a new view of lupus anticoagulants and other "antiphospholipid antibodies". Blood 1994;84:2854–2867.
32. Arvieux J, Roussel B, Jacob MC, Colomb MG. Measurement of anti-phospholipid antibodies by ELISA using β_2-glycoprotein I as an antigen. J Immunol Methods 1991;143:223–229.
33. Viard JP, Amoura Z, Bach JF. Association of anti-β_2 glycoprotein I antibodies with lupus-type circulating anticoagulant and thrombosis in systemic lupus erythematosus. Am J Med 1992;93:181–186.
34. Haga HJ, Christopoulos C, Machin SJ, Khamashta M, Hughes GR. Lack of specific binding of anticardiolipin antibodies to intact platelets. Lupus 1992;1:387–390.
35. Shi W, Chong BH, Chesterman CN. Beta 2-glycoprotein I is a requirement for anticardiolipin antibodies binding to activated platelets: differences with lupus anticoagulants. Blood 1993;81:1255–1262.
36. Rote NS, Ng AU, Dostal-Johnson DA, Nicholson SL, Siekman R. Immunologic detection of phosphatidylserine externalization during thrombin-induced platelet activation. Clin Immunol Immunopathol 1993;66:193–200.
37. Arvieux J, Roussel B, Pouzol P, Colomb MG. Platelet activating properties of murine monoclonal antibodies to beta 2-glycoprotein I. Thromb Haemost 1993;70:336–341.
38. Arnout J. The pathogenesis of the antiphospholipid syndrome: a hypothesis based on parallelisms with heparin-induced thrombocytopenia. Thromb Haemost 1996;75:536–341.
39. Robbins DL, Leung S, Miller-Blair DJ, Ziboh V. Effect of anticardiolipin/β_2-glycoprotein I complexes on production of thromboxane A_2 by platelets from patients with the antiphospholipid syndrome. J Rheumatol 1998;25:51–56.
40. Ford I, Urbaniak S, Greaves M. IgG from patients with antiphospholipid syndrome binds platelets without induction of platelet activation. Br J Haematol 1998;102:841–849.
41. Forastiero R, Martinuzzo M, Carreras LO, Maclouf J. Anti-β_2 glycoprotein I antibodies and platelet activation in patients with antiphospholipid antibodies: association with increased excretion of platelet-derived thromboxane urinary metabolites. Thromb Haemost 1998;79:42–45.
42. Joseph JE, Donohoe S, Harrison P, Mackie IJ, Machin SJ. Platelet activation and turnover in the primary antiphospholipid syndrome. Lupus 1998;7:333–340.
43. Peaceman AM, Rehnberg KA. The effect of aspirin and indomethacin on prostacyclin and thromboxane production by placental tissue incubated with immunoglobulin G fractions from patients with lupus anticoagulant. Am J Obstet Gynecol 1995;73:1391–1396.
44. Shoenfeld Y, Blank M. Effect of long-acting thromboxane receptor antagonist (BMS 180,291) on experimental antiphospholipid syndrome. Lupus 1994;3:397–400.
45. Moncada S, Vane JR. Unstable metabolites of arachidonic acid and their role in haemostasis and thrombosis. Br Med Bull 1978;34:129–135.
46. Habib A, Martinuzzo ME, Carreras LO, Levy-Toledano S, Maclouf J. Increased expression of inducible cyclooxygenase-2 in human endothelial cells by antiphospholipid antibodies. Thromb Haemost 1995;74:770–777.
47. Moatter T, Gerritsen ME. Fibroblast growth factor upregulates PGG/H synthase in rabbit microvascular endothelial cells by a glucocorticoid-independent mechanism. J Cell Physiol 1992;151:571–578.

48. Murakami M, Matsumoto R, Austen KF, Arm JP. Prostaglandin endoperoxide synthase-1 and -2 couple to different transmembrane stimuli to generate prostaglandin D2 in mouse bone marrow-derived mast cells. J Biol Chem 1994;269:22269–22275.
49. Habib A, Martinuzzo M, Lebret M, Levy-Toledano S, Carreras LO, Maclouf J. Lupus anticoagulant IgGs do not depend on serum for the induction of cyclooxygenase-2 by human endothelial cells. In: Samuelson B, Paoletti R, Granstrom E, Ramwell PW, Folco G, Nicosia S, editors. Advances in prostaglandin, thromboxane, and leukotriene research. New York: Raven Press, 1993;42–48.
50. Del Papa N, Raschi E, Catelli L et al. Endothelial cells as a target for antiphospholipid antibodies: role of anti-β_2 glycoprotein I antibodies. Am J Reprod Immunol 1997;38:212–217.
51. Del Papa N, Guidali L, Sala A et al. Endothelial cells as target for antiphospholipid antibodies. Arthritis Rheum 1997;40:551–561.
52. George J, Blank M, Levy Y et al. Differential effects of anti-β_2 glycoprotein I antibodies on endothelial cells and on the manifestations of experimental antiphospholipid syndrome. Circulation 1998;97:900–906.
53. Minuz P, Andrioli G, Degan M et al. The F2-isoprostane 8-epiprostaglandin F2a increases platelet adhesion and reduces the antiadhesive and antiaggregatory effects of NO. Arterioscler Thromb Vasc Biol 1998;18:1248–1256.
54. Hörkkö S, Miller E, Branch DW, Palinski W, Witztum JL. The epitopes for some antiphospholipid antibodies are adducts of oxidized phospholipids and β_2 glycoprotein I (and other proteins). Proc Natl Acad Sci USA 1997;94:10356–10361.
55. Iuliano L, Praticò D, Ferro D et al. Enhanced lipid peroxidation in patients positive for antiphospholipid antibodies. Blood 1997;90:3931–3935.
56. Ames PRJ, Nourooz-Zadeh J, Tommasino C, Alves J, Brancaccio V, Anggard EE. Oxidative stress in primary antiphospholipid syndrome. Thromb Haemost 1998;79:447–449.

35 Family Studies and the Major Histocompatibility Complex

W. A. Wilson

Introduction

Approximately one-third of the close relatives of antiphospholipid syndrome (APS) patients have antiphospholipid antibodies (aPL) in serum, sometimes in association with clinical features of APS [1–3]. Several other autoantibodies and autoimmune diseases also cluster among family members of APS patients (Fig. 35.1). Family studies provide evidence that genetic factors underlie APS, and are also useful to the clinician in identifying family members of APS patients who may require monitoring or treatment for APS or associated autoimmune diseases. The following patient illustrates some of these points.

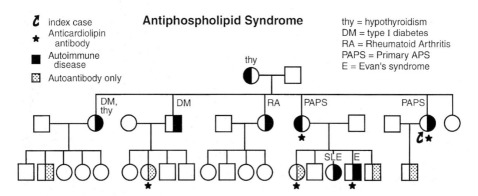

Figure 35.1. Family of index case with PAPS showing autoimmune diseases and autoantibodies. thy = hypothyroidism, DM = diabetes mellitus, RA = rheumatoid arthritis, PAPS = primary antiphospholipid antibody syndrome, SLE = systemic lupus erythematosus, E = Evans' syndrome (autoimmune hemolytic anemia and thrombocytopenia). Autoantibodies included antinuclear antibodies and/or rheumatoid factor. The family members who have SLE and Evans' syndrome developed these diseases 2 and 3 years after entry into the study, respectively. Reproduced in modified form, with permission [1].

Case

A 36-year-old woman is being successfully treated with warfarin for primary APS, characterized by recurrent syncope, near-syncope and right optic nerve ischemia. She has a positive VDRL (syphilis test) with negative fluorescent treponemal antibodies (FTA) detected on routine testing 16 years ago prior to her marriage. She has had two normal pregnancies, but stated that her son, age 13 years, bruises somewhat after contact sports. Evaluation of her son confirmed autoimmune thrombocytopenia with platelet count of 6000. The patient also has a sister, age 34, who has had two episodes of calf vein thrombosis while on oral contraceptives. A cousin, aged 31, is receiving low-dose aspirin for presyncopal spells associated with moderately elevated IgM anticardiolipin antibodies (aCL).

The process of identifying the specific genetic origins of aPL and APS and differentiating them from those of other autoimmune diseases is in its early stages. This chapter summarizes recent studies of familial APS, and the possible contribution of the major histocompatibility complex genes to the origins of APS. As illustrated by the above patient, biologic false positive treponemal serology (BFP-STS) has long been recognized as a harbinger of autoimmune diseases in persons with chronic BFP-STS [4, 5], and among close family members. Among the family members of persons with primary APS, overt autoimmune diseases tend to occur among adult family members, whereas younger family members may exhibit autoantibodies only (Fig. 35.2). However, during prolonged follow-up, some of these younger family

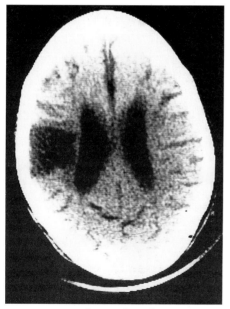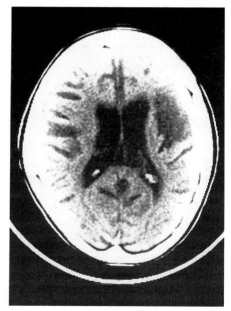

the proband   the proband's sister

Figure 35.2. Computerized axial tomography scans in the proband and her sister, ages 25 and 39 years respectively at onset of primary APS. The proband was hospitalized with left cerebral infarction, thrombocytopenia (69 000/mm³) and BFP-STS. Her history included one episode of calf vein thrombosis and two spontaneous second trimester miscarriages. Five months later she developed a right parietal lobe infarct.

members develop autoimmune diseases indicating that full expression of auto-immunity is often delayed. Important questions that remain to be resolved concern: (a) the relative contribution of specific environmental and genetic factors to this familial autoimmunity; (b) whether retroviruses that induce autoimmunity might confound the search for genetic causes of APS, through their transmissibility either in the human genome (for endogeneous retroviruses) or perinatally in maternal blood or breast milk.

Family Studies (Table 35.1)

Family members of systemic lupus erythematosus (SLE) patients, like those of APS patients, often exhibit various autoantibodies as well as autoimmune diseases such as autoimmune thyroid disease, autoimmune thrombocytopenia and/or hemolytic anemia, rheumatoid arthritis, type I diabetes mellitus, Sjögren's syndrome, and overlap connective tissue disease [6–8]. Analysis of this wide spectrum of auto-immune syndromes among SLE family members and led Bias and her colleagues to suggest that an autoimmunity trait occurred in these families and that the inherit-ance of this trait was along Mendelian autosomal dominant lines [8]. A significant genetic contribution to risk of developing SLE is also suggested by the higher con-cordance for SLE among monozygotic twins (25–30%) than among dizygotic twins (5–10%) [9]. To date the only report of monozygotic twins with aPL or APS is that of an 18-year-old woman with primary APS who had BFP-STS, IgG and IgM aCL, IgG anti-β_2-glycoprotein I (anti-β_2GPI) and lupus anticoagulant (LA) [10]. Her monozygotic twin sister was concordant for the antibodies, but was asymptomatic [10]. Familial aPL or APS has been the subject of several reports of one or more families, in which the index cases were chosen for a variety of features, including LA, SLE or SLE-like illnesses, aPL with thrombocytopenia, stroke, Graves disease and Sneddon's syndrome [11–17]. Larger family studies of APS have confirmed a high aCL prevalence (about 30%) among family members [1–3]. In one of these studies, the low aCL prevalence (5%) among spouses of index cases was consistent with a genetic rather than an environmental effect [2].

Table 35.1. Some family studies of APS.

Reference	Subjects	Conclusion
Mackworth-Young 1987 [36]	101 first degree relatives of 22 SLE patients	aCL* prevalence high in relatives
Wilson 1995 [1]	38 first and second degree relatives of 3 PAPS patients	aCL* prevalence high (30%) in relatives. C4 null alleles HLA DQB₁ allele associated with aCL
Goldberg 1995 [2]	87 family members and 18 spouses of 23 APS patients (mainly secondary APS)	aCL* present in 33% of family members. Low aCL prevalence in spouses
Goel 1999 [3]	101 family members of 7 PAPS patients	Autosomal dominant or codominant model deduced

* aCL = IgG or IgM anticardiolipin antibody.

A recent study of APS features or aPL in 101 family members of seven primary APS patients was consistent with an autosomal dominant or codominant model [3]; in this study none of several genetic markers including human leukocyte antigen (HLA), segregated with APS or aPL among family members [3]. By analogy with SLE, it is possible that APS is multigenic with each gene having only a modest contribution to risk, necessitating more powerful, larger genetic studies than have been done so far. As discussed below, population studies of APS patients, which are less rigorous than segregation analysis, suggest an association of HLA loci with risk of APS or aPL.

The possibility that APS breeds true in some families is also of great interest, because genetic studies in such families are less likely to be confused by secondary associations, as may occur in studies of APS secondary to SLE. A pedigree of a patient with primary APS demonstrated a remarkable absence of autoantibodies other than aCL [16]. In another report, Goel et al studied seven families of probands with primary APS, with each family having at least one other family member affected by APS [3]; they found that 31 of 101 family members had clinical or serologic evidence of aPL of APS, , but that only one family member had another autoimmune disease (undifferentiated connective tissue disease) [3].

MHC Class II Associations of Primary aPL Syndrome

Studies of genetic risk factors for APS have largely focussed on demonstrating associations of various HLA alleles with aPL or APS in various populations (Tables 35.2–35.4). These studies vary considerably in the methods used and the types and groups of subjects. Alleles have been studied by phenotyping or by genotyping (RFLP), with some studies including the more rigorous pedigree analysis of MHC alleles and haplotypes. All isotypes (IgG, M, A) of aPL were assayed in some studies, whereas IgG aCL, or LA only were studied in others.

Table 35.2. MHC Class II studies of primary aPL Syndrome PAPS.

Reference	Patient group (n)	Controls	Techniques	Association
Goldstein et al 1990 [19]*	PAPS (12)	n = 360	Phenotyping	DR53
Trabace et al 1991 [28]	Recurrent miscarriage (49) 25 aCL pos 24 aCL neg	n = 100	Phenotyping	DR7
Asherson et al 1992 [18]	PAPS (13)	n = 69	RFLP Oligotyping	DR53 DR4 (DQ7)
Wilson et al 1995 [1]	Family study of PAPS (38) 10, aCL pos 28, aCL neg	n = 26 (local) n = 191 (workshop)	RFLP oligotyping Pedigree analysis	TRAELDT[†]
Camps et al 1995 [20]	PAPS (19)	n = 261	Phenotyping	DR4, DR7 DR53
Vargas-Alarcon et al 1995 [21]	PAPS (17)	n = 100	Phenotyping and RFLP oligotyping	DR5[‡]

* Published in abstract form.
[†] All DR5 – bearing haplotypes also contained DQ7.
[‡] Combination of DQB1*0301 (DQ7) and other TRAELDT-bearing alleles.

Table 35.3. MHC Class II Studies of aPL in SLE and other diseases.

Reference	Patient group (n)	Controls	Techniques	Association
Canoso et al 1982 [29]	Chlorpromazine-treated patients (97) 57% LA pos.	n = 150	Phenotyping	B44*
Savi et al 1988 [25]	SLE, (80) 45% aCL pos	n = 318 n = 633	Phenotyping, HLA A,B,C, DR	DR7*
McHugh et al 1989 [25][†]	SLE (46) 17% IgG aCL pos	British Transplant Service	Phenotyping	DR4
McGregor et al 1990 [38][‡]	SLE (67) 27% IgG or M aCL pos		Phenotyping	None
McNeil et al 1990 [27][†]	Coronary artery disease (28) 18 aCL pos 10 aCL neg	n = 241	Phenotyping DR4	DR53
Sebastiani et al 1990 [26][†]	SLE (44) 48% IgG aCL pos 32% IgM aCL pos	n = 58 n = 360	Phenotyping Phenotyping	None DR7
Goldstein et al 1990[19][‡]	SLE (72) 28% IgG aCL pos			
Arnett et al 1991 [32][§]	SLE (9), PAPS (8), Sjogrens (2), PSS (1)	n = 139	Genotyping DR5, DR52	DQ7*
Hartung et al 1992 [23]	SLE (314) > 50% aCL pos	Workshop	Phenotyping DR4	DR53
Gulko et al 1993 [22]	SLE (97) 31% IgG aCL pos 18% IgM aCL pos 14% IgA aCL pos	Internal	RFLP Genotyping	None[¶]

* Significant after correction for multiple comparisons.
[†] Published as a letter to the editor.
[‡] Published in abstract form.
[§] aPL present as lupus anticoagulant only, 20 patients.
[¶] DQ7 was negatively correlated with survival.

Table 35.4. Primary APS pedigrees exhibited four MHC Haplotypes containing C4B deficiency as well as TRAELDT alleles.*

Haplotype	DRB1	DQB1	DQA1	C4A	C4B
1	1301	0603	0103	3[†]	Q0 silent
2	1101	0301	05012	3	Q0 deleted
3	1301	0603	0103	3	Q0 deleted
4	1501	0602	0102	3	Q0 deleted

* Highlighted are putative risk factors that are deleted or silent (nonexpressed) C4 genes or one of the DQB1 alleles that encode the TRAELDT sequence (03, 06 series). The silent C4B gene was a gene conversion, that is, it was a structural C4B gene that also contained C4A-specific nucleotide sequences.
[†] Electrophoretic phenotype of C4 allele.

It will not be easy to ascertain which major histocompatibility complex (MHC) genes are true causes of APS, and which genes are innocent bystanders, because many of the MHC risk factors associated with primary or secondary APS are often carried in linkage disequilibrium within similar haplotypes. In 13 primary APS patients studied by Asherson et al using restriction fragment length polymorphism (RFLP) genotyping techniques[18], increased frequencies were found of MHC class II alleles HLA-DR4, DR53, DQB1* 0301 (DQ7) and DQB1*0302. The findings in this small number of subjects are very similar to those of other studies of primary APS patients. Thus Goldstein et al [19] and Camps et al [20], who studied 13 and 19 primary APS patients from Canada and Spain respectively, also showed increased frequencies of DR4 and DQ7. However, among 17 Mexican patients with primary APS, Vargas-Alarcon and colleagues found that HLA-DR5 was increased [21]; it is interesting however, that in this study, all haplotypes that contained -DR5 also contained HLA-DQ7. Larger studies of primary APS are needed to confirm the findings in these groups of primary APS subjects.

MHC Class II Associations of Secondary APS

SLE

In SLE, the MHC associations of aPL are to some extent influenced by the MHC associations of SLE itself; in spite of this, the results of MHC class II studies of aPL in SLE patients are generally consistent with those found in primary APS patients. In agreement with most studies of primary APS, a very large European multicenter study of 314 SLE patients reported that HLA-DR53, DR4 and DR7 phenotypes were associated with aCL [23].

Smaller populations of SLE patients from England [24], Italy [25, 26] and a study of aCL in ischemic heart disease from Australia [27] also showed increases or trends towards increases in DR4 and/or DR7. An Italian study of 49 women with unexplained recurrent miscarriages also showed a trend for HLA DR7 to be associated with aCL [28]. An American study of 46 Caucasian and 45 African–American SLE patients found no significant MHC class II associations of aPL antibodies, although in this study, -DQ7 was negatively and independently correlated with survival in SLE [22]. Early studies by Canoso and her colleagues of chlorpromazine-induced LA reported an association with the HLA-B44 phenotype [29], which is known to be linked on the same haplotype with DR4, DQ7 and a C4B deficiency allele, in general agreement with some of the above studies.

Although the above associations of HLA genes with aCL appear to be multiplex, it must be borne in mind that many of the putative risk factors discussed above, including HLA DR4 or DR7 and DQB1*0301, DQB1*0302 or DQB1*0303 are often carried in linkage disequilibrium, in the same MHC haplotypes [30, 31]. Accordingly, these alleles may in fact be surrogates or markers that are closely linked to the genes that are true contributors to the cause of APS.

MHC-DQB1 Alleles: a Unifying Hypothesis

Arnett et al have suggested that one such true risk factor for aPL may be a MHC-DQB1 oligonucleotide allele that encodes seven consecutive residues (71–77, TRAELDT) in the third hypervariable region, located in the DQB1 outer domain; in this location this putative epitope is positioned to influence immune responses, by affecting presentation of antigens to the T lymphocyte receptor [32]. From their analysis of autoantibody profiles and MHC genotypes (RFLP) in 20 patients with a variety of connective tissue diseases, Arnett et al found that HLA-DQ7 was associated with the presence of the LA [32]. An analysis of the alleles that contribute to the HLA-DQ7 specificity showed that LA was most strongly associated with DQB1*0301 [32]. Moreover, among patients who had LA but not DQ7, all possessed DQB1*0302 or *0602 alleles.32 All the foregoing DQB1 alleles (*0301, *0302, *0303, *0602) encode the same sequence in the 71–77 (TRAELDT) region of the third hypervariable DQB1 region described above [32].

In agreement with the above findings, pedigree analysis by Wilson et al of MHC class II and III genotypes and haplotypes among family members of primary APS patients, confirmed an increase in the DQB1 TRAELDT alleles, especially among family members who had aCL in serum [1]. In addition, among seven APS probands studied by Goel et al 11 out of 13 HLA-DBQ alleles were DQB1*03- or *06- (i.e., TREALDT) [3]. A recent study of anti β_2GPI antibodies in three ethnic groups by Arnett and colleagues is also consistent with the TRAELDT hypothesis [33]; they found anti β_2GPI to be associated with HLA-DQB1*03-alleles and to a lesser extent *DQB1*06-alleles [33].

The size of the relative risk of aPL associated with these alleles is modest (2–3) [2, 32], since about 50% of HLA-DQB1 genes in disease-free control populations encode the TRAELDT sequence in the DQB1 outer domain. Accordingly, other unknown risk factors must be important in aPL production.

Complement (C4) Deficiency Alleles

With respect to other MHC putative risk factors, there is evidence that aPL are also associated with haplotypes containing deficiency alleles of the fourth complement component, C4. Deficiency alleles of C4 are of interest in relation to APS because the haplotypes that contain C4 deficiency alleles have been associated with familial SLE and several other autoimmune diseases [6–8]. In addition, Stephansson and her colleagues have shown a high prevalence of C4A null alleles among persons with chronic BFP-STS, some of whom developed autoimmune diseases (including APS) on prolonged follow-up [5]. Accordingly, HLA haplotypes that include C4 null alleles may contribute to a non-specific autoimmunity trait that includes aPL production.

Primary APS

Among 38 Caucasian family members of index cases selected for PAPS, Wilson et al, using RFLP genotyping as well as phenotyping techniques, reported that MHC haplotypes containing deficiency alleles of C4A and C4B were associated with aCL [1]. There was great variation in the haplotypes that contained these deficiency alleles of C4 (Table 35.4). Some deficiency alleles were C4A or C4B gene deletions, while others were C4B gene conversions (structural C4B genes that contained C4A-specific nucleotide sequences) that had no C4 gene product in serum [1]. However, all deficiency alleles appeared to be true deficiency alleles that generated no C4 gene product in serum [1]. This is consistent with the hypothesis that reduced C4 production and function causes an immunologic deficit that is a primary risk factor for autoimmunity; it has been suggested that C4 deficiency states cause deficits in the opsonization and clearance of antigens and this leads to the persistence of antigens in the circulation, thus producing autoimmunization. Bentolia et al, using pheno-typing techniques only, also found a high prevalence of C4A and C4B null alleles among 20 primary APS patients [34]. Asherson et al [18] did not find an increased prevalence of C4 gene deletions among 13 primary APS patients, but these authors identified C4 null alleles by Taq 1 RFLP only, and Taq 1 RFLP does not detect all C4 null alleles, especially null alleles of C4B.

In view of the linkage disequilibrium within the MHC, the MHC haplotypes that contain C4A or C4B deficiency alleles are of interest, and have been analyzed in rel-ation to the TRAELDT sequence discussed above [1]. Among family members of primary APS patients, MHC DQB1 alleles that encode the TRAELDT sequence were present in four out of five haplotypes that contained C4B deficiency alleles (Table 35.4). This raises the possibility that coexistent MHC risk factors may interact with one another and thereby have additive or multiplicative effects on risk of devel-oping APS, but this possibility has not been evaluated. In contrast, alleles encoding TRAELDT were not present in any haplotypes that contained C4A gene deletions (including the very common C4A null-containing ancestral haplotype [1]). Thus, any risk for primary APS or aPL associated with C4A deletions would appear to be independent of the TRAELDT alleles.

Secondary APS

C4A and C4B null phenotypes were also reported to be associated with aCL among African–Americans with active SLE [35]. However, studies among Caucasian SLE patients have not shown this association [23] or were inconclusive [36] and C4A null alleles were not associated with polyclonal aCL among SLE patients studied by Petri et al [37]. This difference may relate to interethnic variation in SLE and/or the nega-tive linkage disequilibrium described above between C4A gene deletions (which occur in 40–50% of Caucasian SLE patients) and the MHC-DQB1 alleles that encode TRAELDT [1]. This lack of association between C4A deletions and aPL in Caucasian SLE patients also suggests that in Caucasians, as further discussed below, TRAELDT alleles may be stronger or more specific risk factors for aPL than C4A gene deletions.

Familial Aggregation of Autoimmunity

Associations of C4 deficiency alleles with primary APS are of additional interest as this may partly account for familial aggregation of several autoimmune diseases with primary APS, discussed above. This is because the MHC ancestral haplotypes that contain C4A deficiency alleles have been associated with several autoimmune diseases including SLE, autoimmune thyroid diseases, type I diabetes mellitus and Sjögren's syndrome [38]. As discussed above, these diseases aggregate among family members of patients with primary APS, and sometimes coexist with each other in patients with aPL antibodies (Fig. 35.1).

Summary

The class II and especially the DQB1 locus of MHC genes, as well as C4 deficiency alleles appear to be associated with genetic risk for developing aPL. The extensive linkage disequilibrium among some of these risk factors makes it difficult to assign a causal role for any of these alleles by means of previous population studies of patients with APS; studies of patients with primary APS, in particular, have involved relatively few patients. Although there appear to be some overall similarities between the known MHC associations of primary APS and those of secondary APS, only a modest relative risk of APS is associated with these MHC alleles, as discussed above, and other unknown risk factors must also be important. Whether these unknown risk factors for primary APS are different from those in secondary APS is an area for further investigation. In addition, new genes continue to be identified in the MHC class II and III regions that appear to have important roles in antigen processing and recognition [31]. Interethnic studies of these and other alleles in large cohorts would be informative since ethnic groups of African, Japanese or Caucasian backgrounds often exhibit differing allelic linkage disequilibria within the MHC. Interethnic studies of linkage relationships in various MHC haplotypes have, for example, helped to clarify the role of MHC alleles in rheumatoid arthritis [31]. Further clarification of the roles of these MHC alleles will also depend on functional studies in laboratory models to assess the roles of these risk factors in aPL production. The roles of non-MHC risk factors and of environmental agents that are operative within families also warrant further studies.

References

1. Wilson WA, Scopelitis E, Michalski JP et al. Familial anticardiolipin antibodies are associated with C4 deficiency genotypes that coexist with MHC DQB risk factors. J Rheumatol 1995;22:227–235.
2. Goldberg SN, Conti-Kelly AM, Greco TP et al. A family study of anticardiolipin antibodies and associated conditions. Am J Med 1995;98:473–479.
3. Goel N, Ortel TL, Bali D et al. Familial antiphospholipid antibody syndrome. Arthritis Rheum 1999;43:318–327.
4. Harvey AM, Shulman LE. Connective tissue disease and the chronic biologic false positive test for syphilis. Med Clin N Am 1966;50:1271–1279.
5. Stephansson EA, Koskimies S, Lokki M-L. HLA antigens and complement C4 allotypes in patients with chronic biologic false positive seroreactions (CBFP) for syphilis: a follow up study of SLE patients and CBFP Reactors. Lupus 1993:2;77–81.
6. Lippman SM et al. Genetic factors predisposing to autoimmune diseases: autoimmune hemolytic anemia, chronic thrombocytopenic purpura, and systemic lupus erythematosus. Am J Med 1982;73:827–840.
7. Reveille JD, Arnett FC, Wilson RW et al. Null alleles of the fourth component of complement and HLA haplotypes in familial systemic lupus erythematosus. Immunogenetics 1985;21:299–311.
8. Bias WB, Reveille JD, Beatty TH et al. Evidence that autoimmunity in man is a mendelian dominant trait. Am J Hum Genet 1986;39:584–602.
9. Deapen D, Escalante A, Weinrib L et al. Revised estimate of twin concordance in systemic lupus erythematosus. Arthritis Rheum 1992;35:311–318.
10. Cevallos R, Darnige L, Arvieux J et al. Antiphospholipid and β_2 glycoprotein-1 antibodies in monozygotic twin sisters. J Rheumatol 1994;21:70–71.
11. Mackie IJ, Colaco CB, Machin SJ. Familial lupus anticoagulants. Br J Haematol 1987;67;359–363.
12. Matthey F, Walshe K, Mackie IJ, Machin SJ. Familial occurrence of the antiphospholipid syndrome. J Clin Pathol 1989;42:495–497.
13. Peettee AD, Wasserman BA, Adams NL et al. Familial Sneddons syndrome. Neurology 1994;399–405.
14. Ford P, Brunet D, Lillicrap DP et al. Premature stroke in a family with lupus anticoagulant and antiphospholipid antibodies. Stroke 1990;21:66–71.
15. May KP, West SG, Moulds J, Kotzin BL. Different manifestations of the antiphospholipid antibody syndrome in a family with systemic lupus erythematosus. Arthritis Rheum 1993;36:528–533.
16. Dagenais P, Urowitz MB, Gladman DD, Norman CD. A family study of the antiphospholipid syndrome associated with other autoimmune diseases. J Rheumatol 1992;19:1393–6.

16. Bansal AS, Hogan PG, Gibbs H, Grazer IH. Familial primary antiphospholipid antibody syndrome. Arthritis Rheum 1996;39:705–706.
17. Motta C, Meyer O. Childhood-onset SLE: antiphospholipid antibodies in 37 patients and their first degree relatives. Pediatrics 1993;92:849–853.
18. Asherson RA, Doherty DG, Vergani D et al. Major histocompatibility complex associations with primary antiphospholipid syndrome. Arthritis Rheum 1992;35:124–125.
19. Goldstein B, Smith CD, Sengar DPS. MHC class II studies of primary antiphospholipid antibody syndrome and of serum antiphospholipid antibodies in systemic lupus erythematosus. Arthritis Rheum 1990;33:S125.
20. Camps MT, Cuadrado MJ, Ocon P et al. Association between HLA class II antigens and primary antiphospholipid syndrome from the South of Spain. Lupus 1995;4:51–55.
21. Vargas-Alarcon G, Granados J, Bekker C et al. Association of HLA-DR5 (possibly DRB1*1201) with the primary antiphospholipid syndrome in Mexican patients. Arthritis Rheum 1995,38:1340–1343.
22. Gulko PS, Reveille JD, Koopman WJ et al. Anticardiolipin antibodies in systemic lupus erythematosus: clinical correlates, HLA associations and impact on survival. J Rheumatol 1993;20:1684–1693.
23. Hartung K, Coldewey R, Corvetta A et al. MHC gene products and anticardiolipin antibodies in systemic lupus erythematosus. Results of a multicenter study. Autoimmunity 1992;13:95–99.
24. McHugh NJ, Maddison PJ. HLA-DR antigens and anticardiolipin antibodies in patients with systemic lupus erythematosus. Arthritis Rheum 1989;32:1623–1624.
25. Savi M, Ferraccioli GF, Neri TM et al. HLA-DR antigens and anticardiolipin antibodies in northern Italian systemic lupus erythematosus. Arthritis Rheum 1988;31:1568–1570.
26. Sebastiani GD, Lulli P, Passiu G et al. Anticardiolipin antibodies: their relationship with HLA-DR antigens in systemic lupus erythematosus. Br J Rheumatol 19 ;30:156–157.
27. McNeil HP, Gavaghan TP, Krilis SA et al. HLA-DR antigens and anticardiolipin antibodies. Clin Exp Rheumatol 1990;8:425–427.
28. Trabace S, Nicotra M, Cappellacci S et al. HLA-DR and DQ antigens and anticardiolipin antibodies in women with recurrent spontaneous abortions. Am J Reprod Immunol 1991;26:147–149.
29. Canoso RT, Lewis ME, Yunis EJ. Association of HLA-BW44 with chlorpromazine-induced autoantibodies. Clin Immunol Immunopathol 1982;25:278–282.
30. Arnett FC, Reveille JD. Genetics of systemic lupus erythematosus. Rheum Dis Clin N Am 1992;18:865–892.
31. Nepom BS, Nepom GT. Polyglot and polymorphism: an HLA update. Arthritis Rheum 1996;38:1715–1721.
32. Arnett FC, Olsen ML, Anderson KL, Reveille JD. Molecular analysis of major histocompatibility complex alleles associated with the lupus anticoagulant. J Clin Invest 1991;87:1490–1495.
33. Arnett FC, Thiagarajan P, Ahn C, Reveille JD. Associations of anti β_2-glycoprotein I autoantibodies with HLA class II alleles in three ethnic groups. Arthritis Rheum 1999;42:268–274.
34. Bentolia S. High prevalence of C4 "null" alleles in primary antiphospholipid syndrome. Arthritis Rheum 1995;38(9):S171.
35. Wilson WA, Perez MC, Michalski JP, Armatis PE. Cardiolipin antibodies and null alleles of C4 in black Americans with systemic lupus erythematosus. J Rheumatol 1988;15:1768–1772.
36. Petri M, Watson R, Winkelstein JA, McLean RH. Clinical expression of systemic lupus erythematosus in patients with C4A deficiency. Medicine 1993;72:236–244.
36. Mackworth-Young CG, Chan J, Harris N et al. High incidence of anticardiolipin antibodies in relatives of patients with systemic lupus erythematosus. J Rheumatol 1987;14:723–726.
38. Citera G, Wilson WA: Ethnic and geographic perspectives in SLE. Lupus 1993;2:351–353.

36 Monoclonal Antiphospholipid Antibodies and their Sequences

A. Rahman and D. Isenberg

Introduction

The antiphospholipid antibody syndrome (APS) is a disorder in which the presence of antiphospholipid antibodies (aPL) is associated closely with the tendency to develop venous and/or arterial occlusion, recurrent fetal loss and thrombocytopenia [1, 2]. The clinical consequences of high levels of these antibodies are described elsewhere in this book and will not be considered in detail in this chapter.

There are two broad categories of phospholipids, negatively charged and neutral. The neutral phospholipids include phosphatidylethanolamine, phosphatidylcholine, platelet-activating factor, and sphingomyelin. Negatively charged phospholipids include phosphatidylglycerol, phosphatidylserine, phosphatidic acid, phosphatidylinositol and cardiolipin.

aPL have been detected in 1.5–5% of the population [3] but they are found much more frequently in patients with infections or autoimmune diseases, in particular systemic lupus erythematosus (SLE) and the primary and secondary antiphospholipid syndromes. It has been estimated that aPL are present in 25–50% of patients with SLE [reviewed in 4]. By definition, all patients with primary antiphospholipid antibody syndrome (PAPS) must possess these antibodies.

aPL found in patients with clinical features of APS tend to show preferential binding to negatively charged phospholipids and this binding is dependent on the presence of the protein cofactor β_2-glycoprotein I (β_2-GPI). aPL found in patients with infections do not show this cofactor dependence, bind both negatively charged and neutral phospholipids and are not associated with the clinical features of the syndrome.

The clinical features of the syndrome are related more closely to the levels of IgG than IgM aPL. This has been shown for both venous thromboembolic disease [5] and fetal loss [reviewed in 6]. This distinction resembles that observed with anti-double stranded DNA antibodies (anti-dsDNA) in systemic lupus erythematosus. Thus there is considerable evidence [7, 8] to show that levels of IgG anti-dsDNA correlate more closely with clinical features of SLE, particularly nephritis, than do levels of IgM anti-dsDNA antibodies.

Stimulus to aPL Generation

Phospholipids are ubiquitous components of cell membranes that are known to undergo functional redistribution in different pathophysiological conditions [discussed in detail elsewhere, 9]. Phospholipid exposure is known to occur during the course of apoptosis and may be a key factor in the pathogenesis of APS. Indeed, as Casciola-Rosen et al [10] have proposed, apoptosis may represent a common pathway by which autoantibodies against several self-antigens are produced. The work of these authors demonstrated that keratinocyte cell lines exposed to ultraviolet radiation underwent notable changes by which molecular structures, restricted normally to nuclear or cytoplasmic components or to the inner side of plasma membranes, were shown to accumulate on the outer surface of newly generated blebs or particles, such as the apoptotic bodies [11]. Thus, in the context of APS, phosphatidylserine, a potent surface proagglutinant that is restricted normally to the inner surface of the membrane bilayer, may become exposed as a consequence of apoptosis. It may thereby represent an antigenic stimulus to APL production [discussed in 9].

It has been further speculated that the reactive oxygen species (ROS) may activate the apoptotic process through ROS-dependent signal transduction pathways. These reactive oxygen species may also be involved in phospholipid oxidation which is crucial in the unveiling of phospholipid epitopes against which most aPL are directed. Hokko et al [12] showed that aPL are actually directed against neoepitopes of oxidized phospholipids or neoepitopes generated by adduct formation between breakdown products of oxidized phospholipids and associated proteins. Perhaps linked to this is the knowledge that β_2GPI–phospholipid interaction induces the formation of highly immunogenic phospholipids or protein epitopes. Thus, Hokko et al [12] also showed that sera from patients with the APS or affinity purified IgG did not bind efficiently to a cardiolipin analog that is incapable of undergoing liquid peroxidation. A full account of the potential connections between apoptosis and aPL has been published recently [9].

The Role of Sequence Analysis in the Study of aPL

The IgG aPL found in patients who have clinical features of APS tend to bind specifically to negatively charged phospholipids and this binding is dependent on the presence of β_2GPI. Sequence analysis of aPL can be used to investigate the molecular features which differentiate antibodies possessing these clinically important binding properties from antibodies lacking these properties. Knowledge of these features may lead to a better understanding of the way in which they develop. It may also allow the production of a clearer image of the antibody–PL–β_2GPI interaction.

In order to relate the properties of a particular aPL antibody to its sequence, it is necessary to obtain appreciable quantities of both the immunoglobulin itself and the mRNA which encodes it. This is most conveniently achieved by studying monoclonal antibodies (mAb) produced from Epstein–Barr virus-transformed cells or from hybridomas. In order to analyze sequences of mAb, it is necessary to understand the way in which antibody sequences are encoded.

The Genetic Origin of Antibody Sequences

An immunoglobulin molecule consists of two identical heavy chains and two identical light chains, as shown in Fig. 36.1. There are two types of light chain, designated
kappa and lambda. Each chain consists of a constant region and a variable region.
The constant regions have the same sequence in all antibodies of a given isotype,
regardless of binding specificity. The variable regions (designated V_H and V_L for the

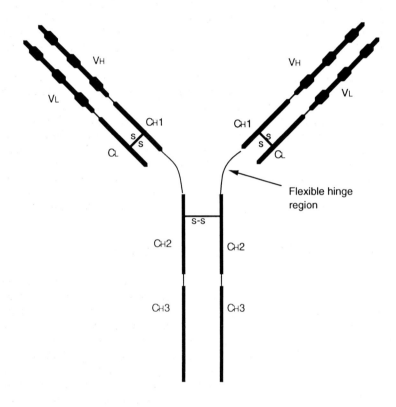

In each V region CDRs and FRs are distinguished as shown
below.

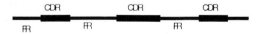

Figure 36.1. The figure shows the arrangement of constant and variable regions in the light and heavy chains
and the disulfide bonds linking the chains. The positions of complementarity-determining regions (CDRs) and
framework regions (FRs) within the variable domains are also shown. V_H = variable region of the heavy chain;
V_L = variable region of the light chain; C_L = constant region of the light chain; C_H1, C_H2 and C_H3 are the three
domains making up the constant region of the heavy chain; S-S = disulfide bond.

heavy and light chains, respectively) differ in sequence in antibodies which bind different antigens. Within these regions, three areas of very high variability, known as the complementarity determining regions (CDRs) are separated by less variable framework regions (FRs) (see Fig. 36.1). Evidence from crystallographic studies suggests that the FRs form a scaffolding, from which loops encoded by the CDRs extend to make contact with the antigen [13]. Thus, the sequences of the CDRs of V_H and V_L are particularly important in determining the antigen-binding properties of an antibody.

Both the V_H and V_L sequences are produced by fusion of gene segments which are separate in germline DNA but brought together in B lymphocytes. The V_L domain is encoded by two segments (the V_L and J_L genes) and the V_H domain by three segments (the V_H, D_H and J_H genes). The gene segments are brought together by a site-specific recombination process [14].

The overall effect of this recombination process is to provide each B cell with a large potential repertoire of variable domain sequences [15]. This large repertoire arises partly because there are a relatively large number of V_H, D_H, J_H, V_L and J_L gene segments from which those expressed can be chosen. In addition, the junctions between the segments are somewhat flexible. Nucleotides can be lost from one or both genes at a junction, or new nucleotides can be added by the enzyme terminal deoxynucleotidyltransferase. CDR3 of the heavy chain is especially variable because most of it is encoded by the D_H genes. D_H genes can be fused together or inverted during the recombination process and some are capable of encoding productive amino acid sequences in all three reading frames. (reviewed in 15).

The Importance of Somatic Hypermutation

Once a B lymphocyte has rearranged gene segments to produce both a productive (i.e., without premature termination codons or frameshifts) $V_H D_H J_H$ sequence and a productive $V_L J_L$ sequence, it can secrete a complete antibody molecule. The lymphocyte is stimulated to divide and produce a clone of cells by interactions between antibody molecules on its surface and antigen. The sequences, and thus the properties, of the immunoglobulin molecules secreted by different members of the clone can be altered by a process known as somatic hypermutation [16]. Somatic mutations are those which are not inherited through the germline and are not present in all cells of the body. Somatic mutations developing in a single cell are passed on to its descendants. In B lymphocytes, the frequency of somatic mutation has been shown to be far higher in the gene segments encoding immunoglobulin variable regions than in the rest of the genome [17].

It has been argued that somatic mutations are particularly important in the development of IgG antibodies which bind to antigens with high affinity [17, 18]. When monoclonal antibodies (mAb) to a particular antigen are derived from mice, the IgG mAb tend to show more specificity, more somatic mutations and higher affinity for the antigen than IgM mAb [19]. Somatic mutations in these high affinity antibodies tend not to be distributed randomly. Replacement mutations, which alter the amino acid sequence of the antibody, are concentrated in the CDRs. Silent mutations, which do not alter the amino acid sequence, are not concentrated in this way. The explanation for this is that, in the presence of antigen, those antibody secreting cells which develop mutations enhancing the affinity of antibody for antigen are stimulated to divide faster than other clones [17, 18] and therefore undergo selective expansion. Clearly, the mutations most likely to alter binding affinity in this way will be replacement mutations in the CDRs. Therefore, a finding of a high ratio of replacement to silent (R : S) mutations in the CDRs but not the FRs of the sequence of an antibody may be taken as evidence that this sequence arose as the result of such an antigen driven process [18, 20].

By comparing the sequences of different mAb that bind phospholipids, it is possible to deduce the extent to which particular variable region gene segments are used preferentially to encode these antibodies and the extent to which monospecific and/or high-affinity binding is dependent on the presence of somatic mutations in these genes. However, these deductions can only be accurate if it is possible to be sure which gene segments have been used to encode each antibody. This has not been possible for human mAb until very recently, because the complete repertoire of human V_H, V_κ and V_λ genes was not known until the publication of comprehensive maps of these loci during the last few years [21–24].

The Repertoire of V_H, V_κ and V_λ Gene Segments in Humans and Mice

Functional V_H, V_κ and V_λ genes are found on human chromosomes 14, 2 and 22, respectively. In all three of these loci there are a large number of pseudogenes (genes which cannot give a functional product), as well as functional genes. The genes can be classified into families on the basis of sequence homology. Two V_H genes belong to the same family if they share the same nucleotide sequence at more than 80% of positions. Similar rules can be applied to the classification of V_κ and V_λ genes. In humans, there are seven V_H, seven V_κ and 10 V_λ families. The families are not equal in size. For example, the majority of V_H genes belong to just three families, V_H 1,3 and 4. Similarly, three V_κ families (V_κ I–III) and three V_λ families (V_λ 1–3) are larger than the others.

The potential repertoire of functional variable region gene segments available to a human antibody secreting cell comprises approximately 50 V_H [21, 22], 40 V_κ [23] and 30 V_λ [24] genes. However, not all of these genes are equally likely to be expressed. Brezinschek et al [25] estimated that a group of just eight genes from three families (V_H1,3 and 4) accounted for over 50% of all productive rearrangements in IgM-secreting peripheral B cells. Similarly, Cox et al [26] have reported that just 11 of the 40 potentially functional V_κ genes account for 90% of expressed V_κ sequences.

It is important to note that this preferential rearrangment of certain V_H and V_L gene segments is independent of antigen specificity. It appears to be a bias intrinsic to the rearrangement process, and it is important to allow for this when attempting to decide whether particular genes or families are used preferentially to encode aPL.

The Importance of Allelic Polymorphism

Allelic polymorphism leads to small differences in sequence between alleles of the same gene in different haplotypes. This observation is important in the interpretation of sequences of mAb because it can lead to uncertainty in determining the site and nature of somatic mutations. This uncertainty is reduced where the germline gene in question is known to display little or no polymorphism, i.e., it is likely to have practically the same sequence in everyone.

For most human V_H, V_κ and V_λ genes, polymorphism does indeed appear to be very limited. Review of all published alleles of V_H genes [27] shows that the majority of alleles differ by only one to two nucleotides. It seems reasonable to assume, therefore, that where the V_H sequence of a mAb differs at many positions from all published alleles of the most similar germline gene, these differences result from mutation rather than polymorphism. Similar conclusions can be reached from review of published alleles of human V_κ [27] and V_λ [24] genes.

Principles of Analysis of mAb Sequences

In order to draw meaningful conclusions from the published V_H and V_L sequences of a monoclonal aPL it is first necessary to compare each to the most similar allele of the most similar known germline gene. Differences between the germline and V_H (or V_L) sequences can then be considered sites of somatic mutations, the number and positions of which can be noted. By carrying out this process for a number of different aPL, varying in properties such as specificity and affinity for anionic phospholipids, one may seek to answer the following questions.

1. *Are particular variable region genes used preferentially to encode aPL?* This would be suggested if many different aPL were encoded by a particular gene or family of genes to an extent which could not readily be explained by the inbuilt preference for rearrangement of certain genes noted above.
2. *Do high-affinity IgG aPL contain more somatic mutations than lower-affinity or IgM aPL, as would be expected on theoretical grounds?*
3. *Does the pattern of mutation suggest that such high affinity aPL arise due to antigen-driven selection of mutations?* The major evidence suggesting this would be a high R : S ratio in CDRs but not FRs. In addition, some workers have reported the isolation of distinct, but clonally related, mAb from an individual mouse or patient. Clonally related mAb are those descended from the same original B cell. They can be recognized by their V_H CDR3 sequences, which will be essentially identical, even at the V–D and D–J junctions. Because the potential for diversity in this CDR is so great, it is very unlikely that identical V_H CDR3 sequences would develop in cells derived from different clones. The process of hybridoma formation is inefficient, so that if two clonally related hybridomas are produced, the implication is that the clone from which they were derived had a very large number of members. This is evidence for clonal expansion as suggested by the theory of antigen drive.
4. *Do particular sequence features in the CDRs seem to occur commonly in aPL?* In both murine [28] and human [29] anti-DNA antibodies, the presence of positively charged and/or basic amino acids including arginine, asparagine and lysine in the CDRs is a recurring feature. The presence of such residues in V_HCDR3 seems particularly common in anti-dsDNA mAb, particularly in the mouse [19, 28]. Such amino acids often occur at sites of somatic mutation, suggesting that their presence is selected due to their ability to form charge interactions or hydrogen bonds

with the negatively charged phosphodiester backbone of the DNA molecule. Because the aPL found in patients with APS commonly bind strongly to negatively charged but not neutral phospholipids, similar reasoning would suggest that monoclonal aPL might also show accumulations of positively charged amino acids in their CDRs.

Sequences of Monoclonal aPL Derived from Mouse Models of APS

MRL *lpr/lpr* mice frequently produce aPL. Apart from a relatively high incidence of myocardial infarction these mice do not develop clinical features suggestive of thrombosis. Kita et al [30] analyzed 14 monoclonal aPL from MRL *lpr/lpr* mice. Sequence analysis showed that different aPL from a single mouse tended to be clonally related, suggesting that clonal expansion had occurred. Allowing for this, the 14 antibodies could be shown to derive from nine different clones. Six of these clones used V_H genes of the largest murine V_H family, designated J558. It is not clear, however, whether this represents a true preference for use of these genes in encoding APL. It has been estimated that almost 50% of spontaneously activated B cells in MRL *lpr/lpr* mice express J558 genes, regardless of antigen specificity [31]. Mutations in these 14 monoclonal APL were almost all found in FRs. Though some of the antibodies had V_H CDR 3 regions which were rich in arginine, there was no apparent relationship between arginine content and affinity for cardiolipin.

The (NZW × BXSB) F_1 mouse may be a better autoimmune model of APS. Male (NZW × BXSB) F_1 mice develop some features characteristic of human APS, such as thrombocytopenia and vascular disease. Mice of both sexes produce serum aPL, some of which are of IgG isotype and show binding to cardiolipin which is enhanced by β_2GPI. These binding properties were used to distinguish two of six monoclonal aPL derived from mice of this strain as "pathogenic" [32]. These two antibodies also induced thrombosis when injected into mice. Sequence analysis showed that both used J558 V_H genes. The other four "non-pathogenic" antibodies were less likely to use genes from this family. The degree of somatic mutation in these six mAb is uncertain as the germline genes of origin have not been assigned definitely. As with MRL *lpr/lpr*-derived aPL, there was no relationship between the CDR arginine content and binding to cardiolipin. Indeed, neither pathogenic aPL had any positive residues in V_HCDR 3.

Monestier et al [33] described a further nine monoclonal IgG aPL from (NZW × BXSB) F_1 mice. All but one used genes from the J558 family. There was no preference for any V_L family. Two mAb from a single mouse were clonally related. Two mAb from a different mouse would only bind cardiolipin in the presence of β_2GPI but the sequence characteristics of these mAb did not differ markedly from those of the other seven. Although replacement mutations appeared to cluster in the CDRs of V_H but not V_L, the authors did not comment upon this. Eight of the antibodies had arginine, asparagine or both in V_HCDR 3. The only exception, however, was the antibody which behaved most like a pathogenic APL in that it was completely dependent on β_2-GPI for binding to cardiolipin and would bind β_2-GPI alone on irradiated plates.

Overall, the evidence from murine monoclonal aPL is equivocal. There may be preferential use of genes from the J558 family and clonal expansion does seem to occur in the development of these antibodies. The extent to which antigen driven somatic mutation and the presence of basic residues in CDRs are important remains unclear.

Sequences of Monoclonal Human aPL

Sequences of almost 30 human mAb that bind phospholipids have been reported. Many of the early reports, however, referred to polyreactive IgM antibodies that had been selected for binding to a different antigen (usually single stranded or double-stranded DNA), and which were then noted to bind cardiolipin (or another phospholipid) as well. These antibodies typically showed relatively low affinity for phospholipid. In common with other polyreactive IgM antibodies they had V_H and V_L sequences containing relatively few somatic mutations.

As interest in aPL and the APS has grown, several groups have sought to produce and study mAb that only bind phospholipids. These may be more representative of the antibodies involved in the pathogenesis of APS than the polyreactive antibodies that were referred to above. The mAb most relevant to pathogenesis would be IgG antibodies that showed specific binding to negatively charged but not neutral phospholipids, particularly if this binding were dependent on the presence of β_2GPI. No sequences of antibodies with all of these properties have been reported, but monospecific IgM and IgG human aPL have been studied, and some of these have been shown to induce pathological changes in immunodeficient mice.

Thus, the human monoclonal aPL that have been described so far can be conveniently considered in three groups, polyreactive IgM antibodies, specific IgM aPL, and IgG aPL. The differences in sequence characteristics between these three groups provide some clues as to the molecular characteristics important at the phospholipid-binding site.

Sequences of Polyreactive IgM Human Monoclonal aPL

The sequence and binding characteristics of these antibodies are summarized in Table 36.1 [34–39]. The majority of these antibodies were obtained from cells derived from healthy individuals. Four antibodies (18/2, 1/17, C119 and C471) were derived by immortalizing lymphocytes from patients with SLE, but these patients did not have features of APS. Thus, the 15 mAb listed in this table may be representative of natural autoantibodies [40], which tend to be of IgM isotype, polyreactive and are present without ill effect in healthy individuals.

There is no evidence for preferential use of particular genes or families in these polyreactive antibodies. 12 of the 15 mAb use genes from the largest V_H families, V_H 1,3 and 4, and the most commonly used gene is V3-23 which is the most commonly rearranged V_H gene in IgM secreting B cells regardless of antigen specificity [25]. Of the light chains which have been sequenced, all use genes which are members of the three largest V_κ or V_λ families. Three of the 15 antibodies used the V_H 6 family gene 6-01. However, this apparently high prevalence of 6-01-derived aPL is misleading, because these antibodies were isolated in an experiment which expressly set out to produce mAb encoded by this gene [37].

Table 36.1. Sequence characteristics of human polyreactive IgM aPL.

mAb	Origin	V$_H$ gene[*]	V$_H$ homology	V$_L$ family	V$_L$ gene	V$_L$ homology	High R:S in CDR	Basic residues in CDR[†]	Ref.
18/2	SLE PBL	3–23	100%	NP	NP	NP	No	No	34
1/17	SLE PBL	3–23	100%	NP	NP	NP	No	No	34
C6B2	Sickle cell spleen	4–61	97%	NP	NP	NP	No	No	35
Kim 4.6	Healthy tonsil	3–30	100%	V$_λ$1	1b	100%	No	No	36
A10	Healthy PBL	6–01	99%	NP	NP	NP	No	No	37
A431	Healthy PBL	6–01	98%	NP	NP	NP	No	No	37
L16	Fetal liver	6–01	100%	NP	NP	NP	No	No	37
C119	SLE PBL	3–23	96%	V$_κ$III	L6	100%	Yes	No	38
C471	SLE PBL	3–64	99.6%	V$_κ$III	L2	100%	No	No	38
B122	Healthy PBL	1–18	97%	V$_κ$I	L12	98%	No	No	38
B6204	Healthy PBL	3–23	97%	V$_κ$III	A27	99.7%	No	No	38
H3	Healthy PBL	1–46	97%	V$_κ$3	3I	97%	No	No	39
H5	Healthy PBL	4–30	96%	NP	NP	NP	Yes	Yes	39
A5	Healthy PBL	3–23	100%	V$_λ$3	3p	97%	Yes	No	39
Bou53.6	Healthy tonsil	3–23	100%	V$_κ$I	L12	99%	No	No	39

* The family to which a V$_H$ gene belongs is given by the first digit of its name. Thus V3-23 belongs to the V$_H$3 family, V4-61 to the V$_H$4 family, etc.

† In this column, an accumulation of basic residues is taken to occur where there are at least three such residues within V$_H$CDR3 or three basic residues occur within a run of four successive amino acids in any other CDR. The reasons for choosing these limits are described in reference 29.

SLE, systemic lupus erythematosus; PBL, peripheral blood lymphocytes; CLL, chronic lymphocytic leukemia; PAPS, primary antiphospholipid antibody syndrome.

The majority of these mAb show very few somatic mutations. In mathematical terms, the degree of sequence homology between the V$_H$ or V$_L$ sequences and the germline genes from which they were derived is very high. As noted previously, a relative lack of somatic mutations is a common rule in IgM antibodies. B122 and B6204 [38], derived from peripheral blood lymphocytes (PBL) of healthy people do carry many mutations in V$_H$, but these are not clustered in the CDRs suggesting that they have not been accumulated due to antigen drive. Only one of the mAb, H5, shows an accumulation of positively charged residues in a CDR, since it has three successive arginines in V$_H$CDR3 [39].

Sequences of More Specific Human IgM aPL

The five IgM aPL shown in Table 36.2 [41–45] have different phenotypic and sequence characteristics from those in Table 36.1 and are likely to be more representative of pathogenic aPL found in APS. All except one (REN) bind specifically to phospholipids and not to DNA. However, the mAb REN, described by Mariette et al [42] is the only one of these five whose binding to cardiolipin is enhanced by $β_2$GP1. REN, BH 1 [43] and RSP 4 [45] were all produced from cells of patients who had serum aPL, and the patients from whom REN and BH-1 were obtained also had clinical features of APS.

Table 36.2. Sequence characteristics of more specific human IgM aPL.

mAb	Origin	V_H gene[*]	V_H homology	V_L family	V_L gene	V_L homology	High R:S in CDR	Basic residues in CDR[†]	Ref.
Kim 13.1	Healthy tonsil	1–69	99.7%	V_κIII	L6	100%	No	Yes	41
REN	CLL	4–61	100%	V_λ8	8a	99.7%	No	Yes	42
BH1	PAPS PBL	3–30	100%	V_λ3	3r	99%	No	Yes	43
STO 103	Healthy tonsil	4–61	100%	V_κIV	B3	100%	No	Yes	44
RSP 4	SLE PBL	3–30	97%	V_λ1	1e	98%	No	Yes	45

[*] The family to which a V_H gene belongs is given by the first digit of its name. Thus V3-23 belongs to the V_H3 family, V4-61 to the V_H4 family, etc.
[†] In this column, an accumulation of basic residues is taken to occur where there are at least three such residues within V_HCDR3 or three basic residues occur within a run of four successive amino acids in any other CDR. The reasons for choosing these limits are described in reference 29.
SLE, systemic lupus erythematosus; PBL, peripheral blood lymphocytes; CLL, chronic lymphocytic leukemia; PAPS, primary antiphospholipid antibody syndrome.

Like the polyreactive IgM listed in Table 36.1, these more specific aPL contain very few somatic mutations in either chain. A striking difference, however, is that they all have accumulations of basic or positively charged residues in the CDRs. In four of the antibodies (REN, BH 1, Kim 13.1 [41] and RSP 4) these residues were in V_HCDR3, similar to findings previously noted in some anti-DNA antibodies [reviewed in 29]. In STO 103 [44], there are four successive basic residues in V_LCDR1. These results suggest that where rearrangements of germline genes create highly positively charged V_HCDR3 sequences, it may sometimes be possible for the resulting antibodies to bind specifically to negatively charged phospholipids without accumulating many somatic mutations. Such unmutated, yet monospecific IgM aPL may be important in the pathogenesis of APS. It should be stressed, however, that many other human mAb have been described which also have accumulations of basic residues in the CDRs but which do not bind to phospholipids at all [29]. Other sequence features must therefore play a role in the formation of a phospholipid binding site.

Sequences of Human Monoclonal IgG aPL

Three groups have reported sequences of human monoclonal IgG aPL [46–48] and these are listed in Table 36.3. R149 [46], LJ-1, AH-2, DA-3 and UK-4 [all 47] were all produced from PBL of patients with SLE. Though these patients all had serum aPL or lupus anticoagulant they did not have definitive features of APS. LJ-1, AH-2, DA-3 and UK-4 bind specifically to anionic phospholipids whereas R149 also binds ssDNA. 516 [48] was derived from a patient with PAPS but is polyreactive. 519 [48] was derived from a healthy adult who had no circulating aPL but it is a monospecific phospholipid binder. None of these seven mAb shows β_2GP1 dependent binding to phospholipids, which raises doubts about their clinical relevance to APS. However, 516 and 519 may be representative of pathogenic aPL because they have been shown to induce fetal resorption when infused into healthy strain pregnant mice [48].

Table 36.3. Sequence characteristics of monoclonal human IgG aPL.

mAb	Origin	V_H gene*	V_H homology	V_L family	V_L gene	V_L homology	High R:S in CDR	Basic residues in CDR[†]	Ref.
R149	SLE PBL	1–69	97%	V_κII	A3	99.4%	Yes	Yes	46
LJ-1	SLE PBL	NP	NP	V_λ3	3h	98%	No	No	47
AH-2	SLE PBL	5–51	94%	V_λ1	1e	99%	Yes	Yes	47
DA-3	SLE PBL	5–51	94%	V_λ1	1e	99%	Yes	Yes	47
UK-4	SLE PBL	3–74	95%	V_λ2	2a2	94%	Yes	Yes	47
516	PAPS PBL	1–69	97%	V_κI	L19	97%	No	No	48
519	Healthy PBL	4–34	98%	V_κIII	L2	99%	No	No	48

* The family to which a V_H gene belongs is given by the first digit of its name. Thus V3-23 belongs to the V_H3 family, V4-61 to the V_H4 family, etc.

[†] In this column, an accumulation of basic residues is taken to occur where there are at least three such residues within V_HCDR3 or three basic residues occur within a run of four successive amino acids in any other CDR. The reasons for choosing these limits are described in reference 29.

SLE, systemic lupus erythematosus; PBL, peripheral blood lymphocytes; CLL, chronic lymphocytic leukemia; PAPS, primary antiphospholipid antibody syndrome.

The IgG antibodies in Table 36.3 generally show more mutations than the IgM antibodies in Tables 36.1 and 36.2. Thus, there are no unmutated V_H or V_L sequences in any of these mAb. With the exception of UK-4, the V_H sequences tend to be more mutated than the V_L sequences. This is also a common finding amongst human monoclonal anti-DNA antibodies [29]. In four of the five mAb derived from patients with SLE, there is some clustering of replacement mutations in the CDRs and mutations lead to an increase in the number of basic residues in the CDRs (the exception is LJ-1 for which only the sequence of V_L is available). This is in keeping with the idea that monospecific IgG antibodies develop as a result of antigen-driven accumulation of CDR mutations that increase affinity for the antigen (in this case anionic phospholipid). AH-2 and DA-3 are clonally related aPL derived from a single patient. As noted previously, this suggests that the aPL-secreting clone from which they are descended was highly expanded in this patient, and the large numbers of somatic mutations in AH-2 and DA-3 V_H imply that this expansion was antigen driven.

The antibodies 516 and 519, however, do not show a pattern of mutation suggestive of antigen drive and do not contain accumulations of basic residues in their CDRs. This serves as an example that the general rule linking antigen-driven mutation to IgG isotype and specific binding does not always apply. Similarly, it is possible for a polyreactive IgM antibody to carry many mutations, with high R:S ratios in CDRs. The antibody C119, described by Rioux et al (38) and shown in Table 36.1, is an example of such an antibody.

Gene usage in these IgG antibodies is unremarkable. All the major V_κ and V_λ families are represented. Members of the three largest V_H families are also used. The use of the gene V5-51 to encode the clonally related mAb AH-2 and DA-3 is interesting as this is one of only two members of the small V_H5 family which has rarely been shown to be expressed in functional antibodies. These two antibodies contain a cluster of replacement mutations in FR3, as does the mAb 519, which is derived from a different

V_H gene 4-34. In fact, these mutations lead to the production of the same sequence motif, threonine–alanine–isoleucine–tyrosine–phenylalanine (TAIYF) in both DA-3 and 519. Perhaps this FR motif may play a role in binding to phospholipids.

Summary

Both human and murine monoclonal aPL have been produced. Analysis of the sequences of these antibodies is useful in trying to determine the molecular features which correlate with clinically important binding properties. There is no evidence that particular genes or families of genes are used preferentially to encode human aPL, though there may be a preference for J558 V_H genes in murine aPL.

In human monoclonal aPL, there seems to be a link between specificity for negatively charged phospholipids and the presence of accumulations of positively charged or basic amino acids in CDRs. In IgG, but not IgM, aPL these concentrations probably arise due to antigen-driven somatic mutation. It is possible, though unproven, that the driving antigen may be phosphatidylserine exposed on apoptotic blebs and oxidized by ROS. However, the link between antigen-driven mutation and specific, high-affinity binding must not be overemphasized. Not all IgG aPL are heavily mutated whereas some polyreactive IgM antibodies do carry clusters of replacement mutations in CDRs.

Little is known about the sequence features required to confer β_2GPI-dependent binding to phospholipids, as few murine and no human mAb showing this dependence have been sequenced. The production and analysis of such antibodies is likely to be a major advance in the next few years.

Computer based methods now exist for creating three-dimensional models of monoclonal antibodies from their V_H and V_L sequences [49, 50]. Such models are likely to be useful in creating hypotheses about the sequence motifs important at the phospholipid-binding site. Comparison of sequences of different aPL may also be used to create such hypotheses (for example, suggesting that the TAIYF motif shared between DA-3 and 519 may be important). The hypotheses may then be tested by altering the supposedly crucial residues by site-directed mutagenesis, expressing the mutated sequences in bacteria or eukaryotic cells, and checking whether the properties of the altered antibodies produced have changed. Such methods are well established in the study of anti-DNA antibodies [51] and are likely to be applied to the study of monoclonal aPL in the near future.

References

1. Harris EN. A re-assessment of the antiphospholipid syndrome. J Rheumatol 1990;17:733–735.
2. Levy RA. Clinical manifestations of the aPL syndrome. Lupus 1996;5:393–397.
3. Harris EN, Spinnato JA. Should anticardiolipin tests be performed in otherwise healthy pregnant women? Am J Obstet Gynecol 1991;165:1272–1277.
4. Morrow WJW, Nelson L, Watts R, Isenberg DA. Autoimmune rheumatic disease, 2nd edn. Oxford: Oxford University Press, 1999.
5. Alarcon-Segovia D, Deleze M, Oria CV et al. Antiphospholipid antibodies and the anti-phospholipid syndrome in systemic lupus erythematosus: a prospective analysis of 500 consecutive patients. Medicine 1989;68:353–365.

6. Khamashta MA, Hughes GRV. The antiphospholipid syndrome. In: Maddison PJ, Isenberg DA, Woo P, Glass DN, editors. Oxford textbook of rheumatology, 2nd edn. Oxford: Oxford University Press, 1998;1202–1216.

7. Okamura M, Kanayama Y, Amastu K et al. Significance of enzyme linked immunosorbent assay (ELISA) for antibodies to double stranded and single stranded DNA in patients with lupus nephritis: correlation with severity of renal histology. Ann Rheum Dis 1993;52:14–20.

8. Isenberg DA, Ravirajan CT, Rahman A, Kalsi J. The role of antibodies to DNA in systemic lupus erythematosus – a review and introduction to an international workshop on DNA antibodies held in London, May 1996. Lupus 1996;6:290–304.

9. Pittoni V, Isenberg DA. Apoptosis and antiphospholipid antibodies. Semin Arthritis Rheum 1998;28:163–176.

10. Casciola-Rosen L, Rosen A, Petri M, Schlissel M. Surface blebs on apoptotic cells are sites of enhanced pro-coagulant activity. Implication for coagulation events and antigenic spread in systemic lupus erythematosus. Proc Natl Acad Sci USA 1996;93:1624–1629.

11. Casciola-Rosen LA, Anhalt G, Rosen A. Autoantigens targeted in systemic lupus erythematosus are clustered in two populations of surface structures on apoptotic keratinocytes. J Exp Med 1994;179:1317–1321.

12. Hokko S, Miller E, Dudl E et al. Antiphospholipid antibodies are directed against epitopes of oxidized phospholipids. J Clin Invest 1996;98:815–825.

13. Amzel LM, Poljak RJ, Saul F, Varga JM, Richards FF. The three-dimensional structure of a combining region-ligand complex of immunoglobulin New at 3.0A resolution. Proc Natl Acad Sci USA 1987;71:1427–1430.

14. Alt FW, Blackwell TK, Depinho RA, Reith MG, Yancopoulus GD. Regulation of genome rearrangement events during lymphocyte differentiation. Immunol Rev 1986;89:5–30.

15. Tonegawa S. Somatic generation of antibody diversity. Nature 1983;302:575–581.

16. Neuberger MS, Milstein C. Somatic hypermutation. Curr Opin Immunol 1995;7:248–254.

17. Berek C, Milstein C. The dynamic nature of the antibody repertoire. Immunol Rev 1988;105:5–26.

18. Shlomchik MJ, Marshak-Rothstein A, Wolfowicz CB, Rothstein TL, Weigert MG. The role of clonal selection and somatic mutation in autoimmunity. Nature 1987;328:805–811.

19. Tillman DM, Jou NT, Marion TN. Both IgM and IgG anti-DNA antibody are the products of clonally selective B cell stimulation in (NZB × NZW) F1 mice. J Exp Med 1993;176:361–380.

20. Chang B, Casali P. The CDR1 sequences of a major proportion of human germline Ig V_H genes are inherently susceptible to amino acid replacement. Immunol Today 1994;15:367–373

21. Matsuda F, Shin EK, Nagaoka H et al. Structure and physical map of 64 variable segments in the 3′ 0.8-megabase region of the human immunoglobulin heavy chain locus. Nat Genet 1993;3:88–94.

22. Cook GP, Tomlinson IM, Walter G et al. A map of the human immunoglobulin V_H locus completed by analysis of the telomeric region of chromosome 14q. Nat Genet 1994;7:162–168.

23. Schable KF, Zachau HG. The variable genes of the human immunoglobulin κ locus. Biol Chem Hoppe-Seyler 1993;374:1001–1022.

24. Williams SC, Frippiat JP, Tomlinson IM, Ignatovitch O, Lefranc M-P, Winter G. Sequence and evolution of the human germline $V_λ$ repertoire. J Mol Biol 1996;264:220–232.

25. Brezinschek H-P, Foster SJ, Brezinschek RI, Dorner T, Domiati-Saad R, Lipsky PE. Analysis of the human V_H gene repertoire: differential effects of selection and somatic hypermutation in human peripheral CD5+/IgM+ and CD5-/IgM+ B cells. J Clin Invest 1997;97:2488–2501.

26. Cox JPL, Tomlinson IM, Winter G. A directory of human germline $V_κ$ segments reveals a strong bias in their usage. Eur J Immunol 1994;24:827–836.

27. Tomlinson IM, Williams SC, Corbett SJ, Cox JPL, Winter G. V BASE: a database of human immunoglobulin variable region genes. Cambridge UK: MRC Centre for Protein Engineering, 1996.

28. Radic MZ, Weigert M. Genetic and structural evidence for antigen selection of anti-DNA antibodies. Annu Rev Immunol 1994;2:487–520.

29. Rahman A, Latchman DS, Isenberg DA. Immunoglobulin variable region sequences of human monoclonal anti-DNA antibodies. Semin Arthritis Rheum 1998;28:141–154

30. KitaY, Sumida T, Ichikawa K et al. V gene analysis of anticardiolipin antibodies from MRL lpr/lpr mice. J Immunol 1993;151:849–856.

31. Foster MH, MacDonald M, Barrett KJ, Madaio MP. VH gene analysis of spontaneously activated B cells in adult MRL lpr/lpr mice. J558 bias is not limited to classic lupus antibodies. J Immunol 1991;147:1504–1511

32. Kita Y, Sumida T, Iwamoto I, Yoshida S, Koike T. V gene analysis of anticardiolipin antibodies from (NZW × BXSB) F1 mice. Immunology 1994;82:494–501.

33. Monestier M, Kandiah DA, Kouts S et al. Monoclonal antibodies from (NZW × BXSB) F1 mice to $β_2$-glycoprotein I and cardiolipin. J Immunol 1996;156:2631–2641.

34. Dersimonian H, Schwartz RS, Barrett KJ, Stollar BD. Relationship of human variable region heavy chain germ-line genes to genes encoding anti-DNA autoantibodies. J Immunol 1987;139:2496–2501.

35. Hoch S, Schwaber J. Identification and sequence of the V_H gene elements encoding a human anti-DNA antibody. J Immunol 1987;139:1689–1693.

36. Siminovitch KA, Misener V, Kwong PC, Song QL, Chen PP. A natural autoantibody is encoded by germline heavy and lambda light chain variable region genes without somatic mutation. J Clin Invest 1989;84:1675–1678.

37. Logtenberg T, Young FM, Van Es JH, Gmelig-Meyling FHJ, Alt FW. Autoantibodies encoded by the most J_H-proximal human immunoglobulin heavy chain variable region gene. J Exp Med 1989;170:1347–1355.

38. Rioux JD, Zdarsky E, Newkirk MM, Rauch J. Anti-DNA and anti-platelet specificities of SLE-derived autoantibodies: evidence for CDR 2H mutations and CDR 3H motifs. Mol Immunol 1995;32:683–696.

39. Hohmann A, Cairns C, Brisco M, Bell DA, Diamond B. Immunoglobulin gene sequence analysis of anticardiolipin and anticardiolipin idiotype (H3) human monoclonal antibodies. Autoimmunity 1995;22:49–58.

40. Avrameas S. Natural autoantibodies: from horror autotoxicus to "gnothi seauton". Immunol Today 1991;121:154–159.

41. Siminovitch KA, Misener V, Kwong PC et al. A human anticardiolipin antibody is encoded by developmentally restricted heavy and light chain variable region genes. Autoimmunity 1990;8:97–105.

42. Mariette X, Levy Y, Dubreuil M-L, Intrator L, Danon F, Brouet JC. Characterization of a human monoclonal autoantibody directed to cardiolipin/β_2 glycoprotein I produced by chronic lymphocytic leukaemia B cells. Clin Exp Immunol 1993;94:385–390.

43. Harmer IJ, Loizou S, Thompson KM, So AKL, Walport MJ, Mackworth-Young C. A human monoclonal antiphospholipid antibody that is representative of serum antibodies and is germline encoded. Arthritis Rheum 1995;38:1068–1076.

44. Denomme GA, Mahmoudi M, Cairns E, Bell DA. Immunoglobulin V region sequences of two human antiplatelet monoclonal antibodies derived from B cells of normal origin. J Autoimmunity 1994;7:521–535.

45. Demaison C, Ravirajan CT, Isenberg DA, Zouali M. Analysis of variable region genes encoding anti-Sm and anti-cardiolipin antibodies from a systemic lupus erythematosus patient. Immunology 1995;86:487–494

46. van Es J, Aanstoot H, Gmelig-Meyling FHJ, Derksen RHWM, Logtenberg T. A human systemic lupus erythematosus-related anti-cardiolipin/single stranded DNA autoantibody is encoded by a somatically mutated variant of the developmentally restricted 51P1 V_H Gene. J Immunol 1992;149:2234–2240.

47. Menon S, Rahman MAA, Ravirajan CT et al. The production, binding characteristics and sequence analysis of four human IgG monoclonal antiphospholipid antibodies. J Autoimmunity 1997;10:43–57.

48. Ikematsu W, Luan F-L, La Rosa L et al. Human anticardiolipin monoclonal antibodies cause placental necrosis and fetal loss in BALB/c mice. Arthritis Rheum 1998;41:1026–1039.

49. Chothia C, Lesk AM, Tramontano A et al. Conformations of immunoglobulin variable regions. Nature 1989;342:877–883.

50. Kalsi JK, Martin ACR, Hirabayashi Y et al. Functional and modelling studies of the binding of human monoclonal anti-DNA antibodies to DNA. Mol Immunol 1996;33:471–483.

51. Rahman A, Latchman DS, Isenberg DA. The role of in vitro expression systems in the investigation of antibodies to DNA. Semin Arthritis Rheum 1998;28:130–139 .

37 Apoptosis and Antiphospholipid Antibodies

K. B. Elkon

Introduction and Personal Note

In the early 1980s, a motley crew of itinerants strove to discover the cause of systemic lupus erythematosus (SLE) in Graham Hughes' laboratory at the Hammersmith Hospital, London. The crew included myself, Azzudin Gharavi, Bernie Colaco and others. Having presented a stimulating paper by Robert Schwartz at a journal club demonstrating that some murine anti-DNA monoclonal antibodies cross react with phospholipids [1], Aziz, Bernie and I decided to test the same idea in human SLE and Graham decided to re-explore the clinical associations of anticardiolipin (aCL) autoantibodies. The resulting publications [2, 3] were a start and led to the subsequent collaboration between Aziz and Nigel Harris, development of the quantitative solid-phase immunoassay for antiphospholipid antibodies (aPL) that transformed the field.

In this brief review, I will provide an outline of apoptosis and discuss its potential relevance to aPL and systemic autoimmunity.

What Is Apoptosis?

The modern era of apoptosis began with the electron microscopic descriptions, first by Kerr, that ischemia of the liver led to morphologic changes characterized by shrinkage of hepatocytes (shrinkage necrosis). The name "apoptosis" was coined by Kerr, Wyllie and Currie in 1972 to describe the form of death characterized by cell shrinkage, nuclear condensation and cell blebbing [4]. This term also conveyed the concept that apoptosis reflected a common form of cell death that was similar to leaves falling from a tree ("apo" means from and "ptosis", a fall, in Greek).

Necrosis is distinguished from apoptosis predominantly by morphologic appearances. Necrotic cells are swollen and electron microscopy reveals disorderly fragmentation of chromatin as well as severe damage to the mitochondria. The distinction between apoptosis and necrosis remains important from a number of perspectives. In contrast to the genetic and biochemical programs that regulate apoptosis, necrotic cells usually result from death "by accident", e.g., thermal or drug injury, infection or infarction of an organ. The immune response to necrotic cells is usually proinflammatory (release of tumor necrosis factor-α (TNF-α), interleukin (IL)-1, IL-6) whereas apoptotic cells usually elicit an anti-inflammatory response (transforming growth factor-β (TGF-β), prostaglandin E_2 (PGE$_2$)) [5].

The distinction between apoptosis and necrosis is, however, not watertight. The same inducers (e.g., ischemia, hydrogen peroxide) may produce either apoptosis or necrosis depending on the dose and, consequently, the severity of the injury. The cell fate decision is determined, in part, by cellular energy reserves such as ATP [6]. Some inducers may initially cause apoptosis followed by necrosis (postapoptotic necrosis). This is likely to occur if there is a delay in removal of the apoptotic cells.

How Does Apoptosis Occur?

A schematic diagram of an apoptotic cell and the key pathways that regulate apoptosis are shown in Fig. 37.1. For detailed discussion of the biochemistry of apoptosis, the reader is referred to a recent series of reviews in *Science* (vol 281, pp 1298–1326, 1998). Death of a cell may forced upon the cell by a receptor mediated pathway such as Fas/ APO-1/ CD95 (Fig. 37.1a) or be the result of an intrinsic program that works through the mitochondria (Fig. 37.1b). In either event, cysteine-rich proteases (caspases) that have specificity for aspartic acid residues become activated (caspase 8 or 10 in the case of Fas) or caspase 9 in the case of mitochondrial pathways. These initiator caspases induce a cascade that activates the effector caspases such as caspase 3, 6 and 7. The caspase cascade results in the cleavage of a number of substrates that include certain autoantigens (e.g., chromatin (through the cleavage of the inhibitor of caspase-activated Dnase (ICAD) releasing CAD [7],U1-RNP, DNA-protein kinase) as well as structural proteins within the cytosol, nuclear and plasma membranes. Of particular interest to autoimmunity is the cleavage of chromatin into nucleosome fragments and the translocation of negatively charged phospholipids from the inside to the outside of the cell membrane (Fig. 37.1).

What Happens to Dying Cells in Vivo?

Within the immune system alone, more than 10^8 apoptotic cells are removed from the body each day. These apoptotic cells are generated in vast numbers in the central lymphoid organs such as the thymus and bone marrow by out of frame rearrangements of antigen receptors, negative selection or simple "neglect". In addition, a significant load of apoptotic cells is also produced in the peripheral immune system due to the relatively short life span of lymphocytes and myeloid cells as well as specialized sites of secondary selection of high affinity B cells in germinal centers. The specialized sites of selection (thymus, bone marrow and lymphoid follicles) have remarkably efficient phagocytes that remove the dying cells rapidly.

Key alterations occur in the cell membrane of the dying cell that alert macrophages to phagocytose the cell and degrade it in a non-inflammatory fashion. Amongst the ligands expressed on apoptotic cells is the negatively charged phospholipid, phosphatidylserine (PS), that binds to a receptor on macrophages and induces phagocytosis [8] (Fig. 37.2). PS is also known to bind to β_2-glycoprotein (β_2GP), a protein abundant in serum, so it is not yet clear whether the ligand is PS

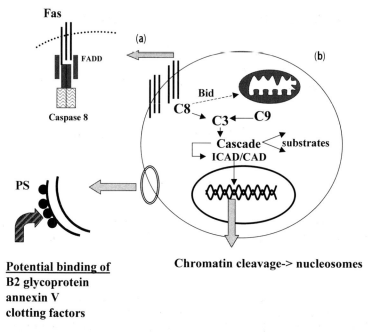

Potential binding of
B2 glycoprotein
annexin V
clotting factors

Figure 37.1. The fundamental pathways of apoptosis. Biochemical pathways leading to cell death may be initiated by a death ligand such as Fas Ligand **a**. Fas is clustered and recruits the adaptor molecule, FADD. This, in turn, leads to recruitment and autoprocessing of caspase 8 and 10 followed by the effector caspases, 3, 6 and 7. In addition, caspase 8 cleaves a proapoptotic molecule, Bid which causes release of cytochrome c from mitochondria and amplification of the caspase cascade. **b** Apoptosis may also be initiated by stimuli such as growth factor withdrawal leading to cytochrome c release from the mitochondria. In the presence of cytochrome c and ATP, the protein Apaf-1 cleaves caspase 9 which promotes the caspase cascade. Caspases cleave a large number of substrates within the cell, amongst them ICAD, an inhibitor of the DNase CAD. Once cleaved, CAD moves into the nucleus and cleaves chromatin into nucleosomes (hence the characteristic ladder observed on gel electrophoresis). Caspases also cleave some lupus protein autoantigens such as 70k RNP and DNA protein kinase. A very early and almost universal event following the induction of apoptosis is the "flip-flop" of phosphatidylserine (PS) from the inside to the outside of the cell membrane. As discussed in the text, this alteration is important as PS may serve as a possible immunogen for anti-phospholipid autoantibodies and potential co-factor for the coagulation cascade.

alone or a PS–protein conjugate [9]. Similarly, certain sugars may be selectively exposed on the membrane triggering their phagocytosis [10].

A number of other receptors have been implicated in the uptake of apoptotic cells by phagocytes in vitro (Fig. 37.2). These include the integrins, $\alpha_v\beta_5$ on dendritic cells [11] and $\alpha_v\beta_3$ on macrophages [12] as well as class A and class B scavenger receptors [13–15]. CD36, a single chain transmembrane type B scavenger receptor [16] appears to collaborate with $\alpha_v\beta_3$ via a thrombospondin bridge to effect phagocytosis (Fig. 37.2). Other receptors implicated in phagocytosis of apoptotic cells include the ATP-binding cassette transporter ABC1 [17] and CD14, a glycophospholipid receptor known to bind to lipopolysaccharide (LPS) [18]. The relative importance of each of these receptors, their interactions (positive and negative) as well as their ligands remain to be fully defined (Fig. 37.2).

Apoptotic Cell   **Phagocyte**

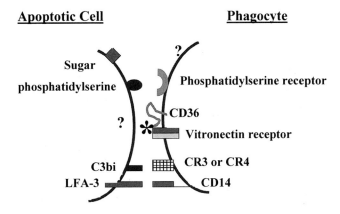

Figure 37.2. Ligands and receptors implicated in phagocytosis of apoptotic cells. See text for discussion. * is thrombospondin, that forms a bridge between CD36 and the vitronectin receptor, $\alpha_v\beta_3$.

Our laboratory has recently observed that, when serum is included in the medium with apoptotic cells, complement is activated and C3bi is deposited on the surface of the apoptotic cell [19]. C3bi is a ligand for CR3 and CR4 and phagocytosis of apoptotic cells could be significantly inhibited by blocking antibodies to these receptors. These findings suggest a potentially important link between complement and processing of apoptotic cells.

Why Is Apoptosis Relevant to aPL and Systemic Autoimmunity?

Six clinical observations have focussed attention on the products of apoptotic cells as antigens or immunogens in SLE.

1. Nucleosomes are detected in the circulation of SLE patients with active disease [20].
2. Nucleosomes, are more strongly antigenic than DNA or histones alone and antibodies to nucleosomes precede those to DNA and histones [21, 22].
3. Nucleosomes, but not isolated DNA or histones, deposit in the glomeruli suggesting that it is in situ fixation of nucleosomes, rather than DNA/anti-DNA immune complexes that causes lupus nephritis [23, 24].
4. SLE antigens are redistributed to apoptotic blebs when cells such as keratinocytes undergo programmed cell death [25]. Some, but not all, of these antigens undergo modification, including cleavage and phosphorylation [26–28].
5. An increase in apoptosis of SLE peripheral blood mononuclear cells (PBMC) in vitro has been observed [29], which has been correlated with lymphopenia in the patient [30]. Freshly isolated lymphocytes from patients show high annexin V binding [31] and elevated caspase 3 functional activity [32] indicating that accelerated apoptosis occurs in vivo.

6. SLE macrophages *may* have a reduced uptake of apoptotic cells, in vitro [33, 34]. These results, should however, be interpreted with caution in view of the rapid death of SLE macrophages in culture (unpublished observations)].

The fact that autoantibodies target many of the products of apoptotic cells does not necessarily mean that the apoptotic cells *induced* the immune response. To address whether apoptotic cells can be immunogenic, our laboratory injected apoptotic thymocytes in the absence of adjuvant into normal syngeneic mice and quantified autoantibody production. The results of these studies showed that low levels of autoantibodies against ss-DNA and negatively charged phospholipids can be generated following immunization with apoptotic cells, but autoantibodies against protein antigens were not [35]. Of considerable interest, IgG was detected in the glomeruli of the injected mice. Although it is possible that the dose, duration or mode of administration may not accurately mimic exposure that occurs in spontaneous disease, it appears that a large load of apoptotic cells can initiate humoral autoimmunity but does not lead to long-standing autoimmunity.

The generation of low titers of aPL in these studies is intriguing. We have speculated that exposure of a multivalent antigen on the cell surface may be sufficient to break B- (see Fig. 37.3), but not T-cell tolerance accounting for the transient nature of the immune response [35]. Important questions for the future are whether exposure to large numbers of apoptotic cells can lead to protracted autoimmunity, if uptake of apoptotic cells is impaired or macrophage responses are altered in other ways (cytokine production, antigen processing) or if additional T cell defects are present.

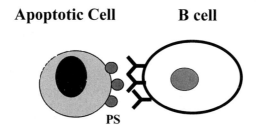

Figure 37.3. Phosphatidylserine (PS) exposure on the cell surface of apoptotic cells may activate B lymphocytes. PS exposure may act as a polyvalent, T-independent antigen capable of cross-linking surface immunoglobulin on the surface of B lymphocytes. As discussed in the text, additional factors are required to induce protracted loss of tolerance and establishment of an autoimmune state.

Conclusions

There is no doubt that impaired Fas mediated apoptosis results in systemic autoimmunity in humans [see 36, 37] but that only rare cases of SLE have Fas or Fas ligand mutations [38, 39]. Similarly, there seems to be considerable evidence that SLE patients have enhanced lymphocyte apoptosis in vitro and probably in vivo. The data summarized here provides circumstantial evidence to support the argument that antigen selection, particularly autoantibodies to negatively charged phospholipids in SLE, may be explained by B-lymphocyte responses to apoptotic cells.

In an Editorial on apoptosis published a number of years ago we asked whether there was "too little or too much apoptosis?" in SLE [40]. Perhaps that was not the right question since abundant apoptosis occurs in Fas deficient mice – presumably by alternative pathways. What we need to know is whether apoptotic signal transduction pathways are fully functional in SLE patients and whether the processing and response to cell corpses is appropriate.

References

1. Lafer E, Rauch J, Andrzejewski C et al. Polyspecific monoclonal lupus autoantibodies reactive with both polynucleotides and phospholipids. J Exp Med 1981;153:897–904.
2. Colaco CB, Elkon KB. The lupus anticoagulant, a disease marker in ANA negative lupus, yet cross reactive with autoantibodies to ds DNA. Arthritis Rheum 1985;28:67–74.
3. Boey ML, Gharavi AE, Elkon KB, Loizou S, Hughes GRV. Thrombosis in SLE, striking association with the presence of circulating "lupus anticoagulant". Br Med J 1983;287:1021–1023.
4. Kerr JFR, Wyllie AH, Currie AR. Apoptosis: a basic biological phenomenon with wide-ranging implications in tissue kinetics. Br J Cancer 1972;26:239–257.
5. Fadok VA, Bratton DL, Konowal A, Freed PW, Westcott JY, Henson PM. Macrophages that have ingested apoptotic cells in vitro inhibit proinflammatory cytokine production through autocrine/paracrine mechanisms involving TGF-beta, PGE$_2$, and PAF. J Clin Invest 1998;101:890–898.
6. Leist M, Single B, Castoldi AF, Kuhnle S, Nicotera P. Intracellular adenosine triphosphate (ATP) concentration: a switch in the decision between apoptosis and necrosis. J Exp Med 1997;185:1481–1486.
7. Enari M, Sakahira H, Yokoyama H, Okawa K, Iwamatsu A, Nagata S. A caspase-activated DNase that degrades DNA during apoptosis, and its inhibitor ICAD. Nature 1998;391:43–50.
8. Fadok VA, Voelker DR, Campbell PA, Cohen JJ, Bratton DL, Henson PM. Exposure of phosphatidylserine on the surface of apoptotic lymphocytes triggers specific recognition and removal by macrophages. J Immunol 1992;148:2207–2216.
9. Balasubramanian K, Schroit AJ. Characterization of phosphatidylserine-dependent beta-2 glycoprotein I macrophage interactions. J Biol Chem 1998;273:29272–29277.
10. Duvall E, Wyllie AH, Morris RG. Macrophage recognition of cells undergoing programmed cell death. Immunology 1985;56:351–358.
11. Albert ML, Pearce SFA, Francisco LM et al. Immature dendritic cells phagocytose apoptotic cells via alpha-v-beta-5 and CD36, and cross-present antigens to cytotoxic T lymphocytes. J Exp Med 1998;188:1359–1368.
12. Savill J, Dransfield Hogg N, Haslett C. Vitronectin receptor-mediated phagocytosis of cells undergoing apoptosis. Nature 1990;343:170–173.
13. Platt N, Suzuki H, Kurihara Y, Kodama T, Gordon S. Role for the class A macrophage scavenger receptor in the phagocytosis of apoptotic thymocytes in vitro. Proc Natl Acad Sci USA 1996;93:12456–12460.
14. Sambrano GR, Steinberg D. Recognition of oxidatively damaged and apoptotic cells by an oxidized low density lipoprotein receptor on mouse peritoneal macrophages: role of membrane phosphatidylserine. Proc Natl Acad Sci USA 1995;92:1396–1400.
15. Fukasawa M, Adachi H, Hirota K, Tsujimoto M, Arai H, Inoue K. SRB1, a class B scavenger receptor, recognizes both negatively charged liposomes and apoptotic cells. Exp Cell Res 1996;222:246–250.
16. Ren Y, Silverstein RL, Allen J, Savill J. CD36 gene transfer confers capacity for phagocytosis of cells undergoing apoptosis. J Exp Med 1995;181:1857–1862.
17. Luciani M-F, Chimini G. The ATP binding cassette transporter, ABC1, is required for the engulfment of corpses generated by apoptotic cell death. EMBO J 1996;15:226–235.
18. Devitt A, Moffatt OD, Raykundalia C, Capra JD, Simmons DL, Gregory CD. Human CD14 mediates recognition and phagocytosis of apoptotic cells. Nature 1998;392:505–509.
19. Mevorach D, Mascarenhas J, Gershov DA, Elkon KB. Complement-dependent clearance of apoptotic cells. J Exp Med 1998;188:2301–2311.
20. Rumore PM, Steinman CR. Endogenous circulating DNA in systemic lupus erythematosus, occurrence as multimeric complexes bound to histone. J Clin Invest 1990;86:69–74.
21. Burlingame RW, Rubin RL, Balderas RS, Theofilopoulos AN. Genesis and evolution of anti-chromatin autoantibodies in murine lupus implicates T-dependent immunization and self antigen. J Clin Invest 1993;91:1687–1696.

22. Amoura Z, Chabre H, Koutouzov S et al. Nucleosome restricted antibodies are detected before anti-ds DNA and/ or anti-histone antibodies in serum of MRL-Mp *lpr/lpr* and +/+ mice, adn are present in kidney eluates of lupus mice with proteinuria. Arthritis Rheum 1994;37:1684–1688.
23. Termaat RM, Assmann KJ, Dijkman HB, van Gompel F, Smeenk RJ, Berden JH. Anti DNA antibodies can bind to the glomerulus via two distinct mechanisms. Kidney Int 1992;42:1363–1371.
24. Kramers C, Hylkema MN, van Bruggen MCJ et al. Anti-nucleosome antibodies complexed to nucleosomal antigens show anti-DNA reactivity and bind to rat glomerular basement membrane in vivo. J Clin Invest 1994;94:568–577.
25. Casciola-Rosen LA, Anhalt G, Rosen A. Autoantigens targeted in systemic lupus erythematosus are clustered in two populations of surface structures on apoptotic keratinocytes. J Exp Med 1994;179:1317–1330.
26. Casciola-Rosen LA, Anhalt GJ, Rosen A. DNA-dependent protein kinase is one of a subset of autoantigens specifically cleaved early during apoptosis. J Exp Med 1995;182:1625–1634.
27. Utz PJ, Hottelet M, Schur PH, Anderson P. Proteins phosphorylated during stress-induced apoptosis are common targets for autoantibody production in patients with systemic lupus erythematosus. J Exp Med 1997;185:843–854.
28. Casiano CA, Martin SJ, Green DR, Tan EM. Selective cleavage of nuclear autoantigens during CD95 (Fas/APO-1)-mediated T cell apoptosis. J Exp Med 1996;184:765–770.
29. Emlen W, Niebur J-A, Kadera R. Accelerated in vitro apoptosis of lymphocytes from patients with systemic lupus erythematosus. J Immunol 1994;152:3685–3692.
30. Georgescu L, Vakkalanka RK, Elkon KB, Crow MK. Interleukin-10 promotes activation-induced cell death of SLE lymphocytes mediated by Fas ligand. J Clin Invest 1997;100:2622–2633.
31. Perniok A, Wedekind F, Herrmann M, Specker C, Schneider M. High levels of circulating early apoptotic peripheral blood mononuclear cells in systemic lupus erythematosus. Lupus 1998;7:113–118.
32. Ohsako S, Elkon KB. Increased caspase-like activity in freshly isolated lymphocytes from SLE patients. Arthritis Rheum 1998;41:S70.
33. Mevorach D, Song X, Elkon KB. Decreased phagocytosis of apoptotic cells in patients with systemic lupus erythematosus. Arthritis Rheum 1996;39S:143.
34. Herrmann M, Voll RE, Zoller OM, Hagenhofer M, Ponner BB, Kalden JR. Impaired phagocytosis of apoptotic cell material by monocyte-derived macrophages from patients with systemic lupus erythematosus. Arthritis Rheum 1998;41:1241–1250.
35. Mevorach D, Zhou J-L, Song X, Elkon KB. Systemic exposure to irradiated apoptotic cells induces autoantibody production. J Exp Med 1998;188:387–392.
36. Vaishnaw AK, Orlinick JR, Chu JL, Krammer PH, Chao MV, Elkon KB. Molecular basis for the apoptotic defects in patients with CD95 (Fas/Apo-1) mutations. J Clin Invest 1999;103:355–363.
37. Martin DA, Zheng L, Siegel RM et al. Defective CD95/APO-1/Fas signal complex formation in the human autoimmune lymphoproliferative syndrome, type Ia. Proc Natl Acad Sci USA 1999;96:4552–4557.
38. Vaishnaw AK, Toubi E, Ohsako S et al. Both quantitative and qualitative apoptotic defects are associated with the clinical spectrum of disease, including systemic lupus erythematosus in humans with Fas (APO-1/CD95) mutations. Arthritis Rheum 1999;42:1833–1842.
39. Wu J, Wilson J, He J, Xiang L, Schur PH, Mountz JD. Fas ligand mutation in a patient with systemic lupus erythematosus and lymphoproliferative disease. J Clin Invest 1996;98:1107–1113.
40. Elkon KB. Apoptosis in SLE-Too little or too much? Clin Exp Rheumatol 1994;12:553–559.

38 The Contribution of Experimental Models to our Understanding of Etiology, Pathogenesis and Novel Therapies in the Antiphospholipid Syndrome

M. Blank, I. Krause and Y. Shoenfeld

Animal models are of great value in the evaluation of pathogenic mechanisms as well as novel and experimental treatments, that cannot be tested directly on patients. Considerable progress has been made in recent years in developing in vivo experimental models for antiphospholipid syndrome (APS), either of spontaneously occurring disease or which may be actively induced in naive mice. The APS models served as a valuable tool for assessing the efficacy of various modalities of treatment, in different stages of the disease. In this chapter we summarize the spectrum of murine models for APS and therapeutic interventions which have been studied employing those models, many of them showed promising potential for application in human patients.

Animal Models of Spontaneously Occurring APS

Among the autoimmune strain of mice, the MRL/lpr was the first to be reported as an animal model for APS. The MRL/lpr mouse strain was first proposed as a model for an accelerated membranoproliferative glomerulonephritis associated with anti-DNA production [1]. It was later shown by Gharavi et al [2] that the mice develop, at the age of 2 months, high levels of autoantibodies including anticardiolipin (aCL), in association with thrombocytopenia and reduced litter size. The disease could be accelerated by immunization with β_2-glycoprotein I (β_2GPI) [3]. The mice may also have significant vasculopathy in the central nervous system, including vascular occlusions and perivascular infiltrates in the choroid plexus [4], hence may serve as a model for neurological complication of APS [5].

A hybrid strain derived by mating the NZB with the NZW mouse, resulting in the (NZW×B×SB)F1 males, has been described as another model for APS [6]. The mice develop a systemic lupus-like disease and several autoantibodies, circulating immune complexes, lupus nephritis, thrombocytopenia and a high rate of myocardial infarction, resulting in death before 6 months of age. Elevated titers of aCL are increasingly developed with age, which were shown to be β_2GPI-dependent.

Abnormal immune responses were demonstrated, such as defective T-cell immune responses and polyclonal B-cell activation. The autoimmune state of the (NZW×B×SB)F1 is associated with decreased expression of interleukin-2 (IL-2) and increase in IL-4 production, implying decreased T helper 1 (Th1) cell response and activation of Th2 cells [7].

Animal Models of Experimental APS in Naive Mice

In Vivo Thrombosis

Pierangeli et al [8–13] employed a mouse model of induced venous thrombosis to elucidate the thrombogenic role of antiphospholipid antibodies (aPL) in vivo. The model allows continuous and quantitative monitoring of focally-induced, non-occlusive mural thrombus of a mouse femoral vein. The animal is anesthetized, femoral vein minimally mobilized and subjected to a standardized "pinch" injury to induce thrombosis. The vessel is transilluminated using acrylic optical fibers connected to a light source, and clot formation and dissolution are visualized by a standard surgical microscope equipped with a video camera, video recorder, and computer assisted analysis system. Employing this model, CD1 mice were intraperitoneally injected with either immunoglobulins derived from APS patients or healthy controls, while monitoring the size and dynamics of thrombus formation or disappearance [8, 9]. It was found that immunoglobulins from APS patients, or affinity-purified aCL of IgG and IgM isotypes and aCL monoclonal antibodies, enhanced significantly the thrombus area and the mean disappearance time, indicating that aCL play a role in thrombus formation [9, 10] should start after thrombus formation [9, 10]. Immunization of mice with β_2GpI induced production of aPL, which were thrombogenic in-vivo [11]. Furthermore, mice injected with anti-GDKV monoclonal antibodies enhanced thrombosis and endothelial cell activation in-vivo and in-vitro [12]. GDKV synthetic peptide, mimics an epitope located at the fifth domain of human β_2GpI which is a phospholipid-binding site. It was also shown that mice treated with hydroxychloroquine had significantly smaller thrombi that persisted for a shorter period of time compared with animals treated with placebo [13].

Passive Transfer of Pathogenic aPL

Branch et al [14] were the first to report on the pathogenicity of aPL in normal mice. Human aPL taken from women with the APS and a history of fetal loss caused fetal loss in pregnant BALB/c mice upon intraperitoneal injection of IgG–aCL on day 8 of pregnancy. Histologic examination of the uteroplacental interface showed decidual necrosis an intravascular deposition of IgG and fibrin. The pathogenic role of aPL in pregnant mice was confirmed by Blank et al [15] who reported on a passive induction of APS in ICR mice by infusion of aCL through the tail vein. A polyclonal IgG fraction derived from a patient with primary APS, or a mouse aCL monoclonal antibody (mAb) was administered on different days of pregnancy, resulting in lower fecundity rate, increased absorption index of embryos (the equivalent of human fetal loss), lower number of embryos per pregnancy, and lower mean weights of embryos and placentae. The above findings were accompanied by a prolonged activated partial thromboplastin time (aPTT) and thrombocytopenia [15]. The results of this study provided the evidence for a direct effect of aCL upon pregnancy outcome. The same protocol was used by other investigators, to show the pathogenicity of aPL [16], which was also demonstrated by infusion of aCL mAbs derived from mice with APS, or antiphosphatidylserine (aPS) from APS patients into naive mice at different stages of the pregnancy, yielding similar results [17]. Ikematsu et al [18] injected β_2GPI-independent human aCL IgG mAbs into mated female BALB/c mice, to study their effect on pregnancy outcome. The mice injected with aCL displayed a significantly higher rate of fetal resorptions and a significant reduction in fetal and placental weight. These findings were accompanied by a placental human IgG deposition and necrosis. The results of the study indicate that human aCL IgG that are β_2GPI independent can induce pathology. Nevertheless, experimental APS can also be induced by passive transfer of anti-β_2GPI Abs, as was shown by George et al [19]. Anti-β_2GPI mAbs, cloned from a patient with APS, were passively administered to pregnant BALB/c mice resulting in clinical findings consistent with APS (increased fetal resorptions, reduced platelet counts, and prolonged aPTT).

Induction of Experimental APS in Naive Mice by Idiotypic Immunization

This model is based on Jerne's theory of the idiotypic network [20]. Immunization of naive mice with an autoantibody (Ab1) results in generation of anti-idiotypic antibody (i.e., Ab2) and 2–3 months later the mice develop anti-anti-idiotypic antibodies (i.e., Ab3). Ab3 may simulates Ab1 in its binding properties [21]. The generation of Ab3 is followed by the emergence of the full-blown serological, immunohistochemical and clinical manifestations of the respective autoimmune disease. Immunization of naive mice with a human pathogenic monoclonal aCL (H-3) [22] or aPS [23] in the footpads emulsified in complete Freund's adjuvant (CFA), followed by a booster injection 3 weeks later, led to the generation of Ab$_2$, namely an antiautoantibody (anti-Id), and later to a mouse Ab$_3$ (antiantiautoantibody, i.e., mouse-aCL), which simulates the original autoantibody. The mice also exhibited thrombocytopenia and their aPTT was prolonged, indicating the existence of lupus anticoagulant. When mated, the immunized female mice had low fecundity and increased rate of fetal resorptions. The live fetuses and their compatible placentas were smaller than those of mice immunized with irrelevant Ig. Immunization of mice with a special human anti-DNA (16/6 Id$^+$) mAb led to the induction of APS secondary to experimental systemic lupus erythematosus (SLE) [24]. In addition, mice having experimental APS induced by immunization with H-3 aCL mAb, displayed impaired neurological abilities and behavior [25]. Vasculopathy of microvessels in the brain of the APS mice was demonstrated by immunofluorescence and electron microscopy. The results of this study point to the central role of aPL in neurological dysfunctions associated with APS. Active induction of primary APS was also conducted by utilizing IgG fraction derived from a patient with monoclonal gammopathy, monospecific and with high affinity for CL [26]. The pathogenic role of aPL in the development of heart valve lesions (Libman–Sacks endocarditis) was confirmed by demonstrating deposits of immunoglobulins including aCL, and of complement components, in affected valves [27].

In order to clarify which part of the aCL immunoglobulin molecule has the pathogenic potential, we constructed and expressed single chain Fv aCL, exchanging heavy and light chains between the pathogenic and non-pathogenic Abs [28]. Single chain Fv (scFv) were prepared from four aCL mAbs, either pathogenic or non-pathogenic. All four scFv$_s$ showed the same antigen binding properties as the original mAbs. Replacement of the pathogenic VH domain with a non-pathogenic VH, decreased the binding and avidity of the scFv to CL and completely abrogated the anticoagulant activity. Exchanging the pathogenic aCL VH with anti-DNA VH resulted in shift from aCL to anti-DNA binding of the scFv. Replacement of the pathogenic aCL VL with a non-pathogenic VL did not affect the avidity of the scFv for CL nor its anticoagulant activity. BALB/c mice were immunized with either aCL scFv$_s$, or scFv resulting from the replacement of the heavy and the light chains. The mice which were immunized with scFv$_s$ developed the same clinical manifestations, as the mice immunized with the original mAbs (elevated titers of mouse aCL (β_2GPI-dependent), associated with lupus anticoagulant activity, thrombocytopenia, prolonged aPTT and high percentage of fetal resorptions). Immunization with a non-pathogenic aCL-scFv did not lead to any clinical findings. Replacement of heavy/light chains between the pathogenic and non-pathogenic Abs point to the importance of the heavy chain variable domains in the pathogenic potential of aCL.

Immunization with β_2GPI

Gharavi et al demonstrated two non-cross-reactive populations of anti-β_2GPI and aPL Abs, following active immunization of normal rabbit or mice with purified β_2GPI. The aPL had binding specificities indistinguishable from autoantibodies obtained from human and murine lupus [29]. Similar results were obtained by Pierangeli et al using a lipid-free adjuvant, thus excluding the possibility that antibody induction occurred because β_2GPI formed complexes with PL in the CFA [30]. Blank et al described the emergence of a full-blown APS disease in naive BALB/c mice immunized with β_2GPI in CFA [31], manifested by elevated levels of antibodies directed against negatively charged phospholipids (cardiolipin, phosphotidylserine, phosphatidylinositol), followed by prolonged aPTT, thrombocytopenia, and a high percentage of fetal resorptions. The data point to the ability of β_2GPI to induce pathogenic aCL following active immunization.

Bone Marrow Transplantation

Abnormal autoimmune function is increasingly recognised to be T-cell mediated. To investigate the potential of bone marrow (BM) cells from mice with primary APS to transfer the disease to naive mice, and to determine the importance and the role of T cells in the APS, whole-population or T cell-depleted BM cells from mice with experimental primary APS were infused into total body-irradiated naive BALB/c recipients [32]. BM cells (in the presence of T cells) had the potential to induce experimental APS in naive mice, which resulted in: high serum titers of aCL, antiphosphatidylserine, and antiphosphatidylinositol antibodies; an increased number of antibody-forming cells specific for each of the above phospholipids; a positive lymph node cell proliferative response to aCL mAb; and clinical features of primary APS, including thrombocytopenia, prolonged aPTT, and a high frequency of fetal resorptions. T-cell-depleted BM cells did not transfer the disease, pointing to the important role of T cells in the development and transfer of experimental primary APS.

Therapeutic Interventions in Murine Models for APS

Antithrombotic Treatments

Aspirin has significant antithrombotic properties, and regimens using aspirin were suggested to be effective in protecting against fetal loss associated with APS. Employing the model of passively-induced APS it was found that aspirin treatment, especially in low doses, significantly improved pregnancy outcome [33]. This was manifested by fewer fetal resorptions and higher mean embryo weights. In a later study it was shown that treatment of APS mice with thromboxane receptor antagonist causes significant reduction in fetal resorption rate, as well as increase in platelet count and decrease in aPTT [34]. Anticoagulation with heparin has already been used to prevent fetal loss in pregnant women with APS. A potentially better preparation for use in pregnancy is low-molecular-weight heparin (LMWH). In comparing the effectiveness of LMWH with regular heparin in the prevention of fetal resorption in mice with experimental APS, it was found that although heparin treatment decreased the degree of fetal loss, LMWH was much more effective in that respect [35].

Immunomodulation of Experimental APS

Oral Tolerance

Systemic tolerance to various antigenscan be achieved by feeding with pathogenic proteins [36]. Feeding of BALB/c mice with low dose β_2GPI at certain time points of experimental APS development, had different effect on disease improvement [37]. The serological and clinical markers of experimental APS were prevented when the mice received orally β_2GPI before disease induction upon immunization with the autoantigen. The treated group was characterized by low titers of serum anti-β_2GPI and aCL in the sera, lack of fetal resorptions, low incidence of thrombocytopenia and normal values of aPTT. β_2GPI given at an early stage of the disease reduced the clinical manifestations. However, administration of β_2GPI 70 days postimmunization had less significant effect on disease expression. Tolerized mice exhibit diminished T-lymphocyte proliferation response to β_2GPI in comparison to β_2GPI immunized mice fed with ovalbumin (OVA). When non-tolerant β_2GPI-primed T-lymphocytes were mixed with CD8+ T cells from the tolerized mice, a significant inhibition of proliferation upon exposure to β_2GPI was observed. The induction of suppression was β_2GPI-specific and driven, as well as transforming growth factor-β (TGF-β) mediated. The β_2GPI specific response of T-lymphocytes from the β_2GPI fed mice was reversed by anti-TGF-β Abs. The tolerance was adoptively transferred by CD8+ T cells from the tolerized mice into naive mice. Those CD8+ cells were major histocompatibility complex (MHC) class I restricted, found to secrete TGF-β and had no cytolytic activity. Oral administration of β_2GPI suppressed priming of

CTLs in the recipient mice. Finally, β_2GPI-induced oral tolerance has an immuno-modulating effect in experimental APS, demonstrating the importance of β_2GPI in the pathogenesis of the disease.

Feeding of Mice with Gammaglobulin

Strains of lupus mice, BSB, MRL/*lpr* and NZB, differ in their capacity to become orally tolerant after feeding with bovine gammaglobulin and casein [38, 39]. The mechanisms of tolerance in lupus-prone mice seems to be affected by multiple factors, not present in normal strains of mice, and the reasons for such a difference remains unclear. Preliminary studies in feeding with intravenous immunoglobulins (IVIG) prevented the appearance of aCL and anti-β_2GPI Abs in the IVIG fed mice, immunized with pathogenic aCL (data not published).

Synthetic Peptides

Employing an hexapeptide-phage-display-library we identified three hexapeptides which bind specifically to anti-β_2GPI mAbs, causing endothelial cell activation and experimental APS [40]. The following synthetic peptides were used: peptide A: NTLKTPRVGGC, peptide B: KDKATFGTHDGC and peptide C: CATLRVYKGG. Peptides A, B and C inhibited specifically the biological functions of the corresponding anti-β_2GPI mAbs in vitro and in vivo. Exposure of endothelial cells to anti-β_2GPI mAbs, and their corresponding peptides, led to inhibition of endothelial cell activation as shown by decreased expression of adhesion molecules (E-selectin, intracellular adhesion molecule-1 (ICAM-1), vascular cell adhesion molecule-1 (VCAM-1)) and monocyte adhesion. In vivo infusion of the anti-β_2GPI mAbs followed by administration of the specific peptides into BALB/c mice, resulted in prevention of the peptide-treated mice from developing experimental APS.

Immunomodulation by Antibodies

Administration of specific anti-idiotypic Abs was found to be effective, resulting in attenuation of clinical and serological manifestation of experimental APS [41]. The anti-idiotypic treatment was associated with a shift from Th2 to Th1 immune response, characterized by a rise in the level of Th1-related cytokines in the sera of the treated mice and decrease in Th2-relalated cytokines. Furthermore, elevation in the number of IL-2 and interferon-g (IFN-g) secreting cells (Th1) and elimination of the IL-4 and IL-6 secreting cells (Th2), was noticed in the APS treated mice, supporting the role of Th1 cytokines in suppression of idiotypic-induced APS manifestations. Similarly, treatment with anti-CD4 mAbs prevented the appearance of clinical manifestations of experimental APS, especially when the antibodies were administered early in the course of the disease [42]. The effect of anti-CD4 Abs was studied also in the (NZWBSB)F1 model [43]. Prolongation of survival rate and reduction of severity of autoimmune diseases were observed after treatment with anti-CD4 mAb, while, anti-CD8 mAb treatment accelerated the diseases, suggesting that CD4$^+$ cells are involved in the development of autoimmune diseases and CD8$^+$ cells have a suppressive effect in (NZWBSB)F1 mice. IVIG have been reported to be effective in treating several autoimmune diseases. Treatment of APS mice with IVIG resulted in a complete clinical, serological and pathological remission that lasted as long as the treatment was given. Inhibition studies pointed to the presence of anti-idiotypic activity to aCL in the IVIG preparation [44].

Interleukin-3

The role of IL-3 was studied by Fishman et al [45]. Treatment with murine recombinant IL-3 on pregnant mice induced with the experimental APS resulted in abrogation of fetal loss, as well as by normal platelet count. Ciprofloxacin, a potent antibiotic agent of the quinolone family, which enhances production of IL-3 in irradiated mice, was found to prevent pregnancy loss, as well as other clinical manifestations of APS [46]. The effect was probably mediated via increased IL-3 and granulocyte–monocyte colony-stimulating factor (GM-CSF) expressions, manifested by elevated levels of IL-3 in the sera and increased IL-3 mRNA transcription in splenocytes. GM-CSF increased expression was documented by elevated titers in the sera and enhanced number of colony forming cells in the bone marrow.

Bromocriptine

Bromocriptine (BRC), which inhibits the secretion of prolactin and has immunoregulatory properties [47], was found to suppress experimental APS, leading to a marked reduction of autoantibodies level accompanied by disappearance of clinical and pathological manifestations of the disease. The effect of BRC was mediated through the induction of natural non-specific CD8 suppressor cells [48]. This effect was related to enhancement of IL-3 expression, since high level of the cytokine was found in the sera of ciprofloxacin-treated mice, compared to control group.

Bone Marrow Transplantation (BMT)

APS mice which were transfused with BM cells (T-cell depleted) from syngeneic naive mice had reduced titers of aPL, which was related to depletion of antibody-forming cells in vivo, and reduced proliferative response of lymph node cells to aCL mAbs. The recipients showed improvement in clinical parameters following syngeneic BMT [49]. The effect of BMT was also examined using the (NZWBSB)F1 model for APS [50]. It was found that in contrast to non-treated mice, who died of myocardial infarction or renal failure at the age of 7 months, the treated mice showed no evidence of myocardial infarction even 1 year after BMT. This was associated with lower levels of aCL. Those results provide a theoretical background to exploit the use of autologous T-cell depleted BMT for patients with severe and extreme disease .(e.g., catastrophic APS) resistant to other therapeutic modalities in clinical practice.

Conclusions

The availability of animal models for APS has provided experimental data important in the elucidation of this complicated disease. In this chapter we have presented our own and others experience with various experimental models for murine APS. Many treatment modalities were highly effective in ameliorating clinical, serological and histological manifestations of the disease. Promising approaches for the treatment of APS patients include the use of oral tolerance, specific synthetic peptides, immunomodulation with anti-idiotypic Abs, anti-CD4 antibodies, administration of cytokines like IL-3 or IL-3 inducer (ciprofloxacin), IVIG, bromocriptine, aspirin and/or LMW-heparin. Bone-marrow transplantation might be useful in extreme cases of the disease. The results might promote the handling of controlled clinical trials to evaluate the application of those treatments in APS patients.

References

1. Gutierrez Ramos JC, Andreu JL, Moreno de Alboran I et al. Insights into autoimmunity: from classical models to current perspectives. Immunol Rev 1990;118:73–101.
2. Gharavi AE, Mellors RC, Elkon KB. IgG anti-cardiolipin antibodies in murine lupus. Clin Exp Immunol 1989;78:233–238.
3. Aron AL, Cuellar ML, Brey RL et al. Early onset of autoimmunity in MRL/++ mice following immunization with beta 2 glycoprotein I. Clin Exp Immunol 1995;101:78–81.
4. Smith HR, Hansen CL, Rose R, Canoso RT. Autoimmune MRL-1pr/1pr mice are an animal model for the secondary antiphospholipid syndrome. J Rheumatol 1990;17:911–915.
5. Hess DC. Models for central nervous system complications of antiphospholipid syndrome. Lupus 1994;3:253–257.
6. Hashimoto Y, Kawamura M, Ichikawa K et al. Anticardiolipin antibodies in NZW x BXSB F1 mice. A model of antiphospholipid syndrome. J Immunol 1992;149:1063–1068.
7. Yoshii H, Yamamoto K, Okudaira H et al. Age-related differential mRNA expression of T cell cytokines in NZB/NZW F1 mice. Lupus 1995;4:213–216.
8. Pierangeli SS, Barker JH, Stikovac D et al. Effect of human IgG antiphospholipid antibodies on an in vivo thrombosis model in mice. Thromb Haemost 1994;71:670–674.
9. Pierangeli SS, Liu XW, Barker JH, Anderson G, Harris EN. Induction of thrombosis in a mouse model by IgG, IgM and IgA immunoglobulins from patients with the antiphospholipid syndrome. Thromb Haemost 1995;74:1361–1367.
10. Olec T, Pierangeli SS, Handly HH, et al. A monoclonal IgG anticardiolipin antibody from a patient with the antiphospholipid syndrome is thrombogenic in mice. Proc Natl Acad Sci USA 1996;93:8606–8611.
11. Gharavi AE, Pierangeli SS, Gharavi EE et al. Thrombogenic properties of antiphospholipid antibodies do not depend on their binding to beta2 glycoprotein 1 (beta2GP1) alone. Lupus 1998;7:341–346.
12. Gharavi AE, Pierangeli SS, Colden-Stanfield M, Liu XW, Espinola RG, Harris EN. GDKV-induced antiphospholipid antibodies enhance thrombosis and activate endothelial cells in vivo and in vitro. J Immunol 1999;163:2922–2927.
13. Edwards MH, Pierangeli S, Liu X, Barker JH, Anderson G, Harris EN. Hydroxychloroquine reverses thrombogenic properties of antiphospholipid antibodies in mice. Circulation 1997;96:4380–4384.
14. Branch DW, Dudley DJ, Mitchell MD et al. Immunoglobulin G fractions from patients with antiphospholipid antibodies cause fetal death in BALB/c mice: a model for autoimmune fetal loss. Am J Obstet Gynecol 1990;163:210–216.
15. Blank M, Cohen J, Toder V, Shoenfeld Y. Induction of anti-phospholipid syndrome in naive mice with mouse lupus monoclonal and human polyclonal anti-cardiolipin antibodies. Proc Natl Acad Sci USA 1991;88:3069–3073.
16. Piona A, La Rosa L, Tincani A et al. Placental thrombosis and fetal loss after passive transfer of mouse lupus monoclonal or human polyclonal anti-cardiolipin antibodies in pregnant naive BALB/c mice. Scand J Immunol 1995;41:427–432.
17. Blank M, Tincani A, Shoenfeld Y. Induction of experimental antiphospholipid syndrome in naive mice with purified IgG antiphosphatidylserine antibodies. J Rheumatol 1994;21:100–104.
18. Ikematsu W, Luan FL, La Rosa L et al. Human anticardiolipin monoclonal autoantibodies cause placental necrosis and fetal loss in BALB/c mice. Arthritis Rheum 1998;41:1026–1039.
19. George J, Blank M, Levy Y et al. Differential effects of anti-beta2-glycoprotein I antibodies on endothelial cells and on the manifestations of experimental antiphospholipid syndrome. Circulation 1998;97:900–906.
20. Jerne NK, Roland J, Cazenave PA. Recurrent idiotopes and internal images. EMBO J 1982;1:243–247.
21. Shoenfeld Y. Idiotypic induction of autoimmunity: a new aspect of the idiotypic network. FASEB J 1994;8:1296–1301.
22. Bakimer R, Fishman P, Blank M, Sredni B, Djaldetti M, Shoenfeld Y. Induction of primary antiphospholipid syndrome in mice by immunization with a human monoclonal anticardiolipin antibody (H-3). J Clin Invest 1992;89:1558–1563.

23. Yodfat O, Blank M, Krause I, Shoenfeld Y. The pathogenic role of anti-phosphatidylserine antibodies: active immunization with the antibodies leads to the induction of antiphospholipid syndrome. Clin Immunol Immunopathol 1996;78:14–20.

24. Blank M, Krause I, Ben Bassat M, Shoenfeld Y. Induction of experimental anti-phospholipid syndrome associated with SLE following immunization with human monoclonal pathogenic anti-DNA idiotype. J Autoimmunity 1992;5:495–509.

25. Ziporen L, Shoenfeld Y, Levy Y, Korczyn AD. Neurological dysfunction and hyperactive behavior associated with antiphospholipid antibodies. A mouse model. J Clin Invest 1997;100:613–619.

26. Cohen J, Bakimer R, Blank M, Valesini G, Shoenfeld Y. Pathogenic natural anti-cardiolipin antibodies: the experience from monoclonal gammopathy. Clin Exp Immunol 1994;97:181–186.

27. Ziporen L, Goldberg I, Arad M et al. Libman-Sacks endocarditis in the antiphospholipid syndrome: immunopathologic findings in deformed heart valves. Lupus 1996;5:196–205.

28. Blank M, Waisman A, Mozes E, Koike T, Shoenfeld Y. Pathogenic role of anti-cardiolipin single chain Fv domains: induction of experimental APS. International Immunol 1999;11:1917–1926

29. Gharavi AE, Sammaritano LR, Wen J, Elkon KB. Induction of antiphospholipid autoantibodies by immunization with beta 2 glycoprotein I (apolipoprotein H). J Clin Invest 1992;90:1105–1109.

30. Pierangeli SS, Harris EN. Induction of phospholipid-binding antibodies in mice and rabbits by immunization with human beta 2 glycoprotein 1 or anticardiolipin antibodies alone. Clin Exp Immunol 1993;93:269–272.

31. Blank M, Faden D, Tincani A et al. Immunization with anticardiolipin cofactor (beta-2-glycoprotein I) induces experimental antiphospholipid syndrome in naive mice. J Autoimmunity 1994;7:441–455.

32. Blank M, Krause I, Lanir N et al. Transfer of experimental antiphospholipid syndrome by bone marrow cell transplantation. The importance of the T cell. Arthritis Rheum 1995;38:115–122.

33. Krause I, Blank M, Gilbrut B, Shoenfeld Y. The effect of aspirin on recurrent fetal loss in experimental antiphospholipid syndrome. Am J Reprod Immunol 1993;29:155–161.

34. Shoenfeld Y, Blank M. Effect of long-acting thromboxane receptor antagonist (BMS 180,291) on experimental antiphospholipid syndrome. Lupus 1994;3:397–400.

35. Inbar O, Blank M, Faden D, Tincani A, Lorber M, Shoenfeld Y. Prevention of fetal loss in experimental antiphospholipid syndrome by low-molecular-weight heparin. Am J Obstet Gynecol 1993;169:423–426.

36. Weiner HL, Friedman A, Miller A et al. Oral tolerance: immunologic mechanisms and treatment of animal and human organ-specific autoimmune diseases by oral administration of autoantigens. Annu Rev Immunol 1994;12:809–837.

37. Blank M, George J, Barak V, Tincani A, Koike T, Shoenfeld Y. Oral tolerance to low dose beta 2-glycoprotein I: immunomodulation of experimental antiphospholipid syndrome. J Immunol 1998;161:5303–5312.

38. Carr RI, Tilley D, Forsyth S, Etheridge P, Sadi D. Failure of oral tolerance in (NZB NZW)F1 mice is antigen specific and appears to parallel antibody patterns in human systemic lupus erythematosus (SLE). Clin Immunol Immunopathol 1987;42:298–310.

39. Miller ML, Cowdery JS, Laskin CA, Curtin MF, Jr., Steinberg AD. Heterogeneity of oral tolerance defects in autoimmune mice. Clin Immunol Immunopathol 1984;31:231–240.

40. Blank M, Shoenfeld Y, Cabilly S, et al. Prevention of experimental antiphospholipid syndrome and endothelial cell activation by synthetic peptides. Proc Natl Acad Sci USA 1999;96:5164–5168.

41. Krause I, Blank M, Levi Y, Koike T, Barak V, Shoenfeld Y. Anti-idiotype immunomodulation of experimental anti-phospholipid syndrome via effect on Th1/Th2 expression. Clin Exp Immunol 1999; in press.

42. Tomer Y, Blank M, Shoenfeld Y. Suppression of experimental antiphospholipid syndrome and systemic lupus erythematosus in mice by anti-CD4 monoclonal antibodies. Arthritis Rheum 1994;37:1236–1244.

43. Adachi Y, Inaba M, Sugihara A et al. Effects of administration of monoclonal antibodies (anti-CD4 or anti-CD8) on the development of autoimmune diseases in (NZW BXSB)F1 mice. Immunobiology 1998;198:451–464.

44. Krause I, Blank M, Kopolovic J et al. Abrogation of experimental systemic lupus erythematosus and primary antiphospholipid syndrome with intravenous gamma globulin. J Rheumatol 1995;22:1068–1074.

45. Fishman P, Falach-Vaknine E, Zigelman R et al. Prevention of fetal loss in experimental antiphospholipid syndrome by in vivo administration of recombinant interleukin-3. J Clin Invest 1993;91:1834–1837.

46. Blank M, George J, Fishman P et al. Ciprofloxacin immunomodulation of experimental antiphospholipid syndrome associated with elevation of interleukin-3 and granulocyte-macrophage colony-stimulating factor expression. Arthritis Rheum 1998;41:224–232.

47. Buskila D, Sukenik S, Shoenfeld Y. The possible role of prolactin in autoimmunity. Am J Reprod Immunol 1991;26:118–123.
48. Blank M, Krause I, Buskila D et al. Bromocriptine immunomodulation of experimental SLE and primary antiphospholipid syndrome via induction of nonspecific T suppressor cells. Cell Immunol 1995;162:114–122.
49. Blank M, Tomer Y, Slavin S, Shoenfeld Y. Induction of tolerance to experimental anti-phospholipid syndrome (APS) by syngeneic bone marrow cell transplantation. Scand J Immunol 1995;42:226–234.
50. Adachi Y, Inaba M, Amoh Y et al. Effect of bone marrow transplantation on antiphospholipid antibody syndrome in murine lupus mice. Immunobiology 1995;192:218–230.

Section 4

Therapy

39 Management of Thrombosis in the Antiphospholipid Syndrome

M. A. Khamashta

Introduction

Despite the enormous amount of work focussed on the pathogenesis and clinical manifestations of the antiphospholipid syndrome (APS), there has been surprisingly little published on the management of thrombosis associated with antiphospholipid antibodies (aPL) and there are only limited data from prospective clinical trials on which to base treatment decisions [1].

Long-term prognosis in APS is most influenced by the risk of recurrent thrombosis. The thrombotic complications of aPL are unpredictable and the mechanisms triggering these events in individual patients are ill-defined. Despite the development of newer assays such as anti-β_2-glycoprotein I and antiprothrombin antibodies, the serological "fingerprint" of the patient most at risk for arterial (especially stroke) or venous thrombosis, remains elusive.

A number of management questions keep recurring (Table 39.1). Useful data are beginning to emerge which serve as a guide to optimal management of thrombosis in APS. These are reviewed in this chapter.

Table 39.1. Thrombosis in APS – management dilemmas.

- Does the patient with venous thrombosis and aPL require "conventional" short-term anticoagulation or long-term treatment?
- How does one manage a patient with recurrent thrombosis despite high-intensity warfarin therapy and the concurrent use of low-dose aspirin?
- What is the risk–benefit analysis of using high-dose warfarin in a 65-year-old with aPL-associated stroke?
- What is the best management strategy for patients on warfarin because of aPL-associated thrombosis with severe thrombocytopenia?
- Should asymptomatic individuals (increasingly being identified) with circulating aPL who have never, as yet, suffered thrombosis be treated and, if so, with what?

Thromboprophylaxis of aPL-positive Subjects but no Previous Thrombosis

Available data from clinical studies suggest that the thrombotic risk associated with aPL may be substantial. In a prospective study of healthy men, those with aPL suffered 5 times the risk for venous thrombosis or pulmonary embolus [2]. Women initially referred to an obstetrical group for pregnancy-related aspects of APS had 15.7 thromboses per 100 patient-years in an average of 3 years of follow-up [3]. Finazzi et al [4] designed a large prospective study in 360 unselected patients with aPL and showed that high titer IgG anticardiolipin antibody (aCL) was a significant predictor for thrombosis. Vaarala et al [5] showed that patients with high levels of aCL had a higher risk of myocardial infarction and that this risk was independent of any other factors. While there have been few rigorously designed epidemiological studies, available data suggest that the stroke risk associated with aPL may be substantial, especially in young adults [6]. A study of lupus patients with aPL but no thrombosis, showed that no less than one half (52%) had developed the syndrome over 10 year follow-up [7]. Recently, Gomez-Pacheco et al [8] have suggested that the detection of antibodies directed against β_2-glycoprotein I may predict the risk of thrombosis in asymptomatic individuals with aPL.

Despite the accumulating data that aPL is a serious risk factor for thrombosis, to date, no study has attempted to address the prophylactic management of the aPL-positive individuals. In treating patients with aPL it is important to remove or reduce other risk factors for thrombosis. Patients are advised to stop smoking, and women are counselled against the use of estrogen-containing oral contraceptive pills. Although low-dose aspirin (75 mg/day) has been considered to be a logical prophylaxis, the Physician Health study showed that low-dose aspirin use in men with aCL did not protect against deep venous thrombosis or pulmonary embolus [2]. Hydroxychloroquine has well-documented antiplatelet effects and has been shown to reduce the risk of thrombosis in both SLE patients [9, 10] and animal models of APS [11]. However, the need for regular eye-checks for the early detection of retinal toxicity is a limiting factor for the long-term use of antimalarials in the primary thromboprophylaxis of aPL-positive individuals. Low-intensity oral anticoagulation with target International Normalized Ratio (INR) around 1.5, has been shown to be effective in other prothrombotic states including central venous catheterization [12], stage IV breast cancer [13] and ischaemic heart disease in men at increased risk [14]. A prospective randomised trial comparing low-dose aspirin with low-intensity warfarin in subjects with SLE and/or an adverse pregnancy history is currently in progress in the United Kingdom. Until these results are available, we suggest that individuals with a persistently positive aCL or positive lupus anticoagulant (LA) take low-dose aspirin (75 mg/day) indefinitely. Furthermore, high risk situations such as surgery should be covered with subcutaneous heparin prophylaxis.

Prevention of Recurrent Thrombosis in APS

Treatment of the acute thrombotic event, if identified, is no different in APS than in the general population. Patients are anticoagulated with heparin followed by warfarin. Fibrinolytic therapy has been used successfully in patients with APS [15].

The risk of recurrent thrombosis in patients with APS is high. The level of this risk has been variously reported ranging between 22–69% [16–20]. The type of thrombosis is predictive; retrospective analysis of patients with APS and recurrent thrombosis showed that a venous thrombosis is followed by another venous thrombosis in more than 70% of cases, and an arterial thrombosis is followed by another arterial thrombosis in more than 90% of cases [16, 17].

The description of APS by Hughes in 1983 [21] provided a new insight into vascular aspects of neurological disease. Here for the first time, was a common prothrombotic disorder which resulted in arterial as well as venous thrombosis. The cerebral circulation appears to be particularly targeted, with strokes and transient ischemic attacks, movement disorders, epilepsy, myelopathy and migraine being major manifestations. Anecdotally, the initiation of adequate anticoagulant therapy coincide with rapid, often dramatic, amelioration of symptoms. A controlled trial of aspirin versus warfarin prophylaxis for recurrent stroke is still under way. Meanwhile, most experts in the field of APS agree that those with arterial events should have long-term anticoagulation. However, the length of anticoagulation is those with APS and venous thromboembolism has been debated [22]. Two recent large and prospective long-term follow up studies of patients with venous thromboembolism, have confirmed that the risk of recurrence in APS patients is significantly much higher than in patients without aPL [19, 20]. They also showed the benefit of long-term oral anticoagulation in these patients. Thus, the current recommendations once a patient has had a thrombosis associated with aPL is long-term (possibly life-long) warfarin therapy (Table 39.2). It is not clear, however, whether prolonged anticoagulation is necessary in APS patients whose first thrombotic episode developed in association with surgery, oral contraceptive pill, pregnancy or other circumstantial thrombotic risk factors.

Most patients requiring long-term anticoagulant therapy respond well to warfarin targeted to an INR of 2.0–3.0. However, the optimal intensity of anticoagulation therapy is uncertain for patients with aPL-associated thrombosis. There are reports based on retrospective analyses of observational studies, that patients with APS and thrombosis are inadequately protected from recurrent thrombotic episodes if treated

Table 39.2. Thromboprophylaxis of aPL-positive individuals: recommendations.

Asymptomatic subjects:
  Low-dose aspirin
  Hydroxychloroquine/chloroquine (SLE)
  Low-intensity warfarin (INR around 1.5)

Thrombosis:
  Long-term warfarin
    Venous: INR 2.5–3.0
    Arterial: INR $\geq$ 3.0

Recurrent thrombosis:
  Warfarin INR $\geq$ 3.0 + low-dose aspirin

Difficult (resistant) cases with recurrent thrombosis
  Warfarin $\geq$ 3.0 +
    Immunosuppressive drugs
    Corticosteroids
    Intravenous immunoglobulins
    Plasmapheresis

at a targeted INR of 2.0–3.0 [16, 17]. In our series, which is the largest retrospective study of 147 aPL-associated thrombosis followed-up for a mean of 6 years, a recurrent thrombosis occurred in 69% of patients. High-intensity warfarin (INR ≥ 3.0) with or without low-dose aspirin, was the most effective therapeutic option in the secondary prevention of venous and arterial thrombosis in these patients [17]. Some dispute this and prefer to advocate an INR of 2.0–3.0 for those with venous thrombosis, reserving intensive anticoagulation (INR 3.0–4.0) for those with recurrent venous thrombosis or arterial thrombosis [18, 19, 22]. Discontinuation of warfarin can lead to major recurrent thrombosis, and the highest rate of recurrence of thrombosis was found in the first 6 months after cessation of warfarin therapy [17, 20]. Low-dose aspirin alone does not prevent recurrent thrombosis in these patients [16, 17]. Some patients with APS continue to have recurrent thrombotic events despite an INR of 3.0–4.0. Whether additional therapy with low-dose aspirin is efficacious in this situation is not known, but the risk of haemorrhage is increased when aspirin is used alongside oral anticoagulant therapy [23].

Oral anticoagulation therapy carries an inevitable risk of serious hemorrhage. The rate of life-threatening bleeding in subjects taking warfarin, based on a prospective study, is at least 0.25% per annum [24]. This rises rapidly when the INR exceeds 4.0. In APS, serious bleeding complications may occur, but their risk is not higher than that observed in other thrombotic conditions warranting oral anticoagulation [25]. However, it should be kept in mind that these data have been obtained from series of young patients with primary or SLE-related APS. Age has been demonstrated to be a risk factor for severe bleeding episodes in patients placed on long-term anticoagulation [24] and Piette and Cacoub have recently reported similar experience in their elderly patients with APS [26].

It is increasingly evident that many patients have uncontrollable fluctuations of INR. It is not uncommon for patients with APS to "know" precisely when their INR has fallen – the headaches, dysarthria, memory disturbance and neurological features predictably returning when the INR drops, for example, below 2.8. Concerns exist over the validity of the INR in control oral anticoagulant dosing if LA is present. The inhibitor occasionally increases the prothrombin time and, in turn, the INR, which may thus not reflect the true degree of anticoagulation [27]. This phenomenon seems to be more likely when certain recombinant thromboplastin reagents are used and can usually be circumvented by careful selection of the thromboplastin to be used for the prothrombin time test [28, 29]. One of the features of APS is that many patients are relatively resistant to warfarin, some requiring up to 25 mg daily to maintain adequate anticoagulation. In our experience, most of these patients were receiving other drugs and, notably, azathioprine at the same time as warfarin therapy. Azathioprine interacts with warfarin, reducing its efficacy by possible hepatic enzyme induction [30]. Conversely, patients on warfarin who stop azathioprine may be at risk of bleeding and should be monitored carefully.

The role of steroids and immunosuppressive drugs in the treatment of patients with aPL and thrombosis is uncertain. Such drugs have severe side effects when given for prolonged periods and aPL are not always suppressed by these agents. Furthermore, in our series of patients with APS, corticosteroids and immunosuppressive therapy, prescribed in some patients to control lupus activity, did not prevent further thrombotic events [17]. The use of these drugs is probably justified only in patients with life-threatening conditions with repeated episodes of thrombosis despite adequate anticoagulation therapy, namely catastrophic APS. In this rare but life-threatening condition, plasmapheresis has also been used [31]. It is tempting to speculate that more targeted immunosuppressive therapy may be a future option in this antibody-mediated disease.

Autoimmune thrombocytopenia is an accompanying problem in 25% of individuals with APS [32]. Generally, it is mild (platelet counts between $50-150 \times 10^9$ l), but occasionally severe thrombocytopenia occurs. The treatment of choice is corticosteroids. The treatment of thrombosis and thrombocytopenia in the same patient is a difficult clinical problem and requires careful management. It is worth noting that thrombocytopenia does not necessarily protect patients against thrombosis [18] and platelet counts of $50-100 \times 10^9$ l in APS should not modify the treatment policy of thrombosis with warfarin. If the platelet count falls below 50×10^9 l then this is an indication to start corticosteroids. In these patients, the intensity of anticoagulation should be reduced because of the increased risk of bleeding. Splenectomy has been safely and successfully performed in APS patients with steroid-resistant thrombocytopenia [33].

References

1. Khamashta MA. Management of thrombosis and pregnancy loss in the antiphospholipid syndrome. Lupus 1998;7 (suppl 2): S162–S165.
2. Ginsburg KS, Liang MH, Newcomer L et al. Anticardiolipin antibodies and the risk for ischemic stroke and venous thrombosis. Ann Intern Med 1992;177:997–1002.
3. Silver RM, Draper ML, Scott JR, Lyon JL, Reading J, Branch DW. Clinical consequences of antiphospholipid antibodies: an historic cohort study. Obstet Gynecol 1994;83:372–377.
4. Finazzi G, Brancaccio V, Moia M et al. Natural history and risk factors for thrombosis in 360 patients with antiphospholipid antibodies: a four year prospective study from the Italian registry. Am J Med 1996;100:530–536.
5. Vaarala O, Manttari M, Manninen V et al. Anticardiolipin antibodies and risk of myocardial infarction in a prospective cohort of middle-aged men. Circulation 1995;91:23–27.
6. Kittner S, Gorelick PB. Antiphospholipid antibodies and stroke: an epidemiological perspective. Stroke 1992;23:I19–I22.
7. Shah N, Khamashta MA, Atsumi T, Hughes GRV. Outcome of patients with anticardiolipin antibodies: a 10 year follow-up of 52 patients. Lupus 1998;7:3–6.
8. Gomez-Pacheco L, Villa AR, Drenkard C, Cabiedes J, Cabral AR, Alarcon-Segovia D. Serum anti-β_2-glycoprotein I and anticardiolipin antibodies during thrombosis in systemic lupus erythematosus patients. Am J Med 1999;106:417–423.
9. Wallace DJ, Linker-Israeli M, Metzger AL, Stecher VJ. The relevance of antimalarial therapy with regard to thrombosis, hypercholesterolemia and cytokines in SLE. Lupus 1993; 2(Suppl):S13–S15.
10. Petri M. Hydroxychloroquine use in the Baltimore lupus cohort: effects on lipids, glucose and thrombosis. Lupus 1996;5 (Suppl):S16–S22.
11. Edwards MH, Pierangeli S, Liu X et al. Hydroxychloroquine reverses thrombogenic properties of antiphospholipid antibodies in mice. Circulation1997;96:4380–4384.
12. Bern MM, Lokich JJ, Wallach SR et al. Very low doses of warfarin can prevent thrombosis in central venous catheters: a randomized prospective trial. Ann Intern Med 1990;112:423–428.
13. Levine M, Hirsh J, Gent M et al. Double-blind randomised trial of very low-dose warfarin for prevention of thromboembolism in stage IV breast cancer. Lancet 1994;343:886–889.
14. The Medical Research Council's General Practice Research Framework. Thrombosis prevention trial: randomised trial of low-intensity oral anticoagulation with warfarin and low-dose aspirin in the primary prevention of ischaemic heart disease in men at increased risk. Lancet 1998;351:233–241.
15. Julkunen H, Hedman C, Kauppi M. Thrombolysis for acute ischemic stroke in the primary antiphospholipid syndrome. J Rheumatol 1997;24:181–183.
16. Rosove MH, Brewer PMC. Antiphospholipid thrombosis: clinical course after the first thrombotic event in 70 patients. Ann Intern Med 1992;117:303–308.

17. Khamashta MA, Cuadrado MJ, Mujic F, Taub N, Hunt BJ, Hughes GRV. the management of thrombosis in the antiphospholipid antibody syndrome. N Engl J Med 1995;332:993–997.
18. Krnic-Barrie S, O'Connor CR, Looney SW, Pierangeli SS, Harris EN. A retrospective review of 61 patients with antiphospholipid syndrome. Analysis of factors influencing recurrent thrombosis. Arch Intern Med 1997;157:2101–2108.
19. Schulman S, Svenungsson E, Granqvist S and the Duration of Anticoagulation Study Group. Anticardiolipin antibodies predict early recurrence of thromboembolism and death among patients with venous thromboembolism following anticoagulant therapy. Am J Med 1998;104:332–338.
20. Kearon C, Gent M, Hirsh J et al. A comparison of three months of anticoagulation with extended anticoagulation for a first episode of idiopathic venous thromboembolism. N Engl J Med 1999;340:901–907.
21. Hughes GRV. Thrombosis, abortion, cerebral disease and the lupus anticoagulant. Br Med J 1983;287:1088–1099.
22. Ginsberg JS, Wells PS, Brill-Edwards P et al. Antiphospholipid antibodies and venous thromboembolism. Blood 1995;86:3685–3691.
23. Meade TW, Miller CJ. Combined use of aspirin and warfarin in primary prevention of ischemic heart disease in men at risk. Am J Cardiol 1995;75:23B–26B.
24. Palareti G, Leali N, Cocheri S et al. Bleeding complications of oral anticoagulant treatment: an inception-cohort, prospective collaborative study (ISCOAT) Italian study on complications of oral anticoagulant therapy. Lancet 1996;348:423–428.
25. Al-Sayegh FA, Ensworth S, Huang S, Stein HB, Kinkhoff AV. Hemorrhagic complications of long-term anticoagulant therapy in 7 patients with systemic lupus erythematosus and antiphospholipid syndrome. J Rheumatol 1997;24:1716–1718.
26. Piette JC, Cacoub P. Antiphospholipid syndrome in the elderly: caution. Circulation 1998;97:2195–2196.
27. Moll S, Ortel TL. Monitoring warfarin therapy in patients with lupus anticoagulant. Ann Intern Med 1997;127:177–185.
28. Robert A, Le Querrec A, Delahousse B et al. Control of oral anticoagulation in patients with the antiphospholipid syndrome: influence of the lupus anticoagulant on International Normalized Ratio. Thromb Haemost 1998;80:99–103.
29. Lawrie AS, Purdy G, Mackie IJ, Machin SJ. Monitoring of oral anticoagulant therapy in lupus anticoagulant positive patients with the antiphospholipid syndrome. Br J Haematol 1997;98:887–892.
30. Rivier G, Khamashta MA, Hughes GRV. Warfarin and azathioprine: a drug interaction does exist. Am J Med 1993;95:342.
31. Asherson RA, Cervera R, Piette JC et al. Catastrophic antiphospholipid syndrome. Clinical and laboratory features of 50 patients. Medicine (Baltimore) 1998;77:195–207.
32. Cuadrado MJ, Mujic F, Munoz E, Khamashta MA, Hughes GRV. Thrombocytopenia in the antiphospholipid syndrome. Ann Rheum Dis 1997;56:194–196.
33. Galindo M, Khamashta MA, Hughes GRV. Splenectomy for refractory thrombocytopenia in the antiphospholipid syndrome. Rheumatology 1999;38:848–853.

40   The Management of Antiphospholipid Syndrome in Pregnancy

L. Lakasing, S. Bewley and C. Nelson-Piercy

Introduction

Antiphospholipid syndrome (APS) predominantly affects young women and there has been a growing awareness of this condition amongst obstetricians and gynecologists over the last decade. In this chapter we discuss the association between APS and recurrent pregnancy loss, and present some of the dilemmas in the management of on-going pregnancies in women with APS. Knowledge of the pathogenesis of adverse pregnancy outcome in APS is incomplete and some of the numerous hypotheses and areas of research in this rapidly evolving field are outlined.

The Effect of Pregnancy on APS

Pregnancy is a hypercoagulable state and women with APS are at increased risk of thrombosis unless thromboprophylaxis or anticoagulation is adequate. Some studies show a significant proportion of patients still have thrombotic episodes despite thromboprophylaxis [1, 2]. Pregnancy may also exacerbate pre-existing thrombocytopenia, and this may be further compounded by medication since aspirin and heparin administered during pregnancy may cause thrombocytopenia (see Table 40.2). Thromboprophylaxis, full anticoagulation and the management of thrombocytopenia in pregnant women with APS are discussed in more detail below.

The Effect of APS on Pregnancy

APS and Early Pregnancy Complications

Many cases of APS are diagnosed following investigation for recurrent miscarriage. The association between APS and recurrent miscarriage is well known [3–6], with second trimester loss being particularly common [7]. The prospective fetal loss rate in primary APS is reported to be 50–75% [8, 9]. In patients with systemic lupus erythematosus (SLE) and secondary APS some studies suggest this may be over 90% [10, 11], although this is likely to be an overestimate. It has been suggested that the risk of fetal loss is directly related to the antibody titer [12, 13], but this is certainly not true in all cases. Some studies have shown maternal IgG aCL levels to be particularly reliable predictors of miscarriage [14, 15]. Although this makes theoretical sense, as this subclass of antibodies can cross into the fetoplacental circulation [16], many women with recurrent miscarriage have IgM aCL antibodies only. It is impossible to predict which women will develop complications in pregnancy and some women with persistently elevated aPL titers and a history of thromboses ± thrombocytopenia will have no complications at all. Previous poor obstetric outcome remains the most important predictor of future risk [17–19].

APS and Late Pregnancy Complications

In pregnancies that do not end in miscarriage or fetal loss, there is a high incidence of early onset pre-eclampsia (PET) [20–23] and intrauterine growth restriction (IUGR) [17, 24], placental abruption [25] and premature delivery [26, 27]. Because patients with APS form a heterogeneous group, the incidence of these complications varies between units. Those units which manage patients with systemic manifestations of APS inevitably have a higher incidence of complications in pregnancy [1, 28], whilst those that recruit women predominantly from recurrent miscarriage clinics will have a lower incidence of these complications [29, 30]. It is essential to appreciate these differences in order to critically appraise the literature, and indeed to advise patients. Table 40.1 shows a summary of the main studies in this field. In our own unit, the majority of APS cases have previously been identified by rheumatology and hematology colleagues, and despite enthusiastic multidisciplinary team management, there is a 70% live birth rate, 18% incidence of PET, 31% babies are born with birth weights less than the 10th centile for gestational age, and 43% of infants are delivered prematurely with a mean gestation of approximately 34 weeks [1]. Approximately 70% of these women are delivered by Caesarean section, and 7% of babies die in the neonatal period due to problems related to prematurity [1]. Regular ultrasound scanning for fetal growth is recommended in these patients, and in specialist units assessment of uterine artery Doppler waveforms is performed in the mid-trimester [31, 32]. The presence of mid-trimester uterine artery notches in high-risk pregnancies is associated with PET, IUGR and intrapartum asphyxia with a sensitivity of 68% and a positive predictive value of 42% [33]. In high risk pregnancies, abnormal uterine artery Doppler velocimetry is also of some value in predicting placental abruption, a common feature of APS pregnancies, but gives no indication as to the timing of this

Table 40.1. Pregnancy complications in different populations of women with APS.

Study	Utah [28]	St. Thomas [1]	Liverpool [29]	St. Mary's [30]
Pregnancies (*n*)	82	60	53	150
Population	Predominantly systemic	Predominantly systemic	Predominantly recurrent miscarriage	All recurrent miscarriage
PET (%)	51	18	3	11
IUGR (%)	31	31	11	15
Preterm delivery (%)	37	43	8	24

Adapted from Ref. 36.

event [34]. Histological evidence of impaired trophoblast migration in placental bed biopsies from women showing these high resistance Doppler waveforms has been reported [35], although the extent of uteroplacental pathology does not always correlate with the severity of maternal / fetal disease.

Therapeutic Options in APS Pregnancies

Many therapeutic options have been tried in APS pregnancies and the risks and benefits of each form of therapy continue to be an active area of debate [37]. The most commonly used are aspirin, heparin, warfarin and steroids. A summary of the side-effects of these drugs is shown in Table 40.2. Preconceptual review of medication is useful as it allows clinicians to place each patient in a risk category and treat her accordingly. These individualised treatment regimes limit the problems associated with polypharmacy in pregnancy and enable resources to be used appropriately.

Aspirin

Women with APS are advised to take low-dose aspirin (75 mg daily) during pregnancy. The rationale for this is aspirin-mediated inhibition of thromboxane, increased vasodilation and subsequent reduced risk of thromboses in the placenta and elsewhere. However, the use of aspirin in APS pregnancies has never been subjected to a randomized trial, although several non-randomized studies suggest this is beneficial [38–40], and there are animal data to support this [41]. In low risk APS pregnancies, i.e., no previous thromboses or miscarriages, a randomized controlled trial of aspirin versus no aspirin failed to show any benefit of treatment [42]. Damage to the developing trophoblast occurs early in pregnancy, and therefore if aspirin is used it is likely to be of most benefit if administered from the preconceptual period.

Table 40.2. Therapeutic options in APS pregnancies.

	Maternal side effects	Fetal side effects	Breastfeeding
Aspirin	GI disturbances	Safe	Safe
Warfarin	GI disturbances Hypersensitivity Hemorrhage	Teratogenic Hemorrhage Miscarriage	Safe
Heparin	Osteoporosis Thrombocytopenia Hemorrhage/bruising Hypersensitivity	Safe	Safe
Prednisolone	Infection Diabetes Hypertension Osteoporosis Peptic ulceration Muscle wasting Cushing's syndrome Depression/psychosis	Safe	Safe ?adrenal suppression (very rare, only if > 30 mg daily)

Treatment is usually continued at least until delivery if not into the puerperium. Low-dose aspirin does not affect the use of regional anaesthesia during labor. Renal and hepatic impairment does not occur with this dose of aspirin and bronchospasm is exceptionally rare affecting a minority of asthmatics.

Heparin

Women with APS and a previous history of thromboembolism are treated with heparin as thromboprophylaxis in pregnancy. For those with recurrent pregnancy loss but without a history of thromboembolism, there is as yet no consensus [43], and some studies have suggested that heparin therapy in addition to aspirin may contribute to improved fetal outcome [7, 44]. One group has shown improved fetal outcome using heparin alone [45]. Most specialist units caring for pregnant women with APS use aspirin and heparin together in women with a history of previous thrombosis or second trimester loss, and there is accumulating evidence for a role for heparin in women with recurrent first trimester loss [46, 47]. However, the potential benefits of heparin should be balanced against the risk of heparin-induced osteoporosis [48–50]. The problem of osteoporosis is compounded by concomitant use of steroid medication, and indeed by pregnancy itself [51–54]. Low-molecular-weight heparins (LMWH) are commonly used in APS patients because of the convenience of once-daily administration, the improved antithrombotic (αXa) to anticoagulant (αIIa) ratio, the decreased risk of heparin-induced thrombocytopenia and the probable decreased risk of heparin-induced osteoporosis [54]. Although factor Xa levels may be used to monitor LMWH use [55], experience has shown that doses are virtually never altered as a result [56], and therefore it is no longer our advice to measure factor Xa levels routinely. LMWH administration is omitted at least 12 hours prior to elective delivery, but in case urgent delivery is necessary reversal with protamine sulfate is possible. The molecular weight of unfractionated heparin ranges from 12–15 kDa and that of LMWH from 4–5 kDa therefore neither preparation is able to cross the placenta. Heparin and LMWH are not excreted into breast milk [57].

Warfarin

When there has been a thrombotic event in the index pregnancy despite heparin thromboprophylaxis, or in patients with a history of previous cerebrovascular thromboses, the risk of recurrence is sufficiently high to consider antenatal administration of warfarin [58]. In practice the use of warfarin is avoided in the first trimester unless a woman develops transient ischemic attacks or other thromboembolic events at that time. This is because, unlike heparin, warfarin does cross the placenta and is potentially teratogenic, producing a typical embryopathy characterized by nasal hypoplasia, stippled epiphyses, rhizomelia, digital dysplasia, eye anomalies and developmental delay [59]. The exact incidence of these anomalies is unknown largely due to case-reporting bias. Review of the literature suggests that it is between 2–4% [60]. Patients require close supervision and regular international normalized ratio (INR) estimates maintaining an INR between 2.0–2.5. It must be remembered that the maternal INR may not accurately reflect the fetal coagulation status and animal studies show that the risk of fetal intraventricular hemorrhage is still present despite optimum maternal control [61]. The fetus is therefore at risk throughout pregnancy during the period of warfarin administration [62]. Warfarin is discontinued and intravenous infusion of unfractionated heparin is commenced a fortnight before planned delivery to allow clearance of warfarin by both mother and fetus. Every attempt should be made to avoid rapid reversal of warfarin anticoagulation with vitamin K at the time of delivery as this makes subsequent anticoagulation in the postnatal period difficult. There is no evidence to suggest that fetal outcome is improved with the use of warfarin. There is no significant excretion of warfarin into breast milk [63, 64].

Steroids

In the past high-dose steroids ($\geq$ 60 mg daily) were used to suppress LA and aCL and some studies reported improved fetal survival [65, 66]. However, these therapeutic regimes resulted in considerable maternal morbidity including gestational diabetes, hypertension and sepsis, and subsequent studies failed to show an improvement in pregnancy outcome [39, 67]. Cowchock et al. demonstrated that aspirin and heparin gave equivalent fetal outcomes when compared with aspirin and steroids with significantly less maternal morbidity [44] and more recently there have been suggestions that steroid use may be detrimental to fetal outcome by promoting preterm delivery [68]. Therefore, the use of steroids in APS pregnancies has been abandoned except for the treatment of maternal thrombocytopenia or coexistent systemic lupus erythematosus for which prednisolone is still first-line therapy. Regular blood glucose monitoring is required with long-term administration of steroids. Patients requiring > 7.5 mg prednisolone daily prior to delivery should be given intrapartum intravenous hydrocortisone. Breastfeeding is rarely contraindicated, although patients on $\geq$ 30 mg prednisolone with healthy term babies may consider bottle-feeding because of the theoretical risk of neonatal hypothalamic-pituitary-adrenal axis suppression at these high doses.

Others

Immunosuppression with azathioprine, intravenous immunoglobulin [69–71], plasma exchange [72] and interleukin-3 therapy [73] have all been tried in APS pregnancies. The variable course of the disease and the small numbers of patients in these studies have made it impossible to draw any conclusions about these treatments but clinical trials continue. Immunoglobulin therapy is probably the most promising of these, but because this treatment is expensive and as yet of unproven benefit, its use is limited to salvage therapy in women who develop complications despite treatment with aspirin and heparin [74]. A 2 g/kg course of intravenous immunoglobulin administered in divided doses over 2–5 days in the second or early third trimester in pregnancies complicated by IUGR has been shown to temporarily improve uteroplacental Doppler waveforms [75]. This may allow prolongation of intrauterine life and subsequent improvement in neonatal outcome but more research is needed in this area.

Management of APS Pregnancies at St. Thomas' Hospital

St. Thomas Hospital is a national referral center for APS and there are weekly high-risk antenatal clinics for women with APS. Women from all over the UK are referred and many are well known to the rheumatology and hematology services. This affords us the privilege of preconceptual counseling in most cases. At this visit women undergo a risk assessment and future therapy is planned. Many women have related disorders which are also addressed at this time, e.g. SLE or thrombocytopenia. Apart from standard prepregnancy advice, e.g. folic acid, women who are not already taking aspirin are advised to start from the preconceptual period onwards until after delivery. LMWH is offered to women who are taking long-term oral anticoagulation, those with previous thrombotic events, those with one or more previous second trimester losses, and those with recurrent (three or more) first trimester losses. LMWH is administered from the time of a positive pregnancy, but not preconceptually in order to limit the time of heparin usage. An early ultrasound scan is recommended to confirm the presence of a fetal heart and accurately date the pregnancy. Patients are seen regularly by the multidisciplinary team. The frequency of visits depends on the presence of any complications and practical issues such as the commuting distance.

As well as routine aspects of antenatal care offered to all pregnant women e.g. serum screening and the 20-week anomaly ultrasound examination, women with APS are offered Doppler analysis of uterine artery waveforms at 20 and 24 weeks' gestation. Heparin is discontinued in APS patients with recurrent first trimester miscarriage alone and normal uterine artery Dopplers at 20 weeks' gestation as we consider the risks of long-term heparin to outweigh the benefits in this subgroup of patients. In the others, heparin is continued for a variable time up to and after delivery depending on the initial risk assessment, e.g. women who have had a previous second trimester loss alone can discontinue treatment immediately following delivery, whereas those with previous thromboses are advised to continue use for 6 weeks following delivery or transfer back to warfarin after delivery. In the third trimester, ultrasound scans to assess fetal growth are offered at 28 and 34 weeks' gestation, or more frequently if indicated. In cases with IUGR, ultrasound biophysical profiles may be used to obtain further information about fetal well-being. These specialist scans are conducted at the Fetal Medicine Unit at Guy's Hospital.

Patients have direct access to hospital 24 hours a day and inpatients are regularly reviewed by the multidisciplinary team. Women who develop PET are managed according to the standard hospital protocol. A specialist team of midwives care for these high-risk pregnancies and this provides continuity of care. Anesthetists are involved when planning delivery especially in women who are fully anticoagulated, and a bereavement counseling service is provided by consultant obstetricians and neonatologists where appropriate.

Pathogenesis of Adverse Pregnancy Outcome in APS

The safe and successful treatment of pregnant women with APS lies in understanding the etiology of this condition, and the mechanism by which complications in pregnancy may arise. As yet there are many more questions than answers [76]. Most research has been in the form of drug trials and conclusions have been largely unconvincing due to small numbers, poor study design and variable entry criteria and outcome measures. More recently there has been a shift in emphasis to more laboratory-based research using models for trophoblast development and molecular biological techniques to determine various aspects of antibody–endothelial interactions [77].

Early Pregnancy Failure

Impaired development of the trophoblast and failure to establish an effective fetopla-cental circulation may result in early pregnancy failure. The factors governing tro-phoblast invasion and early placental development are multiple and complex. Some factors specific to APS pregnancies have been well characterized, in particular β_2-glycoprotein I (β_2GpI) [78], but many others are also involved. It is likely that growth factors [79, 80], cytokines [81], integrins [82, 83], cell adhesion molecules [84, 85], and class I major histocompatibility complex antigens [86] are all instrumental. The effect of aPL on the function of these molecules has yet to be established.

Late Pregnancy Complications

Late pregnancy complications are likely to arise from damage to the uteroplacental vasculature. After 15 weeks' gestation the vasculosyncytial membrane is porous enough for IgG antibodies to be able to cross into the fetal circulation. High concen-trations of IgG antibodies have been eluted from placentas from women with aPL-positive sera with poor pregnancy outcomes [16]. Whether these aPL antibodies themselves are directly responsible for structural and/or functional damage to the placental vessels or whether they act indirectly via another secondary mechanism is unclear. It has been difficult to extrapolate antibody data from animal studies to clin-ical experience in humans [87, 88]. It is clear, however, that in order to recognize endothelial cells, aPL antibodies require the presence of certain cofactors [89, 90], the best characterized of which are β_2GPI [91] and prothrombin [92]. Much work has been done in this area but few conclusions drawn.

Histological examination of placentae from APS pregnancies often show throm-boses of the uteroplacental vasculature and placental infarction [93]. There may be decidual vasculopathy characterized by fibrinoid necrosis and atherosis of decidual vessels [94]. These findings suggest thrombotic damage to the fetoplacental circula-tion, and whilst some groups have published data to support this [95–97], others disagree [98, 99]. Another possibility is that placental dysfunction and subsequent fetal demise in APS pregnancies are secondary to the maternal vasculopathy, which is thought to also affect the placental bed vessels, and not due to primary antibody-mediated fetoplacental events at all.

Summary

Pregnant women with APS are at risk of complications at all stages of pregnancy. They require specialist care and a team approach involving obstetricians, obstetric physicians, rheumatologists, hematologists, anaesthetists, neonatologists and spe-cialist midwives. Close monitoring of the various aspects of this condition may reduce maternal morbidity and improve fetal outcome. Therapeutic options com-monly include aspirin, heparin, warfarin and steroids.

The pathogenesis of the adverse pregnancy outcome in APS has not yet been elu-cidated although there is active research in this field. Until this is ascertained, we must accept that many aspects of management are purely empirical and it is our duty to counsel patients thoroughly such that they understand the risks and benefits of the treatment options they are offered.

References

1. Lima F, Khamashta MA, Buchanan NMM et al. A study of sixty pregnancies in patients with the antiphospholipid syndrome.Clin Exp Rheumatol 1996;14:131–136.
2. Ringrose DK. Anaesthesia and antiphospholipid syndrome – a review of 20 obstetric patients. Int J Obstet Anaesth 1997;6:107–111.
3. Julkunen H. Pregnancy in systemic lupus erythematosus. Contraception, fetal outcome and congenital heart block. Acta Obstet Gynaecol Scand 1994;73:517–520.
4. MacLean M, Cumming G, McCall F et al. The prevalence of lupus anticoagulant and anticardiolipin antibodies in women with a history of first trimester miscarriages. Br J Obstet Gynaecol 1994;101:103–106.
5. Silver RM, Branch DW. Recurrent miscarriage: autoimmune considerations. Clin Obstet Gynaecol 1994;37:745–760.
6. Rai RS, Clifford K, Cohen H et al. High prospective fetal loss rate in untreated pregnancies of women with recurrent miscarriage and antiphospholipid antibodies. Hum Reprod 1995;10:3301–3304.
7. Branch DW, Rodgers GM. Induction of endothelial cell tissue factor activity by sera from patients with antiphospholipid syndrome: a possible mechanism of thrombosis. Am J Obstet Gynecol 1993;168:206–210.
8. Lockwood CJ, Romero R, Feinberg RF et al. The prevalence and biologic significance of lupus anticoagulant and anticardiolipin in a general obstetric population. Am J Obstet and Gynecol 1989;161:369–373.
9. Perez MC, Wilson WA, Brown HL et al. Anti-cardiolipin antibodies in unselected pregnant women in relationship to fetal outcome. J Perinatol 1991;11:33–36.
10. Branch DW, Scott JR, Kochenour NK. Obstetric complications associated with lupus anticoagulant. N Engl J Med 1985;313:1322–1326.
11. Lubbe WF, Butler WS, Palmer SJ et al. Lupus anticoagulant in pregnancy. Br J Obstet Gynaecol 1984;91:357–363.
12. Harris EN, Chan JK, Asherson RA et al. Thrombosis, recurrent fetal loss and thrombocytopenia. Predictive value of the anticardiolpin antibody test. Arch Intern Med 1986;146:2153–2156.
13. Reece EA, Garofalo J, Zheng XZ et al. Pregnancy outcone – influence of antiphospholipid antibody titer, prior pregnancy loss and treatment. J Reprod Med 1997;42:49–55.
14. Lockwood CJ, Reece EA, Romero R et al. Antiphospholipid antibody and pregnancy wastage. Lancet 1986;2:742–743.
15. Lynch A, Marlar R, Murphy J et al. Antiphospholipid antibodies in predicting adverse pregnancy outcome. A prospective study. Ann Inter Med 1994;120:470–475.
16. Katano K, Aoki K, Ogasawara M et al. Specific antiphospholipid antibodies (aPL) eluted from placentae of pregnant women with aPL-positive sera. Lupus 1995;4:304–308.
17. Pattison NS, Chamley LW, McKay EJ et al. Antiphospholipid antibodies in pregnancy: prevalence and clinical associations. Br J Obstet Gynaecol 1993;100:909–913.
18. Buchanan NMM, Khamashta MA, Morton KE et al. A study of 100 high risk lupus pregnancies. Am J Reprod Immunol 1992;28:192–194.
19. Ramsey Goldman R, Kutzer JE, Kuller LH et al. Pregnancy outcome and anticardiolipin antibody in women with systemic lupus erythematosus. Am J Epidemiol 1993;138:1057–1069.
20. Branch DW, Andres R, Digre KB et al. The association of antiphospholipid antibodies with severe pre-eclampsia. Obstet Gynecol 1988;73:541–545.
21. Moodley J, Bhoola V, Duursma J et al. The association of antiphospholipid antibodies with severe early-onset pre-eclampsia. S Afr Med J 1995;85:105–107.
22. Yasuda M, Takakuwa K, Tanaka K. Studies on the association between the anticardiolipin antibody and pre-eclampsia. Acta Med Biol 1994;42:145–149.
23. Dekker GA, de Vries JIP, Doelitzsch PM et al. Underlying disorders associated with severe early-onset preeclampsia. Am J Obstet Gynecol 1995;173:1042–1048.
24. Yasuda M, Takakuwa K, Tokunaga A et al. Prospective studies of the association between anticardiolipin antibody and outcome of pregnancy. Obstet Gynecol 1995;86:555–559.
25. Birdsall MA, Pattison NS, Chamley L. Antiphospholipid antibodies in pregnancy. Aust N Z J Obstet Gynaecol 1992;32:328–330.
26. Kelly T, Whittle MJ, Smith DJ et al. Lupus anticoagulant and pregnancy. J Obstet Gynaecol 1996;16:26–31.
27. Botet F, Romera G, Montagut P et al. Neonatal outcome in women treated for the antiphospholipid syndrome during pregnancy. J Prenat Med 1997;25:192–196.

28. Branch DW, Silver RM, Blackwell JL et al. Outcome of treated pregnancies in women with antiphospholipid syndrome: an update of the Utah Experience. Obstet Gynaecol 1992;80:614–620.
29. Granger K A, Farquharson RG. Obstetric outcome in antiphospholipid syndrome. Lupus 1997;6:509–513.
30. Backos M, Rai R, Baxter N et al. Pregnancy complications in women with recurrent miscarriage associated with antiphospholipid antibodies treated with low dose aspirin and heparin. Br J Obstet Gynaecol 1999;106:102–107.
31. Kerslake S, Morton KE, Versi E et al. Early Doppler studies in lupus pregnancy. Am J Reprod Immunol 1992;28:172–175.
32. Caruso A, De Carolis S, Ferrazzani S et al. Pregnancy outcome in relation to uterine artery flow velocity waveforms and clinical characteristics in women with antiphospholipid syndrome. Obstet Gynecol 1993;82:970–976.
33. Campbell S, Pearce JMF, Hackett G et al. Qualitative assessment of uteroplacental blood flow: early screening test for high-risk pregnancies. Obstet Gynecol 1986;68:649–653.
34. Harrington K, Cooper D, Lees C et al. Doppler ultrasound of the uterine arteries: the importance of bilateral notching in the prediction of pre-eclampsia, placental abruption or delivery of a small-for-gestational-age baby. Ultrasound Obstet Gynecol 1996;7:182–188.
35. Lin S, Shimizu I, Suehara N et al. Uterine artery velocimetry in relation to trophoblast migration into the myometrium of the placental bed. Obstet Gynecol 1995;85:760–765.
36. Langford K, Nelson-Piercy C. Antiphospholipid syndrome in pregnancy. Contemp Rev Obstet Gynaecol 1999;11:93–98.
37. Cowchock FS. Autoantibodies and pregnancy loss. N Engl J Med 1997;337:197–198.
38. Elder MG, de Swiet M, Robertson A et al. Low-dose aspirin in pregnancy. Lancet 1988;1:410–410.
39. Silver R, MacGregor SN, Sholl JS et al. Comarative trial of prednisolone plus aspirin versus aspirin alone in the treatment of anticardiolipin antibody positive obstetric patients. Am J Obstet Gynecol 1993;169:1411–1417.
40. Balasch J, Carmona F, Lopez-Soto A et al. Low-dose aspirin for prevention of pregnancy losses in women with antiphospholipid syndrome. Hum Reprod 1993;8:2234–2239.
41. Krause I, Blank M, Gilbrut B et al. The effect of aspirin on recurrent fetal loss in experimental antiphospholipid syndrome. Am J Reprod Immunol 1993;29:155–161.
42. Cowchock S, Reece EA. Do low-risk pregnant women with antiphospholipid antibodies need to be treated? Am J Obstet Gynecol 1997;176:1099–1100.
43. Lockshin MD. Which patients with antiphospholipid antibody should be treated and how? Rheum Dis Clin N Am 1993;19:235–247.
44. Cowchock FS, Reece EA, Balaban D et al. Repeated fetal losses associated with antiphospholipid antibodies: a collaborative randomized trial comparing prednisolone with low-dose heparin treatment. Am J Obstet Gynecol 1992;166:1318–1323.
45. Ruffati A, Orsini A, Di Lenardo L et al. A prospective study of 53 consecutive calcium heparin treated pregnancies in patients with antiphospholipid antibody-related fetal loss. Clin Exp Rheumatol 1997;15:499–505.
46. Kutteh WH. Antiphospholipid antibody-associated recurrent pregnancy loss – treatment with heparin and low-dose aspirin is superior to low-dose aspirin alone. Am J Obstet Gynecol 1996;174:1584–1589.
47. Rai R, Cohen H, Dave M et al. Randomized controlled trial of aspirin and aspirin plus heparin in pregnant women with recurrent miscarriage associated with phospholipid antibodies (or antiphospholipid antibodies). Br Med J 1997;314:253–257.
48. de Swiet M, Ward PD, Fidler J et al. Prolonged heparin therapy in pregnancy causes bone demineralization. Br J Obstet Gynaecol 1983;90:1129–1134.
49. Dahlman TC. Osteoporotic fractures and the recurrence of thromboembolism during pregnancy and the puerperium in 184 women undergoing thromboprophylaxis with heparin. Am J Obstet Gynecol 1993;168:1265–1270.
50. Nelson-Piercy C Low molecular weight heparin for prophylaxis of thromboembolic disease during pregnancy. In: Garner P, Lee R, editors. St. Louis: Mosby, 1995;147–158.
51. Smith R, Stevenson JC, Winearls CG et al. Osteoporosis of pregnancy. Lancet 1985;1178–1180.
52. Khastgir G, Studd J. Pregnancy-associated osteoporosis. Br J Obstet Gynaecol 1994;101:836–838.
53. Smith R, Athanasou NA, Ostlere SJ et al. Pregnancy-associated osteoporosis. Quart J Med 1995;88:865–878.
54. Nelson-Piercy C. Heparin-induced osteoporosis in pregnancy. Lupus 1997;6:500–504.
55. Hunt BJ, Doughty H, Majumdar G et al. Thromboprophylaxis with low molecular weight heparin (Fragmin) in high risk pregnancies. Thromb Haemost 1997;77:39–43.

56. Nelson-Piercy C, Letsky E, de Swiet M. Low molecular weight heparin for obstetric thromboprophylaxis: experience of 69 pregnancies in 61 high risk women. Am J Obstet Gynecol 1997;176:1062–1068.
57. Nelson-Piercy C. Low molecular weight heparin for obstetric thromboprophylaxis. Br J Obstet Gynaecol 1994;101:6–8.
58. Hunt BJ, Khamashta MA, Lakasing L et al. Thromboprophylaxis in antiphospholipid syndrome pregnancies with previous cerebral arterial thrombotic events: is warfarin preferable? Thromb Haemost 1998;79:1060–1061.
59. Shaul WL, Hall JG. Multiple congenital anomalies associated with oral anticoagulants. Am J Obstet Gynecol 1977;127:191–198.
60. Ginsberg JS, Hirsh J, Turner DC et al. Risks to the fetus of anticoagulant therapy during pregnancy. Thromb Haemost 1989;61:197–203.
61. Howe AM, Webster WS. Exposure of the pregnant rat to warfarin and vitamin K1: an animal model of intraventricular hemorrhage in the fetus. Teratology 1990;42:413–420.
62. Wellesley D, Moore I, Heard M et al. Two cases of warfarin embryopathy: a re-emergence of this condition? Br J Obstet Gynaecol 1998;105:805–806.
63. Orme ML, Lewis PJ, de Swiet M et al. May mothers given warfarin breast-feed their infants? Br Med J 1977;1:1564–1565.
64 McKenna R, Cole ER, Vasan U. Is warfarin sodium contraindicated in the lactating mother? J Paediatr 1983;103:325–327.
65. Kwak JYH, Barini R, Gilman-Sachs A et al. Down-regulation of maternal antiphospholipid antibodies during early pregnancy and pregnancy outcome. Am J Obstet Gynecol 1994;171:239–246.
66. Lubbe WF, Butler WS, Palmer SJ et al. Fetal survival after prednisolone suppression of maternal lupus anticoagulant. Lancet 1983;1:1361–1363.
67. Lockshin MD, Druzin ML, Qamar T. Prednisolone does not prevent recurrent fetal death in women with antiphospholipid antibody. Am J Obstet Gynecol 1989;160:439–443.
68. Laskin CA, Bombardier C, Hannah ME et al. Prednisolone and aspirin in women with autoantibodies and unexplained recurrent fetal loss. N Engl J Med 1997;337:148–153.
69. Spinnato JA, Clark AL, Pierangeli SS et al. Intravenous immunoglobulin therapy for the antiphospholipid syndrome in pregnancy. Am J Obstet Gynecol 1995;172:690–694.
70. Kaaja R, Julkunen H, Ammala P et al. Intravenous immunoglobulin treatment of pregnant patients with recurrent pregnancy losses associated with antiphospholipid antibodies. Acta Obstet Gynaecol Scand 1993;72:63–66.
71. Arnout J, Spitz B, Wittevrongel C et al. High-dose intravenous immunoglobulin of a pregnant patient with an antiphospholipid syndrome: immunological changes associated with a successful outcome. Thromb Haemost 1994;71:741–747.
72. Fulcher D, Stewart G, Exner T et al. Plasma exchange and the anticardiolipin syndrome in pregnancy. Lancet 1989;2:171–171.
73. Fishman P, Falach Vaknine E, Zigelman R et al. Prevention of fetal loss in experimental antiphospholipid syndrome by in vivo administration of recombinant interleukin-3. J Clin Invest 1993;21:1834–1837.
74. Gordon C, Kilby MD. Use of intravenous immunoglobulin therapy in pregnancy in systeric lupus erythematosus and antiphospholipid antibody syndrome. Lupus 1998;7:429–433.
75. Somerset DA, Raine-Fenning N, Gordon C, Weaver JB, Kilby MD. Intravenous immunoglobulin therapy in compromised pregnancies associated with antiphospholipid antibodies and systemic lupus erythematosus. Eur J Obstet, Gynecol Reprod Biol 1998;79:227–9.
76. Branch DW. Thoughts on the mechanism of pregnancy loss associated with the antiphospholipid syndrome. Lupus 1994;3:275–280.
77. Lakasing L, Poston L. Adverse pregnancy outcome in antiphospholipid syndrome: focus for future research. Lupus 1997;6:1–4.
78. Di Simone N, Meroni P L, Del Papa N et al. Antiphospholipid antibodies affect trophoblast gonadotrophin secretion and invasiveness by binding directly and through adhered β2-glycoprotein I. Arthritis Rheum 1999.
79. Lala PK, Hamilton GS. Growth factors, proteases and protease inhibitors in the maternal-fetal dialogue. Placenta 1996;17:545–555.
80. McMaster MT, Bass KE, Fisher SJ. Human trophoblast invasion, Autocrine control and paracrine modulation. Ann N Y Acad Sci 1994;734:122–131.
81. Guilbert L, Robertson SA, Wegmann TG. The trophoblast as an integral component of a macrophage-cytokine network. Immunol Cell Biol 1993;71:49–57.
82. Burrows TD, King A, Loke YW. Trophoblast migration during human placental implantation. Hum Reprod Update 1996;2:307–321.

83. Fisher SJ, Damsky CH. Human cytotrophoblast invasion. Semin Cell Biol 1993;4:183–188.
84. Vicovac L, Aplin JD. Epithelial–mesenchymal transition during trophoblast differentiation. Acta Anat 1996;156:202–216.
85. Aplin JD. The cell biology of human implantation. Placenta 1996;17:269–275.
86. McMaster MT, Librach CL, Yan Zhou, et al. Human placental HLA-G expression is restricted to differentiated cytotrophoblasts. J Immunol 1995;154:3771–3778.
87. Vogt E, Ah-Kau N, Rote NS. A model for the antiphospholipid antibody syndrome: monoclonal antiphosphotidylserine antibody induces intrauterine growth restriction in mice. Am J Obstet Gynecol 1996;174:700–707.
88. Silver RM, Smith LA, Edwin SS et al. Variable effects on murine pregnancy of immunoglobulin G fractions from women with antiphospholipid antibodies. Am J Obstet Gynecol 1997;177:229–233.
89. Roubey RAS. Autoantibodies to phospholipid-binding plasma proteins: a new view of lupus anti-coagulants and other "antiphospholipid" autoantibodies. Blood 1994;84:2854–2867.
90. Lockwood CJ, Rand JH. the immunology and obstetrical consequences of antiphospholipid anti-bodies. Obstet Gynaecol Survey 1994;49:432–441.
91. Galli M, Comfurius P, Maassen C et al. Anticardiolipin antibodies directed not to cardiolipin but to a plasma protein cofactor. Lancet 1990;335:1544
92. Fleck RA, Rapaport SI, Viiaya Mohan Rao L. Anti-prothrombin antibodies and the lupus anticoagulant. Blood 1988;72:512–519.
93. De Wolf F, Carreras LO, Moerman P et al. Decidual vasculopathy and extensive placental infarction in a patient with repeated thromboembolic accidents, recurrent fetal loss, and a lupus anticoagulant. Am J Obstet Gynecol 1982;142:829–834.
94. Erlendsson K, Steinsson K, Johannsson JH et al. Relation of antiphospholipid antibody and placental bed inflammatory vascular changes to the outcome of pregnancy in successive pregnancies of 2 women with systemic lupus erythematosus. J Rheumatol 1993;20:1779–1785.
95. Labarrere CA, Faulk WP. Fetal stem vessel endothelial changes in placentae from normal and abnor-mal pregnancies. Am J Reprod Immunol 1992;27:97–100.
96. Rand JH, Wu XX, Guller S et al. Reduction of annexin V (placental anticoagulant protein-1) on pla-cental villi of women with antiphospholipid antibodies and recurrent spontaneous abortion. Am J Obstet Gynaecol 1994;171:1566–1572.
97. Rand JH, Wu XX, Andree HAM et al. Pregnancy loss in the antiphospholipid-antibody syndrome – a possible thrombogenic mechanism. N Engl J Med 1997;337:154–160.
98. La Rosa L, Meroni PL, Tinicani A et al. β2-glycoprotein I and placental anticoagulant protein I in placentae from patients with antiphospholipid syndrome. J Rheumatol 1994;21:1684–1693.
99. Lakasing L, Campa JS, Poston R et al. Normal expression of tissue factor, thrombomodulin and annexin V in placentas from women with antiphospholipid syndrome. Am J Obstet Gynecol 1999;181:180–189.

41 Management of Thrombocytopenia in Hughes Syndrome

M. Galli and T. Barbui

Introduction

Hughes syndrome is defined by the association between antiphospholipid antibodies (aPL), i.e., lupus anticoagulants (LA) and anticardiolipin antibodies (aCL), and peculiar clinical manifestations, such as arterial and venous thrombosis, recurrent miscarriages, and thrombocytopenia. Two forms of Hughes syndrome have been described: the "primary" syndrome [1], that occurs in the absence of any underlying disease, and the "secondary" syndrome [2], that develops in association with another pathological condition, mainly systemic lupus erythematosus.

Thromboses are the most frequent clinical events in Hughes syndrome, because they occur in approximately 30% of patients [3], with an overall incidence of 2.5% patients/year [4]. Venous thrombosis accounts for about two-thirds of all the thromboembolic events, represented mainly by deep vein thrombosis of the legs, and pulmonary embolism [5]. On the other hand, complete cerebral ischemic strokes and transient ischemic attacks are the most common arterial thrombotic events in patients with Hughes syndrome [5]. Thrombotic events may be recurrent and are often spontaneous. Obstetrical complications include abortion, fetal loss, intrauterine growth retardation and pre-eclampsia [6]. They are reported in about 10–20% of women with Hughes syndrome [5] and are regarded as peculiar types of thrombotic complications involving the placental vessels [7].

A variable degree of thrombocytopenia is reported in as many as 20–40% of patients with antiphospholipid antibodies [3, 5]. Even though thrombocytopenia is a rather common manifestation of Hughes syndrome, uncertainties still exist regarding its pathogenesis, treatment, and influence on the policy of the therapy of thrombosis.

Pathophysiology of Thrombocytopenia

Thrombocytopenia of the Hughes syndrome is classified among the immune thrombocytopenias (Table 41.1). Idiopathic thrombocytopenic purpura – the most common and better known of this group of conditions – has been pathogenetically linked to specific autoantibodies directed against glycoproteins IIb/IIIa and Ib/IX

Table 41.1. Classification of immune thrombocytopenias.

Acute idiopathic thrombocytopenic purpura

Chronic idiopathic thrombocytopenic purpura

Thrombocytopenia associated with:
 Systemic lupus erythematosus and other connective tissue diseases
 Hughes syndrome
 Lymphoproliferative disorders
 Cancer
 Thyroid diseases
 Sarcoidosis
 Systemic infections

Alloimmune thrombocytopenia
 Post-transfusional purpura
 Neonatal purpura

Drug-induced thrombocytopenia
 Heparin
 Gold
 Monoclonal antibodies to platelet glycoproteins
 Quinidine-quinine
 Sulfa-containing antibiotics
 Penicillin, ampicillin, cephalosporins

(less frequently, also glycoproteins Ia/IIa and V) [8]. Upon binding to platelet membrane, these antibodies increase the peripheral destruction of opsonized platelets [9, 10]. Typically, the half-life of platelets becomes very short, and their scavenging from circulation takes place mainly in the spleen and the liver.

Approximately 15 years ago, aPL had been suggested to cause thrombocytopenia, based on the high prevalence of aCL in patients with idiopathic thrombocytopenic purpura [11] and on the interaction between platelet membrane phospholipids and these antibodies (see below). Our group has recently reported that the prevalence of thrombocytopenia is higher in a subgroup of LA positive patients displaying a specific coagulation profile associated with the presence of antiprothrombin antibodies [12] (Table 41.2). This may raise the possibility that antiprothrombin

Table 41.2. Association between antiphospholipid syndrome and caoagulation profiles*: retrospective analysis of 140 patients with lupus anticoagulants.

Clinical events	No. (%)	Coagulation profile*		P
		dRVVT	KCT	
Venous thrombosis	36 (26)	25	11	< 0.02
Arterial thrombosis	29 (21)	18	11	n.s.
Recurrent miscarriages	20 (21)	10	10	n.s.
Thrombocytopenia	51 (42)	19	32	< 0.015

* Coagulation profiles are generated by the comparison of the ratio of the dilute Russell's viper venom time (dRVVT) and the kaolin clotting time (KCT): when the ratio of the former test exceeds that of the latter one, the patient is allocated to the "dRVVT" coagulation profile, when the opposite occurs, the plasma is allocated to the "KCT" coagulation profile.

Table 41.3. Prevalence of antiglycoprotein antibodies in 64 Patients with Hughes syndrome.

Anti-GP IIb/IIIa	Anti-GP Ib/IX	Number	(%)
+	−	6	(9)
+	+	14	(22)
−	+	7	(11)
−	−	37	(58)

antibodies are responsible for the reduction of platelet count in patients with aPL. Even though this hypothesis cannot be excluded, other findings question the direct role of aPL in the pathogenesis of thrombocytopenia. In fact, antibodies directed against glycoproteins IIb/IIIa and Ib/IX are found in about 40% of patients with aPL (Table 41.3) [13], a figure similar to those already known for idiopathic thrombocytopenic purpura [14]. Moreover, antibodies against a 50–70 kDa internal platelet protein have been specifically found in patients with aPL and thrombocytopenia but not in patients with idiopathic thrombocytopenic purpura [15]. Antibodies directed towards platelet glycoproteins Ia/IIa and IV and towards CD9 have also been detected in the serum of patients with primary Hughes syndrome [16]. Finally, it has been observed that immunosuppressive treatment of idiopathic thrombocytopenic purpura increased platelet number and reduced the titers of platelet-associated IgG but not those of aPL [17]. These data would indicate that antiplatelet and aPL comprize different specificities and suggest that platelet-specific antibodies, rather than aPL, appear to play a role in the pathogenesis of thrombocytopenia of Hughes syndrome.

Interaction Between aPL and Platelets: Parallelism with Heparin-induced Thrombocytopenia

aPL react with negatively-charged phospholipids by means of specific protein "cofactors", which have been identified as β_2-glycoprotein I (for most aCL [18–20], prothrombin [21, 22], (activated) protein C [23], protein S [23], annexin V [24], high- and low-molecular-weight kininogens[25]. β_2-glycoprotein I and prothrombin are by far the two best known and characterized antigenic targets of antiphospholipid antibodies. Both proteins bind to anionic (phospholipid) surfaces: this binding is stabilized by the respective aPL [26, 27].

Anionic phospholipids are an essential constituent of cell membranes. In platelets, they are located in the inner leaflet of the plasma membrane [28]; thus, they are not available for interaction with aPL. However, under physiological conditions, this asymmetric distribution can be lost, resulting in exposure of anionic phospholipids on the outer leaflet of platelet membrane[28]. For platelets, this phenomenon occurs upon activation by different agonists and is accompanied by shedding of microvesicles [28]. Since both activated platelets and platelet-derived microvesicles represent an important in vivo procoagulant surface [28], the interaction between aPL and cellular membranes may be relevant for the pathogenesis of the thrombotic complications of Hughes syndrome (Fig. 41.1).

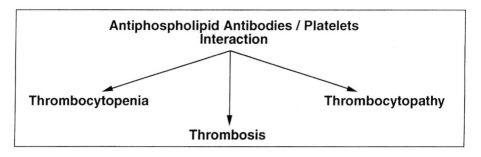

Figure 41.1. Possible consequences of the interaction between antiphospholipid antibodies and activated platelets.

Limited evidence is available on the interaction between aPL and platelets in vivo. Although impairment of the thromboxane A_2/prostacyclin balance [29], and increased urinary excretion and plasma levels of the platelet-specific β-thromboglobulin [30] have been reported, pointing towards a condition of in vivo platelet activation, neither elution of aPL from platelet membrane [31], nor clear evidence for circulating activated platelets have been demonstrated by flow cytometry studies. Fanelli et al [32] found a statistically significant increase in the expression of CD62p above the normal cut-off in the platelet-rich-plasma of nine out of 16 patients with primary Hughes syndrome. No differences were observed for CD63 expression. Joseph et al [33] analyzed a cohort of 20 patients with primary Hughes syndrome for the expression of CD62p, CD63, percentage of circulating reticulated platelets, and levels of soluble P-selectin, taken as indicators of platelet activation. These authors found an increased expression of CD63 and higher median level of soluble P-selectin in the patients' group when compared to the control group. Conversely, other groups failed to find signs of platelet activation both in patients with primary [34, 35] or with with systemic lupus erythematosus-related Hughes syndrome [34].

The presence of microvesicles has been investigated in patients with aPL [36]. By means of flow cytometry, employing specific antiplatelet glycoprotein antibodies, pathological levels of circulating microvesicles were observed in approximately half of the patients. By retrospective analysis, this finding was statistically associated with thrombosis.

The interaction of aPL with platelets has been investigated mainly by in vitro experiments. Even though binding of aPL to resting platelets has been occasionally reported [36, 37], activation and/or damage appear a prerequisite for the binding of aPL [38–40]. Elegant studies with murine monoclonal antibodies to β_2-glycoprotein I were performed by Arvieux et al [41]. These authors demonstrated that the IgG1 antibodies by themselves were unable to activate resting platelets, but that they greatly stimulate platelet activation and secretion induced by subthreshold concentrations of ADP or epinephrine. The effect was blocked by a specific inhibitor of the FcγRII receptor. A similar pattern of reactivity was observed when platelets were substituted by neutrophils [42]. Again, the monoclonal anti-β_2-glycoprotein I antibodies interact with neutrophil surface via the FcγRII receptor, inducing activation, degranulation and adherence of neutrophils to endothelial cells.

Nojima et al [43] showed that plasma and IgG fractions displaying both anticardio-lipin and LA activities were able to enhance CD62p expression of ADP-stimulated platelets. Conversely, plasmas and IgG immunoglobulins containing aCL only or LA activity only failed to induce such a stimulatory effect.

This in vitro behavior of aPL is remarkably similar to that already reported for heparin-induced thrombocytopenia (HIT) [44], another autoimmune thrombo-cytopenia characterized by a high rate of arterial and venous thromboembolic complications [45]. Upon recognition of the complex of heparin bound to platelet factor 4 on the surface of slightly activated platelets [46, 47], the antibodies interact with the FcγRII receptor, in this way enhancing platelet activation, secretion, and shedding of platelet-derived microvesicles [48–50]. Recently, a single base polymorphism of the FcγRII receptor has been reported at position 131, that changes the native arginine to histidine: the FcγRII $^{His\ 131}$ was found to be associated with a predisposition to HIT, since its prevalence was higher than in normal controls [51]. Compared to the FcγRII$^{Arg\ 131}$ isoform, the FcγRII$^{His\ 131}$ allele has a higher affinity for IgG2 [52], which is the major IgG subtype of both heparin-induced antibodies [53] and aPL [54]. At variance with HIT, the prevalence of the different FcγRII genotypes in patients with antiphospholipid antibodies was similar to that of normal controls [55].

The above reported clinical and laboratory similarities between HIT and Hughes syndrome prompted Vermylen et al [56] to put forward a hypothesis to explain both the high risk of thrombosis and the development of thrombocytopenia in patients with the Hughes syndrome. Following mild platelet activation, phospho-lipid-binding proteins (i.e., β_2-glycoprotein I) would interact weakly with anionic phospholipids exposed on the outer surface; aPL stabilize this binding via complex formation and via additional FcγRII receptor interactions. This interaction results in two main consequences:

1. sensitized platelets are quickly removed from circulation, in this way causing thrombocytopenia;
2. platelets are further activated, leading to an increased risk of thrombosis.

One of the most extensively studied effects of the in vitro interaction between activated platelets and aPL is the ability of the antibodies to interfere with the expression of platelet procoagulant properties. aCL (i.e. anti-β_2-glycoprotein I) and anti-prothrombin antibodies provided with LA activity have been shown to hamper the activation of prothrombin by the prothrombinase complex on the surface of calcium ionophore-activated platelets and platelet-derived microvesicles [57]. An opposite effect is exerted by anticardiolipin antibodies on the Factor Xa generating activity of activated gel-filtered platelets: the antibodies block the inhibition of Factor X activation caused by β_2-glycoprotein I [58]. In a rather complex platelet- and monocyte-dependent system, aCL, but not antiprothrombin antibodies, were able to stimulate thrombin generation, thus displaying a procoagulant, rather than an anticoagulant, effect [59].

Prevalence, Clinical Course and Management of Thrombocytopenia

Thrombocytopenia in the Hughes syndrome rarely requires treatment because it is seldom associated with major bleeding [60, 61]. Among the 293 cases enrolled in the

Italian Registry [5], the prevalence of thrombocytopenia was 26%, 32 patients (11%) had platelet counts below 50 000/mm^3 and only two of them (6%) showed severe hemorrhagic complications. Therefore, the prevalence of major hemorrhagic events in Hughes syndrome does not appear significantly different from that reported for idiopathic thrombocytopenia purpura [62].

Recently, thrombocytopenia has been associated with a high risk of mortality in patients suffering from systemic lupus erythematosus [63]. By univariate analysis, thrombocytopenia and arterial thrombosis were the only antiphospholipid-related manifestations statistically associated with mortality in 658 patients with systemic lupus erythematosus (P < 0.001 and P = 0.02, respectively). Unfortunately, the authors did not state whether and to what extent bleeding complications accounted for the death of their patients; therefore, it is possible that thrombocytopenia was simply associated with a more severe disease.

Some authors have speculated about the possibility that thrombocytopenia selects a population of patients with aPL at particular risk for the development of systemic lupus erythematosus [11], but few data exist to support this. Indeed, the first 4-year follow-up analysis of the patients enrolled in the Italian Registry of Antiphospholipid Antibodies study indicates that the rate of progression to overt systemic lupus erythematosus is low, 0.28% patients/year [4], irrespective of whether thrombocytopenia is present or not. Similar data have been recently reported by Stasi et al [64], who performed a long-term follow-up observation of 208 patients with idiopathic thrombocytopenic purpura. These authors identified only four patients who developed laboratory or clinical features consistent with systemic lupus erythematosus or other overt autoimmune diseases over a median follow-up period of 92 months.

Thrombocytopenia in Hughes syndrome rarely requires treatment. However, when this becomes necessary, the same policy as for idiopathic thrombocytopenic purpura should be considered [65]. Recently, a large series of patients has been retrospectively evaluated for treatment outcome according to their antiphospholipid status [17]: corticosteroids, splenectomy, and intravenous immunoglobulins (IVIG) produced response irrespective of the presence of aCL (Table 41.4). Most of the patients were treated with steroids and splenectomy. As expected, corticosteroids produced a similar low rate of sustained response in patients with or without anticardioplipin antibodies (15 and 17%, respectively). Splenectomy was performed in 23 patients; sustained responses were obtained in approximately 60% in both groups. Therefore, the presence of aPL did not seem to affect the treatment outcome. Surgery in these cases should be considered with caution because of the possible risk of both bleeding and thrombosis.

Acquired defects of platelet function have been estimated to occur in as many as 40% of the patients with aPL [38]. Impairment of platelet aggregation has been found in the course of opportunistic infections in acquired immune deficiency syndrome (AIDS) patients with aPL [66], whereas reduced adhesion to subendothelium has been observed by Orlando et al [67]. Other defects include storage pool disease, isolated defects in response to epinephrine or collagen, and impairment of thromboxane B$_2$ synthesis[38]. In vitro experiments performed with the immunoglobulin fractions isolated from patients' plasma led to the suggestion that aPL might be responsible for these acquired qualitative platelet defects [66, 67]. However, the evidence is inconclusive, because only in a few cases were affinity-purified aCL tested [67]. Even though the bleeding time is generally prolonged, the defects are not associated with significant hemorrhagic complications, unless

Table 41.4. Response to treatments of 149 patients with idiopathic thrombocytopenic purpura in relation to antiphospholipid antibodies.*

Treatment	Antiphospholipid antibodies	
	Positive ($n = 69$)	Negative ($n = 80$)
Prednisone ($n = 83$)		
Initial response	32	35
No response	9	7
Sustained response	6	7
Splenectomy ($n = 23$)		
Initial response	12	9
No response	1	1
Sustained response	8	6
IVIG ($n = 25$)		
Initial response	10	12
No response	2	1
Sustained response	0	1

IVIG, intravenous gammaglobulins.
* modified from ref. 17.

another risk factor coexists. Therefore, defective platelet function need only be sought in case of unexplained bleeding in antiphospholipid-positive patients on antithrombotic treatment. Treatment of hemorrhagic complications not associated with thrombocytopenia remains an open question. Only a few case reports have been published: corticosteroid administration and plasma exchange have been found to be useful anedoctally [68, 69].

Prevalence and Treatment of Thrombosis in Relation to Thrombocytopenia

Thromboembolic events are the most common manifestations of Hughes syndrome. When their prevalence is evaluated according to platelet number, it appears that severe, but not moderate, thrombocytopenia protects, at least in part, against thrombosis [5]. The Italian Registry reported that 32% of moderately thrombocytopenic patients (platelet $50-100 \times 10^9/1$) experienced at least one thrombotic event compared with 40% of patients with normal platelet count. Conversely, severe thrombocytopenia (platelets $< 50 \times 10^9/1$) was associated with a lower prevalence of thrombosis (9%). These retrospective data have been confirmed by the 4-year follow-up analysis of patients enrolled in the Italian Registry of Antiphospholipid Antibodies [4]. No significant differences in the incidence of thrombosis were found between patients with a normal platelet count (2.54% patients/year) and those with moderate thrombocytopenia (3.9% patients/year). Again, a lower incidence (0.95% patients/year) was observed in severely thrombocytopenic patients. This difference did not reach statistical significance, probably because of the relatively low number of patients with thrombosis (seven out of 56 patients with mild thrombocytopenia versus two out of 52 severely thrombocytopenic patients).

Thrombotic complications may occur in spite of a very low platelet count, and a group recently showed the association between thrombocytopenia and arterial thrombosis in patients with antiphospholipid antibodies and systemic lupus erythematosus [43]. This raises concern in the management of thromboembolic events when thrombocytopenia is also present.

By retrospective analysis, two studies [70, 71] showed that long-term high-intensity warfarin therapy (Prothrombin International Normalized Ratio, INR > 3.0) confers better antithrombotic protection than low-intensity warfarin and/or aspirin. Three recent studies analyzed the risk of recurrence of thrombosis of antiphospholipid-positive patients in relation to the intensity and duration of oral anticoagulation [72–74]. Two of them [73, 74] agreed on the benefit from a prolonged secondary prophylaxis with oral anticoagulants aimed at maintaining a PT INR range of 2.0–3.0. The third group [72], conversely, found a similar rate of recurrence of thrombosis in patients with and without aPL after discontinuation of oral anticoagulation.

The decision about the duration and the intensity of oral anticoagulant treatment must be weighted against the risk of hemorrhage. Rosove and Brewer [70] and Khamashta et al [71] reported an incidence of significant hemorrhagic complications of 3.1 and 7.1% patients/year, with an incidence of life-threatening bleeding events of 1.9 and 1.7% patients/year, respectively. These figures are somewhat higher than the 1% patients/year incidence of major bleeding reported in patients with prosthetic heart valve replacement, who are similarly on high intensity oral anticoagulation (PT INR 3.0–4.5) [75]. In anticoagulated patients with Hughes syndrome one cannot exclude the possibility that thrombocytopenia (or, less frequently, a platelet function defect) may play a role, at least in part, in the development of hemorrhagic complications. Unfortunately, neither study specifically addressed this problem, because no statement was made regarding platelet count at the times of bleeding events. The survey of the Italian Registry of Antiphospholipid Antibodies [4] reported major bleeding in three patients under oral anticoagulation: one of them was thrombocytopenic and experienced a fatal cerebral hemorrhage.

In our institution, moderate thrombocytopenia does not modify the policy for the treatment of thrombosis of antiphospholipid-positive patients. Conversely, we do not recommend anticoagulant treatment in case of severe thrombocytopenia. More information regarding the optimal management of oral anticoagulation in thrombocytopenic patients with aPL will be provided by the WAPS (Warfarin in the Antiphospholipid Syndrome) clinical trial, which compares long-term, high-dose warfarin therapy (PT INR $\geq$ 3.0) versus "standard" antithrombotic treatment of arterial and venous thrombosis suffered from patients with Hughes syndrome [76].

In conclusion, moderate thrombocytopenia is frequent in Hughes syndrome and, as a rule, does not modify the policy for treatment of thrombosis. Severe thrombocytopenia is relatively uncommon and is seldom associated with bleeding events. When required, its treatment is similar to that of idiopathic thrombocytopenic purpura. Finally, much clinical and laboratory work is still required to elucidate the role of platelets and aPL in the pathogenesis of the thrombotic complications typical of Hughes syndrome.

References

1. Asherson RA, Khamashta MA, Ordi-Ros J, Derksen RHWM, Machin SI, Barquinero J et al. The "primary" antiphospholipid syndrome: major clinical and serological features. Medicine 1989;68:366–374.
2. Alarcon-Segovia D, Deleze M, Oria CV. Antiphospholipid antibodies and the antiphospholipid syndrome in systemic lupus erythematosus: a review of 500 consecutive cases. Medicine 1989;68:353–365.
3. Lechner K, Pabinger-Fasching I. Lupus anticoagulant and thrombosis. Hemostasis 1985;15:254–62.
4. Finazzi G, Brancaccio V, Moia M, Ciavarella N, Mazzucconi G, Schinco PC et al. Natural history and risk factors for thrombosis in 360 patients with antiphospholipid antibodies. A four-year prospective study from the Italian Registry. Am J Med 1996;100:530–536.
5. Italian Registry of Antiphospholipid Antibodies (IR-APA). Thrombosis and thrombocytopenia in antiphospholipid syndrome (idiopathic and secondary to SLE): first report from the Italian Registry. Haematologica 1993;78:313–318.
6. Barbui T, Cortelazzo S, Galli M, Parazzini F, Radici E, Rossi E, Finazzi G. Antiphospholipid antibodies in early repeated abortions: a case-control study. Fertil Steril 1988;50:589–592.
7. De Wolf F, Carreras LO, Moerman P, Vermylen J, Van Assche A, Renaer M. Decidual vasculopathy and extensive placental infarction in a patient with repeated thromboembolic accidents, recurrent fetal loss and a lupus anticoagulant. Am J Obstet Gynecol 1982;142:829–834.
8. Kuniki TJ, Newman PJ. The molecular immunology of platelet proteins. Blood 1992;80:1386–1404.
9. Harrington WJ, Minnich V, Hollingsworth JW, Moore CV. Demonstration of a thrombocytopenic factor in the blood of patients with thrombocytopenic purpura. J Lab Clin Med 1951;38:1–10.
10. Aster RH, Jandl JH. Platelet sequestration in man. II. Immunological and clinical studies. J Clin Invest 1962;43:856–869.
11. Harris EN, Gharavi AE, Hegde U, Derue G, Morgan SH, Englert H et al. Anticardiolipin antibodies in autoimmune thrombocytopenic purpura. Br J Haematol 1985;59:231–234.
12. Galli M, Finazzi G, Norbis F, Marziali S, Marchioli R, Barbui T. The risk of thrombosis in patients with lupus anticoagulants is predicted by their specific coagulation profile. Thromb Haemost 1999;81:695–700.
13. Galli M, Daldossi M, Barbui T. Anti-glycoprotein Ib/IX and IIb/IIIa antibodies in patients with antiphospholipid antibodies. Thromb Haemost 1994;71:571–575.
14. He R, Reid DM, Jones CE, Shulman NR. Spectrum of Ig classes, specificities and titers of serum antiglycoproteins in chronic idiopathic thrombocytopenic purpura. Blood 1994;83:1024–1032.
15. Fabris F, Steffan A, Cordiano L, Borzini P, Luzzatto G, Randi ML et al. Specific antiplatelet autoantibodies in patients with antiphospholipid antibodies and thrombocytopenia. Eur J Haematol 1994;53:232–236.
16. Godeau B, Piette J-C, Fromont P, Intrator L, Schaeffer A, Bierling P. Specific antiplatelet glycoprotein autoantibodies are associated with the thrombocytopenia of primary antiphospholipid syndrome. Br J Haematol 1997;98:873–879.
17. Stasi R, Stipa E, Sciarra A, Perrotti A, Olivieri M et al. Prevalence and clinical significance of elevated antiphospholipid antibodies in patients with idiopathic thrombocytopenic purpura. Blood 1994;84:4203–4207.
18. McNeil HP, Simpson RJ, Chesterman CN, Krilis SA. Antiphospholipid antibodies are directed against a complex antigen that includes a lipid-binding inhibitor of coagulation: $\beta2$-glycoprotein I (apolipoprotein H). Proc Natl Acad Sci USA 1990;87:4120–4124.
19. Galli M, Comfurius P, Maassen C, Hemker HC, de Baets MH, van Breda Vriesman PJC et al. Anticardiolipin antibodies (ACA) directed not to cardiolipin but to a plasma protein cofactor. Lancet 1990;334:1544–1547.
20. Matsuura E, Igarashi Y, Fujimoto M, Ichikawa K, Koike T. Anticardiolipin cofactor(s) and differential diagnosis of autoimmune disease. Lancet 1990;335:177–178.
21. Loeliger A. Prothrombin as co-factor of the circulating anticoagulant in systemic lupus erythematosus? Thromb Diathes Haemorrh (Stuttg) 1959;3:237–256.
22. Bevers EM, Galli M, Barbui T, Comfurius P, Zwaal RFA. Lupus anticoagulant IgG's (LA) are not directed to phospholipids only, but to a complex of lipid-bound human prothrombin. Thromb Haemost 1991;66:629–632.
23. Oosting JD, Derksen RHWM, Bobbink IWG, Hackeng TM, Bouma BN, de Groot PG. Antiphospholipid antibodies directed against a combination of phospholipids with prothrombin, protein C or protein S: an explanation for their pathogenetic mechanisms. Blood 1993;81:2618–2625.

24. Matsuda J, Saitoh N, Goihci K. Anti-annexin V antibody in systemic lupus erythematosus patients with lupus anticoagulant and/or anticardiolipin antibody. Am J Hematol 1994;47:56–61.
25. Sugi T, McIntyre JA. Autoantibodies to phosphatidylethanolamine (PE) recognize a kininogen–PE complex. Blood 1995;86:3083–3088.
26. Willems GM, Janssen MP, Pelsers MMAL, Comfurius P, Galli M et al. Role of divalency in the high-affinity binding of anticardiolipin antibody-β_2-glycoprotein I complexes to lipid membranes. Biochemistry 1996;35:1383–1342.
27. Rao LVM, Hoang AD, Rapaport SI. Mechanism and effects of the binding of lupus anticoagulant IgG and prothrombin to surface phsopholipid. Blood 1996;88:4173–4182.
28. Zwaal RFA, Schroit AJ. Pathophysiologic implications of membrane phospholipid asymmetry in blood cells. Blood 1997;89:1121–1132.
29. Martinuzzo ME, Maclouf J, Carreras LO, Levy-Toledano S. Antiphospholipid antibodies enhance thrombin-induced platelet activation and thromboxane formation. Thromb Haemost 1993;70:667–671.
30. Galli M, Cortelazzo S, Viero P, Finazzi G, de Gaetano G, Barbui T. Interaction between platelets and lupus anticoagulant. Eur J Haematol 1988;41:88–94.
31. Biasiolo A, Pengo V. Antiphospholipid antibodies are not present in the membrane of gel-filtered platelets of patients with IgG anticardiolipin antibodies, lupus anticoagulant and thrombosis. Blood Coagul Fibrinol 1993;4:425–428.
32. Fanelli A, Bergamini C, Rapi S, Caldini A, Spinelli A, Buggiani A, Emmi L. Flow cytometric detection of circulating activated platelets in primary antiphospholipid syndrome. Correlation with thrombocytopenia and anticardiolipin antibodies. Lupus 1997;6:261–267.
33. Joseph JE, Harrison P, Mackie IJ, Machin SJ. Platelet activation markers and the primary antiphospholipid syndrome (PAPS). Lupus 1998;7:S48–S51.
34. Out HJ, de Groot P, van Vliet M, de Gast GC, Niewenhuis HK, Derksen RHWM. Antibodies to platelets in patients with antiphospholipid antibodies. Blood 1991;77:2655–2659.
35. Shechter Y, Tal Y, Greenberg A, Brenner B. Platelet activation in patients with antiphospholipid syndrome. Blood Coagul Fibrinol 1998;9:653–657.
36. Galli M, Grassi A, Barbui T. Platelet-derived microvesicles in patients with antiphospholipid antibodies. Thromb Haemost 1993;69:541 (abstract).
37. Khamashta MA, Harris EN, Gharavi AE, Derue G, Gil A, Vasquez JJ et al. Immune mediated mechanism for thrombosis: antiphospholipid antibody binding to platelet membranes. Ann Rheum Dis 1988;47:849–852.
38. Hasselaar P, Derksen RHWM, Blokzijl L, de Groot P. Cross-reactivity of antibodies directed against cardiolipin, DNA, endothelial cells and blood platelets. Thromb Haemost 1990;63:169–173.
39. Mikhail MH, Szczech LAM, Shapiro SS. The binding of lupus anticoagulant (LACs) to human platelets. Blood 1988;72:333 (abstract).
40. Shi W, Chong BH, Chesterman CN. β_2-glycoprotein I is a requirement for anticardiolipin antibodies binding to activated platelets: differences with lupus anticoagulants. Blood 1993;81:1255–1262.
41. Arvieux J, Roussel B, Pouzol P, Colomb MG. Platelet activating properties of murine monoclonal antibodies to beta 2-glycoprotein I. Thromb Haemost 1993;70:336–341.
42. Arvieux J, Jacob MC, Roussel B, Bensa JC, Colomb MG. Neutrophil activation by anti-b2 glycoprotein I monoclonal antibodies via Fcγ receptor II. J Leukoc Biol 1995;57:387–394.
43. Nojima J, Suehisa E, Kuratsune H, Machii T, Koike T, Kitani T et al. Platelet activation induced by combined effects of anticardiolipin and lupus anticoagulant IgG antibodies in patients with systemic lupus erythematosus. Thromb Haemost 1999;81:436–441.
44. Arnout J. The pathogenesis of the antiphospholipid syndrome: a hypothesis based on parallelisms with heparin-induced thrombocytopenia. Thromb Haemost 1997;75:536–541.
45. George JN, Alving B, Ballem P. Immune heparin-induced thrombocytopenia and thrombosis. Nashville TN: Educational Program of American Society of Hematology, 1994;66–68.
46. Green D, Harris K, Reynolds N, Roberts M, Patterson R. Heparin immune thrombocytopenia: evidence for a heparin–platelet complex as the antienic determinant. J Lab Clin Med 1978;91:167–175.
47. Greinacher A, Michel I, Mueller-Eckhardt C. Heparin-associated thrombocytopenia: the antibody is not heparin specific. Thromb Haemost 1992;67:545–549.
48. Chong BH, Pitney WR, Castaldi PA. Heparin-induced thrombocytopenia: association of thrombotic complications with heparin-dependent IgG antibody that induces thromboxane synthesis and platelet aggregation. Lancet 192;2:1246–1249.
49. Kappa JR, Fisher CA, Addonizio VP Jr. Heparin-induced platelet activation: the role of thromboxane A_2 synthesis and the extent of platelet granule release in two patients. J Vasc Surg 1989;9:574–579.
50. Warkentin TE, Hayward CP, Boshkov LK, Santos AV, Sheppard JA, Bode AP et al. Sera from patients with heparin-induced thrombocytopenia generate platelet-derived microparticles with procoagulant

activity: an explanation for the thrombotic complications of heparin-induced thrombocytopenia. Blood 1994;84:3691–3699.

51. Burgess JK, Lindeman R, Chesterman CN, Chong BH. Single amino acid mutation of Fcγ receptor is associated with the development of heparin-induced thrombocytopenia. Br J Haematol 1995;91:761–756.

52. Warmerdam PAM, van de Winkel JGJ, Vlug A, Westerdaal NAC, Capel PJA. A single amino acid in the second Ig-like domain of the human Fcγ receptor II is critical for human IgG2 binding. J Immunol 1991;147:1338–1343.

53. Arepally G, Poncz M, McKanzie SE, Cines D. Characterization of antibody subclass specificity and antigenic determinants in heparin-associated thrombocytopenia. Blood 1994;84:181 (abstract).

54. Arvieux J, Roussel B, Ponard D, Colomb MG. IgG2 subclass restriction of anti β_2 glycoprotein I antibodies in autoimmune patients. Clin Exp Immunol 1994;95:310–315.

55. Atsumi T, Caliz R, Amengual O, Khamashta MA, Hughes GRV. Fcγ receptor IIa H/R 131 polymorphism in patients with antiphospholipid antibodies. Thromb Haemost 1998;79:924–927.

56. Vermylen J, Hoylaerts MF, Arnout J. Antibody-mediated thrombosis. Thromb Haemost 1997;78:420–426.

57. Galli M, Bevers EM, Comfurius P, Barbui T, Zwaal RFA. Effect of antiphospholipid antibodies on procoagulant activity of activated platelets and platelet-derived microvesicles. Br J Haematol 1993;83:466–472.

58. Shi W, Chong BH, Hogg PJ, Chesterman CN. Anticardiolipin antibodies block the inhibition by β_2-glycoprotein I of the factor Xa generating activity of platelet. Thromb Haemost 1993;70:342–345.

59. Hoffman M, Monroe DM, Roubey RSA. IgG from two patients with the antiphospholipid syndrome increase thrombin generation in an "in vitro" cell-based model of coagulation. XVIth Congress of the International Society of Thrombosis and Haemostasis, Florence, Italy, June 6–12, 1997. Thromb Haemost 1997;1 (suppl): abstract 2.

60. Barbui T, Finazzi G. Clinical trials on antiphospholipid syndrome: what is being done and what is needed? Lupus 1994;3:303–307.

61. Machin SJ. Platelets and antiphospholipid antibodies. Lupus 1996;5:386–387.

62. Cortelazzo S, Finazzi G, Buelli M, Molteni A, Viero P, Barbui T. High risk of severe bleeding in aged patients with chronic idiopathic thrombocytopenic purpura. Blood 1991;77:31–33.

63. Drenkard C, Villa AR, Alarcon-Segovia D, Perez-Vazquez ME. Influence of the antiphospholipid syndrome in the survival of patients with systemic lupus erythematosus. J Rheumatol 1994;21:1067–1072.

64. Stasi R, Stipa E, Masi M, Cecconi M, Scimò MT, Oliva F et al. Long-term observation of 208 adults with chronic idiopathic thrombocytopenic purpura. Am J Med 1995;98:436–442.

65. Galli M, Finazzi G, Barbui T. Thrombocytopenia in the antiphospholipid syndrome. Br J Haematol 1996;93:1–5.

66. Cohen AJ, Philip TM, Kessler CM. Circulating coagulation inhibitors in the acquired immunodeficiency syndrome. Ann Int Med 1986;104:175–180.

67. Orlando E, Cortelazzo S, Marchetti M, Sanfratello R, Barbui T. Prolonged bleeding time in patients with lupus anticoagulant. Thromb Haemost 1992;68:495–499.

68. Manoharan A, Gottlieb P. Bleeding in patients with lupus anticoagulant. Lancet 1984;2:171 (letter)

69. Ordi J, Vilardel M, Oristell J, Valdes M, Knobel A, Alijotas J et al. Bleeding in patients with lupus anticoagulant. Lancet 1984;2:868–869 (letter)

70. Rosove MH, Brewer PMC. Antiphospholipid antibodies: clinical course after the first thrombotic event in 70 patients. Ann Intern Med 1992;117:303–308.

71. Khamashta MA, Cuadrado MJ, Mujic F, Taub NA, Hunt BJ, Hughes GRV. The management of thrombosis in the antiphospholipid antibody syndrome. N Engl J Med 1995;332:993–997.

72. Ginsberg JS, Wells PS, Brill-Edwards P, Donovan D, Moffatt K, Johnston M et al. Antiphospholipid antibodies and venous thromboembolism. Blood 1995;86:3685–3691.

73. Prandoni P, Simioni P, Girolami A. Antiphospholipid antibodies, recurrent thromboembolism, and intensity of warfarin anticoagulation. Thromb Haemost 1996;75:859 (letter)

74. Shulman S, Svenungsson E, Granqvist S, and the Duration of Anticoagulation Study Group. Anticardiolipin antibodies predict early recurrence of thromboembolism and death among patients with venous thromboembolism following anticoagulant therapy. Am J Med 1998;104:332–338.

75. Cortelazzo S, Finazzi G, Viero P, Galli M, Remuzzi A, Parenzan L, Barbui T. Thrombotic and hemorrhagic complications in patients with mechanical heart valve prosthesis attending an anticoagulation clinic. Thromb Haemost 1993;69:316–320.

76. Finazzi G on behalf of the members of the Italian Registry. The Italian Registry of antiphospholipid antibodies. Haematologica 1997;82:101–105.

42 The Role of Antiphospholipid Syndrome in Critical Illness

F. M. K. Williams, G. R. V. Hughes and R. M. Leach

Lupus patients admitted to the intensive care unit (ICU) are often very sick with multiorgan dysfunction and are thought to do poorly. The prevalence of antiphospholipid, or Hughes', syndrome (APS) in lupus patients seen in outpatients is variously reported in different series but is approximately 30% [1]. APS is reported to be associated with increased mortality in patients with systemic lupus erythematosus (SLE) independent of other variables [2]. The prevalence of APS in critically ill lupus patients might, therefore, be expected to be higher than in the outpatient population. However this prevalence has not been ascertained and despite evidence of increasing survival in lupus patients [3], the outcome of lupus patients following critical illness requiring ICU admission has not been established. In fact, there is only one report examining presenting features, prognostic factors and outcome after ICU admission in lupus patients [4]. Based in two South African teaching hospitals, 30 patients were included who were admitted to ICU between 1982 and 1993. Admissions were required for a number of different indications, the most common being infection (37%). Prognosis was shown to be poor, with a 53% mortality on or shortly after discharge from ICU. Only the presence of renal disease was identified as a poor prognostic marker, significantly reducing the survival from the time of diagnosis of SLE. Unfortunately, lack of antiphospholipid antibody data precluded analysis of their effect on outcome. Thus the effect of APS on ICU mortality and long-term survival has not hitherto been investigated.

We studied the clinical features and outcome of 84 admission episodes to ICU by 65 patients with SLE, APS or both, over a 15-year period from 1994 to 1998 inclusive. Of particular interest was the effect of APS on admitting diagnosis, course, outcome of admission and long-term survival. All patients with SLE and/or APS admitted to the ICU of St Thomas' Hospital over a 15-year period from January 1984 to December 1998 were included, with data being collected prospectively for the last 5 years. Only patients who fulfilled the American College of Rheumatology criteria for the classification of lupus [5] and those having APS were included in the study. APS was diagnosed if there was a well documented history of venous or arterial thrombosis, or recurrent fetal loss in the presence of either anticardiolipin antibodies or lupus anticoagulant [6].

The following information was obtained from hospital, ICU and other hospitals' notes as well as microfiched records: date of birth, race, gender, duration of SLE and/or APS, time in hospital before ICU admission, time on ICU and whether admission was emergency or elective. Details of clinical, hematological and serological features and treatment before hospital admission were also obtained, so that the diagnosis of SLE or APS could be confirmed. The primary diagnostic reason for admission to ICU was identified. However, many of the patients had multisystem disorders so "accompanying" diagnoses were also recorded. A diagnosis (primary or accompanying) of infection was made if, in patients with clinical features of focal or systemic infection, there were supporting radiological and/or laboratory data. A primary diagnosis of renal disease was made if patients required initiation of renal replacement therapy. An accompanying diagnosis of renal disease was made in those normally requiring renal replacement, and those with biopsy-proven lupus nephritis, pre-admission proteinuria greater than 1 g/24 hr, or a stable creatinine greater than 200 µmol/l. Patients were categorized as "cardiovascular" (CVS) if they had cardiac arrest or circulatory collapse (not due to sepsis) or heart valve disease requiring surgery. A diagnosis of coagulopathy was used to describe any patient requiring management of hemorrhage, acute thrombosis or disseminated intravascular coagulation. A small number of remaining diagnoses were assigned to a single group (neurological/other). The admissions were recorded as emergency or elective.

We also documented the clinical features and laboratory results obtained on admission to ICU including full blood count, erythrocyte sedimentation rate (ESR), C-reactive protein (CRP), biochemical profile, liver function tests, coagulation screen, arterial blood gases and, more recently, lactate levels. We recorded how the patients were managed on ICU, including whether there was a requirement for mechanical ventilation, renal replacement therapy, anticoagulation, antimicrobial and immunosuppressive therapy. Severity of illness was ascertained using the Acute Physiology and Chronic Health Evaluation (APACHE II) score. Deaths on ICU and in hospital were recorded. Survival after discharge from hospital was ascertained from hospital records and by contacting the patient or their general practitioner by telephone. In order to examine the effect of APS, comparisons were made between patients with APS and those with SLE alone. However, six patients had clinical features strongly suggestive of APS but confirmatory laboratory results could not be found; these six were excluded from the comparative analyses. Data were collected and analysed using Microsoft Excel™ and Unistat. Groups were compared using χ-squared, Fisher's exact and Mann–Whitney tests as appropriate. Survival analysis was performed using Kaplan–Meier survival curves.

Table 42.1 shows the characteristics of the 65 patients with SLE and/or APS admitted to ICU during the study period. Sixty-four patients had SLE, the diagnosis having been established at least 1 month (but up to 26 years) before admission to ICU. Caucasians accounted for 53% of the patient cohort. APS was diagnosed in 33

Table 42.1. Characteristics of patients.

Total number of patients	65
Median (range) age/years	33(16–70)
Male : female	13 : 52
Caucasian : Asian : Afro-Caribbean	34 : 15 : 16
Median(range) time since diagnosis of SLE/years	6(0.1–26)
SLE : SLE+APS : primary APS	32 : 32 : 1

of the 65 patients (51%), 32 with coexisting SLE and one with primary APS. Lupus anticoagulant was present in 31 and anticardiolipin antibody in 20 cases. Fifteen patients had had APS diagnosed prior to ICU admission, of whom 14 were antico-agulated on admission to ICU. One had had anticoagulation stopped due to pregnancy and was admitted with bilateral renal vein thrombosis. An additional two patients with previous coagulopathies were referrals from abroad and the diagnosis of APS was made during ICU admission. The remaining 16 patients had not been diagnosed as having APS, of which nine were admitted to ICU with primary coagulopathies. As described above, six patients had histories strongly suggestive of APS but confirmatory antiphospholipid antibodies (aPL) test results could not be found. One patient who was not tested had a previous history of multiple pulmonary emboli (PE) and deep venous thromboses (DVT). Four patients were negative for antiphospholipid antibodies when tested on a single occasion, but antibody levels are known to wax and wane, so repeated testing is recommended. Their histories were two with DVT and PE, one with Libman–Sachs endocarditis and one with multiple arterial thrombi. The last patient was negative for antiphospholipid antibodies on several occasions and had severe coagulation problems, with recurrent femoral emboli requiring bilateral lower limb amputations.

The 65 patients were admitted on 84 occasions. Seven (8%) admission episodes were elective and 77 (92%) were emergency admissions. The elective admissions included five cardiac valve replacements (four Libman–Sachs endocarditis, one mitral valve prolapse) and two elective hemofiltrations in patients with chronic renal failure. Four of the elective admissions had been preceded by emergency admissions. Many of the emergency admissions were seriously unwell on admission to hospital and were transferred to ICU rapidly: the median length of hospital stay prior to ICU admission was 1 (range 0–180) day. Length of ICU stay was very variable with a median time of 3 (range 0–51) days.

Table 42.2 gives the primary admitting and accompanying diagnoses in 46 admission episodes of patients without APS and the 38 admission episodes with APS. Infective causes accounted for 31 (37%), renal 18 (21%), cardiovascular 18 (21%) and coagulopathies 11 (13%) of primary admitting diagnoses. Renal impairment was the most frequently assigned accompanying diagnosis, accounting for 50%. In total, 47 of the 84 (56%) admissions had a renal diagnosis (either primary or accompanying), of which 42 admissions (89%) required hemofiltration. Thirteen of these admissions (by 10 patients) had required dialysis previously for established chronic

Table 42.2. Primary and accompanying diagnoses for both SLE and APS patients and those with SLE alone, for a total of 84 admissions.

	Infection	CVS	Coagulopathy	Renal	Neuro/other	Total
SLE + APS						
Primary	13	9	8	7	1	38
Accompanying	2	1	4	13	6	26
SLE alone						
Primary	18	9	3	11	5	46
Accompanying	8	3	3	16	2	32
Total patients						
Primary	31	18	11	18	6	84

renal failure. Of the primary diagnoses of infection, 58% were septicaemia and 35% were pneumonia. Where microbiological results were available, the commonest organisms isolated were *Staphylococcus aureus* in 29% (one had methicillin resistance), with pneumococcus, *Klebsiella* and *Escherichia coli* each accounting for 10%. The coagulopathies included nine thrombotic episodes, four hemorrhage and five pregnancy-related (thrombosis, hemorrhage or pre-eclampsia). There were significantly more diagnoses of coagulopathy in the APS group than SLE alone ($P = 0.03$).

Table 42.3 summarizes the management of the patients. Mechanical ventilation was required in 51 (63%) admissions, inotropic support in 55 (68%) and renal replacement therapy in 51 (63%). Antibiotics were prescribed in 72 (89%), anticoagulants in 37 (46%) and corticosteroids in 78 (96%) admission episodes. Immunosuppression with cyclophosphamide was prescribed in 30 (37%) and plasmapheresis was used in 11 (14%) admissions. The only difference between patients with and without APS was a trend towards more frequent anticoagulation in the APS patients ($P = 0.09$).

Table 42.4 reports severity of illness, length of ICU stay and ICU, hospital and total mortality to date. As would be expected, severity of illness measured by APACHE II scores was higher in ICU deaths compared to ICU survivors. Seventeen (26%) of the 65 patients died in ICU and a further two died before hospital discharge. Infection as a primary diagnosis was associated with a significantly greater risk of ICU death than other admission diagnoses ($P = 0.03$). Ten of 31 (32%) admission episodes in which infection was the primary diagnosis were associated with ICU death. Overwhelming septic shock (two pneumococcus, one *Staphylococcus* and one *Klebsiella*) caused four deaths within 48 hours of admission. In six admission episodes infection was the primary diagnosis (two *E. coli*, one pneumococcus, one *Staphylococcus*, one *Pseudomonas* and one unknown), which resulted in multiorgan failure and subsequent death over 3–25 days. All 10 patients with primary infections associated with death had secondary acute renal failure and nine were hemofiltered. In the 35 (9%) remaining admission episodes two patients with a

Table 42.3. Management of 65 patients over 84 admissions (parentheses indicate number of admissions for which data available).

Management	Number
Mechanical ventilation	51(81)
Renal replacement	
haemofiltration	41(81)
dialysis	10(81)
Inotropes	
Dopamine alone	27(81)
Other inotropes (+/– dopamine)	28(81)
Total	55(81)
Anticoagulation	37(81)
Antimicrobial agents	72(81)
Immunosuppression	
Corticosteroids	78(81)
Cyclophosphamide	30(80)
Plasmapheresis	11(81)
Methotrexate	2(80)
Immunoglobulin	1(80)

Table 42.4. Severity of illness, mortality, length of ICU stay and mean survival time of those who subsequently died.

	Total
APACHE II (median and range)	22 (8–45)
Median APACHE II of ICU deaths	31 (18–45)
Median APACHE II of ICU survivors	20 (8–33)
ICU mortality	17/65 (26%)
Hospital mortality (inc ICU deaths)	19/65 (29%)
Total mortality to date/total no. of patients	31/65 (48%)
Length of ICU stay in ICU deaths, median (range)/days	4 (0–50)
Mean survival time (+/-SE) from first admission of hospital survivors who subsequently died (months)	28.2 +/– 6.7

renal primary diagnosis and 1 with coagulopathy died. However, infection (two pneumococcus, one *Klebsiella*) was the eventual cause of death in these three patients. We were surprised to find that despite a relatively low ICU and hospital mortality, the long-term survival of these ICU patients was poor. There was a trend towards reduced survival in those with renal disease but this was not statistically significant ($P = 0.09$). The mean survival time of hospital survivors who subsequently died was 28.2 months. Figure 42.1 illustrates that 5-year survival after first ICU admission was less than 25%.

One of our hypotheses was that patients with APS in addition to lupus do less well, but Table 42.5 shows that this was not the case. No significant differences were observed between the two groups for gender, race, age, ICU or hospital mortality, renal disease, severity of illness (APACHE II) or length of ICU stay. This may indicate that the patients with SLE alone had more severe disease. Table 42.2 compares the primary admitting diagnosis in patients with SLE and APS. The coagulopathies included nine thrombotic episodes, four hemorrhage and five pregnancy-related (thrombosis, hemorrhage or pre-eclampsia). There were significantly more diagnoses of coagulopathy in the APS group than SLE alone ($P = 0.03$). A similar proportion of APS patients were admitted with a primary renal problems but there was

Table 42.5. Comparison of 33 APS patients (32 with coexisting SLE, one primary APS) with 26 patients with SLE alone.

	APS	SLE alone	P value
Ratio female : male	27 : 6	21 : 5	NS
Caucasian: Asian:Afro-Caribbean	18 : 8 : 7	11 : 7 : 8	NS
Median age	32	35	NS
Deaths on ICU	9	7	NS
Deaths to date	17/33 (52%)	11/26 (42%)	NS
Median (range) length of ICU stay	2 (0–47)	4 (0–50)	NS
Length of ICU stay in ICU deaths, median (range)/days	2(0–25)	6(0–50)	NS
Mean survival time from first admission of hospital survivors who subsequently died/months	13 (3–31)	47 (19–69)	0.04
Renal disease	21	17	NS
APACHE II	19	23.5	0.09

NS, not significant.

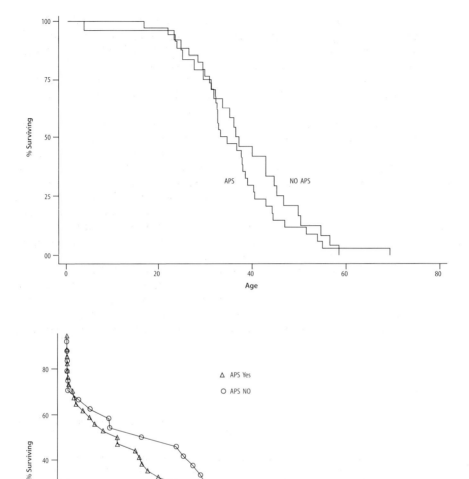

Figure 42.1. Percent survival of APS and non-APS patients by age and time from first ICU admission.

a reduction in infection related admissions compared to SLE patients. Figure 42.1 demonstrates that survival after ICU was not significantly different between the two groups ($P = 0.48$).

This work was undertaken because we were aware of a general belief on ICUs that SLE patients have a worse outcome than other patients of a similar age. This view was supported by the only other study examining ICU admission and outcome in patients with SLE. Unfortunately the authors were unable to examine the effect of APS, or to analyze long-term survival [4]. Our patient numbers allowed us to do that. While ICU mortality in our study (27%) was slightly higher than that quoted for general patients of similar age [7], it was substantially lower than that of the previous lupus study [4]. However, long-term survival in our patients was poor with life expectancy and survival after ICU reduced. Previous studies in patients admitted to ICU with SLE and systemic rheumatic disease have reported a favorable long-term prognosis [8]. Our contrasting results may reflect the severity of the underlying illness in patients referred to a lupus tertiary referral center. The proportion of patients with APS (> 50%) was higher than the expected prevalence of about 30% reported in studies of lupus outpatients [1]. That six patients not confirmed as having APS had clinical histories suggestive of the syndrome hints that the true prevalence may be higher. We found no significant differences between patients with APS and SLE alone except that coagulopathies accounted for a significantly larger proportion of admissions. Long-term survival was not significantly different in our patients with APS, in contrast to outpatient data which suggest patients with APS have increased mortality rates [2].

In conclusion, we should like to emphasize two points. Firstly, that patients with aPL should be identified as early as possible because this alters their management. Secondly, having survived critical illness, patients have a less than 25% 5-year survival. Closely monitored follow-up and ease of access to medical services would surely be prudent in this group of young people who have survived life-threatening illness.

References

1. Cervera R, Khamashta MA, Font J, Sebastiani GD, Gil A et al. Systemic lupus erythematosus: clinical and immunologic patterns of disease expression in a cohort of 1000 patients. Medicine 1993;72:113–124.
2. Drenkard C, Villa AR, Alarcon-Segovia D, Perez-Vazquez ME. Influence of the antiphospholipid syndrome on the survival of patients with systemic lupus erythematosus. J Rheumatol 1994;21:1067–1072.
3. Gladman DD. Prognosis and treatment of systemic lupus erythematosus. Curr Opin in Rheumatol 1996;8:430–437.
4. Ansell SM, Bedhusi S, Ruff B, Mahomed AG, Richards G, Mer M et al. Study of critically ill patients with systemic lupus erythematosus. Crit Care Med 1996;24:981–984.
5. Tan EM, Cohen AS, Fries JF et al. The 1982 revised criteria for the classification of systemic lupus erythematosus. Arthritis Rheum 1982;25:1271–1277.
6. Harris EN, Pierangeli SS, Gharavi AE. Diagnosis of the antiphospholipid syndrome: a proposal for use of laboratory tests. Lupus 1998;7 (Suppl 2):S144–S148.
7. Rowan KM, Kerr JH, Major E, McPherson K, Short A, Vessey MP. Intensive Care Society's APACHE II study in Britain and Ireland I: Outcome by comparisons of intensive cae units after adjustment for case mix by American APACHE II method. Br Med J 1993;307:977–81.
8. Godeau B, Boudjadja A, Dhainaut J-F, Schlemmer B, Chastang C, Brunet F et al. Outcome of patients with systemic rheumatic disease admitted to medical intensive care units. Ann Rheum Dis 1992;51:627–631.

43 Infertility, Oral Contraceptive Pills, Hormone Replacement Therapy and the Antiphospholipid Antibody Syndrome

M. Petri

Infertility

Pathophysiology of Infertility: Role of Autoimmunity

It is now widely accepted that antiphospholipid antibodies (aPL) are one of several mechanisms that can lead to miscarriage. Miscarriages classically associated with aPL occur in the second or third trimester. However, there is a subgroup of patients who lose pregnancies early in the first trimester. It is of great interest whether aPL might also be associated with other gynecologic and fertility issues. For example, Gleicher [1] has reviewed data that aPL can be found in higher than expected frequency in endometriosis [2–6], unexplained fertility [7, 8], sperm antibodies [9], premature ovarian failure [1], failure of in vitro fertilization (IVF) [10], and antitrophoblast antibodies [11]. In the case of endometriosis, two-thirds of women with laparoscopically staged endometriosis exhibit a polyclonal B-cell activation with autoantibodies [2].

It is not at all clear, however, that aPL alone are associated with these other gynecologic and fertility issues. For example, antinuclear antibodies (ANA) and antithyroid antibodies have also been found to be increased in such women [12, 13]. Therefore, Gleicher and others have suggested that it is important to investigate autoimmunity broadly in women with these gynecologic problems.

The field of infertility right now is in great flux. There appear to be multiple mechanisms of infertility, with autoimmunity perhaps playing a role in several of these mechanisms. The fact that there are multiple subgroups of infertility has not been emphasized in many of the articles dealing with aPL and infertility. It is currently unclear whether aPL are involved in all or just in some subgroups of infertility.

It is obviously important to determine whether aPL are representative of the untreated infertile state, or whether they are secondary to treatment or to multiple pregnancy failure, and finally, whether treatment of aPL improves outcome. Each of these issues will be reviewed in this chapter.

Infertility Associated with aPL

The field of infertility is characterized by searches for panels of autoantibodies of multiple isotypes. Laboratory criteria for most of the autoantibodies are not available, making comparisons between different articles impossible. In many studies, patients will have 21 or more assays for aPL. Rarely is any correction done for multiple comparisons, leading to P-values that are probably uninterpretable. In addition, in most studies, the different types of infertility have not necessarily been separately investigated. These issues of study design must be considered in the studies reviewed below and in Table 43.1 [14–35].

Beginning in 1989, multiple cross-sectional studies of autoantibodies and infertility have been published. Gleicher and colleagues in 1989 found that 23 of 26 women with unexplained infertility had one out of 33 potential autoantibody tests positive [7]. Taylor, also in 1989, investigated aPL and anti-smooth muscle antibodies in 41 patients with unexplained infertility and also found an increase in total autoantibodies [8].

In 1994, two controlled studies of multiple autoantibodies in women who were IVF failures were published. Birkenfeld et al in 1994 found that 32.1% of women who had failed IVF had one or more of multiple autoantibodies versus none of those who had had a successful IVF procedure. This article raised the possibility that multiple attempts at IVF might induce autoantibodies because only 10% of women who were candidates for IVF had such autoantibodies [17]. Similarly, in 1994 Geva et al found one or more of multiple autoantibodies in 33% of women who were IVF failures, but no control women. This group studied anticardiolipin, anti-DNA, ANA, lupus anticoagulant and rheumatoid factor [18].

In 1995, multiple groups again looked at the frequency of autoantibodies in infertility, including subtypes of infertility. Aoki and colleagues in 1995 specifically looked at β_2-glycoprotein I-dependent anticardiolipin antibodies. β_2-glycoprotein I dependent anticardiolipin antibodies (aCL) are thought to be the pathogenic aPL in patients who have antiphospholipid antibody syndrome with thrombosis and pregnancy loss. Only 5.4% of women with autoimmune reproductive failure were positive for the β_2-glycoprotein I dependent aCL, versus no controls [19]. The low level of 5.4% is surprising and suggests that what are considered "true" aPL are not very common in women with reproductive failure. Geva et al in 1995 updated their previous report, now looking at 50 women who had three or more IVF failures. Again, looking at all antibodies including ANA, aCL, lupus anticoagulant, anti-DNA and rheumatoid factor, 22% of women had at least one of these autoantibodies as compared to only 2.5% in the IVF control group [21]. Nip et al studied women who had unexplained infertility, endometriosis and tubal factor. Of interest, all three groups had an increase in sperm antibodies. Those with endometriosis had an increase in smooth muscle antibodies and those with tubal factor had an increase in aCL. Importantly, however, the clinical pregnancy rate did not differ among these different groups [22].

In 1996, more cross-sectional studies appeared on autoantibodies and infertility. Balasch and colleagues found only 2.4% positivity for an aPL in a large group of infertile patients. No subgroup of infertile patients stood out in terms of aPL, as opposed to the earlier study of Nip et al. The frequency of aPL was much higher, 10%, in the subgroup that had actually failed IVF, suggesting that IVF itself might lead to aPL production. They also reported that seven infertile women who had aPL had actually had a successful spontaneous pregnancy, raising the question of

Table 43.1. Autoimmunity and infertility.

Study	No. infertile	% Positive	Comparison with controls
Fisch 1991 [14]	35 IVF failure	Higher ANA Higher aPL	$P = $ NS $P \leq 0.0001$
Coulam and Stern 1992 [15]	73 infertile	3% aPL	5%; $P = $ NS
Yron 1992 [16]	35	Higher aCL	$P < 0.001$
Birkenfeld 1994 [17]	IVF failure IVF candidates	32% autoAb 10% autoAb	0% autoAb
Geva 1994 [18]	21 IVF failure	33.3% autoAb 14.2% aCL 4.7% ANA	0% autoAb 0% aCL 0% ANA
Aoki 1995 [19]	65 unexplained infertility 64 endometriosis	4.6% 6.3% anti-β2GPI	0% anti-β2GPI
Fisch 1995 [20]	15 infertile	Higher aCL Higher aPL, but not β2GPI dependent	
Geva 1995 [21]	50 IVF failure	22% autoAb	2.5% autoAb; $P < 0.05$
Nip 1995 [22]	30 unexplained infertility	7% ANA 30% anti-smooth muscle 15% aCL	5% ANA 15% anti-smooth muscle 0% aCL
	20 endometriosis	10% aCL 45% anti-smooth muscle 6% ANA	
	50 tubal infertility	24% aCL 28% anti-smooth muscle	
Balasch [23]	498 infertile 147 endometriosis 102 tubal factor 111 male factor 40 IVF failure	2.4% aPL 1.4% aPL 4.9% aPL 2.7% aPL 10% aPL	
Birdsall 1996 [24]	240 undergoing IVF	15% aPL	
Fichorova 1996 (25)	70 infertile	7% ANA 22.7% aCL	
Kaider 1996 [26]	42 IVF failure	26.2% aPL	4.8%; $P = 0.0$I
Kim 1996 [27]	78 unexplained infertility	20.5% autoAb	3.3% autoAb; $P \leq 0.01$
Roussev 1996 [28]	45 infertility	71% abnormal tests	7% abnormal tests; $P = 0.0001$
Ruiz 1996 [29]	36 infertility	0–43.8% ANA 9.1–6.7% aPL	
Coulam 1997 [30]	312 implant failures	22% aPL 4% aCL	5% aPL 0% aCL
Cubillos 1997 [31]	43	53.5% aPL 37.2% ANA	11.4% aPL 5.7% ANA
Kim 1997 [33]	42 endometriosis + tubal factor 87 tubal factor	38.1% autoAb 2.3% autoAb	
Kutteh 1997 [34]	IVF	18.8% aPL	5.5% aPL
Ulcova-Gallova 1997 [32]		26.5% aCL (IgG)	
Sher 1998 [35]	89 IVF failure	42% aPL	

ANA, antinuclear antibody; aPL, one of multiple antiphospholipid antibody assays; autoAb, one of multiple autoantibody assays.

whether the aPL might be innocent bystanders [23]. In contrast, a second large study of 240 women undergoing IVF found a much higher proportion, 15%, with aPL [24]. Kaider and colleagues compared women who had an IVF failure versus 42 women who had an IVF success. They did a panel of multiple aPL, looking at all three isotypes of each. Of the 21 different aPL assays, 26.2% of those who were IVF failures had an aPL versus only 4.8% of those who had had an IVF success [26]. Kim and colleagues found that women with unexplained infertility had more autoantibodies than women who had ovulatory factors as the cause of their infertility, 20.5% versus only 3.3% [27]. Roussev and colleagues studied multiple autoantibodies including aPL, lupus anticoagulant, antithyroid antibodies, embryotoxic factor, and CD56 positive/CD16 negative lymphocytes. In their unexplained infertility group, which consisted of multiple subtypes including IVF failures, endometriosis, premature ovarian failure and polycystic ovarian disease, at least 65% had one autoantibody or other abnormal test, versus only 7 % of controls. When they limited the analysis to the subgroup that had unexplained fertility, 42% had aPL, 16% had CD 56 positive/CD 16 negative cells, 16% had embryotoxic factor, and 9% had antithyroid antibodies [28]. Ruiz and colleagues compared women who had had infertility versus those who had had recurrent spontaneous abortions. This is an interesting comparison because some women with recurrent spontaneous abortions would be expected to have aPL. In their infertility group they found a very slight increase in antiphosphatidylethanolamine versus those who had recurrent spontaneous abortion, although the P-value missed being significant at 0.052. When they compared their infertile group with those who had never had a successful pregnancy and with those who had had one successful pregnancy, they found an increase in antiphosphatidic acid in those who had never been pregnant, with a P-value of 0.03 [29]. However, in this study, as in many others in this field, no attempt was made to correct for multiple comparisons. When that is done, none of the results would be considered statistically significant.

In 1997, multiple groups again looked at aPL in infertility. Coulam and colleagues examined 312 women who were implant failures versus 100 fertile controls. They did 21 aPL assays in each patient and found that 22% of the implant failures were positive for at least one, versus 5% of the fertile controls. Looking specifically at aCL alone, only 4% of the implant failures had aCL versus 0% of the normal controls [30]. Cubillos and colleagues examined 43 women who had primary infertility. In these women, 37.2% had ANA and 53.5% had at least one aPL assay. This was increased over the 35 controls of whom only 5.7% were ANA positive and 11.4% had an aPL [31]. Kim and colleagues compared women who had different causes of infertility and found that those who had endometriosis and tubal factors as the cause of their infertility had a 38.1% frequency of autoantibodies, and those with a pure tubal cause had only 2.3%. In fact, they went on to look at some treatment issues and felt that those who had endometriosis and tubal factor together were more likely to have a successful pregnancy with corticosteroids. Specifically, the subgroup who had the autoantibodies had the greatest success with corticosteroids [33]. Kutteh and colleagues also studied multiple aPL in infertile women and found that 18.8% of women with IVF failures have an aPL versus only 5.5% of normal women [34]. Ulcova-Gallova and colleagues studied women with what they called intractable infertility. IgG aCL was found in 26.5%, IgG antiphosphatidylinositol in 24.5%, antiphosphatidylethanolamine in 17.6% and antiphosphatidic acid in 20.6% [32].

It would seem from these multiple cross-sectional studies that women with infertility have both an increase in overall autoantibody positivity and, in most studies, an increase in aPL. The frequency of aPL positivity varies widely in the studies, and "classic" aPL, β_2-glycoprotein I-dependent anticardiolipin and lupus anticoagulant, are either not measured or are infrequent. Some studies, however, found no increase in frequency of aPL in infertility. Coulam and Stern in 1992 found no difference in aPL or antisperm antibody in fertile versus infertile women [15]. Balasch et al in 1996 did not find aPL to be associated with any type of infertility [23]. Birdsall and colleagues in 1996 found that 15% of patients undergoing IVF had aPL, but that these were not associated with failure of IVF or any cause of infertility [24]. Denis et al in 1997 studied multiple aPL assays and found that IVF success was equal in women who were either positive or negative for these antibodies [36]. Branch in 1998 reviewed this controversy of whether aPL are increased in women with infertility and felt that issues of study design, patient selection and multiple assays made it impossible to interpret the studies available in the literature [37].

Does In Vitro Fertilization Cause Autoantibodies?

Geva et al in 1995 [21] and Balasch et al in 1996 [23] found a higher frequency of aPL in women who had had IVF failures. This raised the possibility that the increase in estrogen associated with multiple follicular development might lead to higher levels of aPL. However, when actually examined, Yron found high levels of aPL throughout the cycle, uninfluenced by the change in estrogen levels [16]. In addition, two other groups did not find that IVF was associated with increased autoantibodies [20, 24].

Do Autoantibodies Influence the Outcome of In Vitro Fertilization?

Multiple authors have studied whether autoantibodies are predictors of IVF outcome, with very different results (Table 43.2). Kowalik et al in 1997 found that mid-follicular levels of aCL and antiphospholipid did not correlate with IVF outcome [38]. Similarly, Denis et al in 1997 looked at over 21 aPL assays in a large group of 528 women undergoing IVF, and did not find that IVF success was predicted by the presence or the absence of aPL [36]. Birdsall and colleagues found that about 15% of women undergoing IVF had aPL, but that this was not associated with either previous failures of IVF or the cause of infertility. Specifically, they did not find that the frequency of aPL positivity increased with previous IVF attempts [24]. Beer and colleagues have found that idiopathic infertile women who had multiple prior IVF failures had higher levels of the CD56 positive lymphocytes [39]. However, there are currently no data to suggest that multiple IVF failures increase the level of aPL.

Does Treatment of Autoimmunity or of aPL Increase the Success Rate of In Vitro Fertilization?

Because the field of autoimmune reproductive failure has emphasized doing multiple autoantibody assays, it is very hard to dissect out from the current body of work

Table 43.2. Antiphospholipid antibodies and IVF outcome.

Study	Number infertile	% Positive for autoantibodies	IVF outcome
El-Roeiy 1987 [10]	26	38.5%	–
Birkenfeld 1994 [17]	56 IVF failure 69 infertile	32.1% autoAbs 10% auto Abs	+
Gleicher 1994 [111]	105	25.6%	–
Geva 1995 [21]	90	22%	+
Nip 1995 [22]	100	16%	–
Birdsall 1996 [24]	240	15% aPL	–
Kutteh 1997 [34]	191	18.8%	–
Kowalik 1997 [38]	570	11.2% aPS 7% aCL	–
Denis 1997 [36]	528		–

IVF, in vitro fertilization; autoAbs, one of multiple autoantibodies positive; aPL, one of multiple antiphospholipid antibodies positive; aPS, antiphosphatidyl serine; aCL, anticardiolipin.

whether it would be most important to look at corticosteroid therapy to suppress a broadly based B-lymphocyte dysfunctional problem, or whether it would be more important to look at heparin, aspirin and/or intravenous immunoglobulin as potential treatments of an aPL-mediated process. In addition, it is not possible in the current studies to determine if heparin and aspirin, when used, acted through an endothelial cell effect completely unrelated to the presence of aPL.

Several studies have examined whether corticosteroids improve the outcome of IVF. Kemeter and Feichtinger showed in 1986 that prednisone therapy improved pregnancy rates in in vitro fertilization. However, they did include data on either aPL or other autoimmune antibodies [40]. In 1997 Kim et al showed that patients who had endometriosis and tubal factors as the cause of their infertility were more likely to have a successful pregnancy with corticosteroid treatment, with rates of 42.6% clinical pregnancy versus 22.8% without treatment. The subgroup of women who actually had autoantibodies were the most likely to have a clinical pregnancy on corticosteroids with a frequency of 40.9% versus 14.8% [33].

Several authors have examined treatments that might be considered more specific for aPL (Table 43.3). Birkenfeld et al in 1994 found that 15 of 18 women with embryo transfer failures who were given prednisone and aspirin had a clinical

Table 43.3. Antiphospholipid antibodies, treatment, and IVF outcome.

Study	Number	Treatment	Effect
Birkenfeld 1994 [17]	15	A / P	47% success (no controls)
Sher 1994 [112]	169	A / H	49% success (no controls)
Kim 1996 [27]	38	P	Higher clinical pregnancy rate (45 vs 29%) with P
Schenk 1996 [113]	35	A / H	None
Kutteh 1997 [34]	19	A / H	None

A, aspirin; H, heparin; P, prednisone.

pregnancy [17]. Sher et al in 1998 examined 89 women who had had four or more IVF failures and had no male infertility factors involved. Fifty-two of those women had aPL positivity versus 37 who did not. Treatment with heparin, aspirin and intravenous immunoglobulins (IVIG) led to a 42% rate of clinical pregnancy versus 19% of those who did not have aPL, with a P-value of 0.02. The authors conclude that IVF outcome could be improved by heparin, aspirin and IVIG therapy in the aPL-positive group. However, it is also important to note that they did not examine whether the therapy improved the outcome in women who had other autoimmune antibodies [35]. Kutteh et al, in 1997, showed an increased implantation rate with therapy with heparin and aspirin, but this did not reach statistical significance [34]. Kim et al, in 1996, treated women with infertility from ovulatory factors or unexplained infertility with corticosteroids. The group with ovulatory factor had no improvement in clinical pregnancy rate. However, the unexplained infertility group had more pregnancies with corticosteroids, 45.3% versus 29.3% [27].

Coulam has shown some efficacy of IVIG for IVF failure [41]. In addition, Sher et al found that IVIG improved the success rate of women who had infertility and also had antithyroid antibodies [42].

Conclusion

The field of infertility and autoimmunity remains largely uninterpretable because of issues of patient selection, study design, and laboratory criteria for aPL assays. Women in these studies have not necessarily been well characterized in terms of the type of infertility, whether or not there had been multiple IVF failures, and whether they had other autoantibodies or any other symptoms of autoimmune disease. It has not been clear in most studies whether having any autoantibody is important or whether aPL alone are important. For the most part, studies have used a panel of multiple aPL and have not corrected for multiple comparisons. In studies which examined β_2-glycoprotein I-dependent aCL, the frequency of women with infertility who actually had this autoantibody appeared to be very small.

Given that the underlying frequency of aPL, especially β_2-glycoprotein I-dependent aPL is not established in these patients, the issues of treatment become even more confusing. Articles certainly suggest that treatment with prednisone, heparin, aspirin or IVIG may increase the success rate of in vitro fertilization. Whether this increase in success rate has anything to do with suppressing the action of or titer of aPL is completely unknown. In fact, these treatments might be potentially beneficial for women who had other autoantibodies, as well.

Oral Contraceptive Pills

Pathophysiology of Hypercoagulability in Oral Contraceptive Pill Users

It is accepted that oral contraceptive pills increase the risk of both venous and arterial hypercoagulability. The effects of oral contraceptive pills on coagulation, however, are extremely complex. Both the estrogen and the progestin moieties have affects on coagulation. Oliveri and colleagues found that oral contraceptive pills increased fibrinogen and protein C, decreased protein S, and shortened both the prothrombin time and the partial thromboplastin time. Patients on oral contraceptive pills also had a decrease in their activated protein C (APC) sensitivity ratio. Two of these patients, who had APC resistance due to their oral contraceptives, stopped their oral contraceptive and then had normalization of APC sensitivity [43]. Rosing and colleagues found that oral contraceptive pills decreased the sensitivity to APC, with a *P*-value of 0.001. This acquired APC resistance was equivalent to having a heterozygous state for factor V Leiden. In fact, if a person started out as heterozygous to factor V Leiden, starting oral contraceptive pills would be equivalent to moving them to the range of homozygous carriers of factor V Leiden [44]. Creatsas and colleagues also found that oral contraceptive pills shortened the prothrombin time and increased fibrinogen. They also found a decrease in antithrombin III [45]. These studies leave unanswered which of the many effects of oral contraceptive pills on coagulation is pivotal in thrombotic risk.

A second potential pathophysiological role of oral contraceptive pills in hypercoagulability involves antiestrogen antibodies. Beaumont, in 1991, reported that 33% of healthy users of oral contraceptive pills developed antibodies to estrogen. Of those who had a thrombotic event, 72% had antiestrogen antibodies [46]. In 1992, Beaumont and colleagues reported a case–control study with 100 oral contraceptive users and 100 controls. They found elevated levels of homocysteine, antiestrogen antibodies, older age and smoking were predictors of thrombotic events [47]. Albengres and colleagues in 1991 found that 32% of oral contraceptive users had antibodies to estrogen versus only 13% of controls, but they failed to find a predictive effect on thrombosis [48].

Oral Contraceptive Pill and Venous Thromboembolism

It is very important in the studies of thrombosis and oral contraceptive pills to understand the terminology of oral contraceptive pills. "First generation pills" are considered to be those that had 50 μg of ethinylestradiol. The "second generation pills" contain levonorgestrel or norgestimate. The "third generation pills" contain desogestrel or gestodene. In general, estrogen in higher doses increases the risk of thromboembolism. However, although controversial, the type of progestin is also an important independent variable in the risk of thromboembolism. Younger users of oral contraceptives are at greater risk of venous than arterial thromboembolism, with rates of venous thrombosis about two times higher than that of arterial thrombosis [49]. From the age of 30 onwards the risk of arterial thrombosis increases.

The second-generation oral contraceptives were thought to have a relatively small risk of venous thromboembolism. Other risk factors for venous thrombosis in oral contraceptive pill users include obesity, varicose veins, and family history of thrombosis, including factor V Leiden. A higher risk of arterial thrombosis in oral contraceptive pill users is associated with smoking, diabetes, hypertension, migraine and family history.

The third-generation oral contraceptives were actually designed to reduce the risk of arterial thrombosis. Multiple studies on the third-generation oral contraceptives appeared in the literature in 1995 and 1996 (Table 43.4). They differed slightly in study design, although all are case–control studies. Important differences included the sources of the controls, either hospital or community, and the stringency to which the diagnosis of deep venous thrombosis was confirmed. Bloemenkamp et al in 1995 reported on a case–control study of deep venous thrombosis with 126 cases

Table 43.4. Oral contraceptives and venous thromboembolism.

Study	Design	Incidence	Odds ratio
Bloemenkamp 1995 [50]	Leiden Thrombophilia Study	Incidence	8.7 (3.9–19.3) – 3rd generation OCP
Jick 1995 [51]	United Kingdom General Practice	16.1 / 100000, 2nd generation OCP 29.3 / 100000, desogestrol 28.1 / 100000, gestodene	6.0 (3.7–9.8)
WHO 1995 [114]	WHO (hospital-based case–control)		4.15 (3.09–5.57) Europe 3.25 (2.59–4.08) non-Europe
Spitzer 1996 [53]	Transnational Research Group matched case–control		3.2 (2.3–4.3) 2nd generation OCP 4.8 (3.4–6.7) 3rd generation OCP
Farmer 1997 (115]	United Kingdom General Practice nested case–control	3.10 / 10000, 2nd generation OCP 4.96 / l0000, 3rd generation OCP	
Suissa l997 [54]	Transnational Research Group case–control, first-time users		3.0 (1.3–6.8) 2nd generation OCP 9.0 (4.2–19.2) 3rd generation OCP
Bloemenkamp 1998 [55]	Two diagnostic centers (case–control)		3.2 (2.3–4.5)
Martinelli 1998 [56]	Case–control		22.1 (5.9–84.2) for cerebral vein thrombosis 4.4 (1.1–17.8) for deep vein thrombosis

and 159 controls. This study found that a third-generation oral contraceptive pill containing desogestrel increased the risk of thrombosis 8.7 times. Women with factor V Leiden who took oral contraceptive pills containing desogestrel had a 50-fold increase in the risk of thrombosis [50]. Jick et al, in 1995, reported on a case–control study done within a general practice research database. This would, of course, include community patients. This study also found an increased risk of venous thromboembolism with third-generation oral contraceptive pills [51]. Poulter et al, in 1995, using hospital cases and controls, also found an increased risk [52]. Finally, Spitzer et al, in 1996, reported a hospital case–control study showing a much higher rate of venous thromboembolism in the first year [53]. A re-analysis done by Suissa et al did not find any difference between second- and third-generation pills in this study for first time users. This suggests that the apparent increased risk with third-generation users is at least partially explained by patient selection [54]. In 1998 Bloemenkamp and colleagues reported a case–control study with 120 cases and 413 controls in which the risk of deep venous thrombosis was 3.2, with a very tight 95% confidence interval of 2.3 to 4.5 [55].

Oral contraceptives also increase the risk of specific types of venous thrombosis, including cerebral vein thrombosis. Martinelli and colleagues reported a case–control study of cerebral vein thrombosis in which the odds ratio for oral contraceptives was 22.1. In fact, in this study, the odds ratio for deep-vein thrombosis was also increased at 4.4 [56]. In general, almost any type of venous thrombosis has been reported in oral contraceptive users, including mesenteric vein thrombosis [57] and superior ophthalmic vein thrombosis [58].

Whether there is any true difference between second- and third-generation oral contraceptives remains controversial. It is quite possible that the findings in the reported case–control studies were due to prescribing bias with higher risk women getting the newer generation pills because they were initially thought to be safer. It is also possible that some of these results have been confounded by age and duration of use [59]. However, Rosing et al have suggested that the third generation oral contraceptive users develop acquired APC resistance [44]. Thus, the possibility remains that there is a biological effect of the newer generation oral contraceptives that is responsible. In general, however, the most important finding has been that women who have a hypercoagulable state, especially factor V Leiden [50] are at much greater risk of venous thrombosis if exposed to oral contraceptives. Whether women with hypercoagulable states on third-generation oral contraceptive pills are at greater danger of thrombosis requires further study. However, it is of concern that Lauque et al reported two patients who developed pulmonary embolism shortly after being switched from a second-generation to a third-generation oral contraceptive [60].

The overall risk of venous thromboembolism in the general population has been estimated as 1 out of 10 000. In general, the risk of thrombosis in women on oral contraceptive pills is probably somewhere between 2.3 [51], and 3 [61] per 10 000. In fact, the risk of venous thrombosis in pregnancy is much higher at 6 out of 10 000. Therefore, it is important to keep in perspective that oral contraceptives are safer than pregnancy in terms of the risk of venous thromboembolism. For physicians in the United States the debate on second- and third-generation oral contraceptives has not been given the attention seen in the United Kingdom and in Europe. North American subjects are not represented in most of the studies and the oral contraceptives used are not necessarily available in the United States.

Arterial Thromboembolism In Oral Contraceptive Users

In general, the study of cardiovascular events in oral contraceptive users is difficult because there are no randomized controlled trials, and because the larger studies used older oral contraceptives no longer in wide use. Most of the newer studies are case–control studies, which are vulnerable to bias in selection of both cases and controls (Table 43.5) [62].

Lidegaard and colleagues did a 5-year case–control study of cerebral thrombosis. This study included 219 cases and 1041 controls. They found that the risk of cerebral thrombosis was 1.8 in first-generation oral contraceptive pill users, 2.37 in

Table 43.5. Oral contraceptives and cerebral thrombosis.

Study	Design	Incidence	Odds ratio (95% CI)
Petitti et al [63]	Kaiser Permanente (case–control)	11.3/100000	1.18 (0.54–2.59)
WHO 1996 [64]	WHO Collaborative Study (Hospital-based case–control)		2.99 (1.65–5.40) Europe 2.93 (2.15—4) non-Europe
Heinemann 1997 [65]	Transnational Research Group (Case–control)		3.4 (2.1–5.5) 2nd generation OCP 3.9 (2.3–6.6) 3rd generation OCP
Shwartz 1997 [66]	Washington State (case–control)	4.3/l00000	0.89 (0.27–2.94)
Lidegaard 1998 [49]	Denmark (case–control)		2.37 (1.35–4.16) 2nd generation

second-generation users and 1.32 in third-generation users. Only for second-generation users were the results statistically significant. This study discovered the interesting dichotomy that the third-generation pills might cause more venous thrombosis but less arterial thrombosis. It was clearly shown that the greater the amount of estrogen in the pill, the greater the risk, with levels of 50 μg having a risk of 2.65, 40 μg 1.60 and 20 μg 1.59. The effect of progestins was also examined in this study, and, as indicated above, the highest risk was found with the second-generation progestins, levonorgestrel and norgestimate, with odds ratios of 2.43 and 7.09, respectively, as opposed to the third-generation progestin desogestrel, with 1.62, and gestodene, with 1.24 [49].

Several studies have investigated cerebral thrombosis and oral contraceptives. Petitti in 1996 found an odds ratio of 1.2, which was not significant [63]. In a World Health Organization study in 1996, the risk with second-generation oral contraceptives was 1.5 and that with third-generation oral contraceptives was 1.8, although neither odds ratio reached statistical significance [64]. The Transnational Study reported by Heinemann and colleagues in 1997 found a greater risk of cerebral thrombosis with the third-generation pills. The risk estimates were twice as high with the hospital controls than with the community controls, however, suggesting some problems with the study design [65]. Schwartz and colleagues found an odds ratio of 0.89, which did not reach statistical significance [66].

Additional studies have examined the risk of myocardial infarction with oral contraceptives (Table 43.6). The Transnational Group found a risk of 2.35 with second-generation pills, which was statistically significant, and only 0.82 with the third-generation pills [67]. The WHO study found an odds ratio of 5.01 which was statistically significant [68]. A retrospective case–control study done in a United States HMO setting found an odds ratio of 1.65, which failed to reach statistical significance [69]. In general, although arterial thromboembolic events are more important in terms of case morbidity and mortality, the numbers of such events are small and therefore more difficult to study. Overall, oral contraceptives appear to increase the risk of both cerebral thrombosis and myocardial infarction. In addition, there is some early evidence to suggest that the third-generation oral contraceptives may be slightly safer.

Multiple studies have emphasized the importance of comorbidity in arterial thrombosis. Beaumont et al in 1991 found risk factors for arterial thrombosis to include age, duration, hyperlipidemia and smoking [46]. In 1992 the same group found that homocysteine, antiestrogen antibodies, smokers and older age were risk factors [47].

Table 43.6. Oral contraceptives and myocardial infarction.

Study	Study design	Incidence	Results
			Odds ratio (95% CI)
Jick 1995 [51]	UK General Practice Research Database	15 deaths/303470	
Jick 1996 [99]	UK General Practice Research Database	1.8/100000	
Sidney 1996 [69]	Kaiser Permanente (case–control)	5.2/100000	1.65 (0.45–6.06)
WHO 1997 [68]	WHO Collaborative Study Hospital-based case–control		5.01 (2.54–9.90) Europe 4.78 (2.52–9.07) non-Europe
Lewis 1997 [67]	Transnational Research Group Case–control		2.35 (1.42–3.89) for 2nd generation OCP 0.82 (0.29–2.31) for 3rd generation OCP

The increased risk of arterial thrombosis with oral contraceptives has not been confirmed in animal models. In a monkey model, oral contraceptives did not appear to be associated with arterial thrombosis measured after injury and stenosis [70].

Oral Contraceptive Pills Enhance Hypercoagulability in Patients who Have Genetic Causes of Hypercoagulability

Oral contraceptive pills appear to increase the risk of hypercoagulability in patients who have genetic causes of hypercoagulability (Table 43.7), especially factor V Leiden, the most common genetic cause of hypercoagulability in Caucasians. Waselenko et al in 1998 found that patients with factor V Leiden had a risk of venous thromboembolism between 28 to 50 in 10 000 patient years [71]. The highest risk was in the first year of use of oral contraceptive pills. Martinelli in 1998 studied cerebral vein thrombosis and found that 35% of patients with cerebral vein thrombosis had some cause of hypercoagulability [56]. Patients with factor V Leiden had a risk of 7.8, which was statistically significant. For those on oral contraceptive pills, the risk was 22.1. Rintelen et al in 1996 examined 29 people who were homozygous for factor V Leiden. Twenty-five of those had a venous thromboembolic event. Twelve females in this study had taken oral contraceptive pills 6 to 150 months prior to the venous thromboembolic event. Oral contraceptive pills were found to be the most important precipitating factor for venous thromboembolism in women who had factor V Leiden [72]. Rosendaal et al in 1995 [73] found that 3 of 6 women homozygous for factor V Leiden had used oral contraceptive pills within 1 month of a thromboembolic event. Vandenbrouke et al in 1994 found that oral contraceptive pills increased the risk of thrombosis in women who were heterozygous for factor V Leiden [74]. In 1995 Bloemenkamp et al found that third-generation oral contraceptive pills caused a greatly increased risk of thrombosis in women who had factor V Leiden, with the risk increasing 50-fold [50]. Bauersachs et al in 1996 found that although only 3 of 1000 women with factor V Leiden would have a thrombosis if

Table 43.7. Oral contraceptives and genetic causes of hypercoagulability.

Genetic factor	Study design	Result
Factor V Leiden		
Bloemenkamp 1995 [50]	Leiden Thrombophilia Study, case–control	50-fold increase in thrombosis with 3rd generation OCP
Martinelli 1998 [56]	Case–control of cerebral vein thrombosis	OR 7.8 (1.8–34.1)
Rintelen 1996 [72]	29 homozygous patients	80% with thrombosis took OCPs
Bridey 1995 [116]	Case report	Fatal cerebral venous sinus thrombosis with OCP
Glueck 1997 [117]	Osteonecrosis of jaw	OCPs used more commonly
Prothrombin G20210A		
Martinelli 1998 [56]	Case–control study of cerebral vein thrombosis	OR 10.2 (2.3–31)
Gould 1998 [118]	Case report	Celiac axis and splenic infarction with OCP
Antithrombin III		
Pabinger 1994 [78]	Retrospective controlled cohort study	Significant increase in thrombosis
Protein S		
Villa 1996 [82]	Case report	Low free protein S
Koelman 1992 [81]	Case report	Cerebral sinus thrombosis with OCP

they took oral contraceptive pills, their risk of thrombosis on oral contraceptive pills was increased 35-fold [75].

The second most important genetic cause of hypercoagulability is the prothrombin 20210A polymorphism. The prothrombin 20210A polymorphism is found in 2% of healthy people and 18% of families who have a history of venous thromboembolism. It is thought to cause a threefold increase of thromboembolism in heterozygous carriers [76, 77]. This prothrombin gene mutation has been studied in women taking oral contraceptive pills. Martinelli and colleagues found that women who had this prothrombin gene mutation who took oral contraceptive pills had an astounding odds ratio for cerebral vein thrombosis of 149.3 [56]. In fact, in the group with cerebral vein thrombosis, the most frequent comorbid problem found was the prothrombin gene mutation. It is of interest that both prothrombin 20210A and oral contraceptive pills increase the plasma levels of prothrombin [76].

Protein S deficiency may increase the risk of thrombosis in oral contraceptive pill users. In a retrospective study, 34 patients with protein S type 1 deficiency had no excess risk with oral contraceptive pills [78]. However, thromboembolism with oral contraceptive pills was found in three patients, all of whom had a decrease in free protein S [79–81]. Therefore, it appears that a low free protein S is an increased risk factor for thrombosis in users of oral contraceptive pills [82]. This appears to make sense pathophysiologically since oral contraceptive pills are known to diminish the already low levels of protein S in these patients.

Antithrombin III deficiency also appears to be an additional risk factor for patients who take oral contraceptive pills. Fifteen percent of patients with congenital defects of antithrombin III have a venous thromboembolism triggered by oral contraceptive pills [83]. It is of interest that the thromboembolism appeared to be triggered within one to two cycles of oral contraceptive use.

In one study, two of 11 patients with pulmonary embolism had protein C deficiency [60]. There are several case reports of protein C deficiency in oral contraceptives users leading to thromboembolism [84, 85]. Protein C deficiency increased the risk of thrombosis in oral contraceptive users 15-fold in the study of Bauersachs in 1996 [75].

Oral Contraceptive Pills and Antiphospholipid Antibody Syndrome

Pathophysiology

It is known that estrogen can increase the levels of anti-DNA antibodies [86]. In animal models, estrogen increases the production of aCL [87, 88]. Multiple case reports exist of oral contraceptive use precipitating thrombosis in patients who had antiphospholipid antibody syndrome (Table 43.8) [89, 90]. Asherson in 1988 reported on 10 patients with aPL. Four of the patients with venous thromboembolism and three of the patients with arterial thromboembolism had taken oral contraceptive pills. In addition, chorea has been reported with oral contraceptive use in patients with aPL [91]. In another series, Julkunen in 1991 found that two of 31 patients with venous thromboembolism had been on oral contraceptive pills [92].

Table 43.8. Oral contraceptives and antiphospholipid antibodies.

Study	Study design	Result
Bruneau 1986 [119]	10 patients with thrombosis	No association of aPL with thrombosis
Asherson 1987 [120]	10 patients with thrombosis or chorea	Association with both aCL and LA
Julkunen 1991 [92]	Case report	Malignant hypertension, SLE
Asherson 1993 [121]	Case report	Deep vein thrombosis
Julkunen 1991 [92]	31 SLE patients	Two developed deep venous thrombosis
Girolami 1996 [89]	Case series (3)	All had LA and aCL

aPL, antiphospholipid antibody; aCL, anticardiolipin; LA, lupus anticoagulant.

Oral contraceptive pills may also induce systemic lupus erythematosus, thus leading to secondary antiphospholipid antibody syndrome. The risk of lupus in users, diagnosed using American College of Rheumatology criteria and by an American College of Rheumatology rheumatologist was 1.9, which was statistically significant [93].

Hormone Replacement Therapy

It has been some surprise that hormone replacement therapy is associated with thrombotic risk. For many reasons it was initially thought that hormone replacement therapy should not be an issue in thromboembolic risk, especially because the doses of estrogen used were much less than those used in oral contraceptive pills. Studies done in the early 1990s had not found an increased risk of venous thromboembolism with hormone replacement therapy. This included the study of Devor et al in 1992 [94], a case–control study, and a later study of Forbes et al in 1994 [95]. It was felt that the effects on the coagulation system induced by hormone replacement therapy should be not just less, but different, than those of oral contraceptive pills. It was assumed, therefore, that hormone replacement therapy did not confer the same increased risk as oral contraceptives on hypercoagulability [71]. In support of a lack of thromboembolic risk, Saleh and colleagues did not find any differences in biochemical markers of coagulation, namely, prothrombin fragment and thrombin antithrombin complexes in their study of estrogen replacement therapy [96]. However, Scarabin and colleagues found that oral estrogen supplementation did affect coagulation, but that transdermal use did not [97].

However, in 1996, studies published in the Lancet all showed a two- to fourfold risk of venous thromboembolism, not just with estrogen only but also with combined estrogen and progestin hormone replacement therapy (Table 43.9) [98–100]. Most of the venous thromboembolism seen in the studies of hormone replacement therapy appeared to have occurred in the early years of hormone replacement therapy. The risk was approximately 1 out of 5000 patients [101]. This increased risk of venous thromboembolism was confirmed in the recent HERS secondary prevention trial [102].

Although it now is accepted that hormone replacement therapy does increase the risk of venous thromboembolism, there are also negative studies. A 10-year trial did not find any risk [103]. Studies done using the Boston Collaborative Drug Surveillance Program [104] and the Walnut Creek Contract Drug Study [105, 106] found no risk.

Table 43.9. Estrogen replacement therapy and venous thromboembolism.

Study	Study design	Result (Odds ratio with 95% CI)
Daly 1996 [98]	Hospital Case–control	OR 3.5 (I.8–7)
Jick 1996 [122]	Hospital admission	OR 3.6 (I.6–7.8)
Grodstein I996 [100]	Prospective	OR 2.1 (1.2–3.8)
Devor 1992 [94]	Case–control	No association
Hulley 1998 [102]	Randomized, blinded, placebo-controlled secondary prevention trial	Relative hazard 2.89 (1.50–5.58)

However, both of these case–control studies excluded patients who had other risk factors. It is possible that some of the increased risk seen in thromboembolism with hormone replacement therapy is in subgroups of women with comorbidity.

The most surprising information is that the relative risk of venous thromboembolism among peri- and post-menopausal women is actually larger than that seem among younger women who use oral contraceptives.

The arterial thrombotic risk of hormone replacement therapy has not been widely studied. In a monkey model, neither hormone replacement therapy with estrogen alone nor conjugated equine estrogens with medroxyprogesterone were found to increase the risk of thrombosis within an injury and stenosis model [70]. However, in the HERS study, a secondary prevention trial, an increase in cardiovascular events was found in the first year of hormone replacement therapy. These patients were not screened for other hypercoagulable risk factors including genetic risk factors or antiphospholipid antibody syndrome [102]. One possible explanation is that women with other risk factors for hypercoagulability are more likely to have events during the first year of hormone replacement therapy.

Hormone Replacement Therapy and Systemic Lupus Erythematosus

There has been some concerned based on the Nurse's Health Study that women who use postmenopausal hormone replacement therapy might be at increased risk for systemic lupus erythematosus. An odds ratio of 2.5 was found for current users, which was statistically significant [107]. Thus, hormone replacement therapy could conceivably lead to lupus and then to the secondary antiphospholipid antibody syndrome.

However, most of the studies on hormonal replacement therapy and lupus have been designed to determine whether hormone replacement therapy would increase the activity of lupus. Three studies have suggested that this does not occur. A retrospective case–control study done by Arden and colleagues in 1994 found no increase in lupus flares with hormone replacement therapy. In addition, they found no increase in thromboembolic events [108]. A case–control study done by Kreidstein et al in 1997 examined 16 lupus patients on hormone replacement therapy versus 32 controls. The lupus flare rates were equal in the two groups [109]. Finally, a study done by Mok and colleagues in 1998 followed 34 lupus patients, 11 of whom were on hormone replacement therapy and 23 control patients. The lupus flare rate was 0.12 per year in the hormone replacement therapy group and 0.16 in the control group [110].

The SELENA study (the Study of Estrogen in Lupus Erythematosus National Assessment Study) is an ongoing study of hormone replacement therapy in women with SLE. The co-principal investigators, Michelle Petri and Jill Buyon, determined that women with lupus who had moderate to high titers of aCL or a lupus anti-coagulant should not enter the study because of safety concerns of thrombotic risk. During this study there has been no evidence that hormone replacement therapy induces new production of aPL in lupus patients who either had negative or low levels of aCL at entry into the study.

References

1. Gleicher N, Pratt D, Dudkiewicz A. What do we really know about autoantibody abnormalities and reproductive failure: a critical review. Autoimmunity 1993;16(2):115–140.
2. Gleicher N, El-Roeiy A, Confino E, Friberg J. Is endometriosis an autoimmune disease? Obstet Gynecol 1987;70:115–122.
3. Confino E, Harlow L, Gleicher N. Peritoneal fluid and serum autoantibody levels in patinets with endometriosis. Fertil Steril 1990;52:242–245.
4. Kennedy SH, Nunn B, Cederhold-Williams SA, Barlow DH. Cardiolipin antibody levels in endometriosis and systemic lupus erythematosus. Fertil Steril 1989;52:1061–1062.
5. Kilpatrick DC, Haining REB, Smith SSK. Are cardiolipin antibody levels elevated in endometriosis? Fertil Steril 1991;55:436–437.
6. Taylor PV, Maloney MD, Campbell JM et al. Autoreactivity in women endometriosis. Br J Obstet Gynaecol 1991;98:680–685.
7. Gleicher N, El-Roeiy A, Confino E, Friberg J. Reproductive failure because of autoantibodies: Unexplained infertility and pregnancy wastage. Am J Obstet Gynecol 1989;160:1376–1385.
8. Taylor PV, Campbell JM, Scott JS. Presence of autoantibodies in women with unexplained infertility. Am J Obstet Gynecol 1989;161:377–379.
9. El-Roeiy A, Valessini G, Friberg J et al. Autoantibodies and common idiotypes in sperm antibody positive females and males. Am J Obstet Gynecol 1988;158:596–603.
10. El-Roeiy A, Gleicher N, Friberg J, Confino E, Dudkiewicz AB. Correlation between peripheral blood and follicular fluid autoantibodies and impact on in vitro fertilization. Obstet Gynecol 1987;70:163–170.
11. Grimmer D, Landas S, Kemp JD. IgM antitrophoblast antibodies in a patient with a pregnancy-associated lupus-like disorder, vasculitis, and recurrent intrauterine fetal demise. Arch Pathol Lab Med 1988;112:191–193.
12. Stagnaro-Green A, Roman SH, Cobin R, El-Harazy E, Alvarez-Margany M, Davies TF. Detection of at-risk pregnancy by means of highly sensitive assays for thyroid autoantibodies. JAMA 1990;264:1422–1425.
13. Glinoer D, Fernandez Soto M, Bourdoux P et al. Pregnancy in patients with mild thyroid abnormalities: maternal and neonatal repercussions. J Clin Endocrinol Metab 1991;73:421–427.
14. Fisch B, Rikover Y, Shohat L et al. The relationship between in vitro fertilization and naturally occurring antibodies: evidence for increased production of antiphospholipid autoantibodies [see comments]. Fertil Steril 1991;56(4):718–724.
15. Coulam CB, Stern JJ. Evaluation of immunological infertility. Am J Reprod Immunol 1992;27:130–135.
16. Yron I, Tadir Y, Ovadia J et al. Evidence for increased levels of circulating antiphospholipid autoantibodies in patients undergoing in vitro fertilization treatment. Ann NY Acad Sci 1992;651:599–601.
17. Birkenfeld A, Mukaida T, Minichiello L, Jackson M, Kase NG, Yemini M. Incidence of autoimmune antibodies in failed embryo transfer cycles. Am J Reprod Immunol 1994;31:65–68.
18. Geva E, Yaron Y, Lessing JB et al. Circulating autoimmune antibodies may be responsible for implantation failure in in vitro fertilization. Fertil Steril 1994;62:802–806.
19. Aoki K, Dudkiewicz AB, Matsuura E, Novotny M, Kaberlein G, Gleicher N. Clinical significance of beta 2-glycoprotein I-dependent anticardiolipin antibodies in the reproductive autoimmune failure syndrome: correlation with conventional antiphospholipid antibody detection systems. Am J Obstet Gynecol 1995;172(3):926–931.

20. Fisch B, Fried S, Manor Y, Ovadia J, Witz IP, Yron I. Increased antiphospholipid antibody activity in in-vitro fertilization patients is not treatment-dependent but rather an inherent characteristic of the infertile state. Am J Reprod Immunol 1995;34(6):370–374.
21. Geva E, Amit A, Lerner-Geva L, Azem F, Yovel I, Lessing JB. Autoimmune disorders: another possible cause for in-vitro fertilization and embryo transfer failure. Hum Reprod 1995;10:2560–2563.
22. Nip MM, Taylor PV, Rutherford AJ, Hancock KW. Autoantibodies and antisperm antibodies in sera and follicular fluids of infertile patients; relation to reproductive outcome after in-vitro fertilization. Hum Reprod 1995;10:2564–2569.
23. Balasch J, Creus M, Fabregues F et al. APL and human reproductive failure. Hum Reprod 1996;11:2310–2315.
24. Birdsall MA, Lockwood GM, Ledger WL, Johnson PM, Chamley LW. APL in women having in-vitro fertilization. Hum Reprod 1996;11:1185–1189.
25. Fichorova R, Nakov L, Baleva M, Nikolov K, Gegova I. Sperm, nuclear, phospholipid, and red blood cell antibodies and isotype RF in infertile couples and patients with autoimmune rheumatic diseases. Am J Reprod Immunol 1996;36:309–316.
26. Kaider BD, Price DE, Roussev RG, Coulam CB. Antiphospholipid antibody prevalence in patients with IVF failure. Am J Reprod Immunol 1996;35:388–393.
27. Kim CH, Cho YK, Mok JE. The efficacy of immunotherapy in patients who underwent superovulation with intrauterine insemination. Fertil Steril 1996;65:133–138.
28. Roussev RG, Kaider BD, Price DE, Coulam CB. Laboratory evaluation of women experiencing reproductive failure. Am J Reprod Immunol 1996;35:415–420.
29. Ruiz AM, Kwak JY, Kwak FM, Beer AE. Impact of age on reproductive outcome in women with recurrent spontaneous abortions and infertility of immune etiology. Am J Reprod Immunol 1996;35:408–414.
30. Coulam CB, Kaider BD, Kaider AS, Janowicz P, Roussev RG. APL associated with implantation failure after IVF/ET. J Assist Reprod Genet 1997;14:603–608.
31. Cubillos J, Lucena A, Lucena C et al. Incidence of autoantibodies in the infertile population. Early Pregnancy 1997;3:119–124.
32. Ulcova-Gallova Z, Panzner P, Krauz V, Fialova P. [Profile of aPL in various diagnoses associated with reproduction]. Ceska Gynekol 1997;62:6–9.
33. Kim CH, Chae HD, Kang BM, Chang YS, Mok JE. The immunotherapy during in vitro fertilization and embryo transfer cycles in infertile patients with endometriosis. J Obstet Gynaecol Res 1997;23:463–470.
34. Kutteh WH, Yetman DL, Chantilis SJ, Crain J Effect of aPL in women undergoing in-vitro fertilization: role of heparin and aspirin. Hum Reprod 1997;12:1171–1175.
35. Sher G, Zouves C, Feinman M et al. A rational basis for the use of combined heparin/aspirin and IVIG immunotherapy in the treatment of recurrent IVF failure associated with aPL. Am J Reprod Immunol 1998;39:391–394.
36. Denis AL, Guido M, Adler RD, Bergh PA, Brenner C, Scott RT, Jr. APL and pregnancy rates and outcome in in vitro fertilization patients. Fertil Steril 1997;67:1084–1190.
37. Branch DW. APL and reproductive outcome: the current state of affairs. J Reprod Immunol 1998;38:75–87.
38. Kowalik A, Vichnin M, Liu HC, Branch W, Berkeley AS. Midfollicular anticardiolipin and antiphosphatidylserine antibody titers do not correlate with in vitro fertilization outcome. Fertil Steril 1997;68:298–304.
39. Beer AE, Kwak JY, Ruiz JE. Immunophenotypic profiles of peripheral blood lymphocytes in women with recurrent pregnancy losses and in infertile women with multiple failed in vitro fertilization cycles. Am J Reprod Immunol 1996;35:376–382.
40. Kemeter P, Geichtinger W. Prednisolon verbessert die schwangerschaftsrate der IVF. Eine prospective randomisierte studie. Fertilitat 1986;2:71–76.
41. Coulam CB, Krysa LW, Bustillo M. Intravenous immunoglobulin for in-vitro fertilization failure. Hum Reprod 1994;9:2265–2269.
42. Sher G, Maassarani G, Zouves C et al. The use of combined heparin/aspirin and immunoglobulin G therapy in the treatment of in vitro fertilization patients with antithyroid antibodies. Am J Reprod Immunol 1998;39:223–225.
43. Olivieri O, Friso S, Manzato F et al. Resistance to activated protein C in healthy women taking oral contraceptives. Br J Haematol 1995;91:465–470.
44. Rosing J, Tans G, Nicolaes GA et al. Oral contraceptives and venous thrombosis: different sensitivities to activated protein C in women using second- and third-generation oral contraceptives. Br J Haematol 1997;97:233–238.

45. Creatsas G, Kontopoulou-Griva I, Deligeoroglou E et al. Effects of two combined monophasic and triphasic ethinylestradiol/gestodene oral contraceptives on natural inhibitors and other hemostatic variables. Eur J Contracept Reprod Health Care 1997;2:31–38.
46. Beaumont V, Lemort N, Beaumont JL. Oral contraceptives, sex steroid-induced antibodies and vascular thrombosis: results from 1318 cases. Eur Heart J 1991;12:1219–1224.
47. Beaumont V, Malinow MR, Sexton G,et al. Hyperhomocyst(e)inemia, anti-estrogen antibodies and other risk factors for thrombosis in women on oral contraceptives. Atherosclerosis 1992;94:147–152.
48. Albengres E, Abuaf N, D'Athis P, Guichoux JY, Rotten D, Tillement JP. The significance of circulating antiethinyl-estradiol antibodies (AEEA) in the occurrence of thrombosis in women while taking the pill. Int J Clin Pharmacol Ther Toxicol 1991;29:486–493.
49. Lidegaard O, Kreiner S. Cerebral thrombosis and oral contraceptives. A case–control study. Contraception 1998;57:303–314.
50. Bloemenkamp KWM, Rosendaal FR, Helmerhorst FM, Büller HR, Vandenbroucke JP. Enhancement by factor V Leiden mutation of risk of deep-vein thrombosis associated with oral contraceptives containing a third-generation progestagen. Lancet 1995;346:1593–1596.
51. Jick H, Jick SS, Gurewich V, Myers MW, Vasilakis C. Risk of idiopathic cardiovascular death and nonfatal venous thromboembolism in women using oral contraceptives with differing progestagen components. Lancet 1995;346:1589–1593.
52. Poulter NR, Farley TMM, Chang CL, Marmot MG, Meirik O. Safety of combined oral contraceptive pills [letter]. Lancet 1996;347:547.
53. Spitzer WO, Lewis MA, Heinemann LAJ, Thurogood M, Macrae KD. Third generation oral contraceptives and risk of venous thromboembolic disorders: an international case–control study. Br Med J 1996;312:83–88.
54. Suissa S, Blais L, Spitzer WO, Cusson J, Lewis M, Heinemann L. First-time use of newer oral contraceptives and the risk of venous thromboembolism. Contraception 1997;56:141–146.
55. Bloemenkamp KW, Rosendaal FR, Buller HR, Helmerhorst FM, Colly LP, Vandenbroucke JP. Risk of venous thrombosis with use of current low-dose oral contraceptives is not explained by diagnostic suspicion and referral bias. Arch Intern Med 1998;159:65–70.
56. Martinelli I, Sacchi E, Landi G, Taioli E, Duca F, Mannucci PM. High risk of cerebral-vein thrombosis in carriers of a prothrombin-gene mutation and in users of oral contraceptives [see comments]. N Engl J Med 1998;338:1793–1797.
57. Engelke C, Bittscheidt H, Poley F. Mesenteric vein thrombosis with hemorrhagic infarct of the small intestinal as a complication of oral contraceptives. Chirurg 1995;66:634–637.
58. Jaais F, Habib ZA. Unilateral superior ophthalmic vein thrombosis in a user of oral contraceptives. Med J Malaysia 1994;49:416–418.
59. Thorogood M. Oral contraceptives and thrombosis. Curr Opin Hematol 1998;5:350–354.
60. Lauque D, Mazieres J, Rouzaud P et al. Pulmonary embolism in patients using estrogen-progestagen contraceptives. Presse Med 1998;27:1566–1569.
61. Farmer RD, Preston TD. The risk of venous thromboembolism associated with low oestrogen oral contraceptives. J Obstet Gynecol 1995;15:195–200.
62. Westhoff CL. Oral contraceptives and thrombosis: an overview of study methods and recent results. Am J Obstet Gynecol 1998;179(3 Pt 2):S38–S42.
63. Petitti D, Sidney S, Bernstein A, Wolf S, Quesenberry C, Ziel H. Stroke in users of low-dose oral contraceptives. N Engl J Med 1996;335:8–15.
64. WHO Collaborative Study of Cardiovascular Disease and Steroid Hormone Contraception. Ischaemic stroke and combined oral contraceptives: results of an international, multicentre, case–control study. Lancet 1996;348:498–505.
65. Heinemann LAJ, Lewis MA, Thorogood M et al. Case–control study of oral contraceptives and risk of thromboembolic stroke: results from international study on oral contraceptives and health of young women. Br Med J 1997;315:1502–1504.
66. Schwartz SM, Siscovick DS, Longstreth Jr WT et al. Use of low-dose oral contraceptives and stroke in young women. Ann Intern Med 1997;127:596–603.
67. Lewis MA, Heinemann LAJ, Spitzer WO, MacRae KD, Bruppacher R. The use of oral contraceptives and the occurrence of acute myocardial infarction in young women. Results from the Transnational Study on Oral Contraceptives and the Health of Young Women. Contraception 1997;56:129–140.
68. WHO Collaborative Study of Cardiovascular Disease and Steroid Hormone Contraception. Acute myocardial infarction and combined oral contraceptives: results of an international multicentre case–control study. Lancet 1997;349:1202–1209.
69. Sidney S, Petitti DB, Quesenberry Jr CP, Klatsky AL, Ziel HK, Wolf S. Myocardial infarction in users of low-dose oral contraceptives. Obstet Gynecol 1996;88:939–944.

70. Bellinger DA, Williams JK, Adams MR, Honore EK, Bender DE. Oral contraceptives and hormone replacement therapy do not increase the incidence of arterial thrombosis in a nonhuman primate model. Arterioscler Thromb Vasc Biol 1998;18:92–99.

71. Waselenko JK, Nace MC, Alving B. Women with thrombophilia: assessing the risks for thrombosis with oral contraceptives or hormone replacement therapy. Semin Thromb Hemost 1998;24 (Suppl 1):33–39.

72. Rintelen C, Mannhalter C, Ireland H et al. Oral contraceptives enhance the risk of clinical manifestation of venous thrombosis at a young age in females homozygous for factor V Leiden. Br J Haematol 1996;93:487–490.

73. Rosendaal FR, Koster T, Vandenbroucke JP, Reitsma PH. High risk of thrombosis in patients homozygous for Factor V Leiden (activated protein C resistance). Blood 1995;85:1504–1508.

74. Vandenbroucke JP, Koster T, Briët E, Reitsma PH, Beruna RM, Rosendaal FR. Increased risk of venous thrombosis in oral contraceptive users who are carriers of factor V Leiden mutation. Lancet 1994;344:1452–1457.

75. Bauersachs R, Lindhoff-Last E, Erhly AM, Kuhl H. Significance of hereditary thrombophilia for risk of thrombosis with oral contraceptives. Zentralbl Gynakol 1996;118:262–270.

76. Poort SR, Rosendaal FR, Reitsma PH, Bertina RM. A common genetic variation in the 3′-untranslated region of the prothrombin gene is associated with elevated plasma prothrombin levels and an increase in venous thrombosis. Blood 1996;88:3698–3703.

77. Cumming AM, Keeney S, Salden A, Bhavnani M, Shwe KH, Hay CRM. The prothrombin gene G20210A variant: prevalence in a UK anticoagulant clinic population. Br J Haematol 1997;98:353–355.

78. Pabinger I, Schneider B, The GTH study Group on Natural Inhibitors. Thrombotic risk of women with hereditary antithrombin III-Protein C- and Protein S-deficiency taking oral contraceptive medication. Thromb Haemost 1994;71:548–552.

79. Mannucci PM, Valsecchi C, Krachmalnicoff A, Faioni EM, Tripodi A. Familial dysfunction of protein S. Thromb Haemost 1989;62:763–766.

80. Heistinger M, Rumpl E, Illiasch H et al. Cerebral sinus thrombosis in a patient with hereditary protein S deficiency: case report and review of the literature. Ann Hematol 1992;64:105–109.

81. Koelman JHTM, Bakker CM, Plandsoen WCG, Peeters FLM, Barth PG. Hereditary protein S deficiency presenting with cerebral sinus thrombosis in an adolescent girl. J Neurol 1992;239:105–106.

82. Villa P, Aznar J, Mira Y, Fern·ndez MA, Vay· A. Third-generation oral contraceptives and low free protein S as a risk for venous thrombosis [letter]. Lancet 1996;347:397.

83. Girolami A, Simioni P, Girolami B, Zanardi S. The role of drugs, particularly oral contraceptives, in triggering thrombosis in congenital defects of coagulation inhibitors: a study of six patients. Blood Coagul Fibrinol 1991;2:673–678.

84. Girolami A, Simioni P, Sartori MT, Zanardi S. Oral contraceptives caused thrombosis in a monoovular twin with protein C deficiency, while the other, without medication, remained asymptomatic [letter]. Blood Coagul Fibrinol 1992;3:119–120.

85. Roger N, Pedrol E, Casademont J, Grau JM. Protein C deficiency as the cause of a deep venous thrombosis in a patient under treatment with oral contraceptives [letter]. Med Clin (Barc) 1992;98:119.

86. Kanda N, Tsuchida T, Tamaki K. Estrogen enhancement of anti-double-stranded DNA antibody and immunoglobulin G production in peripheral blood mononuclear cells from patients with systemic lupus erythematosus. Arthritis Rheum 1999;42:328–337.

87. Verthelyi D, Ansar Ahmed S. Characterization of estrogen-induced autoantibodies to cardiolipin in non-autoimmune mice. J Autoimmunity 1997;10(2):115–125.

88. Ahmed SA, Verthelyi D. Antibodies to cardiolipin in normal C57BL/6J mice: induction by estrogen but not dihydrotestosterone. J Autoimmunity 1993;6(3):265–279.

89. Girolami A, Zanon E, Zanardi S, Saracino MA, Simioni P. Thromboembolic disease developing during oral contraceptive therapy in young females with aPL. Blood Coagul Fibrinol 1996;7:497–501.

90. Bacci S, Urquiola G, del Medico P et al. Budd–Chiari syndrome, pulmonary thromboembolism, and deep venous thrombosis associated with "lupus anticoagulant" and recent use of oral contraceptives. G E N 1990;44:237–242.

91. Omdal R, Roalso S. Chorea gravidarum and chorea associated with oral contraceptives – diseases due to aPL? Acta Neurol Scand 1992;86:219–220.

92. Julkunen HA. Oral contraceptives in systemic lupus erythematosus: side-effects and influence on the activity of SLE. Scand J Rheumatol 1991;20:427–433.

93. Sanchez-Guerrero J, Karlson EW, Liang MH, Hunter DJ, Speizer FE, Colditz GA. Past use of oral contraceptives and the risk of developing systemic lupus erythematosus. Arthritis Rheum 1997;40:804–808.

94. Devor M, Barrett-Connor E, Renvall M, Feigal D, Jr, Ramsdell J. Estrogen replacement therapy and the risk of venous thrombosis. Am J Med 1992;92:275–282.
95. Forbes CD, Greer IA. Hormone replacement therapy is not a risk for venous thrombosis [see comments]. Scott Med J 1994;39:165–166.
96. Saleh AA, Dorey LG, Dombrowski MP et al. Thrombosis and hormone replacement therapy in postmenopausal women. Am J Obstet Gynecol 1993;169:1554–1557.
97. Scarabin PY, Alhenc-Gelas M, Plu-Bureau G, Taisne P, Agher R, Aiach M. Activation of blood coagulation and increased fibrinolytic potential induced by oral but not percutaneous estrogen/protesterone replacement therapy in postmenopausal women: a randomised controlled trial [abstract]. Haemostasis 1996;26(Suppl 3):466.
98. Daly E, Vessey MP, Hawkins MM, Carson JL, Gough P, Marsh S. Risk of venous thromboembolism in users of hormone replacement therapy. Lancet 1996;348:977–980.
99. Jick H, Jick SS, Myers MW, Vasilakis C. Risk of acute myocardial infarction and low-dose combined oral contraceptives. Lancet 1996;347:627–628.
100. Grodstein F, Stampfer MJ, Goldhaber SZ et al. Prospective study of exogenous hormones and risk of pulmonary embolism in women. Lancet 1996;348:983–987.
101. Barlow DH. HRT and the risk of deep vein thrombosis. Int. J Gynaecol Obstet 1997;59 (Suppl 1):S29–S33.
102. Hulley S, Grady D, Bush T et al. Randomized trial of estrogen plus progestin for secondary prevention of coronary heart disease in postmenopausal women. Heart and Estrogen/progestin Replacement Study (HERS) Research Group. JAMA 1998;280:605–613.
103. Nachtigall LE, Nachtigall RH, Nachtigall RD, Beckman EM. Estrogen replacement therapy II: a prospective study in the relationship to carcinoma and cardiovascular and metabolic problems. Obstet Gynecol 1979;54:74–79.
104. The Boston Collaborative Drug Surveillance Program. Surgically confirmed gallbladder disease, venous thromboembolism and breast tumors in relation to postmenopausal estrogen therapy. N Engl J Med 1974;290:15–19.
105. Petitti DB, Wingerd J, Pellegrin F, Ramcharan S. Oral contraceptives, smoking, and other factors in relation to risk of venous thromboembolic disease. Am J Epidemiol 1978;108:480–485.
106. Petitti DB, Wingerd J, Pellegrin F, Ramcharan S. Risk of vascular disease in women. JAMA 1979;242:1150–1154.
107. Sanchez-Guerrero J, Liang MH, Karlson EW, Hunter DJ, Colditz GA. Postmenopausal estrogen therapy and the risk for developing systemic lupus erythematosus. Ann Intern Med 1995;122:430–433.
108. Arden NK, Lloyd ME, Spector TD, Hughes GRV. Safety of hormone replacement therapy (HRT) in systemic lupus erythematosus (SLE). Lupus 1994;3:11–13.
109. Kreidstein S, Urowitz MB, Gladman DD, Gough J Hormone replacement therapy in systemic lupus erythematosus. J Rheumatol 1997;24:2149–2152.
110. Mok CC, Lau CS, Ho CT, Lee KW, Mok MY, Wong RW. Safety of hormonal replacement therapy in postmenopausal patients with systemic lupus erythematosus. Scand J Rheumatol 1998;27:342–346.
111. Gleicher N, Liu HC, Dudkiewicz A et al. Autoantibody profiles and immunoglobulin levels as predictors of in vitro fertilization success. Am J Obstet Gynecol 1994;170:1145–1149.
112. Sher G, Feinman M, Zouves C et al. High fecundity rates following in-vitro fertilization and embryo transfer in antiphospholipid antibody seropositive women treated with heparin and aspirin. Hum Reprod 1994;9:2278–2283.
113. Schenk LM, Butler L, Morris JP et al. Heparin and aspirin treatment yields higher implantation rates in IVF patients with antiphospholipid antibody seropositivity compared to untreated seronegative patients. 52nd Annual Meeting of the American Society of Reproductive Medicine. Boston, Nov. 2–6, 1996.
114. WHO Collaborative Study of Cardiovascular Disease and Steroid Hormone Contraception. Venous thromboembolic disease and combined oral contraceptives: results of international multicentre case–control study. Lancet 1995;346:1575–1582.
115. Farmer RDT, Lawrenson RA, Thompson CR, Kennedy JG, Hambleton IR. Population-based study of risk of venous thromboembolism associated with various oral contraceptives. Lancet 1997;349:83–88.
116. Bridey F, Wolff M, Laissy JP, Morin V, Lefebvre M, de Prost D. Fatal cerebral venous sinus thrombosis associated with the factor V Leiden mutation and the use of oral contraceptives [letter]. Thromb Haemost 1995;74(5):1382.
117. Glueck CJ, McMahon RE, Bouquot JE, Triplett D, Gruppo R, Wang P. Heterozygosity for the Leiden mutation of the factor V gene, a common pathoetiology for osteonecrosis of the jaw, with thrombophilia augmented by exogenous estrogens. J Lab Clin Med 1997;130:540–543.

118. Gould J, Deam S, Dolan G. Prothrombin 20210A polymorphism and third generation oral contra-ceptives – a case report of coeliac axis thrombosis and splenic infarction [letter]. Thromb Haemost 1998;79(6):1214–1215.

119. Bruneau C, Intrator L, Sobel A, Beaumont V, Billecocq A. Antibodies to cardiolipin and vascular complications in women taking oral contraceptives [letter]. Arthritis Rheum 1986;29:1294.

120. Asherson RA, Harris EN, Hughes GRV, Farquharson RG. Complications of oral contraceptives and aPL: reply to the letter by Bruneau et al [letter]. Arthritis Rheum 1988;31:575–576.

121. Asherson RA, Buchanan N, Baguley E, Hughes GR. Postpartum bilateral renal vein thrombosis in the primary antiphospholipid syndrome [see comments]. J Rheumatol 1993;20:874–876.

122. Jick H, Derby LE, Myers MW, Vasilakis C, Newton KM. Risk of hospital admission for idiopathic venous thromboembolism among users of postmenopausal oestrogens. Lancet 1996;348:981–983.

Section 5
Differential Diagnosis

44 Antiphospholipid Syndrome: Differential Diagnosis

B. J. Hunt and P. R. J. Ames

Introduction

Reaching the correct diagnosis is the aim of every physician. This chapter is designed to ensure that the correct diagnosis is achieved in patients whose differential diagnosis includes the antiphospholipid syndrome (APS). In the past, APS was often not considered in the differential diagnosis of a thrombotic state, although this has occurred less frequently as the condition has become better known and understood. Lack of understanding of the assays can result in interpretation difficulties, particularly if investigator does not appreciate that both lupus anticoagulant and anticardiolipin antibodies are different facets of the same problem, and that both must be performed to exclude the diagnosis.

If physicians read this particular book, then they will consider APS in the differential diagnosis of thrombotic disease, and should be highly skilled at interpreting the antiphospholipid antibody (aPL) assays. However, there is a possibility of "over-diagnosis", which is as important to avoid as non-recognition, for once a diagnosis of APS has been made, the management of thrombosis in APS is not without recognized morbidity and mortality due to bleeding. Thus, in patients with aPL, it is important to establish from the history, examination and investigations that the associated clinical features are consistent with APS, that the aPL assays are reproducible, and that there is no other explanation for the thrombotic events.

In view of the diverse presentation of APS, we have planned this chapter taking into account the new international consensus statement on preliminary criteria for the classification of the antiphospholipid syndrome [1].

Clinical Criteria

Vascular Thrombosis

One or more clinical episodes of arterial, venous or small vessel thrombosis in any tissue or organ. Thrombosis must be confirmed by imaging or Doppler studies or histopathology, with the exception of superficial venous thrombosis. For histopathological confirmation, thrombosis should be present without significant evidence of inflammation in the vessel wall.

The Differential Diagnosis of Venous Thrombosis

Any part of the venous circulation may undergo occlusion in APS. Deep and super-ficial veins of the lower limbs are most frequently involved, followed by pulmonary embolism and arm vessels. In these instances, and in subjects who are relatively young (< 45 years), the differential diagnosis rests on laboratory tests aiming at the identi-fication of congenital or other acquired thrombophilic states. The current venous thrombophilia screen of 1999, is shown in Table 44.1. aPL seem to be a common etiological factor in venous thrombosis in unusual sites such as the abdominal circul-ation. APS has been described as the second most common cause of Budd–Chiari syndrome [2], after myeloproliferative disorders [3], and thrombosis in other abdom-inal veins are reported in APS. APS should be included in the differential diagnosis of cerebral vein thrombosis, since the presence of aPL in this population ranges from 8 to 55%, and affected patients tend to have younger age at onset and more extensive involvement than patients with conventional thrombophilic states [4, 5]. However the recently described prothrombin 20210 mutation, present in 2% of Caucasian individu-als appears also to predispose to thrombosis in the coronary and cerebral venous vessels. The differential effects of hypercoagulable states in different vascular beds is excellently reviewed by Rosenberg and Aird [6]. In the ophthalmology setting, aPL have been detected from 5 to 47% of subjects presenting with retinal vein occlusion, alongside other thrombophilic factors and vasculitis [7–9]. aPL should be included in the differential diagnosis of thrombotic events causing endocrine abnormalities such as Addison's disease [10–12] and Sheehan's syndrome (hypopituitarism) [13]. Although the differential diagnosis of venous occlusions often relies on detecting a thrombophilic state, some clinical features may point towards systemic disorders with a higher than average risk of venous thrombosis. For example a history of oral and genital ulceration in a young person with venous thrombosis would suggest Behçet's disease, which like APS, does not spare any vascular bed.

The Differential Diagnosis of Arterial Thrombosis

When compared to the potentially recognized risk factors for venous thrombotic disease, there are fewer factors to consider in arterial thrombotic disease. All the

Table 44.1. Differential diagnosis of venous thromboembolism in APS.

Activated protein C resistance/factor V Leiden (heterozygote and homozygous)

Heterozygous deficiencies of
   Antithrombin
   Protein C
   Protein S

Prothrombin 20210 heterozygous or homozygous states

Increased levels of Factor VIII

Myeloproliferative disorders

Dysfibrinogenemia

Paroxysmal nocturnal hemoglobinuria

Possible risk factor
   Hyperhomocysteinemia

Table 44.2. Risk factors for arterial thrombosis.

Hypertension
Smoking
Fibrinogen levels
Hyperhomocystenemia
Hyperlipidemia
Diabetes mellitus
Lipoprotein (a)

other known risk factors for arterial thrombotic disease tend to produce thrombosis on the background of arteriosclerosis, i.e. these patients tend to have recognizable risk factors for atherosclerosis. There is anecdotal evidence that there is an accelerated atherosclerosis in APS, suggesting that in those with APS, that management should include attention to treating conventional risk factors as well as anticoagulation. The risk factors for arterial thrombosis are summarised in Table 44.2.

Special Arterial Situations

Special consideration should be given to stroke where up to 18% of young strokes may have aPL [15]. The neurological manifestations of APS are many (see Chapter 5). Some patients present with multiple cerebral lesions on magnetic resonance imaging, consistent with multiple cerebral infarcts. These types of lesions are also seen in multiple sclerosis and a cerebral autosomal dominant arteriopathy with subcortical infarcts and leukoencephalopathy (CADASIL) [16, 17]. CADASIL is a hereditary cause of stroke, migraine with aura, mood disturbances and dementia. Thus if a patient does present with multiple cerebral lesions, a family history of stroke and dementia should be sought. Postmortem studies of affected patients show multiple small deep infarcts in the brain and a diffuse leukoencephalopathy. The vasculopathy leads to median thickening by an eosinophilic, granular and electron-dense material of unknown origin. The genetic defect has been mapped to chromosome 19 and can now be detected in the majority of major neuroscience centers.

It may be very difficult to differentiate APS from multiple sclerosis. Clues include a past history of venous thrombosis and pregnancy loss, suggesting APS, while the presence of cerebellar lesions on magnetic resonance imaging (MRI) are more suggestive of MS [18]. Both states can produce oligoclonal bands in the cerebrospinal fluid (CSF). Another differential diagnosis of multiple cerebral lesions can be cerebral vasculitis, and in such cases the diagnosis may only become apparent on cerebral biopsy.

Catastrophic APS

This syndrome has a number of clinical similarities to heparin-induced thrombocytopenia. In heparin-induced thrombocytopenia patients develop thrombosis at any site, both arterial, venous and microvascular (especially the skin). This is due to the presence of an antibody which binds to platelet factor 4 and heparin [19]. It usually develops within 10–14 days after starting heparin and the first sign is a falling platelet count. It should be differentiated from a transient fall in platelet count that occurs in the first few days of heparin therapy, which is probably due to heparin causing platelet activation and is not associated with any clinically harmful effects. The differentiation of aPL-related thrombocytopenia from heparin-induced thrombocytopenia would appear almost straightforward, especially from the history, although the differential diagnosis could be tricky on the laboratory side when both conditions coexist [20].

Pregnancy Morbidity

1. One or more unexplained deaths of a morphologically normal fetus at or beyond the 10th week of gestation, with normal fetal morphology documented by ultrasound or by direct examination of the fetus; or
2. One or more premature births of a morphologically normal neonate at or before the 34th week of gestation because of severe pre-eclampsia or eclampsia or severe placental insufficiency; or
3. Three or more unexplained consecutive spontaneous abortions before the 10th week of gestation, with maternal anatomic or hormonal abnormalities and paternal and maternal chromosomal causes excluded.

In studies of populations of patients who have more than 1 type of pregnancy morbidity, investigators are strongly encouraged to stratify groups of subjects according to 1., 2. or 3. above.

In the UK pulmonary thromboembolism is the leading cause of maternal death. Deep vein thrombosis underlies this disorder and is frequently unrecognized. The risk factors for thromboembolism in pregnancy remain the same as those outside of pregnancy: congenital and acquired thrombophilias.

APS has also been identified as a cause of first-, second- and third-trimester losses as well as intrauterine growth retardation and pre-eclampsia. One of the major advances in the field of thrombophilia in the last few years has been the recognition that other thrombophilic states also predispose to second- and third-trimester losses, as well as intrauterine growth retardation and pre-eclampsia. In a recent case–control study [21], factor V Leiden, the prothrombin 20210 mutation and homozygous state for the homocysteine MTHFR mutation C677T were strongly associated with late pregnancy complications of placental abruption, pre-eclampsia and eclampsia and intrauterine growth retardation in a group of women in Israel. Only a subset had aPL. Such studies need to be repeated world-wide to establish the size of the relationship between congenital and acquired thrombophilia and adverse pregnancy outcome. Interestingly a cohort study following a group of women with factor V Leiden during pregnancy, found its presence was unrelated to adverse pregnancy outcome apart from an eightfold increased risk of venous thromboembolism [22]. It is now clear that aPL are also associated with first-trimester losses. It is not clear at the time of writing whether congenital thrombophilia are associated with first-trimester losses. The answers should be available in the next few years.

It is important when considering the late pregnancy morbidity associated with aPL to check that the history concurs with that of placental insufficiency, for in the Lupus Pregnancy clinic at St Thomas' we have a number of women referred with APS on the basis of pregnancy loss and aPL is an incidental finding. These women have proved to have pregnancy loss due to other causes such as premature labor secondary to an incompetent cervix (in these cases the waters break first and labor supervenes and the fetus may be born alive of a normal birthweight). Thus history taking and obtaining the postmortem findings in previous pregnancy losses are very important.

In considering the etiology of first-trimester losses it is also important to ensure that other causes of first-trimester losses have been excluded by a gynecologist. It thus seems imperative to run a joint clinic with an obstetrician and/or obstetric physician before aPL can be attributed to be the cause of the pregnancy loss.

Hyperhomocysteinemia

This condition deserves a special mention, for it is the only other condition which has been related to pregnancy loss, arterial thrombosis and possibly venous thrombosis. High plasma levels of homocysteine are the result of the interplay between congenital and environmental factors. There has been a growing interest on mild or moderate hyperhomocysteinemia as a risk factor for arterial and venous thrombosis.

The commonest cause of severe homocysteinemia (fasting plasma levels greater than 100 μmol/l) is a homozygous deficiency of cystathionine-b-synthase, which has a prevalence of 1 in 335 000. Affected individuals present with premature vascular disease and thromboembolism as well as ectopic lens, skeletal abnormalities and mental retardation [23]. Mild to moderate levels (fasting levels between 15 and 100 μmol/l) are encountered in phenotypically normal subjects with genetic defects in metabolism, acquired conditions, or more frequently a combination of the two. Often, acquired hyperhomocysteinemia may follow deficiencies of folate, cobalamin and pyridoxine [24] essential cofactors for homocysteine metabolism and may develop in chronic renal insufficiency. Drugs are another important remedial cause too. Drugs such as methotrexate interfere with the metabolism of folate, nitrous oxide interferes with the metabolism of cobalamin and theophylline and affect vitamin B_6. [reviewed in 23].

A common genetic defect leading to hyperhomocysteinemia is a C to T substitution at nucleotide 677 in the gene coding for methylenetetrahydrofolate reductase (MTHFR) [25]. The prevalence of the homozygous C677T mutation is between 5 and 20% in subjects of Caucasian origin. These individuals tend not to have elevated plasma levels of homocysteine unless they have an accompanying low serum concentration of folate [26]. Case–control and cross-sectional studies indicate that mild-to-moderate hyperhomocysteinemia is associated with an increased risk of thrombosis [reviewed in 23]. A recent study showed that APS patients with homozygous C667T mutation developed thrombosis at an earlier age than those with APS who were heterozygous or without the mutation [27]. However, prospective studies do not unequivocally show that hyperhomocysteinemia is associated with an increased risk of venous thrombosis. Further studies are also required to fully establish the relationship between homocysteine levels, the C677T MTHFR mutation and late pregnancy complications. Most importantly however, randomized placebo-controlled double-blind trials of the effects of homocysteine-lowering vitamins are urgently needed. They will help define the relationship between mild-to-moderate hyperhomocysteinemia and thrombosis and potentially have an impact on the prevention of thrombosis.

Other Clinical Features of APS

Thrombocytopenia

Thrombocytopenia is a feature in some patients with APS, present in almost 20% of aPL carriers and probably of autoimmune pathogenesis. Thrombocytopenic bleeding is not frequent in APS, unless there is a coexistent factor deficiency, but prolonged bleeding times do occur [28]. Screening for aPL in subjects with thrombocytopenia of uncertain cause is useful, especially in thrombocytopenia of pregnancy, where the risks of hemorrhage from thrombocytopenia and thrombosis and pregnancy morbidity from aPL could jeopardize fetal and maternal outcome. aPL were detected in 60% of thrombocytopenic human immunodeficiency virus (HIV) subjects addicted to parenteral drugs [29], but there does not appear to be a relationship with thrombosis: in HIV anticardiolipin antibodies have no anti-β_2-glycoprotein I (β_2GPI) effect.

Skin Involvement

Livedo reticularis appears in a number of rheumatic conditions and hyperviscosity states. The detection of aPL in a subject with livedo reticularis and a stroke may suggest Sneddon's syndrome, hence the finding of aPL positivity in someone with isolated livedo reticularis could warrant closer follow-up. Likewise, skin necrosis, skin ulcers, chilblains and vasculitis have been associated with aPL [30], and may identify those patients at higher risk of vascular damage. Pyoderma gangrenosum is frequently associated with systemic diseases but there are cases where aPL was the only abnormal laboratory finding [31].

The Effect of aPL on Other Thrombophilic Assays

In the presence of aPL, some of the other assays for thrombophilia may cause false positive results. It is well recognized that functional assays for protein C and activated protein C resistance may yield falsely low values in the presence of aPL [32]. Similarly phospholipid-dependent coagulation assays such as factor XII assays may produce reduced levels . This has been studied by Jones et al [33] who found that factor XII antibodies are present in a significant proportion of lupus anticoagulant positive patients and may lead to an erroneous diagnosis of factor XII deficiency. Reduced levels of free protein S are present in some patients with aPL, and thus could lead to an erroneous diagnosis of genetic protein S deficiency [34, 35]. The mechanism of this reduction of free protein S is obscure. Although this could be caused by antibodies to protein S itself, or autoantibodies to β_2GPI with C4b-binding protein [36, 37].

Conclusions

APS/Hughes syndrome is an increasingly diagnosed condition. This chapter emphasises the need for clinicians to consider the full range of differential diagnoses for each clinical state, so that the correct diagnosis is reached in an individual patient.

References

1. Wilson WA, Gharavi A, Koike T et al. International consensus statement on the preliminary classification criteria for definite antiphospholipid syndrome. Arthritis Rheum 1999;42:1309–1311.
2. Pelletier S, Landi B, Piette JC et al. Antiphospholipid syndrome as the second cause of non-tumorous Budd–Chiari syndrome. J Hepatol 1994;21:76–80.
3. De Stefano V, Teofili L, Leone G, Michiels JJ. Spontaneous erythroid colony formation as the clue to an underlying myeloproliferative disorder in patients with Budd–Chiari syndrome or portal vein thrombosis. Semin Thromb Hemost 1997;23:411–418.
4. Carhuapoma JR, Mitsias P, Levine SR. Cerebral venous thrombosis and anticardiolipin antibodies. Stroke 1997;28:2363–2369.
5. Deschiens MA, Conard J, Horellou MH. Coagulation studies, factor V Leiden, and anticardiolipin antibodies in 40 cases of cerebral venous thrombosis. Stroke 1996;27:1724–1730.
6. Rosenberg RD, Aird WC. Vascular-bed-specific hemostasis and hypercoagulable states. N Engl J Med 1999;340:1555–1564.
7. Coniglio M, Platania A, Di Nucci GD, Arcieri P, Modzrewska R, Mariani G. Antiphospholipid-protein antibodies are not an uncommon feature in retinal venous occlusions. Thromb Res 1996;83:183–188.
8. Abu el-Asrar AM, al-Momen AK, al-Amro S, Abdel Gader AG, Tabbara KF. Prothrombotic states associated with retinal venous occlusion in young adults. Int Ophthalmol 1996;20:197–204.
9. Glacet-Bernard A, Bayani N, Chretien P, Cochard C, Lelong F, Coscas G. Antiphospholipid antibodies in retinal vascular occlusions. A prospective study of 75 patients. Arch Ophthalmol 1994;112:790–795.
10. Gonzalez G, Gutierrez M, Ortiz M, Tellez R, Figueroa F, Jacobelli S. Association of primary antiphospholipid syndrome with primary adrenal insufficiency. J Rheumatol 1996;23:1286–1287.
11. al-Momen AK, Sulimani R, Harakati M, Gader AG, Mekki M. IgA antiphospholipid and adrenal insufficiency: is there a link? Thromb Res 1991;64:571–578.
12. Lenaerts J, Vanneste S, Knockaert D, Arnout J, Vermylen J. SLE and acute Addisonian crisis due to bilateral adrenal hemorrhage: association with the antiphospholipid syndrome. Clin Exp Rheumatol 1991;9:407–409.
13. Pandolfi C, Gianini A, Fregoni V, Nalli G, Faggi L. Hypopituitarism and antiphospholipid syndrome. Minerva Endocrinol 1997;22:103–105.
14. Kuzu MA, Ozaslan C, Koksoy C, Gurler A, Tuzuner A. Vascular involvement in Behçet's disease: 8-year audit. World J Surg 1994;18:948–953.
15. Nencini P, Baruffi MC, Abbate R et al. Lupus anticoagulant and anticardiolipin antibodies in young adults with cerebral ischaemia. Stroke 1992;23:189–193.
16. Chabriat H, Vahedi K, Iba-Zizen MT et al. Clinical spectrum of CADASIL: a study of 7 familes. Lancet 1995;346:934–939.
17. Chabriat H, Levy C, Taillia H et al. Patterns of MRI lesions in CADASIL. Neurology 1998;51:452–457.
18. Cuadrado MJ, Khamashta MA, Ballesteros A et al. Can Hughes (antiphospholipid) syndrome be distinguished from multiple sclerosis. Analysis of 27 patients and review of the literature. Medicine 2000;79:57–68.
19. Warkentin TE, Chong BH, Greinacher A. Heparin-induced thrombocytopenia: towards consensus. Thromb Haemost 1998;79:1–7.
20. Lasne D, Saffroy R, Bachelot C et al. Tests for heparin-induced thrombocytopenia in primary antiphospholipid syndrome. Br J Haematol 1997;97:939.
21. Kupferminc MJ, Eldor A, Steinman N. Increased frequency of genetic thrombophilia in women with complications of pregnancy. N Engl J Med 1999;340:9–13.
22. Lindqvist PG, Svenssson PJ, Marsal K et al. Activated protein C resistance and pregnancy. Thromb Haemost 1999;81:532–537.
23. Cattaneo M. Hyperhomocysteinemia, atherosclerosis and thrombosis. Thromb Haemost 1999;81:165–176.
24. Selhub J, Jacques PF, Wilson PWF, Rush D, Rosenberg JH. Vitamin status and intake as primary determinants of homocysteinemia in an elderly population. JAMA 1993;270:2693–2698.
25. Frosst P, Blom HJ, Milos R et al. A candidate risk factor for vascular disease:a common mutation in methylenetetrahydrofolate reductase. Nature Genet 1995;10:111–113.
26. Ma J, Stampfer MJ, Hennekens CH et al. Methylenetetrahydrofolate reductase polymorphism, plasma folate, homocysteine, and risk of myocardial infarction in US physicians. Circulation 1996;94:2410–2416.
27. Ames PRJ, Tammasino C, D'Andrea G, Iannaccone L, Brancaccio V, Margaglione M. Thrombophilic genotypes in subjects with idiopathic antiphospholipid antibodies-prevalence and significance. Thromb Haemost 1998;79:46–49.

28. Galli M, Finazzi G, Barbui T. Thrombocytopenia in the antiphospholipid syndrome. Br J Haematol 1996;93:1–5.
29. Muniz-Diaz E, Domingo P, Lopez M et al. Thrombocytopenia associated with human immuno-deficiency virus infection. Immunologic study of 60 patients addicted to parenteral drugs. Med Clin (Barc) 1993;101:761–765.
30. Tajima C, Suzuki Y, Mizushima Y, Ichikawa Y. Clinical significance of immunoglobulin A antiphos-pholipid antibodies: possible association with skin manifestations and small vessel vasculitis. J Rheumatol 1998;25:1730–1736.
31. Chacek S, MacGregor-Gooch J, Halabe-Cherem J, Nellen-Hummel H, Quinones-Galvan A. Pyoderma gangrenosum and extensive caval thrombosis associated with the antiphospholipid syndrome – a case report. Angiology 1998;49:157–160.
32. Atsumi T, Khamashta MA, Amengual O et al. Binding of the anticardiolipin antibodies to protein C via beta2 glycoprotein I. Clin Exp Immunol 1998;112:325–333.
33. Jones DW, Gallimore MJ, Winter M. Antibodies to factor XII associated with lupus anticoagulant. Thrombo Haemost 1999;81:387–390.
34. Ames PRJ, Iannaccone L, Tommasino C, Brillante M, Brancaccio V. Coagulation activation and fibrinolytic imbalance in subjects with idiopathic antiphospholipid antibodies. A crucial role for acquired free protein S deficiency. Throm Haemost 1996;76:190–194.
35. Parke AL, Weinstein RE, Bona RD, Maier DB, Walker FJ. The thrombotic diathesis associated with the presence of phospholipid antibodies may be due to low levels of free protein S. Am J Med 1992;93:49–56.
36. Walker FJ, Does beta-2-gylcoprotein I inhibit interaction between protein S and C4b-binding protein? Thromb Haemost 1993;69:930 (abstr).
37. Atsumi T, Khamashta MA, Ames PRJ, Ichikawa K, Koike T. Hughes GRV. Effect of beta-2 glyco-protein I and monoclonal anticardiolipin antibodies on the protein S/C4B binding protein system. Lupus 1997;6:358–364.

Section 6

Prognosis

45 Prognosis and Future Directions

M. D. Lockshin

In October, 1998, in the brisk, clear air of Sapporo, Japan, the world's experts on the Hughes syndrome summarized present knowledge about antiphospholipid antibody. This book presents an updated review of this syndrome. The intent of the current chapter is to outline our future needs.

To try to foretell the future, we have to know where we are today. Our understanding can be categorized as clinical and as biological. Contemporary clinical knowledge of the Hughes syndrome includes:

- Definition of its common and rare elements, such as the catastrophic vascular occlusion syndrome, neurologic complications, pregnancy complications (including placental pathology and infertility), and atherosclerosis;
- Acceptance of a possible relationship of Hughes syndrome to other coagulopathies;
- The concept of "antibody-mediated thrombosis";
- Initial testing of laboratory and clinical diagnostic criteria;
- Publication of the first controlled treatment trials, using heparin, immunoglobulin, and toleragens (treatment trials to date have been small and based only on pregnancy survival); and
- Estimations of prognosis in referral populations, and of recurrence rates of thromboses in treated populations.

Regarding the biology of antiphospholipid antibody, we now have good understanding of:

- β_2-glycoprotein I, including its antigenic epitopes, its molecular and possibly crystal structure, and its allelic and mutated genetic variants;
- Mechanisms of action of β_2-glycoprotein I-dependent lupus anticoagulants;
- Mechanisms of action of antibodies directed against other proteins, such as prothrombin;
- Endothelial cell and platelet biology, including interaction with β_2-glycoprotein I and with antiphospholipid antibody;
- Animal studies on mechanisms of thrombosis;
- Experimental induction of antiphospholipid antibodies; and
- Experimental models to test therapies.

Nonetheless, no patient suffering from Hughes syndrome, nor her physician, can believe that prevailing understanding is adequate or treatment anything but rudimentary. Physicians can neither prevent the syndrome nor predict the occurrence of thrombosis. Many patients still suffer hypercoagulability that is refractory to

459

anticoagulation therapy, and many deliver growth-restricted and premature infants. Many if not most patients develop long-term sequelae, such as valvulopathy and vasculopathy. No patient can yet be cured. The remarkable molecular and cell biology of β_2-glycoprotein I crystallization, determination of its amino acid sequence and tertiary structure, and knowing how cellular events are induced even today remains descriptive phenomenology that does not define clinical disease. For the clinician and for the biologist, many opportunities remain. These opportunities are outlined below.

For clinicians, questions begging resolution are:

- Does Hughes' syndrome differ in any important way from non-immunologic coagulopathies? For instance, do the frequency, course, treatment and prognosis of venous thromboses in antithrombin III, protein C, protein S, factor II or factor V mutations, or of arterial thromboses in hyperhomocysteinemia differ from those associated with anticardiolipin antibody or lupus anticoagulant? Do the differences lend themselves to the devising of definitive diagnostic tests?
- Are recurrent pregnancy loss, recurrent venous thrombosis, and recurrent arterial thrombosis (in patients with antiphospholipid antibody) the same or different diseases?
- Does Hughes' syndrome begin at first identification of antibody, at first symptom, or at some other time? What – an infection – induces antibody?
- What induces thrombosis? Can new thromboses be predicted?
- What is the relationship of Hughes syndrome to systemic lupus erythematosus (SLE)?
- What is the long-term prognosis for recurrent thrombosis, vascular and cardiac valvular disease, and neurologic deterioration in treated unselected populations?
- What is the long-term prognosis for asymptomatic persons with antiphospholipid antibody?

The biologists need:

- To define the critical elements of both the antigen and the antibody. For instance, does pathogenic antiphospholipid antibody recognize one or several epitopes of β_2-glycoprotein I? If several, is there a relationship among the epitopes? Among polyclonal antibodies, does illness result from one narrowly targeted antibody, or are all antiphospholipid antibodies potentially noxious?
- To answer: does antiphospholipid antibody act independently of coagulation, or is dysregulated coagulation a sine qua non for clinical disease?
- To identify the site of antibody attack: endothelial cell, platelet, or fluid phase anticoagulant proteins?
- To understand mechanisms of different disease manifestations? Do the same mechanisms account for pregnancy loss, livedo, thrombocytopenia, venous and arterial thromboses and valvulopathy, or do each of these occur by an unique mechanism?
- To create new animal models, since no current model clearly reflects all components of the illness.
- To study exceptions that prove the rule, such as:
  - Does antiphospholipid antibody-negative Sneddon's syndrome tell us that the antiphospholipid antibody itself is irrelevant to the syndrome?
  - What is the meaning of anti-β_2-glycoprotein I and anticardiolipin antibody discordant patients? Is livedo reticularis a clue to pathogenesis?

- Is thrombocytopenia a clue?
- Among experimental mice with fetal resorptions, only about half of fetuses die, and half remain viable. What protects the latter?
- Does the fetus contribute to its own well being? If so, how? By actively neutralizing a noxious principle? Or by being invulnerable because it possesses a molecular or cellular barrier? Or lacks a receptor? Or is fetal survival a matter of serendipity, or placental anatomy, or delivered (antibody) dose?

The biological questions suggest clean, testable hypotheses and potentially clear answers. The clinical questions are muddier, but they are worth pursuit.

The Workshop on Diagnostic Criteria provided a document for clinicians to use to answer their questions. However, because referral criteria, ethnicity, social status, and comorbidity vary from clinic to clinic, no single clinic will itself be able to answer the most compelling questions. Hence future clinical studies must include:

- *Consortia*, which use consensus diagnostic and outcome criteria. European consortia already exist; they may answer some of the important clinical questions.
- *Prospective controlled treatment trials*, which will be possible if both standard criteria and consortia are employed. Such trials will include tests of anticoagulants, antiplatelet agents, immunomodulation, and specific and novel biologic agents.
- Descriptions of long-term outcomes. For instance:
  - What are the incidence, severity, pathogenesis, and prevention of accelerated atherosclerosis in Hughes syndrome patients? Is accelerated atherosclerosis due to inadequate control of known risk factors, defects of lipid transport, to vascular injury, or to activation of platelets or vascular endothelium?
  - Long-standing livedo suggests that, like diabetic patients, Hughes syndrome patients suffer microvasculopathy. Whether this is purely a skin phenomenon or implies parallel visceral damage is unknown. If patients suffer long-term complications of microvascular disease, can the damage be prevented by anticoagulation therapy?
  - The pathogenesis of cardiac valve disease is unknown.
  - Similarly, the pathogenesis, triggers, and meaning of the catastrophic vascular occlusion are unknown. The understanding of this complication may be a key to unlock mysteries of the entire syndrome.
  - How should we interpret the sometimes transient, minute hyperintense lesions seen on magnetic resonance imaging of the brain? Are there implications for short-term or long-term neurologic function? No detailed studies of cognitive ability have been performed on Hughes syndrome patients.
  - Children born of antiphospholipid antibody-complicated pregnancies, though often weight-restricted, appear generally normal. No group has formally studied them. Do they differ from children of similarly complicated pregnancies? Might specific abnormalities attributable to either specific aspects of placental ischemia or transplacental antibody become apparent by detailed examination and others become apparent as these children reach adulthood?

Despite open questions, knowledge about the Hughes syndrome has come very far in a very short time. In less than two decades there have evolved: the definition of a new syndrome, distinct from SLE; an understanding of mechanisms of pregnancy loss in non-SLE as well as in SLE women; an involvement of disordered coagulation in occlusive vascular, atherosclerotic, and placental disease; a coupling of coagulation and immunological abnormalities in disease causation; the introduction of anti-coagulation as life-saving therapy in recurrent pregnancy loss; the demonstration of new mechanisms for encephalopathy, nephropathy, and valvulopathy; a suggestion that infection triggers pathogenic antibodies in SLE; the elucidation of molecular and cell surface requirements for modulation of cell activation by coagulation proteins; a knowledge of the assembly of pro- and antithrombotic proteins on cell surfaces; the molecular definition of β_2-glycoprotein I, and of other proteins of the coagulation system; and the demonstration of a role for β_2-glycoprotein I and antiphospholipid antibody in induction and removal of apoptotic cells.

These lessons are already extraordinary, but the list of unanswered questions is still large. There is high optimism. At the rate at which new knowledge accrues, patients' lives will certainly soon improve.

Index